Surgical Design for Dental Reconstruction with Implants:
A New Paradigm

Surgical Design for Dental Reconstruction with Implants: A New Paradigm

Martin Chin, DDS

Private Practice
Oral and Maxillofacial Surgery
San Francisco, California

Quintessence Publishing Co, Inc

quintessence books

Chicago, Berlin, Tokyo, London, Paris, Milan, Barcelona, Istanbul,
Moscow, New Delhi, Prague, São Paulo, Seoul, and Warsaw

Library of Congress Cataloging-in-Publication Data

Chin, Martin, author.
Surgical design for dental reconstruction with implants : a new paradigm / Martin Chin.
p. ; cm.
Includes bibliographical references and index.
ISBN 978-0-86715-684-3
I. Title.
[DNLM: 1. Oral Surgical Procedures--methods. 2. Dental Implantation, Endosseous--methods. 3. Dental Implants. 4. Reconstructive Surgical Procedures--methods. WU 600]
RK667.I45
617.6'93--dc23
2015002929

Quintessence Publishing Co, Inc
4350 Chandler Drive
Hanover Park, IL 60133
www.quintpub.com

5 4 3 2 1

Editor: Lisa C. Bywaters
Design: Ted Pereda
Production: Sue Robinson

Printed in China

Contents

Dedication

To James F. Chin (1910–2010)
Inventor, teacher, and beloved father

My father taught me several important lessons:

- There is satisfaction in gaining understanding of how things around us work.
- An invention that does not work is not a failure but part of the process of discovery.
- An inventor's mission is to forge a path to a solution where none existed before.
- There is no greater responsibility than the honor of trust between two people.

Preface

The purpose of this book is to demonstrate a strategy to improve the outcome of oral and maxillofacial reconstruction by combining evolving principles of neurophysiology and tissue engineering with an integrated surgical and laboratory technique. This book should be of special interest to surgical clinicians and orthodontists. The surgical principles presented in the forthcoming chapters are equally applicable to the dental implant surgeon, maxillofacial surgeon, and craniofacial surgeon.

Current surgical texts present solutions to clinical problems in terms of anatomical manipulation. Normalizing the appearance of a deformity becomes a vehicle to establish function. Many thoughtful observers, however, have recognized that the relationship between form and function is more complicated than just an anatomical structure. Wolff[1] first identified the relationship between form and function and suggested that some mechanism promotes anatomical units to form in response to demands placed on them. Moss[2] proposed the functional matrix theory, which noted the dependence of skeletal development on the investing soft tissue. Harvold[3] attempted to define parameters that, if met, would result in successful facial skeletal formation.

Each of the aforementioned theories proposes that external, distant processes determine how a skeletal structure forms and is maintained. What is lacking is a method to combine subjective conclusions that researchers have made about the principles of growth and development with the objective process of surgery. This goal is particularly challenging because modern patients demand precise results that are at the limit of surgical tolerance. The objective of this book, therefore, is to bridge the gap between the routine practice of maxillofacial surgery and theoretical laboratory science. The first mission is to set down specific treatment-planning principles that should be considered in every surgical design in order to optimize healing. The second mission is to define specific laboratory and surgical techniques to make precise skeletal movements predictable. The third mission is to validate the approach with clinical examples, including long-term follow-up.

What follows in this book is a discussion of how emerging biotechnology discoveries can combine the theoretical and the clinical and allow establishment of a working model that can be applied to real problems affecting real patients. This integrated approach offers the potential to solve clinical problems that are known to be resistant to conventional treatments.

References

1. Wolff J. The Law of Bone Remodeling. Maquet P, Furlong R (trans). Berlin: Springer, 1986.
2. Moss ML. The functional matrix. In: Kraus B, Reidel R (eds). Vistas in Orthodontics. Philadelphia: Lea and Febiger, 1962:85–98.
3. Harvold EP. The theoretical basis for the treatment of hemifacial microsomia. In: Harvold EP, Vargervik K, Chierici G (eds). Treatment of Hemifacial Microsomia. New York: Alan R. Liss, 1983.

Acknowledgments

I extend sincere appreciation to the many patients and their families whom I have treated over the past 35 years. There is no greater honor than the privilege of being trusted with the care of a patient or someone's child.

I thank Theodore Ng and William K. Tom for the many years of collaboration in planning, surgery, and follow-up care of our patients.

Galen Wagnild and Kathy Mueller provided prosthodontic treatment for many of the patients in the cases presented. The nature of these disorders often poses substantial technical and patient management challenges for the restorative dentist. I very much appreciate the uncompromising and compassionate manner in which they always treat our patients.

Special acknowledgment is extended to Lisa Bywaters, who guided me through the journey of writing this book with perspective and encouragement. I recognize that her unique understanding of publishing and dentistry was critical in being able to organize my approach to surgical practice into a form that would be clear and useful to other clinicians. Without her trust and confidence, writing this book would not have been possible.

My daughter, Lauren Chin, who is a registered dental hygienist and journalist, deserves special recognition for her many contributions. She is the source of many of the illustrations that distill unfamiliar surgical processes into an understandable form. Most important, she has been steadfast in her support of the project and the value to commit these concepts into a form that clinicians, basic scientists, and patients may benefit from in the future.

1 Introduction to Surgical Design Using Embryologic Processes

Currently, facial bones are created by one of two processes. The first is embryologic development in utero, as part of the complex process termed *embryogenesis*. During this process, the skeletal system forms in unison with the other organ systems. The second is reconstructive surgery, which typically involves grafts or transplants.

Emerging biotechnology has introduced additional methods of skeletal construction, including tissue engineering, stem cell transfers, and gene therapy. These procedures are hybrid technologies that combine processes common to embryologic development with mechanisms of general reconstructive surgery. To best apply these new techniques, the clinician must understand how the regenerative process is affected by both surgery and the underlying embryologic mechanisms.

A note about terminology: The repair of damaged or lost structures is considered to be *reconstructive surgery* because replacement is the goal. The fabrication of a portion of the body that is absent because the embryo did not initially form it is more properly termed *constructive surgery*. Creating an anatomical structure that had no existing precursor is a special challenge that is inherently different from the task of replacement or repair. Studying how the embryo fabricates anatomical structures can provide clues as to how the challenge of constructive surgery can be met.

In this book, the term *reconstructive surgery* will be used generally to refer to the basic principles of both reconstructive and constructive surgery, while *constructive surgery* will be applied specifically to cases of agenesis of the missing tissue. The intent of this chapter is to reconcile the differences between reconstructive surgery and embryologic development to reveal clues about the process of regeneration and its potential application to constructive surgery and reconstructive surgery.

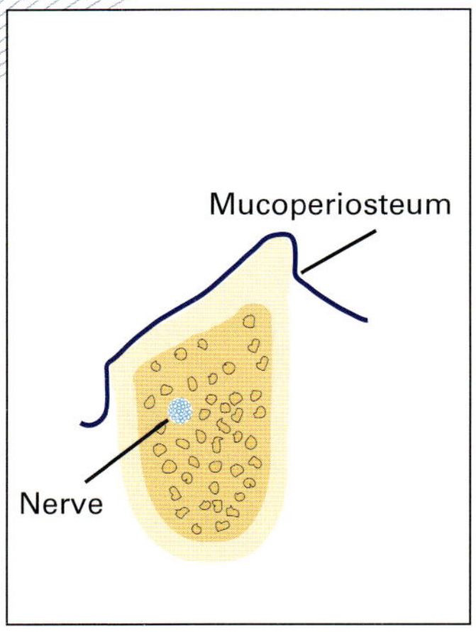

Fig 1-1a Diagram of an alveolar ridge at the mandibular right first molar that lacks bone volume in which to place a dental implant.

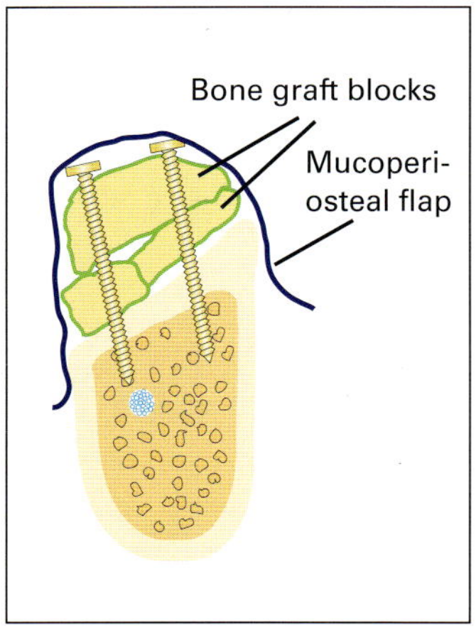

Fig 1-1b Conventional reconstruction of an alveolar ridge deficiency with bone blocks.

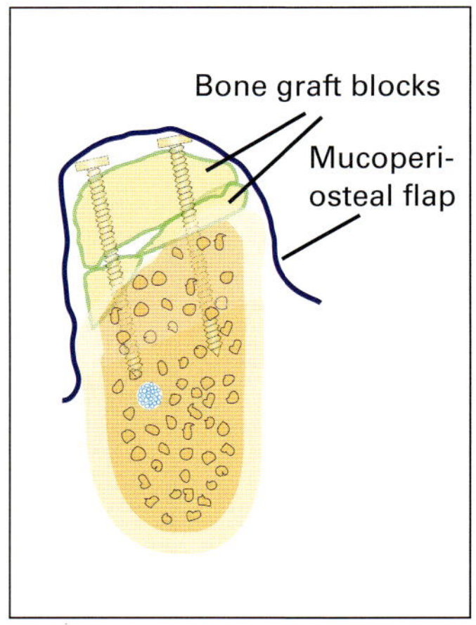

Fig 1-1c As the graft resorbs, vital bone tissue grows vertically into the space created.

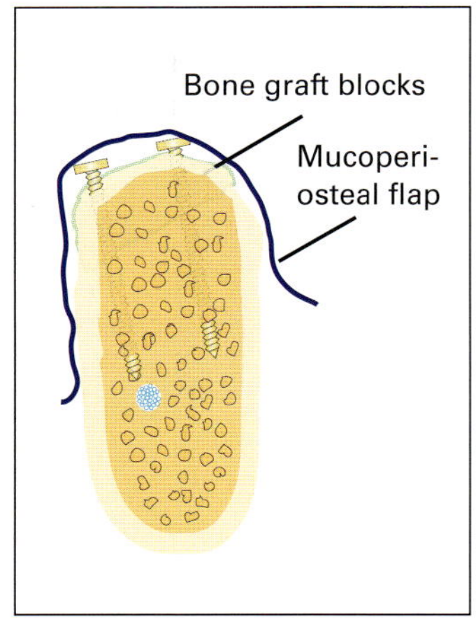

Fig 1-1d Successful alveolar ridge reconstruction by mechanical bone block augmentation.

Goals and Principles of Surgery and Embryogenesis

The creation of functional and esthetic anatomical structures is a basic goal of oral and maxillofacial surgery. To meet this objective, the surgeon is called on to modify existing anatomical structures or to fabricate ones that have been lost or that failed to develop. The task may be to replace a segment of the jaw lost to tumor resection or to create sufficient bone volume in the maxilla to place dental implants. In other cases, patients with congenital clefts request treatment to create portions of the face that did not form. Other patients request placement of osseointegrated implants to anchor a dental prosthesis.

Many different treatment approaches have been developed to address a wide variety of disorders. Whether the task is to place a dental implant or to perform a complex craniofacial procedure, the theoretical basis of the treatment is the same. All of the procedures are based on the basic principles of general reconstructive surgery.

Reconstructive surgery follows a mechanical building model that is superimposed on a background of physiology and an appreciation of wound healing. With this method, a missing anatomical unit is mechanically replaced with grafts or synthetic materials. A successful outcome is thought to depend primarily on local factors, such as the quality of the vascular bed in which the graft is placed and the ability to cover the graft with a tensionless soft tissue closure. The technical precision with which the surgeon executes the intervention is regarded as a critical factor to obtain successful healing.

Augmentation of an alveolar ridge with block bone grafts is a conventional procedure that illustrates this mechanical bone-building strategy. An alveolar ridge that lacks sufficient bone volume to support dental implants exists in a steady state of relative atrophy (Fig 1-1a). A standard surgical strategy for reconstruction is to place some type of bone grafting material onto the alveolar ridge crest and to secure it with screws into the existing cortex (Fig 1-1b). A mucoperiosteal flap is advanced to accommodate the increase in volume. The healing process (Fig 1-1c) involves resorption of the existing cortex of the alveolar ridge, followed by migration of vital bone tissue into the resulting void (Fig 1-1d). The term for this process is *creeping substitution*.

For alveolar ridge reconstruction with bone blocks to be successful, many obstacles must be overcome. The soft tissue closure over the expanded volume is sometimes challenging. The healing process requires resorption of the existing structural anatomy, which must precede the process of simultaneous resorption of the graft and substitution of vital bone tissue. However, the primary problem with reconstructions performed in this manner is the tendency for the site to relapse toward its original phenotype. The volume of bone inserted into the deficiency site cannot be maintained unless it is incorporated into the neuromuscular system, which established and maintains the morphology of the skeleton in a steady state.

The current state of surgical practice is the result of incremental improvements over many years. Prior experience, be it positive or negative, is the main force directing the evolution of surgical science. In current surgical practice, attention is mostly directed at the site of the deformity. How a graft or tissue manipulation is tolerated by the immediately adjacent structures is of primary interest. The effect of distant processes, such as the central nervous system, is considered secondary.

The objectives of embryogenesis and reconstructive surgery are the same: to establish and maintain newly fabricated skeletal structures. Yet the processes of embryogenesis and reconstructive surgery follow unique paths. Developmental anatomists have demonstrated that, prior to formation of the facial skeleton, the facial muscles, fascia, vasculature, and nerves are already in place.[1] The facial skeleton forms last. Thus, in the embryo, the mandible develops within a bed of preexisting soft tissue structures.[2] There is no skeletal or cartilaginous precursor. It does not form by conversion of a cartilage template into an ossified skeletal unit. The mandible forms at the proper site de novo and can be maintained for the life of the individual.

Although developmental anatomists have provided a physical description of how embryologic structures form,[3,4] the underlying mechanisms that control and direct development remain obscure. Most of the important events that regulate this process take place at the molecular level. Communication between and within individual cells operates at the level of the cellular nanostructure. Tissue-formation processes operate on a microscopic level.

Embryogenesis is a dynamic process in which the embryo adds cells, systems, and physical volume at a rapid pace, and a histologic section of an embryo provides a superficial view of development at a single point in time. When many individual sections are considered in series, a simple representation of the continuous development process is illustrated. The method by which the embryo coordinates the process of construction, however, is not revealed by anatomical study.

In the absence of a comprehensive understanding of embryogenesis, theories are the best guide available to scientists and clinicians. Current thinking is that the central nervous system has a primary role in the control and regulation of embryogenesis.[5,6] The response of the local soft tissue systems is thought to play a secondary role. These incompletely understood processes are difficult to apply to clinical treatment but potentially valuable if reconstructive surgeons can exploit the process followed by the developing embryo to form skeletal structures.

Evolutionary Differences in Surgery and Embryogenesis

To appreciate the essential natures of the two skeletal formation systems—embryogenesis and surgery—it is critical to understand how each process came to be. The two systems developed along very different paths.

Differences in temporal scale

The relative lengths of time associated with their development are the first major difference between embryogenesis and surgery. The current state of embryogenesis is the product of a few hundred million years, whereas surgery has developed into its present state over a mere few hundred years. Surgical science and technique improved over this time span in response to incremental advances in the knowledge of physiology. Embryogenesis developed in response to evolution.

Evolution of surgical practice

Historically, surgery was developed by humans to address a problem posed by some type of traumatic injury. When a traumatic defect occurred, management with a simple mechanical solution was the obvious method to try first. If the surgeon encountered a patient with an open wound, the approach would be to dress the wound to allow fibrous connective tissue to replace the missing structures with scar tissue. This approach represents the process of repair, whereby the inherent healing response substitutes scar tissue for the lost specialized tissue. To decrease the size of a large traumatic wound, innovative surgeons used sutures to draw the edges of the remaining tissue closer together. The process of repair remained the same, as scar tissue bridged the remaining deficit.

Prior to the advent of anesthesia and antibiotics, surgery was limited to these types of direct and concise intervention. Without anesthesia, patients were unable to tolerate extensive or elective procedures. Without antibiotics and aseptic techniques, surgeons who extended the scope of surgery increased the risk of uncontrollable infection. The discovery and development of general anesthesia in the 19th century and antibiotics in the 20th century represent major advancements in the practice of reconstructive surgery, allowing surgeons to perform a range of more complex treatments.[7–11] Thus, the modern process of surgical development, assisted by antibiotics and general anesthesia, spans fewer than 175 years.

As the scope of surgery expanded, reconstructive surgery became a logical extension of trauma surgery and was directed at replacement of lost or defective anatomical structures. The goal was to provide a tissue-appropriate replacement that was both functional and esthetic. For example, in the case of a mandibular defect resulting from resection of an odontogenic tumor, the treatment was grafting of the discontinuity defect with an autogenous bone graft from the patient's iliac crest.

Evolution of embryogenesis

Formation of skeletal structures by the embryo follows a path that has been laid out much differently than the development of surgical practice. Hundreds of millions of years saw incremental modifications that gave rise to modern embryogenesis. Molecular evolution and natural selection were forces that drew embryogenesis toward its current state. Despite many years of study, however, full appreciation of this phenomenon will likely remain a work in progress. Answers to the following questions are of interest to surgeons working in the fields of maxillofacial construction and reconstruction:

- By what mechanism does the developing embryo generate a skeletal organ system?
- How does the embryo perform this process?
- What directs the process?
- Is the capability to form bone in this way lost during development or does the latent potential remain?
- Can novel surgeries be engineered that exploit the mechanisms and processes by which the embryo forms skeletal systems in the first place?

Differences in physical scale

Another stark contrast between embryogenesis and surgical reconstruction is the difference of physical scale in which the processes take place. There is a great difference in the physical dimensions of the anatomical structures involved in each of these developmental processes. Surgery involves macroscopic manipulation of tissues by the surgeon's hands, guided by the surgeon's eyes. Even microscope-assisted surgery is performed on structures that are large-scale compared to the environment in which embryogenesis takes place.

The requirement to manipulate tissues by hand is an inherent limitation to the development of advanced surgical technology. Decision-making during surgery is dictated by what the surgeon sees and understands. The operating surgeon cannot directly interact with the processes going on at the cellular and molecular levels.

Embryogenesis, in contrast, is initiated on the level of single cells. Molecular-level mechanisms guide the process of producing and assembling billions of cells into a functioning human. At each moment of each step, all critical organ systems must be functioning individually and maintain coordination with the rest of the body. As cells are added to the developing and growing organism, they must assume their proper role in seamless synchronization with the preexisting and future cells. As the organism transitions dramatically in size, from one cell to billions of cells, all systems must operate in concert. The skeletal system is just one component that needs to be created in the process.

Clinical Application of Embryologic Processes

The task of modern surgeons and scientists is to better understand the processes that the embryo uses to develop and grow. Until that knowledge base is established, clinicians must be satisfied with using theoretical models. Application of an incomplete knowledge of underlying biology to clinical practice is not new. This has always been the challenge of innovative surgeons. The rapid growth of scientific knowledge over the past few hundred years has been substantial. Future research may unlock the hidden mechanisms used by embryos and allow full exploitation of the processes in medical treatment. Until that goal is realized, surgeons will continue to move incrementally forward. Theoretical embryologic models may provide a path to using these mechanisms even though we lack full understanding of the process. Thoughtful planning, objective observation, and long-term follow-up of clinical outcomes will continue to be the method by which surgical science progresses.

Current limitations

Finding ways to apply the principles of embryogenesis and its related processes to patient care is an important frontier in clinical practice. Embryologic development is an elegant process of self-assembly. From basic cell types, complete organ systems are synthesized seamlessly with the surrounding tissue. Having control of this process in a clinical setting would be a very important tool for the reconstructive surgeon. Unfortunately, surgeons cannot reproduce this process with conventional technology.

Because the developmental process is intrinsic to each embryo, the mechanism must be encoded in inherited genetic material—the DNA. The DNA is not simply a blueprint of the finished organism ready for birth. Contained in the DNA is the complex system by which the organism transitions from one living form, a single cell, to an entirely different organism with multiple complex and coordinated systems. Deciphering how the process has been encoded into the DNA is a major challenge of research in regenerative medicine.

After the molecular characterization of DNA by Watson and Crick in 1953 and the subsequent complete mapping of the human genome in 2003, it seemed that widespread clinical application of new biotechnology would follow directly.[12–14] With the full sequence of human DNA revealed, people were hopeful that the key to tissue and organ regeneration was soon to be revealed. Despite substantial energy focused on this pursuit, the underlying processes are revealing themselves slowly.

Even though great potential exists, clinical application of the complex mechanisms of embryogenesis to surgical care has been limited. To date, the most significant development of modern biotechnology has been the revelation that the process of embryogenesis is more complex than first believed. Scientists are trying to penetrate the outer boundaries of the biotechnology "black box" to reveal the underlying processes. Nobody knows if the obstacle to understanding how embryogenesis works is the complexity of the process, the number of mechanisms involved, or both.

Even though our understanding of this field will remain incomplete for many years, there is still an opportunity to improve patient treatments by incorporating these concepts into existing practice. While the current state of relative knowledge remains, the challenge for innovative scientists is to postulate models that may explain the underlying mechanisms. These postulates will become working models that can be tested in the laboratory and clinical setting. If the results of testing and clinical outcomes are consistent, a theory that will provide guidelines for routine treatment planning may evolve. The objective is to establish a path that, when followed, will improve the chances of a good treatment outcome.

Harvold's working model

In the 1970s, orthodontist Egil Harvold (Fig 1-2) and his coworkers developed a series of novel treatment protocols for the management of craniofacial patients.[15] Harvold recognized the potential benefit of modifying existing craniofacial surgery procedures by incorporating treatment techniques that would simulate embryologic processes. The work of Harvold and his associates represents an important early attempt to incorporate embryologic processes into clinical patient care.

Clinical challenge

As director of the Center for Craniofacial Anomalies at the University of California, San Francisco (UCSF), Harvold and his treatment team managed the care of children with a full scope of disorders related to impaired facial growth and development. He recognized that treatment of children with hemifacial microsomia was particularly challenging from both surgical and orthodontic standpoints.[16,17] The ability to lengthen deficient mandibles was challenged by both limited soft tissue and an inability to create a mechanism that would support and regulate the physiology of the newly created ossicle over the long term.

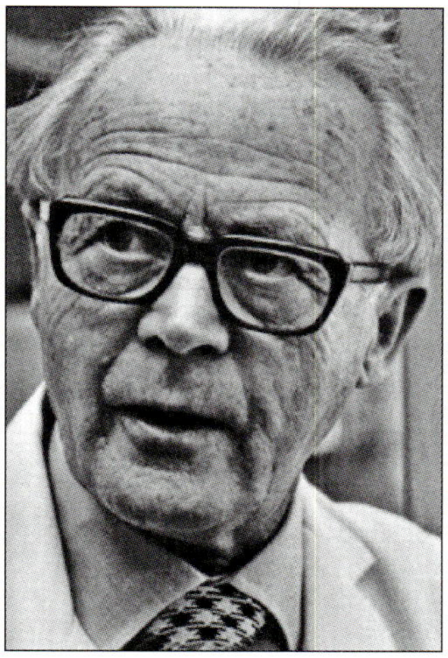

Fig 1-2 Dr Egil Harvold, orthodontist and anatomist, developed novel surgical strategies based on concepts of embryologic development.

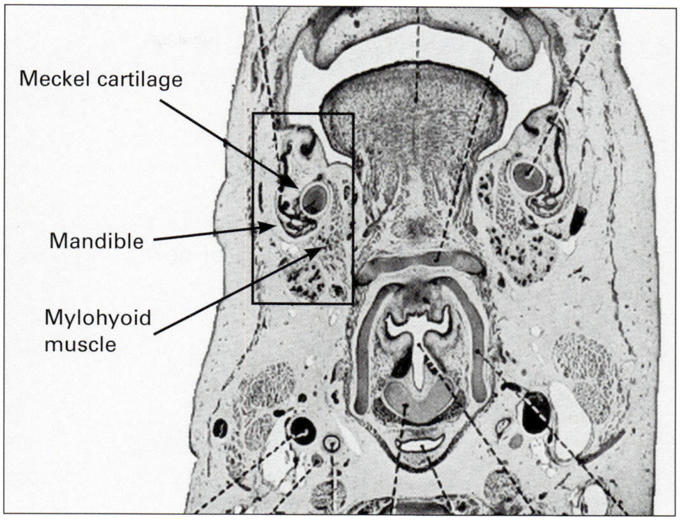

Fig 1-3a Coronal section of a 50-mm human fetus showing the mandible developing within a bone growth–promoting environment established by Meckel cartilage and the mylohyoid muscle. (Adapted from *Human Embryology*[4] with permission from Archie Mossman.)

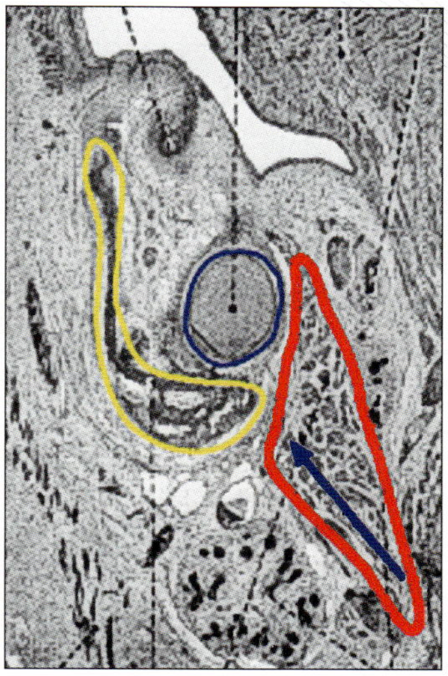

Fig 1-3b *(Inset)* Coronal section of a 50-mm human fetus showing that the mandible *(yellow outline)* develops within a volume stabilized by Meckel cartilage *(blue outline)* and under the mechanical influence of the mylohyoid muscle *(red outline)*. The *blue arrow* indicates the direction of muscle fiber orientation. (Adapted from *Human Embryology*[4] with permission from Archie Mossman.)

At the time, standard treatment of the deficient facial skeletons of these patients followed basic orthopedic principles. Bone grafts harvested from the child's ribs were used to construct the missing anatomical unit. This is the same method that was developed to replace segments of the skeleton lost to trauma or resection. It was not unreasonable for surgeons to apply a technique that was known to remedy a similar physical disorder. The result of this approach, however, was often disappointing. In many cases, the grafted tissue did not heal and was rejected. In other cases, initial healing was observed, but the grafted tissue slowly resorbed and the facial skeleton returned to the original phenotype. These treatment failures were in part due to the failure to recognize that replacement of a lost skeletal unit is a different problem than construction of an anatomical unit that never formed in the first place.

The variety of craniofacial anomalies presenting to the UCSF Craniofacial Center provided an opportunity to study the relationship between abnormal facial skeletal development and abnormal muscle function in a clinical setting. Most reconstructive surgeons focused on fabricating ossicles to fill in the gaps resulting from congenital agenesis or hypoplasia. The impact of deficient muscle development was not considered in the surgical plan. Harvold, in contrast, explored the interaction between muscle function and bone morphology with the objective to design better treatments for facial skeletal deformities.[18]

Harvold and his associates studied bone-muscle interaction by multiple methods. Observations of embryologic and developmental anatomy led to the concept that bone forms in a specialized physical environment and under the regulation of the central nervous system.[19] These theories were tested in animal models.[15] Finally, modifications were made to the existing protocol for surgery, and the results were evaluated for efficacy.[20,21] The research and clinical work performed by Harvold and his associates at the Craniofacial Center attempted to unify two distant disciplines: embryology and reconstructive surgery.

Clues from embryo histology

Serial histology of embryos at various stages of development showed the stepwise formation of organs, including the facial skeleton.[4,15] During the 4th week of development, the mandible can be identified as forming within a space previously occupied by soft tissue (Fig 1-3a). The mandible does not form within a cartilage precursor. It forms de novo within a specific appropriate zone.

Prior to the appearance of the early mandible, Meckel cartilage can be seen just medial to the future site of mandible development. Directed toward this site are the fibers of the mylohyoid muscle (Fig 1-3b). The muscle and its associated branch of the trigeminal nerve are present before the appearance of the mandibular bone to which the muscle will eventually attach.

This anatomical arrangement, the early appearance of the muscle nerve unit, and the adjacent cartilage bar are consistent features of embryologic development. Harvold postulated that the presence of Meckel cartilage results in a region within the mass of facial soft tissue that is partially supported mechanically.[10] The orientation of the mylohyoid muscle into the zone of future mandible development is part of the embryologic self-assembly design.

Harvold further postulated that action by the mylohyoid muscle introduces mechanical signaling to the zone of the future mandible. Cellular activity within this zone is also influenced by the relative mechanical stability afforded by the adjacent Meckel cartilage. The specific action of the mylohyoid muscle is controlled via the trigeminal nerve and its connection through the trigeminal nerve motor nucleus and, eventually, the brain. Possible mechanisms by which muscle activity could control cellular metabolism were not known at the time Harvold was developing his theories. It would take further research by Ingber to define how this process might operate.[22–24]

The specific pattern of muscle activity that would stimulate bone formation has been the subject of further research. Harvold and physiologist Arthur Miller tried to decipher the muscle-stimulation pattern delivered by the brain.[25,26] Nonhuman primates became the test subjects because it was impossible to perform electrophysiologic studies on embryos. These investigations did not reveal the critical signaling pattern that embryos may use to control bone formation. It is likely that using mature animals would not yield the signaling pattern exploited by the embryo. That part of the process remains theoretical.

Clues from clinical observations

The most important and valuable step in determining how to better manage a difficult clinical problem is to improve the quality of the diagnosis. In the case of the craniofacial patient, the diagnosis must extend beyond the obvious physical deficiency to the underlying physiology and etiology. Harvold's team analyzed the relative deficiencies in muscle development.[25,27] Clinical and radiologic features were examined with the specific goal of better understanding the deficiency in the neuromuscular system. When a specific deficiency was identified, a proposal for preoperative muscle conditioning was done. Perioperative muscle conditioning was accomplished with oral functional appliances.[28] This muscle therapy was continued after skeletal surgery to promote healing of the graft and to encourage establishment of a supportive environment for the newly modified skeleton. In these cases, autogenous bone grafts were used to deliver cells to the site of mandibular deficiency. Patients with a hypoplastic temporalis muscle and no lateral pterygoid muscle healed from their surgeries best when the graft was positioned in close proximity to the temporalis tendon. These patients also demonstrated the ability to grow the constructed mandibular ramus when functional appliance therapy was used after surgery.[20] The conclusion was that the temporalis muscle promotes healing of the bone graft when placed within its mechanical signaling reach. The interaction of the muscle and bone continues after graft healing and is important in the maintenance and growth of the constructed skeletal unit.

Clues from the primate laboratory

Extrapolating from findings of embryologic sections, Harvold theorized that bone formed in tissue zones in response to specific mechanical perturbation by muscle function. Clinical and embryologic findings showed a consistency between active muscle and ossicle formation. It followed that there must be a mechanism that initiates and regulates formation of bone in the desired morphology. Because muscle function originates from the central nervous system, the brain must be the ultimate source of construction directions. This concept contrasts with the alternative explanation of local induction, in which the adjacent tissues direct morphologic change that causes a new structure to develop. The lens of the eye, for example, is thought to form under the induction effect of the adjacent tissue.[29]

If the central nervous system is the master control center for anatomical construction, then how is the information transmitted and understood by the individual cells? Because the presence of the muscle and controlling nerve is a consistent finding, it follows that at least part of the regulatory process involves signaling through tissue distortion from muscle contraction. This theorizes a method to translate mechanical cellular distortion into metabolic regulation, resulting in bone formation. It is now understood how physical cellular distortion results in modification and regulation of cellular metabolism.[30–34] Deciphering the specific signaling pattern that the embryo uses to direct cells to form a mandible might yield a method for bone construction that could be used clinically.

To gain some insight into how this process might work, Harvold and Miller devised a series of experiments.[19] The concept was that, if neuromuscular activity controls skeletal formation, the same activity might still be functional in the mature animal to maintain morphology. If muscle activity impacted bone morphology of the mature animal, it might be possible to alter the effect by altering muscle activity.

In their research, techniques of electrophysiology were used to analyze the normal activity of facial muscles. In a second session, the muscles were stimulated with specific frequencies and patterns to determine if the associated muscle attachments or bone grafts would be affected. Unfortunately, no specific pattern of muscle stimulation resulted in de novo bone formation.

The search for mechanical control of cellular processes continues, primarily related to the concept of *tensegrity* as described by Ingber.[23] Ingber used engineering concepts to understand how the cell membrane and organelles were connected with a network of nanostructure fibers. These nanostructures were shown to provide mechanical organization to the cell. Ingber demonstrated that mechanical distortion of the cell resulted in rapid-onset changes in metabolic activity. The theory proposed by Ingber is that the intracellular nanotubules that provide cellular structure are also vectors for communication between organelles. The nanotubules themselves may respond to mechanical force or signals by initiating their own biochemical synthesis. For Harvold's theory to have an anatomical basis, either there must be a route by which mechanical signals are received from the Sharpey fibers of muscle attachments, or else the Sharpey fibers of the periodontal ligament system must enter and direct cellular activity. The mechanisms of tensegrity are a likely vector along which neuromuscular signaling reaches the cell.

Harvold's theory

Based on observations from the embryologic, clinical, and nonhuman primate studies, Harvold developed a working model.[15] He proposed that facial bone surgery should be planned according to a series of guidelines to optimize the healing response. These recommendations followed directly from his theories about how the embryo forms its skeletal system and how muscle deficiencies compromise healing of adult skeletal surgery. When skeletal surgery is to be performed, care should be taken to include the following parameters: a stabilized environment, a source of cells, and neuromuscular input. In addition, the surgery should be performed in an environment that is free of pathologic conditions.

Stabilized environment. The zone or chamber in which the constructed bone is to form must meet specific mechanical conditions. Excessive movement of immature bone interferes with consolidation. Instead of bone formation, the tissue defaults to fibrous connective tissue. If the environment is too stable and will not allow slow tissue movement, bone will not form either. Bone forms best in a zone that meets an ideal balance of stability and mobility. The surgeon must engineer these mechanical zones as potential construction chambers in which new skeletal structures can form and be maintained over the long term.

Source of cells. Having a source of cells with bone-forming potential is a basic prerequisite for construction of an ossicle. At the site of most reconstructive surgeries, cells with bone-forming potential can be recruited from adjacent tissue, including existing native bone. If the number or quality of cells with bone-forming potential is inadequate at the site of ossicle construction, then the procedure should include a method to introduce them. In the past, this condition would be fulfilled by autogenous bone grafting. In the present and future, this requirement could be met with morphogenetic agents, stem cell transfer, or in vitro tissue engineering.

Neuromuscular input. This element provides specific stimulation that regulates cells to form bone. Bone forms within a bed of soft tissue when the environment and stimulating signals are correct. Bone does not form in the absence of a functioning muscle. Because muscle action is involved, the central nervous system is ultimately responsible for generating signals with the proper frequency, pattern, and amplitude. Engineering of a site in which bone will form requires that some muscle system have mechanical (via neural) input in the region. A special condition may occur in the presence of forming and erupting teeth. It seems that bone forms adjacent to developing teeth, creating the alveolar process without an extrinsic muscle attachment. It is possible that the periodontal ligament, with its insertion of fibers into bone, acts similarly to a muscle attachment.

Absence of pathology. Bone will not form if the basic physiology of the environment is compromised. Systemic disorders of the endocrine system or nutritional problems, for example, may prevent bone formation even if the environment is correct. For example, cystic disease or infection of the maxillary sinus will prevent successful healing of sinus elevation grafts, even if the physical environment is appropriate and cells capable of bone formation are present.[15]

Clinical support for Harvold's theory: Lessons from coronoid process regeneration. If skeletal elements form and are maintained when the environment is complete and correct, then clinical examples should be able to confirm this process. Regeneration of the coronoid process after surgical resection illustrates that the adult has not lost the ability to replace a missing anatomical structure without the help of the reconstructive surgeon.[35,36] This shows that the ability for self-assembly is still operating in the adult human. In this case, the process occurs consistently and without input from the surgeon. The process restores the structure with the correct tissue type, correct endosseous tissue architecture, and original external morphology.

Regenerative cycle. The coronoid process serves as the muscle attachment for the temporalis muscle (Fig 1-4a). It is known to grow to a size that interferes with the full range of motion of the mandible. This problem is addressed via resection of the process. The healing course of the coronoid process after resection suggests that regenerative processes are active in the maxillofacial environment.[35,37]

Resection of the coronoid process involves an osteotomy dividing the coronoid process from the mandibular ramus at the level of the sigmoid notch, following reflection of the temporalis muscle attachment (Fig 1-4b). The resected portion of the coronoid process is then removed. The temporalis muscle contracts upward toward its origin, the temporal fossa (Fig 1-4c).

Follow-up radiographs typically show the reappearance of a coronoid process.[35] After the temporalis muscle contracts superiorly into the temporal space, it gradually descends (Figs 1-4d and 1-4e). The detached insertion of the muscle points toward the site of resection. The brain, via the trigeminal nerve, controls the tone and therefore the position of the muscle. Because the tendon occupies a soft tissue compartment that is continuous with the adjacent planes, any muscle movement relays force to the surrounding structures.

The muscle tone oscillates under the direction of the brain. Though the stimulation pattern is poorly defined, it is undeniably important. If the effect of muscle action is blocked or diminished, normal healing does not occur[15,38] (Fig 1-4f). The postulate is that signaling from the brain results in specific, oscillating distortions of the adjacent soft tissues.[15] The region previously occupied by the resected coronoid process succumbs to the influence of this stimulating force. Mechanical distortion of the tissue results in microdistortion of the individual cells in this regenerative zone (Fig 1-4g).

Mechanotransduction by this process is mediated by the nanostructure of the cell through tensegrity.[31] Cells respond to microdistortion by modifying their protein synthesis. The intracellular nanotubular framework is probably the mechanism that translates the mechanical signal into a biochemical one. In this way, the brain controls and directs the regeneration process.

The temporalis tendon continues to descend under the direction of the brain. Cells perform specific metabolic tasks per mechanically signaled instruction. As a result, stem cells are recruited to the regeneration zone and directed to differentiate down an osteoblastic line. Locally produced cytokines direct morphogenesis. In addition to producing the correct cell types, brain-mediated synthesis and remodeling organize the cells into a working community.

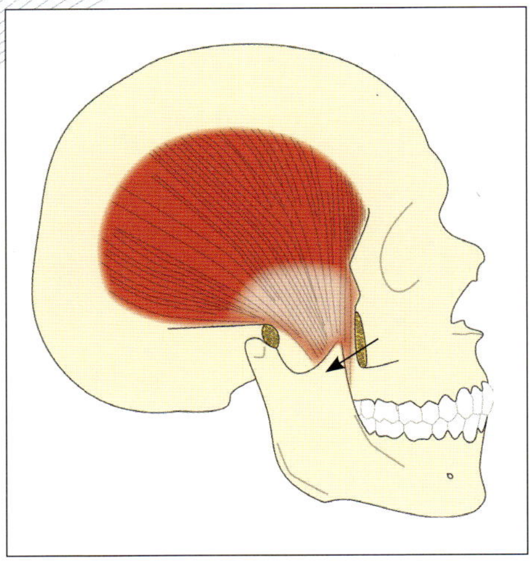

Fig 1-4a The coronoid process *(arrow)* is a familiar anatomical feature of the mandible. It serves as the site of insertion of the temporalis muscle.

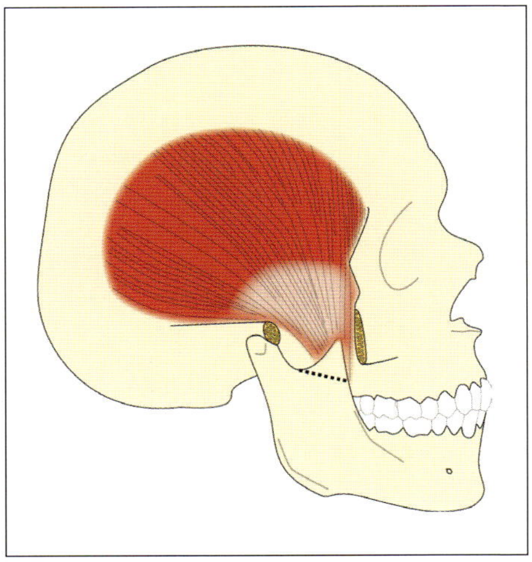

Fig 1-4b Following reflection of the temporalis muscle attachment, an osteotomy *(dotted line)* at the level of the sigmoid notch mobilizes the coronoid process.

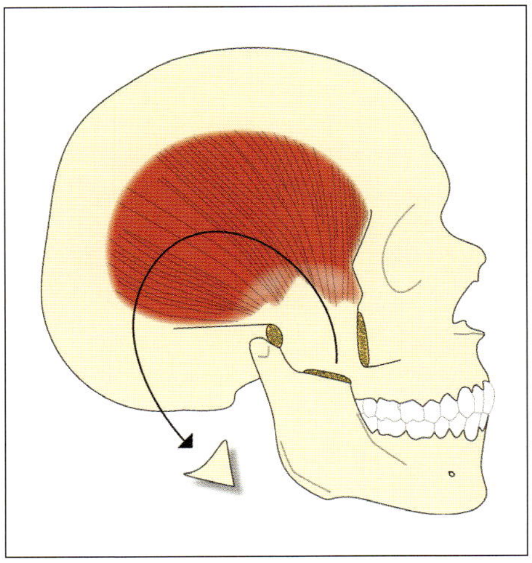

Fig 1-4c The temporalis muscle attachment retracts vertically into the temporal fossa. Removal of the coronoid process *(arrow)* results in an empty space.

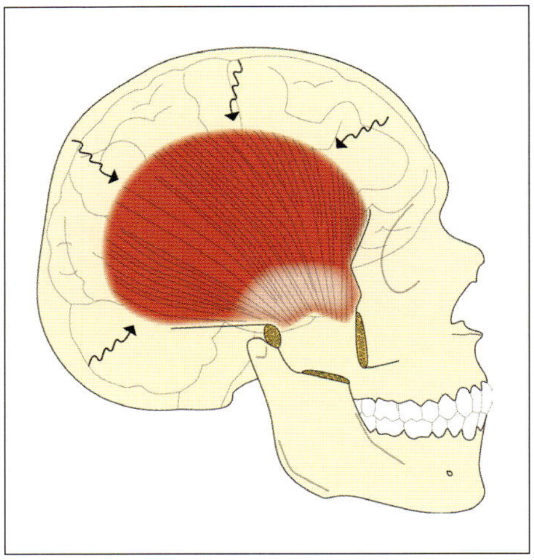

Fig 1-4d Following initial contraction of the temporalis muscle, the tendon descends toward its original position. This may involve active or passive action by the temporalis muscle. The *arrows* denote persistent muscle activity under brain control.

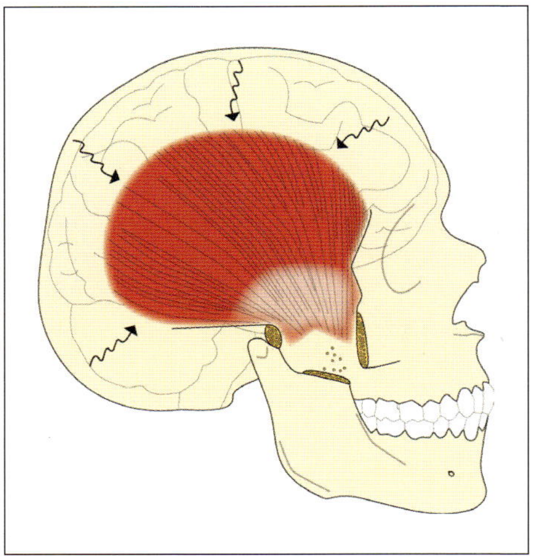

Fig 1-4e The empty space initially created by resection of the coronoid process and contraction of the temporalis muscle is gradually reoccupied. The temporalis muscle descends, and bone begins to form between the osteotomy cut and the Sharpey fiber ends of the tendon.

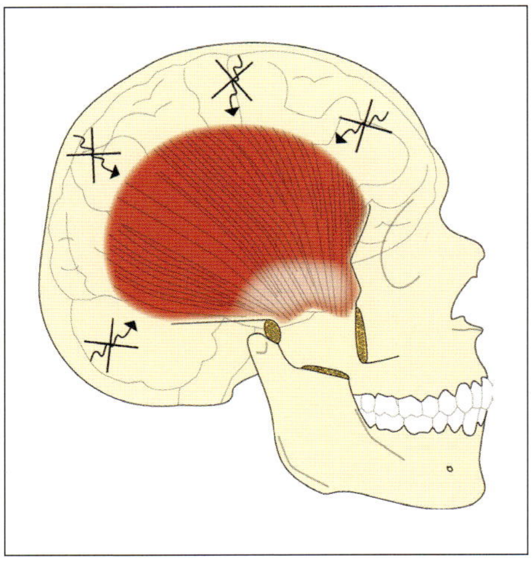

Fig 1-4f If the temporalis muscle is congenitally missing or is surgically disabled, the coronoid process does not re-form. Muscle activity is necessary for the formation, regeneration, and maintenance of a normal skeletal structure.

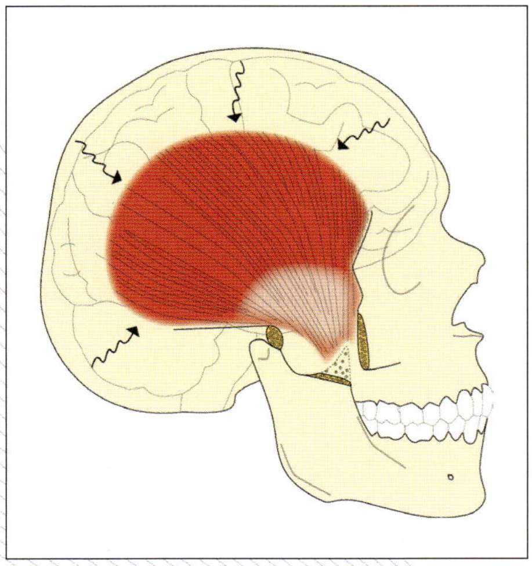

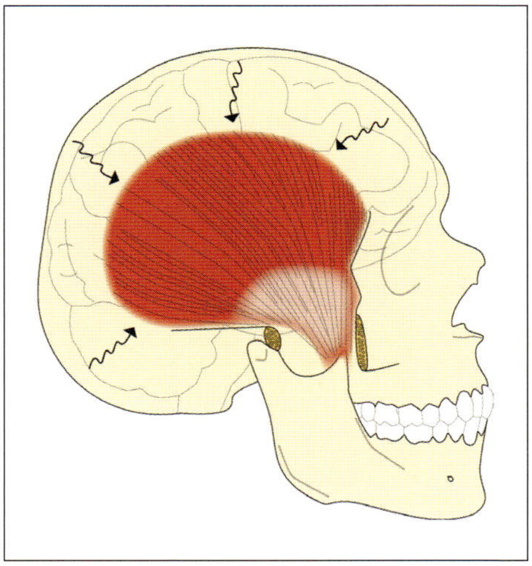

Fig 1-4g *(far left)* Bone formation in the resection void requires participation by a working temporalis muscle. As the muscle tendon descends, the bare Sharpey fibers enter the regeneration site. Interaction between the Sharpey fibers and surrounding cells results in new bone formation. The Sharpey fibers become embedded in the newly formed bone, extending the muscle's mechanical effect on the developing bone.

Fig 1-4h *(left)* The coronoid process regenerates and incorporates a new, working insertion of the temporalis muscle. The structure forms and is maintained, reproducing the original morphology and internal architecture. Regulation by the central nervous system, transmitted through action of the temporalis muscle, is the most likely mechanism directing the process.

The living construct resembles the original coronoid process in both form and function (Fig 1-4h). Its three-dimensional morphology is restored, complete with an intact blood supply, at the same position. The result of this healing sequence is a true replacement for the resected structure. The tissue types are the same as the original. Surgical examination shows the presence of a functional temporalis muscle attachment.[15]

The role of the brain is critical in the process of regeneration. Clinical manifestations of pathology that disrupts the ability of the regeneration site to receive regulatory signals from the brain confirm the importance of this principle.[38] Only recently have modern investigators been able to describe a theoretical anatomical pathway by which signals originating from the brain are delivered to the internal nanostructure of individual cells.[30–33,39]

Discussion

Regrowth of the resected coronoid process is an example of regeneration. The lost structure re-forms, reproducing the correct form and function. Normal bone forms without introduction of grafts or cells. The surgically disconnected temporalis muscle insertion becomes embedded in the newly regenerated ossicle. The end result is complete regeneration without surgical intervention.

This is a process of self-assembly in an adult that follows the pattern of embryologic development. This process occurs because the critical elements needed for bone formation and regulation of morphology are still present even after the ossicle has been removed. The temporalis muscle is associated with the development of the coronoid process in the embryo. The muscle and its associated nerve supply form prior to the formation of the mandible. It introduces the neuromuscular input into the zone of the embryo that will become the coronoid process. Thus, the coronoid process forms under the direction of the temporalis muscle insertion.

In the adult, the forces introduced to the region by muscle function, as directed by the brain, serve to maintain the morphology of the structure despite the dynamics of the remodeling process. Even though the bone turns over many times in a lifetime, the basic shape and function of the coronoid process remain. The process maintains the anatomical unit in a steady state. The specific anatomical form of the coronoid process is most likely derived from information stored in the brain and delivered to the site by the neuromuscular system.

Clinicians observe the structure—whether in a radiograph, surgically, or as a specimen—as a static structure. These views fail to show the underlying complex process in constant play. To be formed by the embryo initially and then be maintained for a lifetime requires a continuous dynamic process. The occurrence of regeneration after resection demonstrates that the process is still active in the adult. Naysayers have argued that the bone simply fills the potential space of the periosteal sleeve left after the coronoid process is removed. Others claim that the remaining local cells sense the loss and simply produce more bone cells to fill the void. Because full appreciation of the underlying mechanisms operating will not be realized for some time, the clinical value of each working theory can only be judged by the efficacy of the results. A scientifically elegant model is not clinically valuable unless it yields better patient outcomes, supported by cases that illustrate poorer outcomes when healing principles are not met, cases that illustrate greater predictability when principles are met, and cases that illustrate initial failure but later healing when the environment is altered to meet the prescribed conditions.

Creation of Construction Chambers as an Alternative Strategy to Reconstructive Surgery

Because the new coronoid process described in the preceding discussion has an analogous precursor, a coronoid that was removed, the phenomenon is properly termed *regeneration*. The logical extension of the theory is to create anatomical structures that never formed in utero by designing and executing surgeries that construct an adequate environment for growth. This advancement in thought and technique surpasses the construction of congenitally missing skeletal units via surgical assembly from grafted tissue. These surgical constructs are best thought of as *construction chambers*. Sites designed and built within the patient would have the capability of assembling the desired skeletal unit and maintaining the structure long term.

Engineering and design of treatment plans that intend to exploit embryologic mechanisms require an appreciation of how the local healing events are influenced by distant processes. The example of coronoid process regeneration illustrates that regulation of cellular behavior at the repair site is related to muscular function that is under the control of the brain. Intact muscle function is necessary for development, regeneration, and maintenance of a skeletal unit.

The precise pattern of muscle activity that directs bone development and organization at the site of regeneration is incompletely understood. It is clearly a refined system that transfers information from the brain to the cells of the repair site by multiple vectors. chemical, electrical, and mechanical methods of information transfer result in efficient and accurate direction of development in the embryo. The embryo has the capability to direct its own assembly. These same mechanisms persist in the growing child and mature adult. Even though understanding of this process is limited, it still can be used to advantage if thoughtfully included in the engineering principles of surgical design.

Although design and construction of bone-forming chambers focus on the local repair site, the underlying engineering involves biology that must consider the mechanisms and pathways that deliver neuromuscular input. Direct control follows known paths from the brain to the site of cellular development (Fig 1-5). The site must support regeneration with the correct physical environment and contain cells that are capable of interpreting the regulatory signals to construct a complex anatomical structure.

In some cases, it is not possible to surgically introduce a direct neuromuscular input unit, such as a functioning muscle attachment, to the site where the skeletal unit is to be formed. In these cases, stimulation of a healing site may be derived from

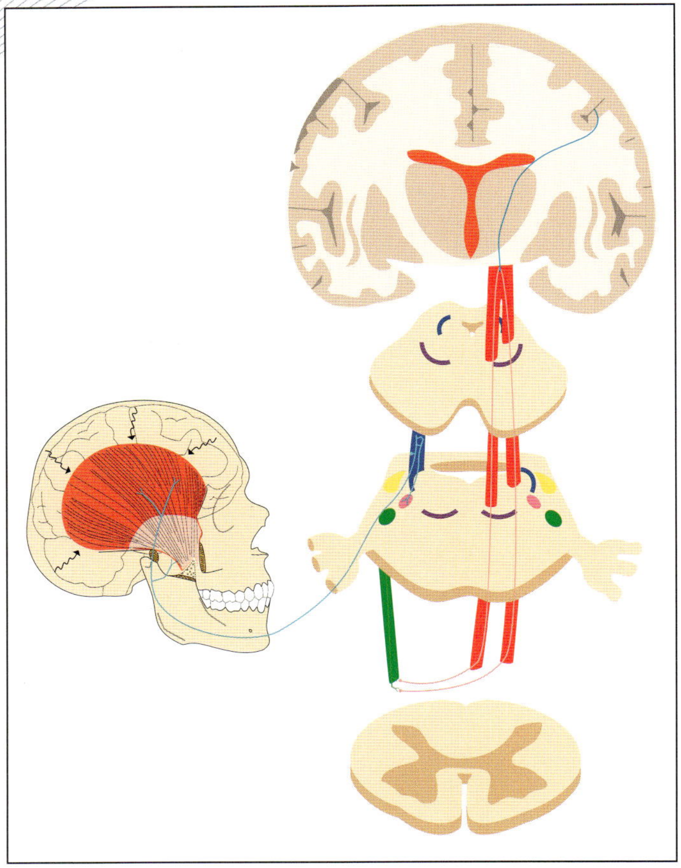

Fig 1-5 The development, maintenance, and regeneration of facial skeletal structures occur within an environment that depends on neuromuscular signaling from the central nervous system. Cellular activity at the coronoid process of the mandible derives regulation from the brain. Temporalis muscle activity is under the control of the trigeminal nerve. Specific mechanical signaling via temporalis muscle function results in modification of local cellular activity. When operating appropriately, the tissues are able to maintain a steady state or to initiate repair or maintenance functions.

adjacent structures. In the case of the mandible, for example, controlling movement of the contralateral side may create a supportive environment on the deficient side.[16] This is possible because the mandible is a bilateral structure; both sides experience movement of a single side.

The general objective is to modify the healing environment by controlling moderate or small movements to stimulate the site toward successful bone formation and organization. In contrast, if a bone graft is placed in a deficient environment that is unchanged, conditions will favor a response of bone resorption as the anatomy reverts back to the original phenotype. If bone augmentation is the objective, the best strategy is to superimpose the grafting procedure on a supportive soft tissue environment.

Conclusion

Knowledge of the biology underlying facial bone development enables the clinician to establish a more accurate diagnosis of the disorder confronted. Reconstructive surgeries are best engineered when these principles are understood and applied. Improved and novel treatment solutions can be developed when clinicians consider the full range of options that will meet the basic engineering requirements for bone formation. The essential requirements for bone formation postulated by Harvold are a starting place from which to begin this process.[15] The design and surgical fabrication of bone-forming constructs will change as new technologies become available.

References

1. Carlson BM. Development of the body systems. In: Carlson BM (ed). Human Embryology and Developmental Biology, ed 3. Philadelphia: Mosby, 2004.
2. Patten BM. Histogenesis of bone. In: Patten BM (ed). Foundations of Embryology. New York: McGraw-Hill, 1964.
3. Carlson BM. Establishment of the basic embryologic body plan. In: Carlson BM (ed). Human Embryology and Developmental Biology, ed 3. Philadelphia: Mosby, 2004.
4. Hamilton WJ, Boyd JD, Mossman HW. Alimentary and respiratory systems, pleural and peritoneal cavities. In: Hamilton WJ, Mossman HW (eds). Hamilton, Boyd and Mossman's Human Embryology, ed 4. Baltimore: Williams and Wilkins, 1972.
5. Carstens MH. Neural tube programming and the pathogenesis of craniofacial clefts, part I: The neuromeric organization of the head and neck. Handb Clin Neurol 2008;87:247–276.
6. Carstens MH. Neural tube programming and craniofacial cleft formation. I. The neuromeric organization of the head and neck. Eur J Paediatric Neurol 2004;8:181–210; discussion 179–180.
7. Morton WT. SMW 100 years ago. William Thomas Green Morton and the discovery of anesthesia [in German]. Schweiz Med Wochenschr 1996;126:2040–2042.
8. Archer WH, William TG. Morton, dentist, who first publicly demonstrated ether anesthesia; a short biography. J Am Dent Assoc 1946;33:1528–1532.
9. Fleming A. On the bacterial action of cultures of penicillin with special reference to the use in the isolation of *B. influenza*. Br J Exp Pathol 1929;10:226–236.
10. Fleming A, Chain E, et al. Penicillin and streptomycin. Lancet 1947;2: 397.
11. Fleming A, Walters W, et al. Penicillin in surgery. Lancet 1947;2: 479.
12. Watson JD, Crick FH. Molecular structure of nucleic acids; a structure for deoxyribose nucleic acid. Nature 1953;171:737–738.
13. Pauling L, Corey RB. A proposed structure for the nucleic acids. Proc Natl Acad Sci U S A 1953;39:84–97.
14. Schmutz J, Wheeler J, Grimwood J, et al. Quality assessment of the human genome sequence. Nature 2004;429:365–368.
15. Harvold EP. The theoretical basis for the treatment of hemifacial microsomia. In: Harvold EP, Vargervik K, Chierici G (eds). Treatment of Hemifacial Microsomia. New York: Alan R. Liss, 1983.
16. Vargervik K. Sequence and timing of treatment phases in hemifacial microsomia. In: Harvold EP, Vargervik K, Chierici G (eds). Treatment of Hemifacial Microsomia. New York: Alan R. Liss, 1983.
17. Ousterhout DK. Skeletal surgery in hemifacial microsomia. In: Harvold EP, Vargervik K, Chierici G (eds). Treatment of Hemifacial Microsomia. New York: Alan R. Liss, 1983.
18. Vargervik K. Assessment of facial and masticatory muscles in hemifacial microsomia. In: Harvold EP, Vargervik K, Chierici G (eds). Treatment of Hemifacial Microsomia. New York: Alan R. Liss, 1983.
19. Miller A. Electromyography as a technique to study neuromuscular characteristics in hemifacial microsomia and other congenital anomalies. In: Harvold EP, Vargervik K, Chierici G (eds). Treatment of Hemifacial Microsomia. New York: Alan R. Liss, 1983.
20. Vargervik K. Treatment of hemifacial microsomia in patients without a functioning temporomandibular joint articulation. In: Harvold EP, Vargervik K, Chierici G (eds). Treatment of Hemifacial Microsomia. New York: Alan R. Liss, 1983.
21. Vargervik K. Treatment of hemifacial microsomia in patients with abnormal, but functioning temporomandibular articulation. In: Harvold EP, Vargervik K, Chierici G (eds). Treatment of Hemifacial Microsomia. New York: Alan R. Liss, 1983.
22. Ingber DE. Integrins, tensegrity, and mechanotransduction. Gravit Space Biol Bull 1997;10:49–55.
23. Ingber DE. Tensegrity: The architectural basis of cellular mechanotransduction. Annual Rev Physiol 1997;59:575–599.
24. Ingber DE. The architecture of life. Sci Am 1998;278:48–57.
25. Vargervik K, Miller AJ. Neuromuscular patterns in hemifacial microsomia. Am J Orthod 1984;86:33–42.
26. Miller AJ, Chierici G. Concepts related to adaptation of neuromuscular function and craniofacial morphology. Birth Defects Orig Artic Ser 1982;18:21–43.
27. Miller AJ, Vargervik K, Chierici G. Sequential neuromuscular changes in rhesus monkeys during the initial adaptation to oral respiration. Am J Orthod 1982;81:99–107.
28. Vargervik K. Appliances utilized in the treatment of hemifacial microsomia. In: Harvold EP, Vargervik K, Chierici G (eds). Treatment of Hemifacial Microsomia. New York: Alan R. Liss, 1983.
29. Carlson BM. Sense organs. In: Carlson BM (ed). Human Embryology and Developmental Biology, ed 3. Philadelphia: Mosby, 2004.
30. Ingber DE. Tensegrity II. How structural networks influence cellular information processing networks. J Cell Sci 2003;116:1397–1408.
31. Ingber DE. Tensegrity I. Cell structure and hierarchical systems biology. J Cell Sci 2003;116:1157–1173.
32. Ingber DE. Tensegrity and mechanotransduction. J Bodyw Mov Ther 2008;12:198–200.
33. Ingber DE. Tensegrity-based mechanosensing from macro to micro. Prog Biophys Mol Biol 2008;97:163–179.
34. Ingber DE, Dike L, Hansen L, et al. Cellular tensegrity: Exploring how mechanical changes in the cytoskeleton regulate cell growth, migration, and tissue pattern during morphogenesis. Int Rev Cytol 1994;150:173–224.
35. Smyth AG, Wake MJ. Recurrent bilateral coronoid hyperplasia: An unusual case. Br J Oral Maxillofac Surg 1994;32:100–104.
36. McLoughlin PM, Hopper C, Bowley NB. Hyperplasia of the mandibular coronoid process: An analysis of 31 cases and a review of the literature. J Oral Maxillofac Surg 1995;53:250–255.
37. Gerbino G, Bianchi SD, Bernardi M, Berrone S. Hyperplasia of the mandibular coronoid process: Long-term follow-up after coronoidotomy. J Craniomaxillofac Surg 1997;25:169–173.
38. Horowitz SL, Shapiro HH. Modifications of mandibular architecture following removal of temporalis muscle in the rat. J Dent Res 1951;30:276–280.
39. Aaron JE. Periosteal Sharpey's fibers: A novel bone matrix regulatory system? Front Endinocrinol 2012;3:98.

2 Establishing and Maintaining Osseointegration Within the Functional Matrix

The ability to design dental implant surgeries that exploit the mechanisms that bone uses to develop and maintain its morphology opens a new range of treatment possibilities. These novel surgical strategies can increase the predictability of current procedures by using the patient's underlying bone-regulation processes to enhance healing. When surgery is engineered properly, challenging reconstructions that have failed previously can be modified to heal successfully. Instead of focusing on placement of the dental implant, this treatment strategy aims to establish an environment that will support the surrounding bone, implant, and osseointegration interface.

The working theory for creation of these bone-forming constructs has been described in chapter 1. That discussion provided basic engineering rules to guide the surgical design of these systems. According to Harvold, successful engineering of bone tissue requires a stabilized environment, a source of cells, neuromuscular input, and an absence of pathology.[1] The nature and role of each essential element of the bone-forming construct must be appreciated and included in surgical design. The omission of one component compromises the healing potential and prevents meaningful evaluation of how well the system performs. How the designer intends to meet the requirements is a matter of creativity. In some cases, surgical plans that appear beyond the capability of normal healing can be made possible and practical for clinical use.

This approach is a departure from the premise that having an existing viable bone unit is a prerequisite for successful healing of a dental implant. In the new strategy, the principal design objective is to fabricate a bone-forming construct at the location of the new skeletal unit. The site may have some preexisting bone or none. If the treatment objective is for the skeletal unit to house a dental implant, then an implant becomes a part of the surgical construct. In these surgeries, osseointegration is achieved by suspending an implant within the regeneration chamber. Bone developing within the regeneration chamber surrounds the dental implant, and an osseointegration interface is created.

This method of establishing and maintaining osseointegration differs from the traditional method in both technique and theory. This approach depends on the underlying regulatory mechanisms that control bone morphology. The concept that local bone metabolism, including the bone securing dental implants, is regulated by local and distant signals challenges conventional assumptions and practice. The proposed theory suggests that osseointegration involves the full hierarchy of bone regulation, extending from brain above to the intracellular nanostructure below, rather than just an interaction between bone and the titanium oxide layer of dental implants. Because these two concepts of osseointegration exist in the same biologic system, they must be parts of a shared physiologic process. Even if the surgeon prefers to remain in the conventional sphere, it is valuable to understand how the processes occurring at the implant site might interact with the global process that maintains the skeleton.

Conventional Concepts of Osseointegration

There is value in comparing and contrasting the two treatment approaches to placement of dental implants. Brånemark's revolutionary work in establishing and maintaining implanted skeletal anchoring devices set dentistry and orthopedics along a new path.[2,3] Early experiences with the original machined-surface titanium implants produced very gratifying results.[4] Subsequent research explored how different materials and titanium surface preparations affected both healing and long-term performance of these devices.[5–7] It seemed clear that, if a typical patient was being treated, predictable healing and long-term service of anchored dental prostheses could be expected. Students today are taught that if a specific technical protocol is followed, the special osseointegration healing response will most often be realized.

Failure to achieve osseointegration is blamed on a litany of issues, including but not limited to *(1)* technical surgical errors, such as excessive heat during drilling or overinstrumentation that compromises the immediate stability of the implant; *(2)* host integrity challenges, such as smoking; *(3)* chronic periodontal disease affecting implants with adverse microflora; and *(4)* prosthesis design and mechanical loading of the implants.

Despite extensive research covering multiple aspects of dental implantology, the current technique and theoretical basis of the treatment remain basically the same as those originally described by Brånemark.[2,3] The surgical process still involves atraumatic creation of a precision osteotomy. Control of friction-generated heat during drilling remains a critical requirement of the surgical technique. Implant shapes and surface preparations have taken on many forms, but titanium remains the most common material.

When the implant is placed in the osteotomy, the surgeon verifies that the device is mechanically stable. In the conventional two-step protocol, the implant is left unrestored until osseointegration has been established. Immediately after the implant has been placed, mechanical stability is maintained by the mechanical wedging of the implant threads against the walls of the cut bone. This condition must be converted to a state in which viable bone grows directly against the titanium oxide layer of the implant surface.

It is important to understand the process occurring in the bone adjacent to the implant surface. When the osteotomy for the implant is made, it does not precisely fit the surface contours of the implant. Drilling, tapping, and placement of self-tapping implants result in substantial gaps between the implant and the bone. The process also creates bone fragments and areas of impaired circulation. Success or failure of the treatment depends on establishment of the osseointegration interface. If fibrous connective tissue forms between the implant surface and bone, the cylinder becomes mobile and is not clinically useful.

The force applied while the implant is torqued in place causes compression of the osteotomy walls and subsequent bone necrosis. Removal of the dead debris by resorption becomes part of the healing process. Demineralization of bone within the osteotomy wall releases sequestered growth factors that are important in the regulation of the healing process. This catabolic phase precedes the formation of new structural bone. During this process, the implant must be maintained in a mechanically stable state. Mobility of the implant is associated with fibrous encapsulation and osseointegration failure.[8,9]

If successful osseointegration is to occur, there must be a mechanism to maintain implant stability while adjacent bone is undergoing resorption and deposition. If all of the bone adjacent to the newly placed implant undergoes resorption as a first step toward healing, the bone loses its mechanical grip on the implant, and mobility develops. A mobile implant tends to develop fibrous encapsulation, and the osseointegrated interface does not form.

Brånemark offered the first and most enduring explanation of the events that occur following placement of the modern dental implant[2] (Fig 2-1).The original Brånemark protocol involved atraumatic creation of a threaded bone preparation to receive the implant. Close fit of the bone preparation and implant was intended to establish continuous physical apposition of the bone and the titanium surface. Even during demineralization of the exposed bone surface, physical contact of bone tissue against the implant surface maintained stability.

Misch revisited the events that occur shortly after implant placement. In his description, the first event is *anabolic modeling*, during which a callus forms between the host bone and the implant surface.[10] The callus fills the voids resulting from the imperfect mating of the implant and the bone preparation site. This action is mediated by cytokines released from local blood clots. Mechanical stability of the implant is maintained by its physical contact with osteotomy walls. Although this bone has been damaged by surgical instrumentation, it still provides

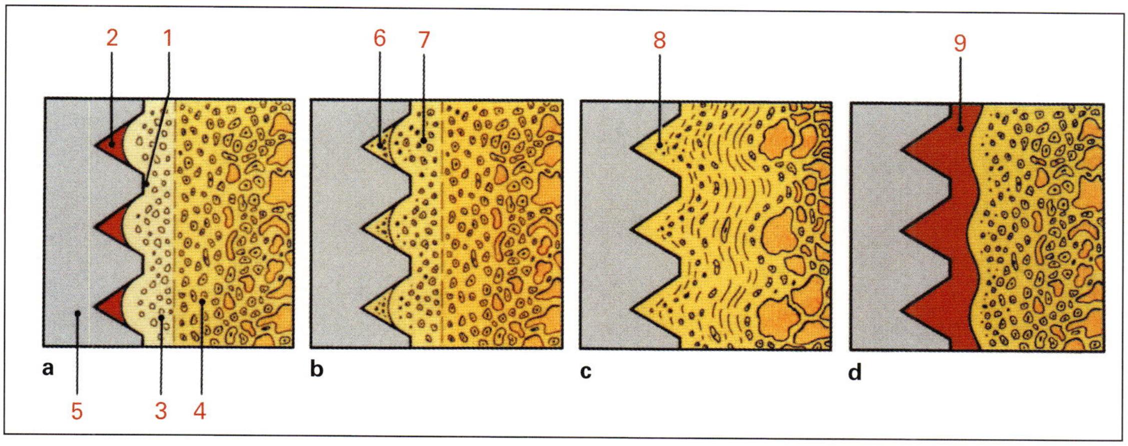

Fig 2-1a In 1977, Brånemark presented this diagrammatic outline of his working theory of bone healing around titanium implants. This method for establishing osseointegration remains standard practice. The threaded bone site cannot be made perfectly congruent to the implant. The object of making a threaded socket in bone is to provide immobilization immediately after placement and during the initial healing period. 1 = contact between implant and bone (immobilization); 2 = hematoma in closed cavity, bordered by implant and bone; 3 = bone that was damaged by unavoidable thermal and mechanical trauma; 4 = original undamaged bone; and 5 = implant.

Fig 2-1b During the unloaded healing period, the hematoma transforms into new bone through callus formation (6). Damaged bone, which also heals, undergoes revascularization, demineralization, and remineralization (7).

Fig 2-1c After the initial healing period, vital bone tissue is in close contact with the implant surface, without any other intermediate tissue. Border zone bone (8) remodels in response to the masticatory load applied.

Fig 2-1d In unsuccessful cases, nonmineralized connective tissue (9), constituting a kind of pseudoarthrosis, forms in the border zone at the implant. This development can be initiated by excessive preparation trauma, infection, loading too early in the healing period before adequate mineralization and organization of hard tissue have taken place, or supraliminal loading at any time, even many years after integration has been established. Once lost, osseointegration cannot be reconstituted. Connective tissue can become organized to a certain degree but is not a proper anchoring tissue because of its inadequate mechanical and biologic capacities, resulting in creation of a *locus minoris resistentiae*. (Reprinted from Brånemark et al[3] with permission.)

mechanical support of the implant, even if the tissue is nonvital. Nonvital bone is later removed by *interface remodeling* until the osseointegration interface is established.

Direct contact of vital bone with the implant is a prerequisite for successful osseointegration treatment. Titanium has endured as the material of choice for dental implants. Many other implant materials had been tried in the past; fibrous encapsulation and implant failure were the most common outcomes. After successful osseointegration of titanium implants in laboratory animals and humans was demonstrated, study focused on why this material seemed to heal better than others. Kasemo described the chemical characteristics of the titanium oxide layer that is the interface between the implant and vital host tissue.[11] His conclusion was that the titanium oxide layer possesses an affinity to form chemical bonds with organic systems and that this affinity results in a phenomenon that maintains the adherence of living bone cells to the implant surface.

Establishment of Osseointegration Within a Bone-Forming Construct

In an ideal clinical situation, a dental implant is placed in a healthy patient in a site with generous bone volume. The site receiving the implant has an uncomplicated history where a natural tooth originally developed but was lost. Periodontal disease has never been a problem. The periodontal phenotype is thick, and the tooth is not visible during smiling. The occlusion is primarily on natural, healthy teeth. In this scenario, a dental implant can be placed and a good outcome expected. There is no need to consider deviating from the standard, familiar protocol. There is no reason to question whether the conceptual understanding accepted in the past is not operating in this case.

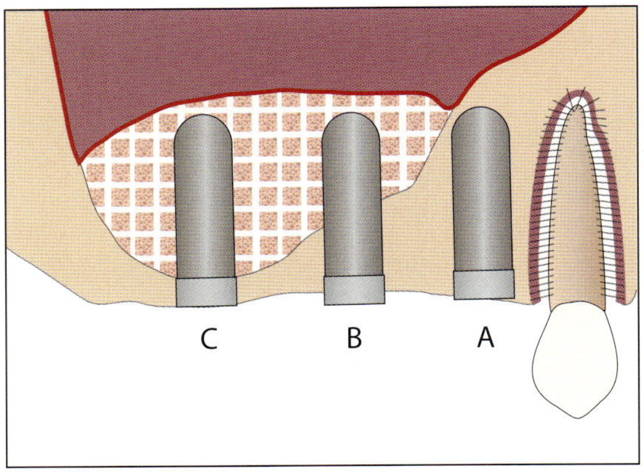

Fig 2-2 Three classes of implant site differ in the amount of native bone that is present. Site A provides full enclosure of the implant and primary stability. Site B provides partial enclosure of the implant but immediate stability. The apical portion of the implant extends into the sinus elevation graft. Site C lacks bone volume to cover any portion of the potential osseointegration surface and possesses no ability to provide primary stability. Only graft material surrounds the implant.

When undesirable outcomes occur, however, identification of a specific cause is important. Blame is directed to defective materials, surgeon error, or host healing deficiency. Often the reason for failure cannot be identified. In other cases, the anatomical defect would seem to preclude a successful outcome, but the procedure is completed anyway. To the surgeon's surprise, the site heals perfectly and goes on to years of useful service.

Exceptions to the predicted outcomes suggest that the physiology of osseointegration requires a more complex explanation than current understanding permits. Some implants will heal successfully even when the basic accepted surgical protocol is not followed. Other implants do not heal despite strict adherence to the protocols in a patient with no healing problems. These contradictions must be explored and understood. An alternative approach to dental implant treatment is to consider how implants interact within the global skeletal physiology. Such an approach would not only help to explain unexpected outcomes that cannot be explained by the current understanding of osseointegration but also reveal how the currently unrecognized processes may be exploited to surgical advantage. In this analysis, the process of osseointegration is examined in how it meets the requirements for bone formation described in chapter 1: a stabilized environment, a source of cells, neuromuscular input, and an absence of pathology.

Stabilized environment

One of the essential elements of a bone-forming construct is a stabilized environment. Managing mechanical movement at the site of bone formation is a theme common to both conventional concepts of osseointegration and fabrication of bone-forming constructs. As mentioned earlier, implant stability is established and maintained by the mechanical mating of the cut bone preparation and the implant surface.

Figure 2-2 depicts implants placed in three implant sites that vary in their amount of native bone. Implant A is fully housed in native bone; there is no need for bone augmentation, and the implant is stable at the time of placement. Implant B is engaged in enough native bone to establish primary stability; the apical portion extends beyond the sinus floor. Implant C is located in the thin sinus floor; there is minimal contact between the implant and bone, and the implant is clearly mobile when it is placed. The thickness of the sinus floor bone is less that the height of the implant's polished collar. No part of the implant surface prepared for osseointegration contacts the native bone. A sinus elevation bone graft covers the exposed implant surfaces of implants B and C.

In the three scenarios depicted, implant A would have the highest likelihood of successfully healing to osseointegration. Even if some areas of the cylinder lack supportive bone-to-implant stabilization, there are other sites that can assume the role of immobilization.

Implant B begins with primary stability. This is despite the imperfect fit of the implant to the bone preparation. Some portion of the mechanical stability obtained through physical wedging of the implant against the cut bone surface is lost when bone adjacent to the cylinder undergoes catabolic demineralization. If too much mechanical support is lost during this catabolic phase, the implant will become mobile and will develop fibrous encapsulation. Some implants in this scenario will be able to maintain stability through the catabolic phase and will go on to develop an osseointegrated interface.

If the cylinder is mobile at the time of placement, as in the case of implant C, successful healing to an osseointegrated surface is unlikely. Most surgeons would elect to defer implant placement at site C and allow the sinus elevation graft to consolidate. The strategy would be to place the implant at site C when there is enough structural bone to stabilize it.

The varying amounts of native bone at the implant site impact *(1)* the ability to establish primary stability, *(2)* the ability to maintain stability through the catabolic healing phase, and *(3)* the availability of osteogenic cells. Implant A should have the highest predictability and implant C the lowest. Implant B may heal but at a compromised rate of success. The failure rate of type B implants is higher than that of type A implants but lower than that of type C implants.

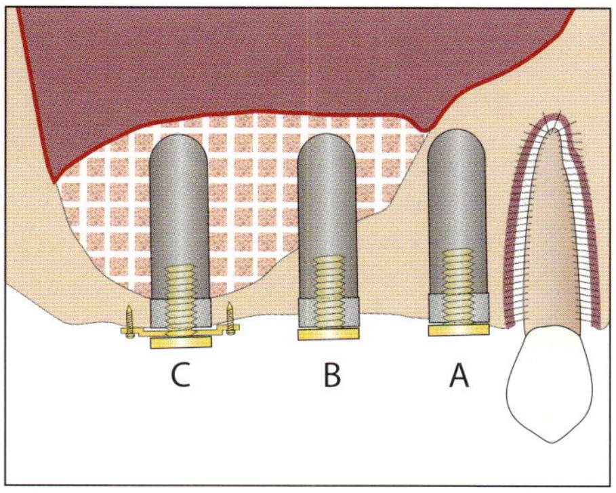

Fig 2-3 A bone plate added to implant C establishes relative mechanical stability. The bone plate is 0.3-mm-thick titanium alloy secured with two microscrews.

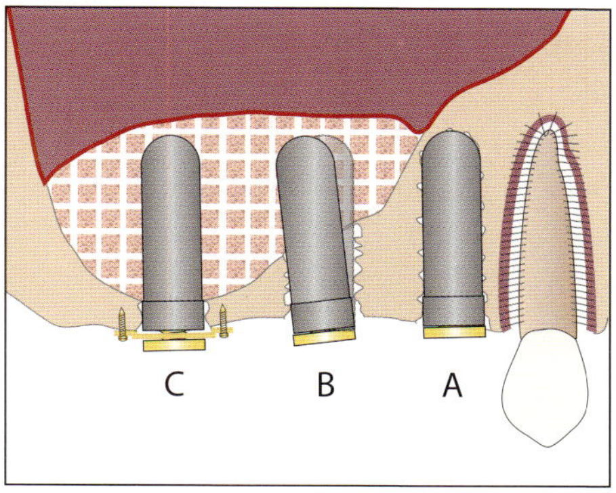

Fig 2-4 The bone adjacent to each implant demineralizes as part of the natural healing sequence. The titanium plate on implant C maintains implant stability despite resorption of surrounding bone. Implant A remains stable because of redundant support provided by the surrounding bone. Implant B is at risk of losing mechanical stability because native bone support is limited.

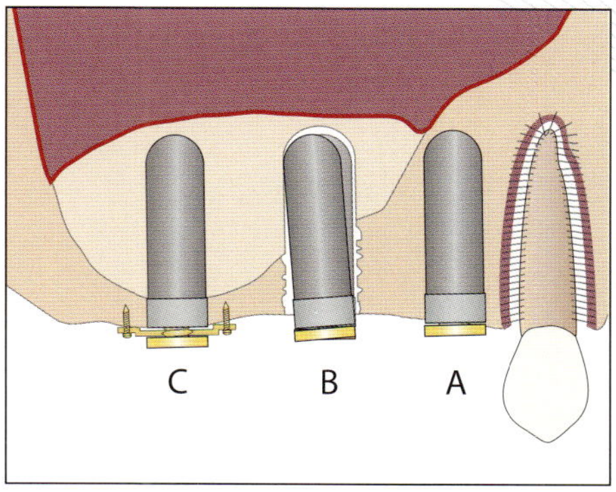

Fig 2-5 Implant B fails to heal because the limited amount of native bone that provided initial mechanical stability is not sufficient to maintain continuous support through the demineralization phase. Implant A heals successfully because its volume of surrounding bone provides redundant mechanical support in the presence of focal, transient demineralization. Implant C heals successfully because the bone plate maintains mechanical stability until the graft consolidates.

Bone plates for added stabilization

In a modification of the scenario, a bone plate has been added to implant C (Fig 2-3). The extension arms of the bone plate reach a distance from the implant site. Two microscrews anchor the bone plate arms to the native bone.

Bone resorption during the catabolic phase of implant healing has a different effect on each implant type (Fig 2-4). Implant A remains stable despite resorption of bone in the walls of the osteotomy. Maintaining the stability of implant B is more challenging because the total amount of stabilizing bone is less and the cylinder is exposed to the same movement forces as the other implants. Implant B is also vulnerable to epithelial migration from two directions, the oral mucosa and the sinus membrane. Implant A, in contrast, only has to confront epithelial downgrowth from the oral side. In the case of implant B, the resorption during the catabolic phase causes implant instability, and the result is fibrous encapsulation.

Implant C experiences total loss of native bone contact. The minimal bone of the atrophic sinus floor is left without a vascular supply when the mucoperiosteum is elevated on the oral side and the sinus membrane is elevated on the superior side. The site is further injured by drilling for placement of the implant. Implant C is therefore suspended by the bone plate and microscrews. The small size of the microscrews and their placement at a distance from the implant osteotomy allows the bone plate to remain stable, maintaining stability of the implant.

The microscrews are implants themselves and should undergo catabolic loosening too. The loosening of the microscrews is delayed compared to the loosening at the implant site. This allows the bone plate–microscrew assembly to stabilize the implant until the graft develops a mechanical grip on the implant.

Without auxiliary stabilization, implant B is vulnerable to low-level forces imparted by bone flexion under function, respiration, and mastication. These forces result in implant movement and fibrous encapsulation. Implant C maintains relative immobility. Thus, osseointegration develops on implants A and C, while implant B fails (Fig 2-5).

The bone plate is fabricated from titanium alloy mesh (Ti-6Al-4V) that is typically used for facial fracture repair. The recommended material is 0.3 mm in thickness. When attached to the dental implant and fixated with small bone screws, the plate provides stability but not rigid immobilization. Clinical experience has shown that the use of bone plates with greater rigidity fails to improve the results, and such plates are much more difficult to place and bend to the contour of the bone. The 0.3-mm-thick titanium material can be bent under the manual pressure of an instrument while remaining attached to the implant.

The ideal degree of immobilization to optimize bone formation is unknown. The embryogenesis process suggests that the ideal environment is one sheltered from major mechanical forces but not rigidly immobilized. In the embryo, the mandible forms at a distance from Meckel cartilage, not immediately adjacent to it. Following the working theory of bone-forming environments, some motion is necessary to allow mechanical signaling to reach precursor cells.[1] Some degree of mobility is thus desirable and necessary.[12–15]

Establishing a degree of physical stability within the bone-forming environment is one of the essential elements for achieving bone formation. An approach that places the dental implant in the center of the construct and then provides auxiliary stabilization satisfies the requirement of a sheltered environment.

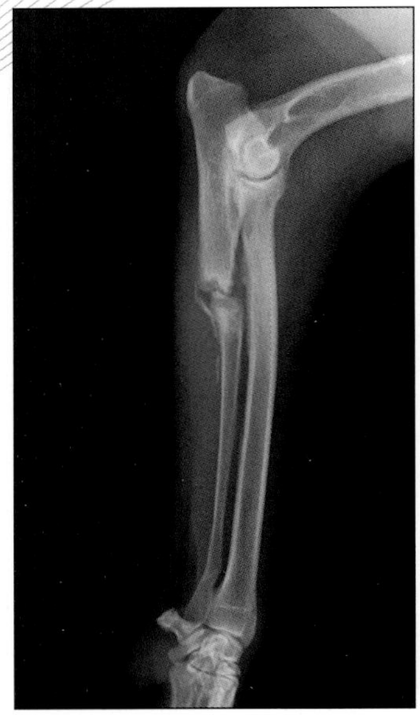

Fig 2-6a Radiograph showing discontinuity of the fibula in a 2-year-old Labrador retriever. The defect occurred when an osteotomy performed to correct a developmental defect failed to heal with an osseous union.

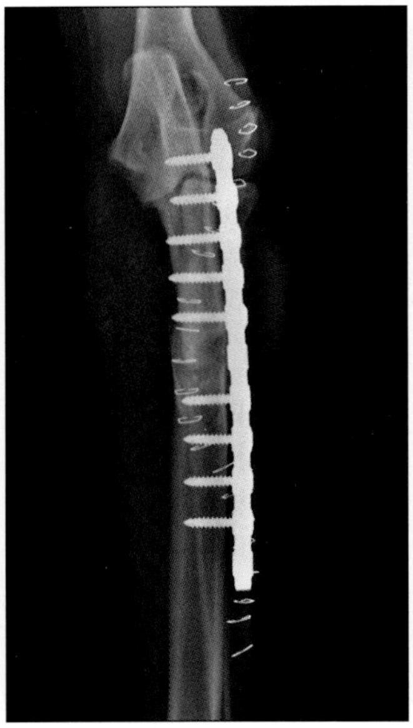

Fig 2-6b Fibula fragments are aligned and stabilized with an 11-hole bone plate and 9 screws. A radiograph confirms that the ends of the bone fragments are in direct contact. The nonunion site has been treated with recombinant human bone morphogenetic protein 2 (rhBMP-2) on absorbable collagen sponges.

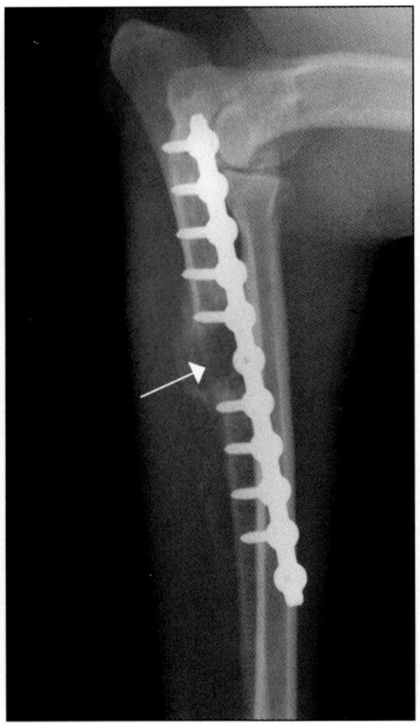

Fig 2-6c Two weeks after surgery, a radiograph shows a large radiolucency *(arrow)* at the repair site. Natural demineralization of the repair site removes structural bone. The bone plate maintains stability during this period. The screws distant from the repair site remain stable. The screws adjacent to the repair site are within the resorption zone.

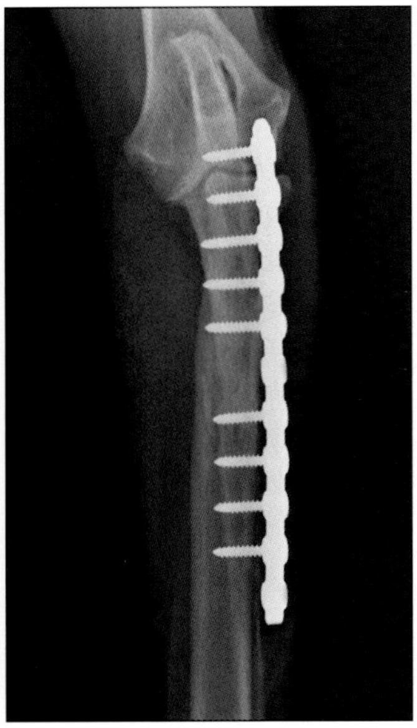

Fig 2-6d Ten weeks after surgery, a radiograph shows that osseous union has restored fibula continuity. (Primary surgeon: Andrew Sams, DVM.)

Lessons from orthopedic practice

The principle of extending anchorage away from the site of catabolic remodeling is common practice in orthopedics. Orthopedic surgeons are trained to extend internal fixation devices a distance from the healing site.

A 2-year-old Labrador retriever developed a nonunion following an osteotomy of the fibula (Fig 2-6a). Following standard orthopedic practice, an 11-hole orthopedic bone plate was contoured to maintain reduction of the osteotomy site (Fig 2-6b). Nine screws were placed extending a distance from the site undergoing repair. No screw was placed at the osteotomy site itself. The repair site was treated with recombinant human bone morphogenetic protein 2 (rhBMP-2) carried on an absorbable collagen sponge. The total dose of rhBMP-2 was 12 mg in 8 mL of sterile water.

Two weeks after surgery, the radiograph revealed a radiolucency extending from the repair site (Fig 2-6c). This represented the catabolic phase of the repair healing, that is, demineralization of bone adjacent to the repair site. The radiolucency reached both the proximal and distal fixation screws. The associated demineralization compromised the mechanical fixation of the screws nearest the repair site. However, multiple screws on the portion of the plate extending from the repair site maintained fixation and immobilization.

Ten weeks after surgical repair of the nonunion, the radiograph of the fibula revealed restoration of the osseous continuity (Fig 2-6d). The zone of demineralization had returned to a normal density.

This case represents the standard treatment of a limb defect by orthopedic surgeons treating humans or animals. Surgical experience has resulted in technical practices that avoid problems related to predictable processes. In this case, the bone at the repair site was expected to undergo resorption as part of the normal healing process. Stabilization that depended on fixation screws located too near the repair site would have resulted in treatment failure as the bone underwent natural resorption in the catabolic phase of healing. The surgeon extended the bone plate to enable placement of fixation screws in bone sites that would not be directly impacted by the demineralization of the repair site. At 2 weeks, dramatic resorption had extended to two of the fixation screws. However, the other screws remained stable until a union of the repair site was achieved.

Source of cells

Surgical designs for dental implant treatment require a source of cells to complete bone formation and osseointegration. The construct will not perform without the presence of cells in adequate quantity and quality.

The surgical designer can introduce cells in different ways. Allowing cells to migrate to the bone-forming chamber from the immediately adjacent tissue can be an effective method. If this source cannot supply enough viable cells, they must be introduced by other means. Use of bone morphogenetic proteins is a very effective way to satisfy the requirement for cells in the construct. Morphogenetic proteins may be delivered to the site on absorbable collagen sponges or a banked allogeneic bone graft. In other cases, autogenous bone may serve to supply cells. Each clinical situation presents a unique challenge for the surgeon in determining how to deliver cells and which carrier provides the best support for healing.

Neuromuscular input

Designing neuromuscular signaling to the bone reconstruction site is an essential component of the treatment. Physical or chemical regulation of cellular activity is needed for both the newly introduced cells and the native tissue. After cells are recruited into the bone-forming environment, they require regulation to direct growth and organization.

Within the jaw systems, teeth can be used to impart regulatory stimulation to bone-forming environments. The periodontal ligament systems transfer mechanical signals from the teeth to the bone. These signals are important in the normal physiology of alveolar bones. Healthy periodontal ligaments originate in the dental roots and insert into the lamina dura. The dental crowns are under constant mechanical challenge while under function. All of the forces borne by the crowns are absorbed by the roots. These forces are delivered to the alveolar bone via the periodontal ligaments. These forces direct formation of the lamina dura and the underlying trabecular architecture of the medullary bone.

The facial muscles exert force on the facial skeleton during their action. The morphology of the facial skeleton reflects the functional stimulation imparted by active facial muscles. If the muscle action is diminished by damage to the motor nerve that supplies it, the affected segment of the facial bone remodels and resorbs. This phenomenon occurs in Parry-Romberg syndrome, affecting both the muscle mass and facial bone morphology. The surgical designer must be aware of how existing muscle action affects the remodeling pattern of the region being reconstructed. In some cases, the surgical designer modifies muscle attachment positions to alter the pattern of stimulation to the benefit of the bone-forming construct.

In some cases, the surgical designer determines that there are no good options for recruiting neuromuscular signaling into an edentulous jaw segment where implants are desired. Because a surgical plan that lacks neuromuscular input will likely result in the failure of a bone graft to heal, an alternative strategy is needed. Bone augmentation and implant reconstruction of a deficient site may not be practical. In these cases, reconfiguration of the alveolar anatomy to eliminate the need for an implant may be the best option.

Absence of pathology

Establishing an environment that is free of pathologic processes is essential to the success of the bone-forming construct. Disease processes may prevent healing by compromising the physical environment, the substrate cell population, or the integrity of the neuromuscular signaling system. When these conditions present as part of the deformity, they must be addressed prior to reconstruction or managed as part of the regeneration process itself. Disease processes that involve alveolar reconstruction are either local or systemic. Typical local disorders include infections that are derived from endodontic, periodontal, or sinus pathology. Systemic disorders cover a wide scope and include healing compromise from medications such as steroids, immunosuppressives, and bisphosphonates. Metabolic disorders such as diabetes may challenge healing. Deficiencies that are related to anomalies of embryogenesis may appear as a local problem but are better considered as systemic disorders.[16]

Management of local pathosis

Infection extending from the maxillary sinus into a sinus elevation graft is an example of local pathosis complicating the healing of a bone-forming construct. This risk is mitigated by careful manipulation of the sinus membrane during sinus grafting procedures to maintain an anatomical barrier between sinus flora and the regeneration chamber. If the maxillary sinus membrane is breached during a sinus elevation procedure, bacteria and secretions penetrate the graft and may result in an infection.

Even with the most careful technique, sinus elevation procedures challenge the existing ventilation and drainage physiology because inflammation is a natural consequence of the surgical process. Use of rhBMP-2 as a graft material may increase the amount of sinus membrane edema.[17] Even if the condition of the sinus is asymptomatic prior to surgery, swelling may obstruct the ostium and prevent clearance of secretions, and sinusitis may result. Patients with a history of sinus infections may benefit from medical or surgical treatment of the sinus prior to sinus elevation grafting.

Management of systemic pathosis

Alveolar deficiencies related to developmental disorders may appear initially as a local problem. It is important to recognize that the underlying pathogenesis of these defects extends beyond the boundaries of the missing part.[18] Even though the anatomy adjacent to a missing skeletal segment appears to be intact, the process that formed the defect impacts the integrity of the adjacent tissue to some degree. As an approximation, the pathogenesis effect within the adjacent tissue volume can be considered to extend radially with the defect as the focus.

If the treatment plan depends on the healing integrity of the adjacent tissue, the surgical designer must take into account the possible compromise in the healing response. In some cases, it is necessary to modify the surgical design in order to remove the pathogenic segment from the regeneration environment.

Conclusion

There are two reasons why the process of osseointegration should be examined from the viewpoint of how implants interact within the global skeletal physiology. First, in some cases there are unexpected outcomes that cannot be explained by the current understanding of osseointegration, and these deserve explanation. Second, if the deficiency in current knowledge can be overcome, the unrecognized processes of osseointegration may be exploited to clinical advantage. With a full understanding of the global mechanisms that regulate bone, the surgeon can engineer an environment that fosters bone growth and osseointegration.

References

1. Harvold EP. The theoretical basis for the treatment of hemifacial microsomia. In: Harvold EP, Vargervik K, Chierici G (eds). Treatment of Hemifacial Microsomia. New York: Alan R. Liss, 1983.
2. Brånemark PI. Osseointegration and its experimental background. J Prosthet Dent 1983;50:399–410.
3. Brånemark PI, Zarb GA, Albrektsson T (eds). Tissue-Integrated Prostheses: Osseointegration in Clinical Dentistry. Chicago: Quintessence, 1986.
4. Albrektsson T. Direct bone anchorage of dental implants. J Prosthet Dent 1983;50:255–261.
5. Albrektsson T. Surface roughness of intraoral dental implant fixtures. Dent Implantol Update 1998;9:73–77.
6. Jungner M, Lundqvist P, Lundgren S. Oxidized titanium implants (Nobel Biocare TiUnite) compared with turned titanium implants (Nobel Biocare Mark III) with respect to implant failure in a group of consecutive patients treated with early functional loading and two-stage protocol. Clin Oral Implants Res 2005;16:308–312.
7. Esposito M, Coulthard P, Thomsen P, Worthington HV. The role of implant surface modifications, shape and material on the success of osseointegrated dental implants. A Cochrane systematic review. Eur J Prosthodont Restorative Dent 2005;13:15–31.
8. Brunski JB, Moccia AF Jr, Pollack SR, Korostoff E, Trachtenberg DI. The influence of functional use of endosseous dental implants on the tissue-implant interface. II. Clinical aspects. J Dent Res 1979; 58:1970–1980.
9. Misch CE. Stress treatment theorem for implant dentistry. In: Misch CE (ed). Contemporary Implant Dentistry, ed 3. St Louis: Mosby Elsevier, 2008:68–91.
10. Misch CE, Misch-Dietsh F. Preimplant prosthodontics: Overall evaluation, specific criteria, and pretreatment prostheses. In: Misch CE (ed). Contemporary Implant Dentistry, ed 3. St Louis: Mosby Elsevier, 2008:233–244.
11. Kasemo B. Biocompatibility of titanium implants: Surface science aspects. J Prosthet Dent 1983;49:832–837.
12. Ingber DE. Integrins, tensegrity, and mechanotransduction. Gravit Space Biol Bull 1997;10:49–55.
13. Ingber DE. Tensegrity and mechanotransduction. J Bodyw Mov Ther 2008;12:198–200.
14. Ingber DE. Tensegrity-based mechanosensing from macro to micro. Prog Biophys Mol Biol 2008;97:163–179.
15. Ingber DE. Cellular tensegrity: Defining new rules of biological design that govern the cytoskeleton. J Cell Sci 1993;104(Pt 3):613–627.
16. Carstens MH. Neural tube programming and craniofacial cleft formation. I. The neuromeric organization of the head and neck. Eur J Paediatric Neurol 2004;8:181–210; discussion 179–180.
17. US Department of Health and Human Services. FDA Public Health Notification: Life-threatening Complications Associated with Recombinant Human Bone Morphogenetic Protein in Cervical Spine Fusion. Issued 1 July 2008. http://www.fda.gov/MedicalDevices/Safety/AlertsandNotices/PublicHealthNotifications/ucm062000.htm. Accessed 17 November 2014.
18. Carstens MH. Neural tube programming and the pathogenesis of craniofacial clefts, part I: The neuromeric organization of the head and neck. Handb Clin Neurol 2008;87:247–276.

3 Engineering Environments for Simultaneous Bone Growth and Osseointegration

The theoretical principles of bone construction can be applied to engineering of environments suitable for placement of dental implants. It is also important to consider how these principles control the osseointegration process itself. When designed and constructed properly, these special environments can extend the potential and predictability of dental implant surgery. Bone can be developed in regions that have poor healing potential. If the conditions for bone construction are met, implants can be placed predictably in situations that initially appear unfavorable.

Clinical Applications

For bone-forming procedures to be successful, the basic conditions required for bone development must exist or be introduced. These conditions include a stabilized environment, a source of cells, neuromuscular input, and an absence of pathology[1] (see chapter 1). Successful bone formation and osseointegration depend largely on how well the surgical design is supported by the regulatory mechanisms already in place. Surgical procedures have the ability to introduce bone-forming cells and to establish a physically stable environment. Control of pathosis related to incursion by bacteria can be achieved through careful soft tissue handling and antibiotics. It is not yet possible to synthesize neuromuscular input. The surgical designer must use the signaling potential of local structures or transport a source from another site. Careful analysis of where neuromuscular signaling is already working is where surgical planning begins.

This chapter presents cases that demonstrate how the theory of bone formation can be applied to management of a clinical problem. These cases show how a slight change in the surgical design can produce a successful and efficient outcome in a compromised site.

Reconstruction of a Failed Implant Site

If the essential elements of bone formation are present, then the site should regenerate without surgical intervention. If a dental implant is suspended within the space in which regeneration is occurring, the device will become embedded, and the bone will osseointegrate with the implant surface. The following case demonstrates the exploitation of the inherent regenerative ability of a site to develop new bone, fill the gaps, and establish an osseointegrated bond with the implant without grafting.

Case description

A patient presented in 1987 for management of several missing posterior teeth. Early machined-surface implants were placed at the site of the maxillary right first and second premolars (Fig 3-1a). The implants were first loaded with a short, splinted hybrid prosthesis.

Additional implants were added to allow placement of prostheses in all four posterior quadrants. The definitive metal-ceramic fixed partial denture restoring the maxillary right first and second premolars was connected to the maxillary right canine with a nonrigid keyway attachment (Fig 3-1b).

Over a period of several months under function, the natural maxillary teeth intruded, resulting in disengagement of the keyway attachment and leaving the implant-borne segment freestanding. The first premolar implant fractured under the occlusal load from the mandibular prosthesis, leaving the apical portion osseointegrated in the maxilla (Fig 3-1c). The second premolar implant lost osseointegration and was removed.

The apical portion of the first premolar implant was removed with a trephine bur (Fig 3-1d). An attempt to separate the core in the area between the implant apex and below the sinus floor was not successful. Instead, the trephine bur penetrated the sinus floor, so the explant, adjacent bone, sinus floor, and sinus membrane were removed as a single unit.

Explantation of the first premolar implant fragment resulted in a large defect that would require placement of a new implant if the quadrant were to be restored with an implant-borne prosthesis (Figs 3-1e and 3-1f). The defect was greater than 5 mm in diameter, and the bone of the osteotomy walls had been instrumented with a trephine bur. The bone on the sinus floor had been removed. In addition, the trephine core had removed a section of the sinus mucosa, which resulted in a large oroantral communication between the sinus and the mouth.

When there is a large perforation of the sinus floor that is continuous with a perforation of the sinus membrane, development of an oronasal fistula is a possible complication. Fistulas develop most often in the posterior molar region and less often in the premolar region. In the premolar region, bone perforations tend to fill with newly generated bone (Fig 3-1g), whereas bone perforations in the molar region tend to epithelialize, resulting in a stable oroantral fistula.

The dynamics of bone healing and remodeling are somewhat different in the premolar and molar regions. The vertical height of native bone is greater in the premolar region than in the posterior or molar region. This natural skeletal morphology is related to the presence of healthy anterior teeth and the proximity to the piriform buttress. The pyramidal region of the maxilla in the canine regions maintains its integrity and volume because it is under the influence of the facial muscle insertions, the nasal airway physiology, and the periodontium of the adjacent teeth. This environment promotes bone growth and filling of the bony tract between the oral cavity and the open maxillary sinus.

If the area were left to heal, the likely outcome would be that the osteotomy created by the trephine bur during explantation would completely fill with viable new bone (Fig 3-1h). This process represents a form of regeneration. In such cases, the defect is filled with appropriate tissue and assumes a normal morphology; no cells, tissue, or grafts are needed. The process exploits a self-assembly capability that formed the structure initially and functions in the adult to maintain its health and integrity.

In this patient, there were many challenges to achieving osseointegration of a new dental implant because of multiple compromising conditions. The defect resulting from removal of the fractured implant was wider than the diameter of the replacement implant so that no native bone contacted the new implant. It is difficult to control heat production when using trephine burs for explantation. Removing the failed implant with this method resulted in damage to the cells that lined the osteotomy wall. The sinus floor and sinus membrane were damaged during removal of the implant, resulting in a patent oroantral communication. All of these factors impair the healing of an implant placed using a conventional protocol.

This case demonstrates that despite substantial challenges to healing, a bone-generating environment engineered in accordance with the principles of bone-formation theory can yield a

Fig 3-1 Bone reconstruction to enable replacement of a failed implant.

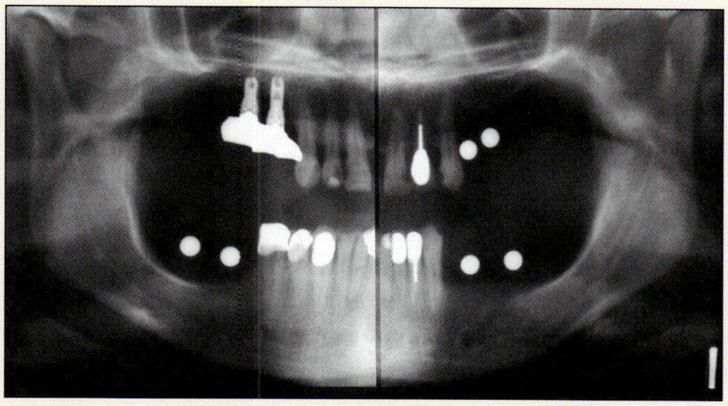

Fig 3-1a The missing maxillary right premolars have been replaced with two original Brånemark implants (Nobel Biocare). The implants placed at the first (3.75 × 7.00–mm) and second (3.75 × 10.00–mm) premolar sites have an external hex design. A cast prosthesis with acrylic resin occlusion is placed initially.

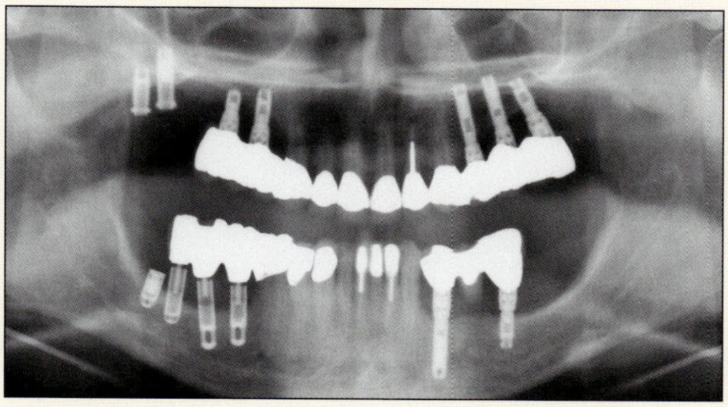

Fig 3-1b As part of a complete dental reconstruction, the maxillary right premolar implants are restored with a fixed prosthesis with metal occlusion.

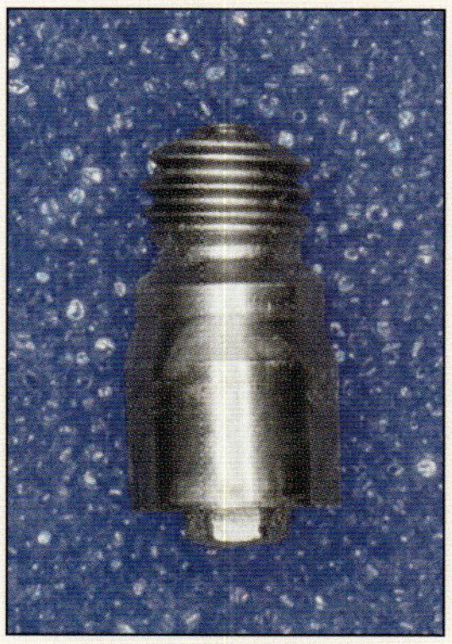

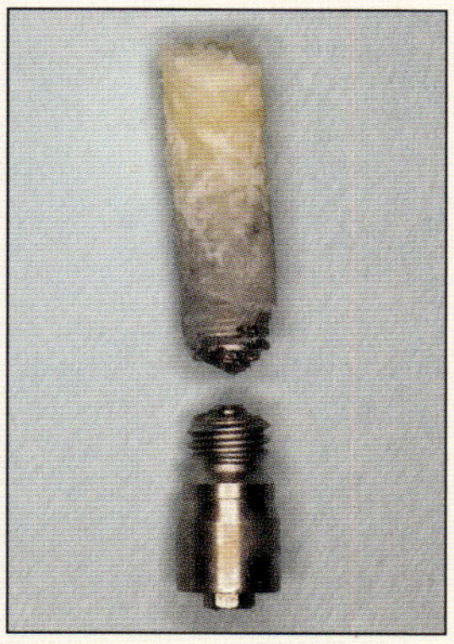

Fig 3-1c *(left)* The maxillary right first premolar implant has fractured and the prosthesis has been removed.

Fig 3-1d *(right)* The apical portion of the implant has been removed with a trephine bur. The osteotomy to remove the fragment included the floor of the maxillary antrum.

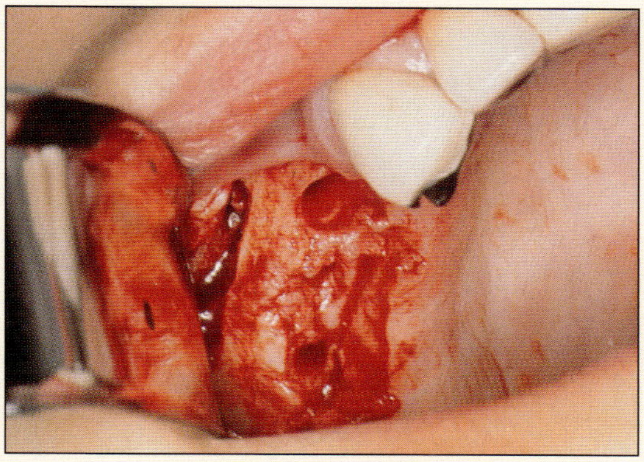

Fig 3-1e The explant procedure results in an osteotomy that is substantially wider and deeper than the original site for implant placement.

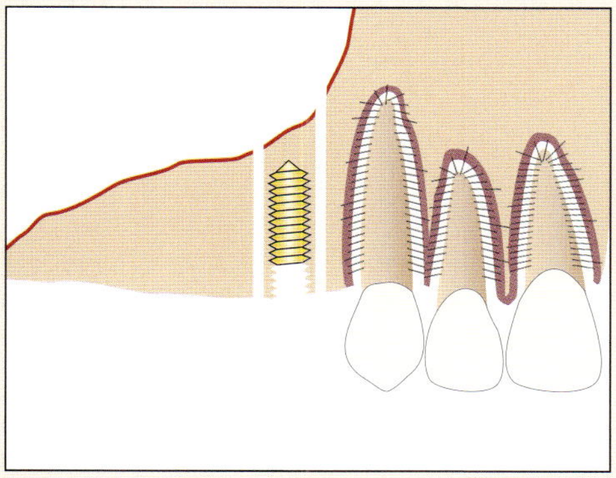

Fig 3-1f The explant site represents the entire vertical dimension of the alveolar process and is 5.5 mm in diameter.

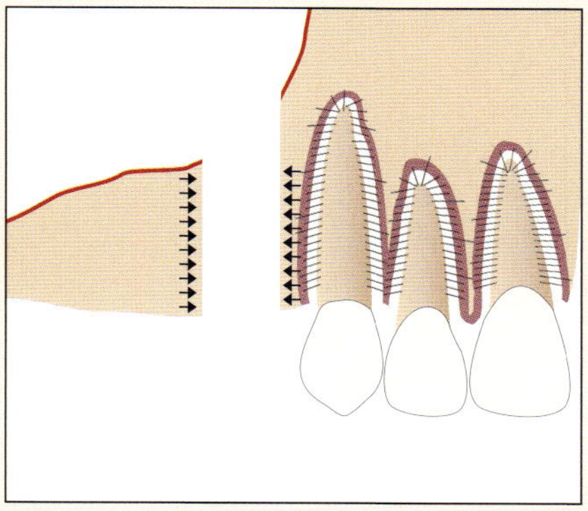

Fig 3-1g In this region of the maxilla, normal healing should fill the osteotomy defect with bone without the need for grafting. Similar defects result from dental extraction, and uncomplicated healing of extraction sites is the familiar and expected outcome.

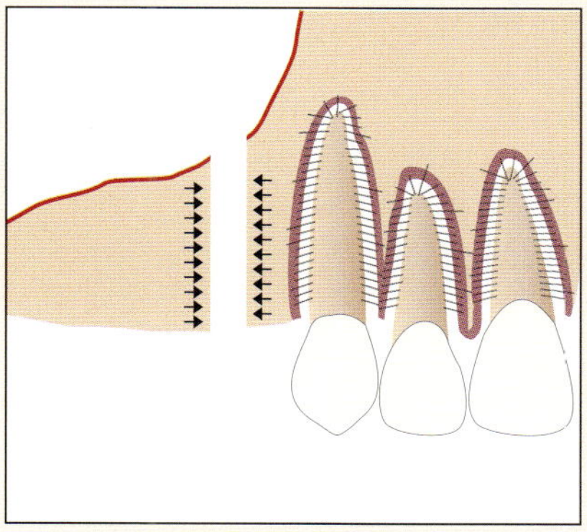

Fig 3-1h One treatment option would be to allow the site to fill with bone and then place a new implant.

→

good outcome. To be successful, the treatment should result in replacement of a dental implant at the prior failure site. The new implant must satisfy the requirements of the restorative treatment plan and serve the patient for many years. The strategy is to take advantage of the natural ability of this area to regenerate. This approach requires an understanding of how the site was formed embryologically and how it is maintained in a steady state as an adult. These conditions must be combined with a surgical objective in such a way that all conditions for bone construction are met.

The working theory of bone formation dictates that an ossicle forms if the conditions are correct. A dental implant interposed in the center of the construction site poses an additional challenge. In this case, a dental implant was suspended in the center of the osteotomy on a titanium plate (Figs 3-1i and 3-1j). No part of the implant was in contact with bone (Fig 3-1k). The titanium plate affixed the implant to the distant stable bone with small bone screws. No grafting material was placed. The sinus membrane remained perforated, so the implant apex was exposed to the open maxillary sinus. The walls of the osteotomy had sustained some instrumentation damage from the trephine bur during explantation.

This is an example of a hybrid construction site. It had both endogenous and artificial components. If designed properly, the site would regenerate the lost bone and achieve osseointegration of the implant simultaneously. In this patient, the requirements of the bone construction theory were met in the following manner:

- *Stabilized environment.* There were two components of the environment to consider. The first component was the osteotomy chamber. This was a channel within the maxilla that was mechanically sheltered from external forces such as the tongue and occlusion. The second component was the implant. If the implant were allowed to move excessively, osseointegration would not have occurred. The titanium plate partially stabilized the implant. The implant was sheltered from excessive force but could still move under low-level forces.
- *Source of cells.* The open medullary bone exposed by the trephine bur was the primary source of cells. If introduced into the chamber, they were not in direct contact with the implant surface.
- *Neuromuscular input.* The premolar and canine region of the maxilla is under the influence of multiple neuromuscular elements. Facial muscles insert in the region and provide the major stimulus to maintain its morphology. Neural input from the nasal cavity and maxillary sinus walls are incompletely understood but contribute to the creation and maintenance of the local skeletal morphology. Additionally, in this patient, the presence of natural teeth and their periodontium stabilized and maintained the surrounding alveolar housing.
- *Lack of pathology.* In this type of situation, infection of the maxillary sinus is the most common source of pathosis. Therefore, good preoperative sinus health and preventive antibiotics were prerequisites to treatment in this patient.

If the treatment is engineered correctly, bone should fill the osteotomy and surround the dental implant (Fig 3-1l). In this patient, the implant became osseointegrated even though no native bone was involved (Fig 3-1m). The entire volume of bone that osseointegrated with the implant was newly constructed (ie, generated) bone. The quality of osseointegration was high because there was no grafting material and there was no mechanical heat damage to the bone involved in implant healing. After 1 year in function, bone surrounded the implant to the polished collar (Figs 3-1n and 3-1o).

Long-term follow-up revealed the success of the treatment. The bone level remained unchanged after 22 years in function (Figs 3-1p to 3-1s).

Discussion

Conventional reconstruction of this failed implant site would typically involve grafting of the explant site as a first stage. After healing and early remodeling of the graft, a dental implant would be placed. Implant surgery protocol would involve an atraumatic osteotomy and then placement of a tightly fitting titanium cylinder. It is believed that close approximation of the bony osteotomy walls to the implant surface is important in achieving osseointegration. Special preparation of the implant surface by abrasives, acid etching, threading, and laser machining is supposed to improve the quality of the healing. The focus is on the space between the bone and the implant surface. Clinicians have come to believe that there is an affinity for bone tissue to bond long term to the titanium surface.[2,3] It is claimed that various mechanical features of the roughened titanium surface enhance the affinity for bone to adhere to the implant.[4–9]

The management of this case contradicts many of the features generally believed to be important in long-term success of the dental implant. In this case, there was less focus on the events taking place at the implant surface. Instead, the focus was on the environment and how the global physiology could be exploited to control and direct the site to develop new bone, fill the gaps, and establish an osseointegrated bond with the implant. No grafting was needed because the inherent regenerative ability of the site supplied new cells and directed three-dimensional assembly of a new ossicle.

In this alternative method for regenerating lost bone and establishing stable osseointegration, the global environment controls the reconstruction site. When an implant device is suspended in a semirigid fashion in the center of the reconstruction environment, the bone surrounds it and creates a stable osseointegrating bond. Local and distant forces regulate recognition and management of the maxillary segment, allowing the design of more efficient and predictable procedures. The utilization of the underlying forces that formed the maxilla during development allows healing to occur despite substantial compromises in the site and staging.

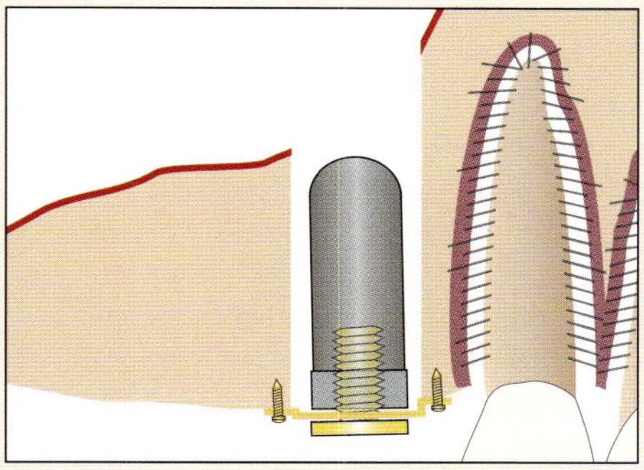

Fig 3-1i In this case, the plan is to suspend an implant into the defect. A titanium bone plate attached to the implant will provide stability. The selected implant is 4.0 mm in diameter and will not engage the walls of the 5.5-mm-wide osteotomy.

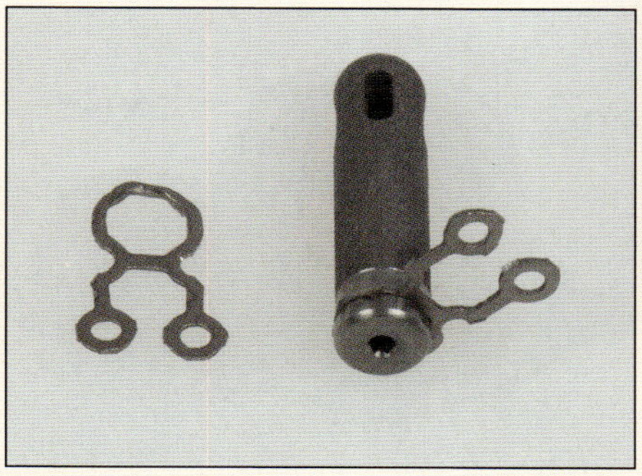

Fig 3-1j The bone plate is 0.3-mm-thick titanium alloy (KLS-Martin). It is attached to the implant by the cover screw.

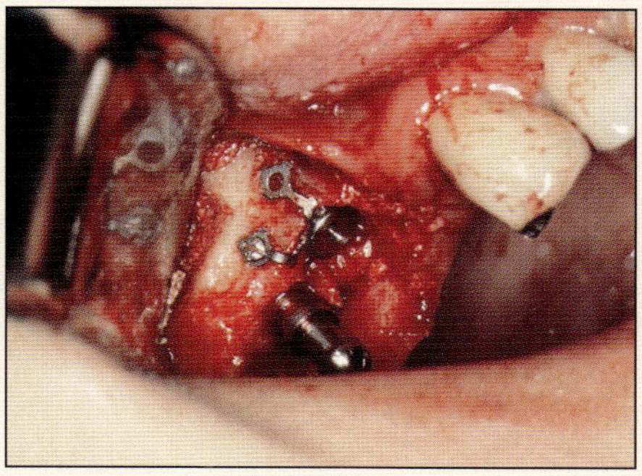

Fig 3-1k The implant (IMZ) is shown with one of two cortex screws securing the bone plate. No part of the implant is in contact with bone. No grafting material has been placed.

Fig 3-1l *(right)* Bone fills the defect and surrounds the dental implant.

Fig 3-1m *(far right)* Four months after explantation of the original implant and placement of the stabilized implant, the site is opened to remove the bone plate and abutment connection. The dental implant is completely surrounded by healthy, viable bone.

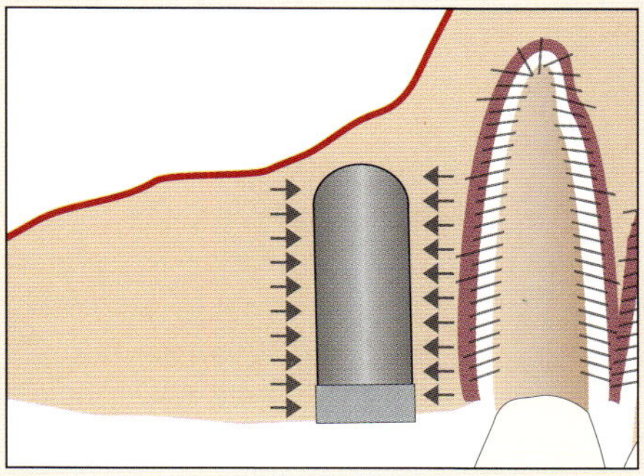

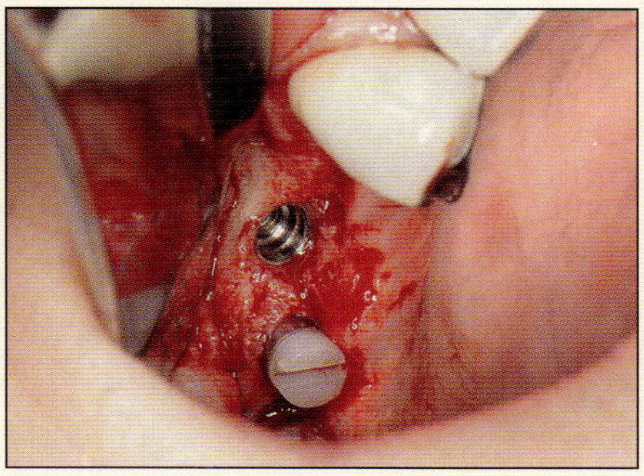

Fig 3-1n *(right)* Implants have been restored and in function for 1 year.

Fig 3-1o *(far right)* Bone surrounds the implant to the polished collar after 1 year. The abutments are IMZ intermobile collars. The implant prosthesis is rigidly connected to the natural tooth splint with a screw-retained T-block.

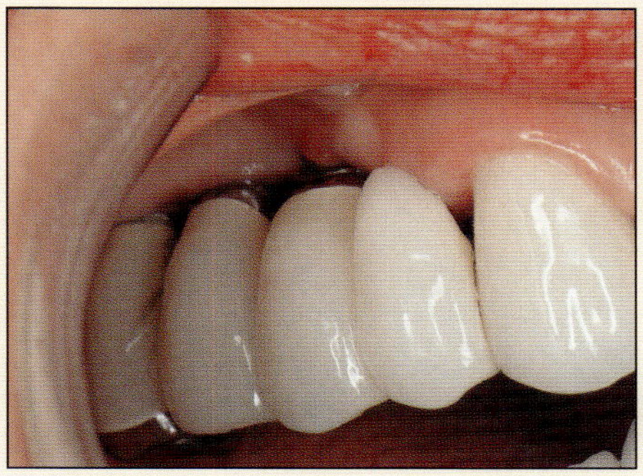

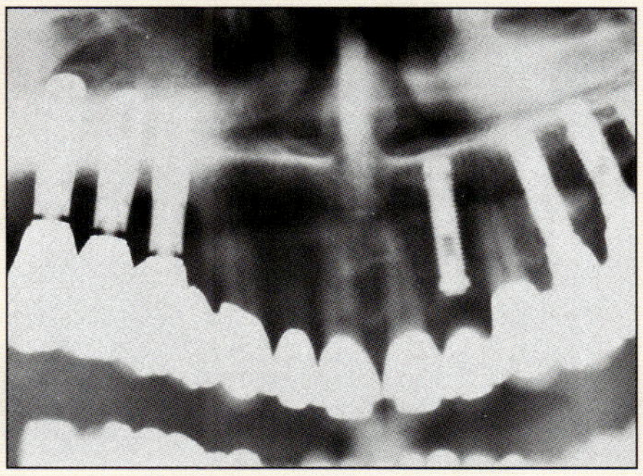

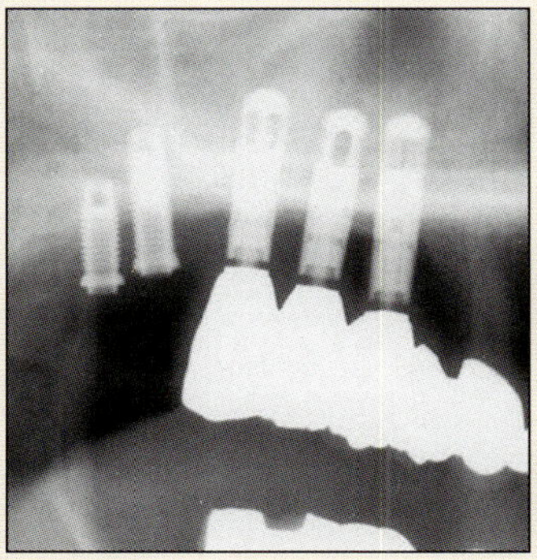

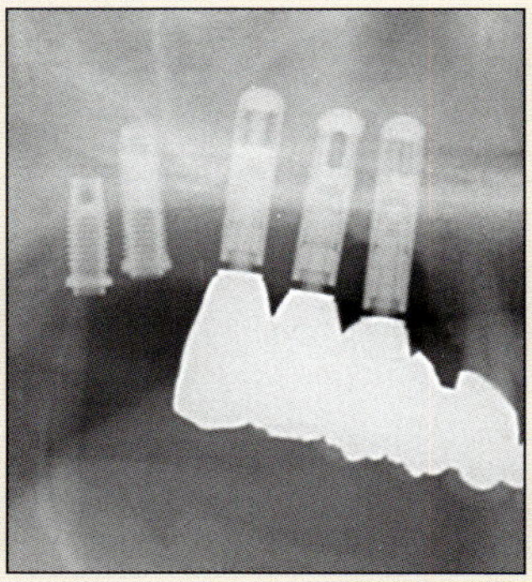

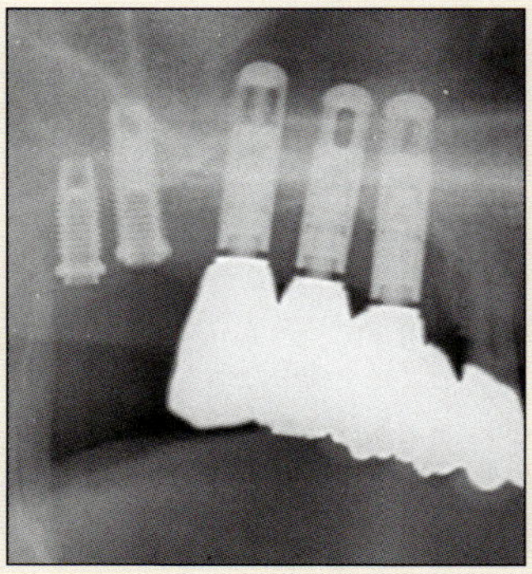

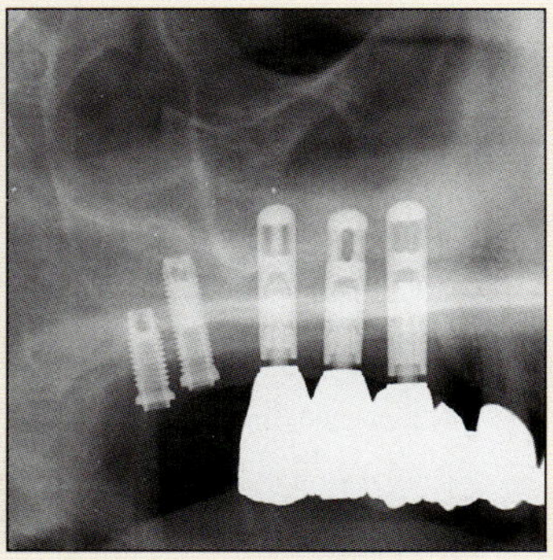

Figs 3-1p to 3-1s Follow-up radiographs after 11 years, 16 years, 19 years, and 22 years, respectively. The bone level remains unchanged.

Bone Reconstruction in a Site Lacking Bone-Forming Cells and a Stabilized Environment

For an engineered bone-forming environment to be successful, each component of the reconstruction system should be considered and optimized. A key factor in the success of bone reconstruction is the availability of bone-forming cells. When cells derived from local bone cannot be delivered to the site in adequate numbers, cells must be introduced through the surgical process. This case predates the clinical availability of recombinant bone morphogenetic proteins and growth factors. To meet the requirement to deliver bone-forming cells, autogenous bone harvested from the iliac crest was used to fill the regeneration chamber.

Another critical element of this system is creation of a stabilized environment. The mechanical and surgical strategy for establishing such an environment is to use dental implants as part of the regenerative construct. This function of the dental implant differs from its familiar role as part of the dental restoration. The implant cylinders serve to establish an area within the chamber in which physical movement is attenuated. A zone that is sheltered from external forces is needed adjacent to the cylinder to promote bone formation.

The role of the stabilized implants is analogous to that performed by Meckel cartilage during embryogenesis of the mandible. The cartilage bar establishes a gradient of stability within the soft tissue volume. Its effect decreases as the distance from the structure increases. The mandible forms at the location where the degree of stabilization is correct for the intensity and pattern of mechanical stimulation from the mylohyoid muscle. The mandible does not form immediately adjacent to Meckel cartilage, suggesting that the region is excessively stabilized. To form bone, the environment needs stability with controlled flexibility. These balanced environments have the potential to form bone rather than fibrous connective tissue.

Some flexibility is also needed to allow the mechanics of neuromuscular signaling to direct cellular metabolism. Neuromuscular input from multiple sources influences the behavior of immature cells occupying the regeneration chamber within bone-forming constructs. Mechanotransduction signaling is part of the communication path between the central nervous system and individual cells. This vector to regulation operates in the developing embryo, and the process is conserved in the mature adult. Following the example of embryogenesis, it is not useful to create an environment within the regeneration chamber that is excessively rigid. This principle influences the design of the bone plates that are used to stabilize implants.

The following case report demonstrates regeneration of bone defects and simultaneous placement of dental implants in a site where the environment lacks a source of bone-forming cells and sufficient bone to achieve primary stability of the implants.

Case description

A 50-year-old patient presented with a failing dentition. He desired a treatment that would result in a fixed prosthesis retained with dental implants. Extensive pneumatization of the maxillary sinuses limited the volume of bone available to establish primary anchorage of dental implants (Fig 3-2a). In addition, the site lacked local bone-forming cells necessary to correct the bone volume deficiency. Radiographs demonstrated the combined inferior and anterior extension of the sinuses that resulted in this mechanical and physiologic deficiency (Fig 3-2b). The thin sinus floor was not adequate to anchor dental implants without external stabilization.

This type of reconstruction requires a comprehensive engineering plan. To be an effective environment stabilizer, the implant must be fixated to bone that will remain mechanically stable during the bone-forming process. If there is adequate existing bone at the implant osteotomy site, it may be enough to provide stability of the implant initially and through the catabolic phase of implant healing. In this patient, the available volume of bone was inadequate to stabilize the implant at the osteotomy site.

Even if there were adequate bone to achieve primary stabilization, this does not necessarily meet the criteria for a stabilizing element. Wedging an implant cylinder in a newly created osteotomy sets in motion a dynamic process. In response to initial implant placement, the bone initially in contact with the implant cylinder undergoes resorption (see chapter 2). Depending on the total surface area anchoring the implant and the rate and distribution of the resorption, the implant cylinder is at risk of losing mechanical stability and failing in its role to shelter the site from excessive mechanical forces (see Figs 2-4 and 2-5). In general, the implant housed completely in native bone has the greatest opportunity to go on to uncomplicated osseointegration.

The use of a bone plate and miniscrews to establish or augment implant stabilization adds to the potential to provide a stable structure and environment. The stability of the device impacts both the healing of the graft and the establishment of osseointegration. Successful healing with this technique is affected by multiple variables. These include the thickness and mass of the bone plate, the size of the stabilizing screws, the shape of the implants, the surface preparation of the implants, the type of graft material used, and the health of the maxillary sinus. In this case, three implants with titanium plasma-sprayed surfaces were placed in the chamber established by sinus membrane elevation (Figs 3-2c and 3-2d). The height of the polished collar was greater than the height of bone in the sinus floor.

An autogenous bone graft harvested from the iliac crest was placed around the implants (Figs 3-2e and 3-2f). The bone graft was needed as a source of cells and as a matrix for new bone formation. The three implants were stabilized with bone plates at the right posterior maxilla. The 0.3-mm-thick plates were secured with 1.0-mm-wide cortex screws. Three implants were also placed at the left posterior maxilla using the same technique. Additional implants were placed in the anterior maxilla and in the right and left posterior mandible. At these sites, the native bone mass was sufficient so that implant placement was performed in a conventional manner. Auxiliary stabilization with bone plates was not needed at these other sites.

Fig 3-2 Bone reconstruction in a site that lacks bone-forming cells and has limited bone volume.

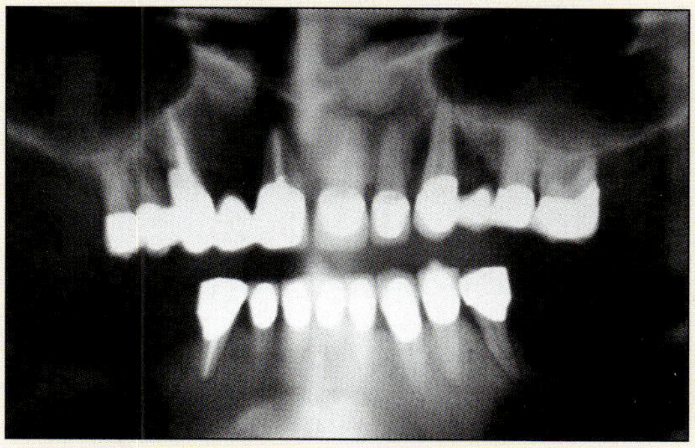

Fig 3-2a A panoramic radiograph prior to treatment shows the failed dentition and extensive pneumatization of the maxillary sinuses.

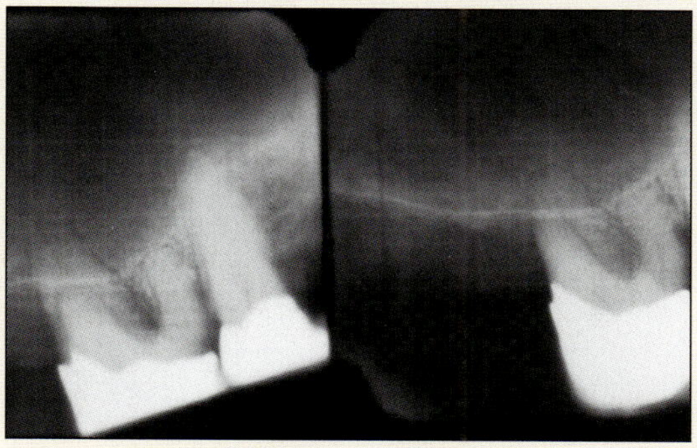

Fig 3-2b Periapical radiographs show the eggshell thickness of the sinus floor.

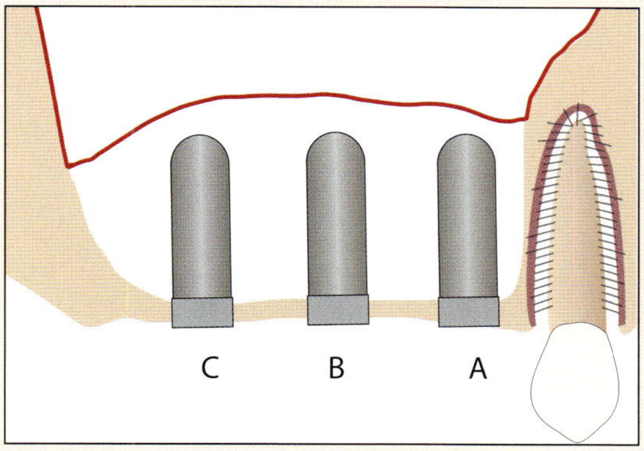

Fig 3-2c When the sinus floor thickness is less than the width of the polished collars on the implants to be used, the titanium plasma-sprayed surface intended for osseointegration is completely without contact with native bone.

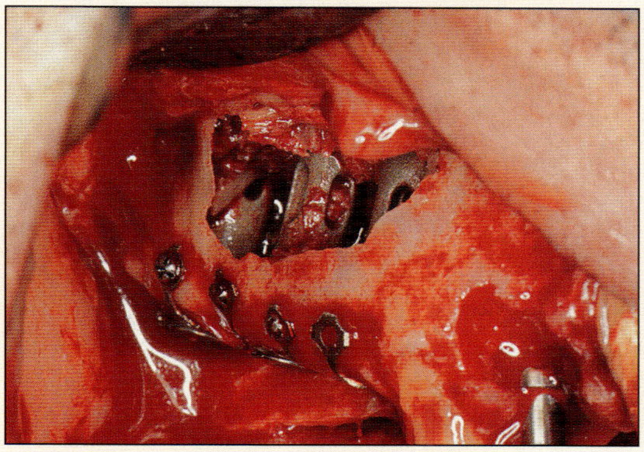

Fig 3-2d Three IMZ implants have been placed under the elevated maxillary sinus membrane. Three titanium bone plates stabilize the cylinders. Microscrews engage the very thin bone of the sinus floor. The implants have no contact with native bone.

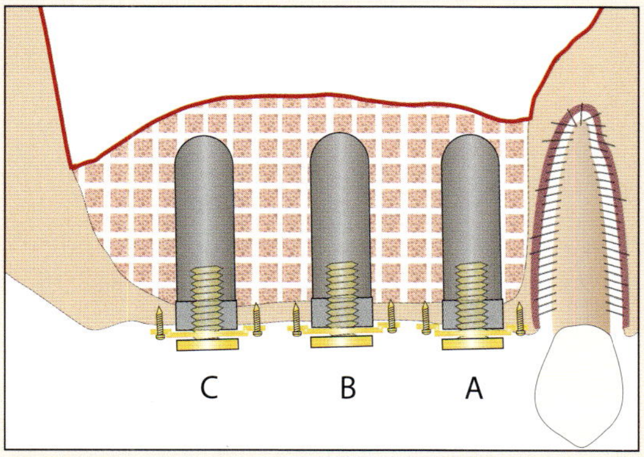

Fig 3-2e Diagram of the bone-forming construct. Three implants provide mechanical stability. The microscrews secure the bone plate to cortical bone located away from the implant osteotomies. The autogenous graft contains natural cytokines that draw cells into the bone-forming environment.

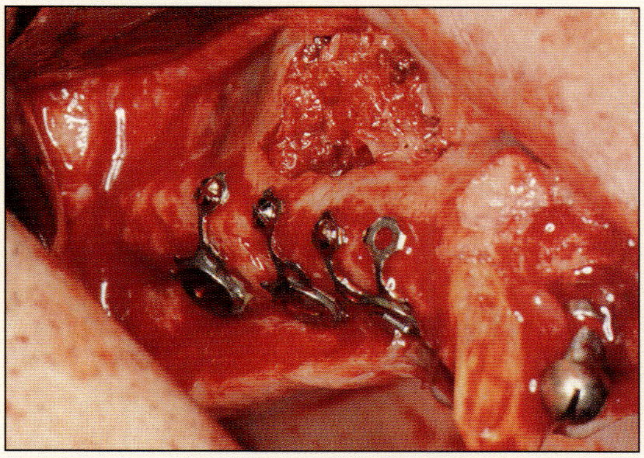

Fig 3-2f Cancellous bone harvested from the patient's iliac crest is positioned to surround the implant bodies.

→

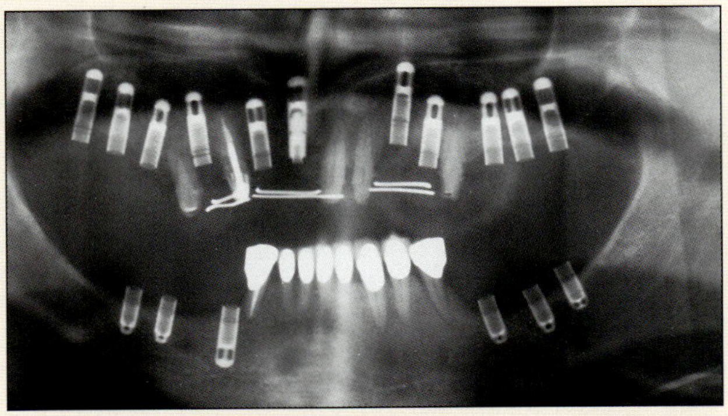

Fig 3-2g Six months after implant placement and grafting, abutments are placed in preparation for restorative procedures. All of the implants have healed successfully. Five natural teeth have been retained for maintenance of a fixed provisional prosthesis.

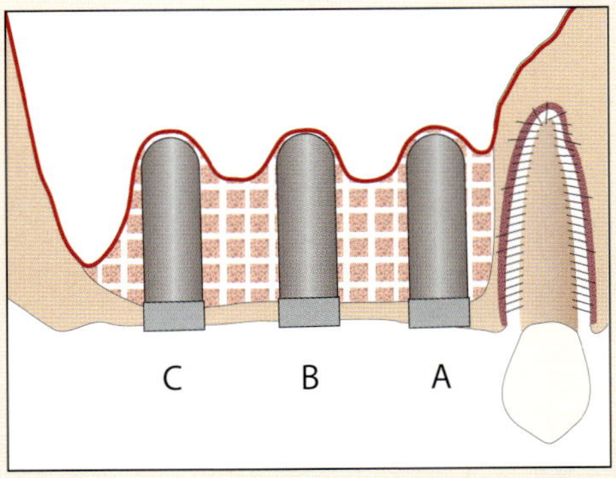

Fig 3-2h Diagram of the remodeling process. The graft resorbs and is replaced by a large volume of vital bone. Remodeling of the graft-derived bone results in vertical collapse of the bone until it meets the apices of the implants.

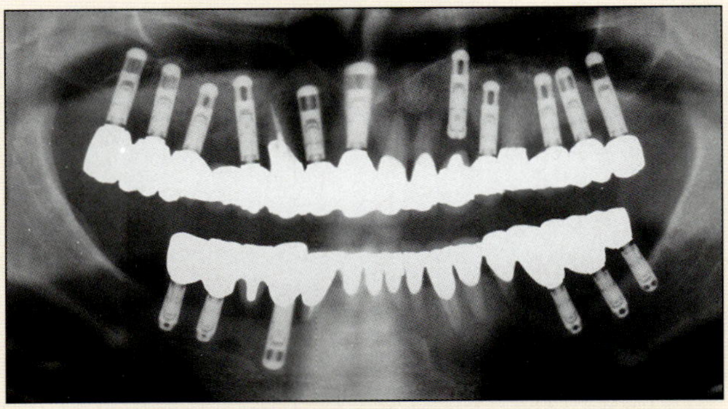

Fig 3-2i A radiograph shows the implants and fixed prosthesis. The abutments are intermobile collars.

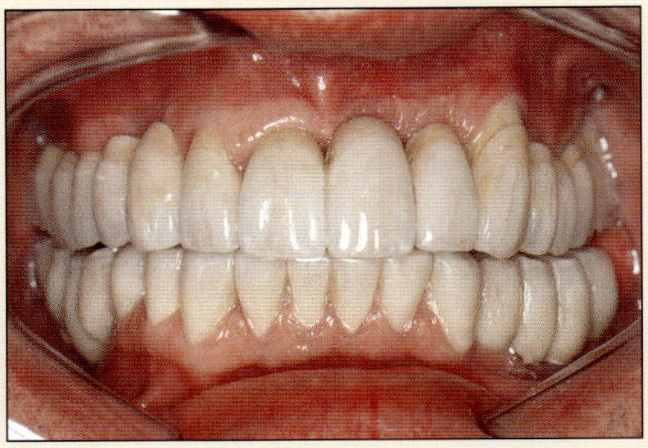

Fig 3-2j Fixed maxillary and mandibular prostheses have been placed.

After 6 months of healing in the maxilla, the bone plates were removed and gingiva formers were placed (Fig 3-2g). When the bone plates are removed and abutments placed, the polished collars of the implants are typically exposed. In this case, the polished collars were positioned above the sinus floor and within the sinus. Because the polished collars were exposed after graft healing, this meant that the entire native sinus floor had been resorbed and replaced with new vital bone (Fig 3-2h).

Fixed implant- and tooth-borne prostheses were then placed to restore the maxillary and mandibular dental arches (Figs 3-2i and 3-2j). The implant-supported segments were rigidly connected to the tooth-borne segments with milled, screw-retained precision attachments.

Follow-up radiographs at 12 years revealed that maxillary bone levels were unchanged (Figs 3-2k and 3-2l). Long-term follow-up at 20 years showed that the prostheses were still in function, but the mandibular implants exhibited some bone loss (Figs 3-2m to 3-2o).

Discussion

When dental implants are suspended within the engineered bone-forming chamber, the new bone will surround and osseointegrate the implants. The new maxillary skeletal segment and the incorporated dental implants in this patient have been fully functional and stable over 20 years of function. The osseointegration interface and the structural mass of bone have shown no sign of resorption. In contrast, bone loss occurred on the mandibular implants that were placed in a conventional manner. This shows that an engineered chamber can generate a new bone segment and promote successful osseointegration of implants in that new bone in a single-stage procedure.

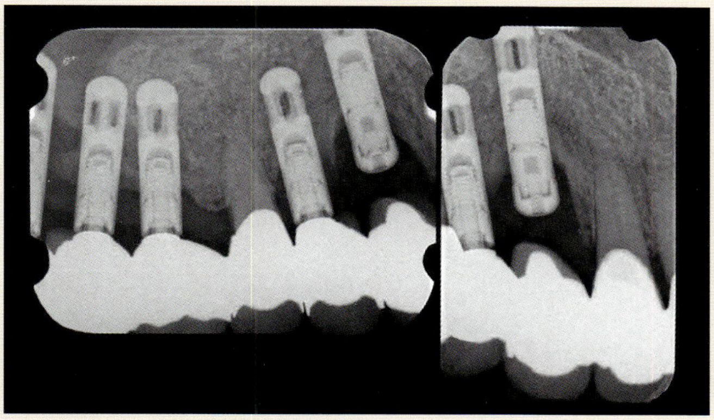

Fig 3-2k Periapical radiographs taken at the 12-year follow-up show that alveolar crest bone levels are unchanged.

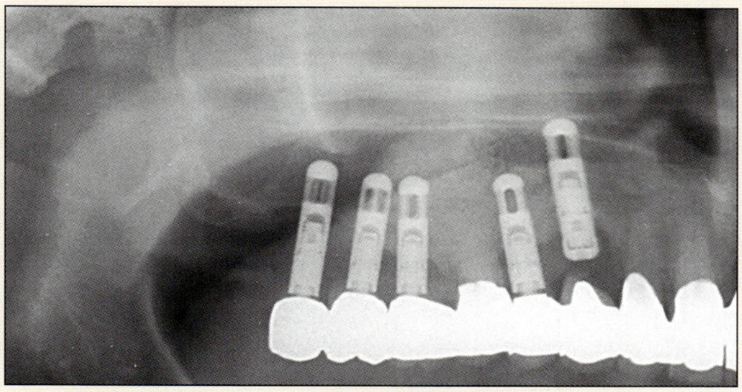

Fig 3-2l A panoramic radiograph taken at the 12-year follow-up shows that the sinus grafts are unchanged.

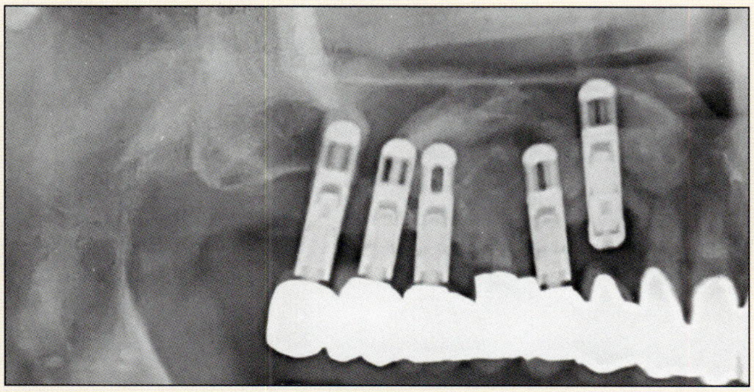

Fig 3-2m A panoramic radiograph at the 20-year follow-up shows that maxillary bone levels are stable.

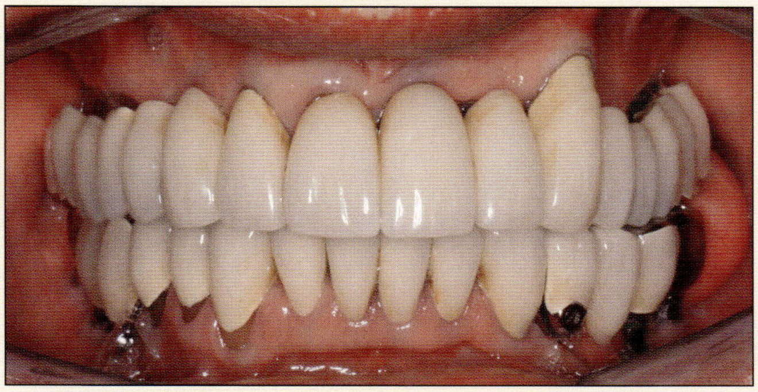

Fig 3-2n After 20 years in function, the maxillary and mandibular prostheses are basically unchanged. No modifications of the prostheses have been required during the 20-year period of service.

Fig 3-2o At the 20-year follow-up, according to the patient, "The teeth feel the same as they did the day they were put in."

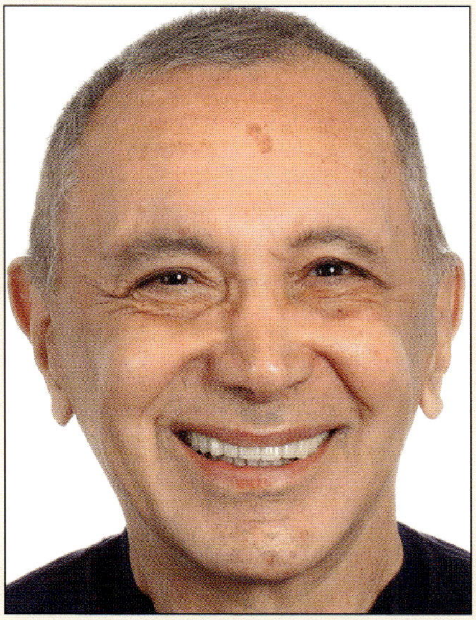

Fig 3-3 Selection of the optimal method for delivery of bone-forming cells based on the needs of the individual site.

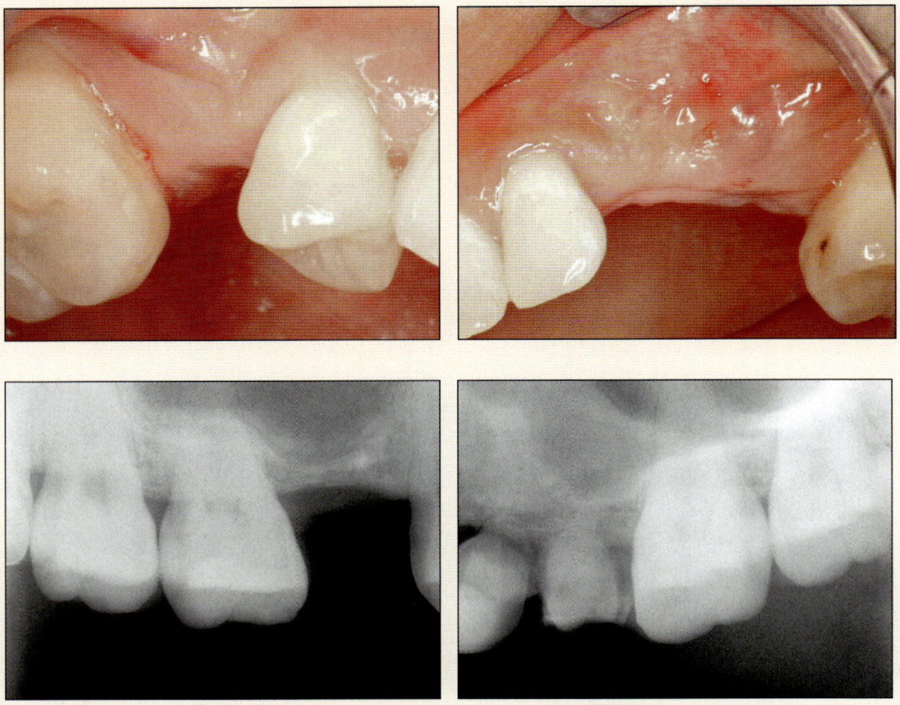

Fig 3-3a *(far left)* Maxillary right posterior dentition at the initial evaluation of a patient aged 19 years.

Fig 3-3b *(left)* Edentulous span in the maxillary left posterior region at the initial evaluation.

Fig 3-3c *(far left)* Pretreatment radiograph of the maxillary right dentition showing the thin sinus floor.

Fig 3-3d *(left)* Pretreatment radiograph of the maxillary left dentition.

Comparison of Carrier Strategies for rhBMP-2

Providing a source of cells with bone-forming potential is an essential element of a successful bone-forming construct. How best to satisfy this requirement depends on how the cells are expected to respond to the other elements of the bone-forming environment. In the following case, a patient was congenitally missing teeth in the right and left sides of the maxilla. Although the clinical problem on the two sides was similar, the specific anatomical features of each site demanded different methods for delivery of bone-forming precursor cells, in this case recombinant human bone morphogenetic protein 2 (rhBMP-2). The case demonstrates the need to choose a cell-delivery method that is specific to the features and demands of each individual regeneration site.

Case description

A 19-year-old man presented for management of congenitally missing teeth in the right and left sides of the maxilla. On the right side, the second premolar had failed to develop. This resulted in a premolar-width space in the dental arch (Fig 3-3a). On the left side, the canine, first premolar, and second premolar had failed to develop. This resulted in a wide edentulous span (Fig 3-3b). Radiographs of the two sites revealed that the sinus had descended into the alveolus, leaving a thin cortex at the ridge crest (Figs 3-3c and 3-3d).

Morphology and physiology of the right side

Before bone-forming constructs could be designed to manage these two defects, it was necessary to understand the forces that were acting to maintain the current morphology. These same forces would act on bone precursor cells introduced as part of the bone-forming construct. On the right side, the anterior and posterior walls of the potential bone construction sites were maintained by the periodontal systems of their respective roots (Fig 3-3e). If a graft were placed in this defect, the bone-forming cells would come under the regulation of the periodontal ligament systems of the adjacent teeth. The posterior wall of the defect was under the regulation of the periodontal ligament system associated with the labial root of the first molar. The palatal root extended further to the apical but was too far medial to exert direct force on the cells introduced by the graft. At the anterior wall of the chamber, the bone extended apically to an area under the influence of the first premolar root and its periodontal system. The potential effect of the periodontal systems on cells introduced by a graft is distance dependent. Given the limited distance between the two teeth, moderate stimulation and regulation of cells could be expected.

Morphology and physiology of the left side

The regulatory parameters operating on the left side created a different situation (Fig 3-3f). Three permanent teeth failed to develop. This resulted in a major defect from anatomical and physiologic standpoints. The existing morphology was maintained by the periodontal systems of the adjacent teeth. Compared to the

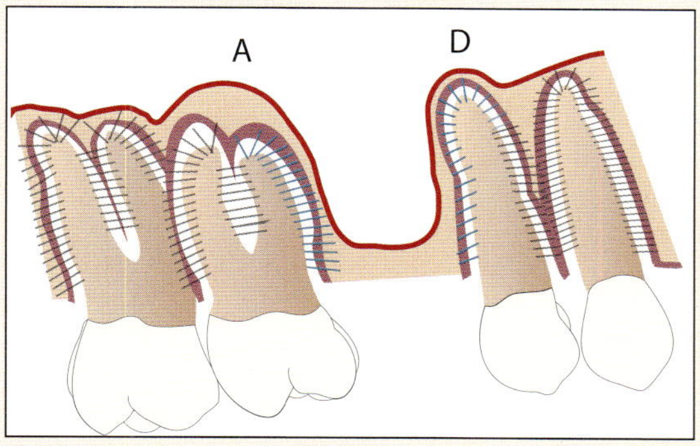

Fig 3-3e Functional analysis of the existing site morphology on the right side. The posterior wall of the defect is under the regulation of the periodontal ligament system associated with the labial root of the first molar (A). At the anterior wall of the chamber, the bone extends apically to a site (D) under the influence of the first premolar root and its periodontal system.

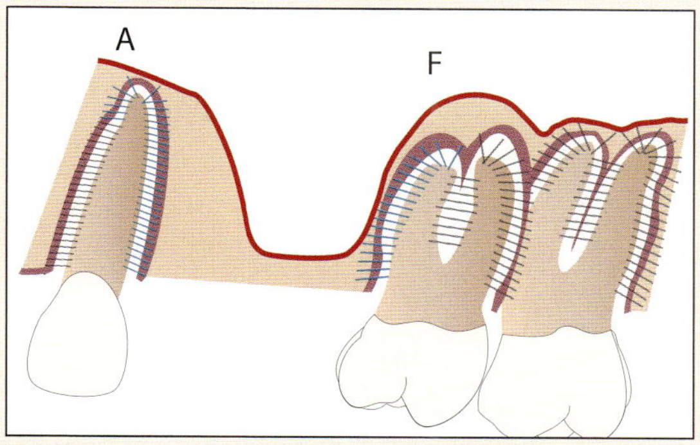

Fig 3-3f Existing regulatory parameters at the left-side defect. The teeth are farther apart than on the right side, and the deficient bone volume is greater. The bone surrounding the root of the lateral incisor (A) and the labial roots of the first molar (F) forms the anterior wall and posterior walls, respectively, of the chamber in which bone is required.

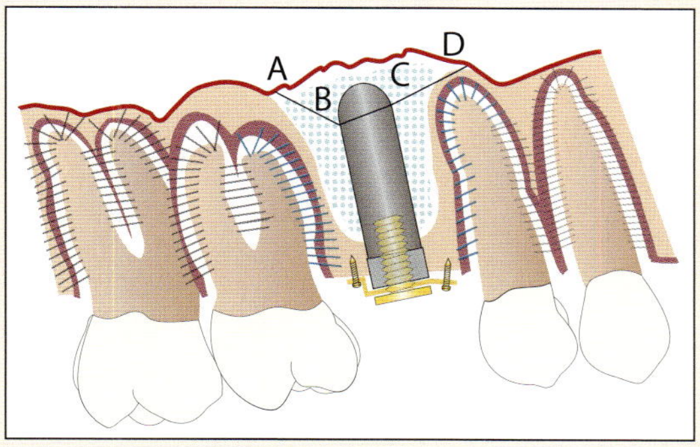

Fig 3-3g Surgical design strategy for the right side. Placement of a dental implant will provide mechanical stability for the bone-forming environment and decrease the volume of bone tissue needed to fill the void *(area below black line)*. Engineering analysis shows the potential bone-forming volume to extend from point A to the junctions between the cylindric body of the implant and its hemispherical apex (points B and C) to point D. This volume defines the amount of bone grafting material needed. The influence of the periodontal systems extending from sites A and D need only reach the surface of the implant to promote bone consolidation and osseointegration. Thus, the graft can be composed of rhBMP-2 carried on an absorbable collagen sponge.

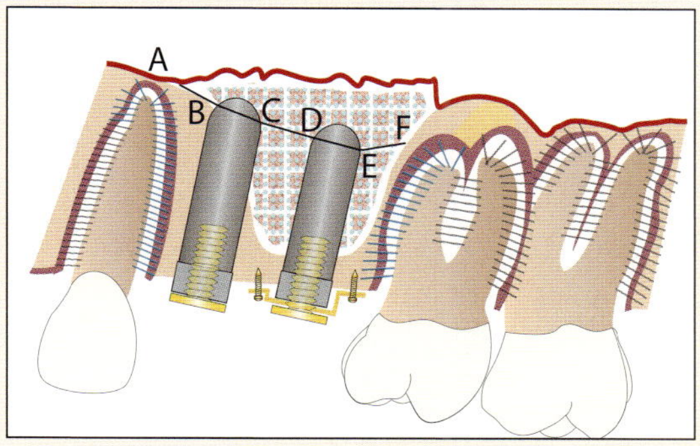

Fig 3-3h Surgical design strategy for the left side. The potential bone-forming environment extends from point A to the junctions between the cylindric body of the implants and their hemispherical apices (B, C, D, and E) to point F. Extending the graft beyond this boundary is not useful. The remaining, minimal chamber volume *(area below black line)* is the only place that needs bone-forming cells.

situation presented on the right side, these teeth were farther apart and the deficient bone volume was therefore greater. As on the right side, the bone surrounding the roots formed the anterior and posterior walls of the chamber in which bone was required. The challenge on the left side was that the distance from the center of the defect to either periodontal system was too great for direct regulation. If a simple rhBMP-2 graft were placed in the left-side defect, the center of that defect would be unlikely to consolidate with viable bone.

Surgical design, right side

The surgical design for the right side is summarized in Fig 3-3g. A dental implant was planned for suspension within the bone construction site. The roles of the implant were to provide mechanical stability for the bone-forming environment, to become the tissue-integrated portion of the dental prosthesis, and to decrease the volume of bone tissue needed to fill the void. Engineering analysis showed the potential bone-forming volume to extend from points A to B to C to D. This volume defined the amount of bone grafting material needed. Extending the graft beyond these boundaries would not have been useful. The influence of the periodontal systems extending from points A and D needed only to reach the surface of the implant to promote bone consolidation and osseointegration.

Because the volume was limited and the distance to the regulating periodontal system was short, the graft could be composed of rhBMP-2 carried on an absorbable collagen sponge (ACS). The advantage of using rhBMP-2 without a particulate carrier is that the void can be directly filled with viable bone. If a particulate carrier is included, the bone construct must resorb the particulate material before the full volume is viable.

Surgical design, left side

The surgical design for the left side is summarized in Fig 3-3h.

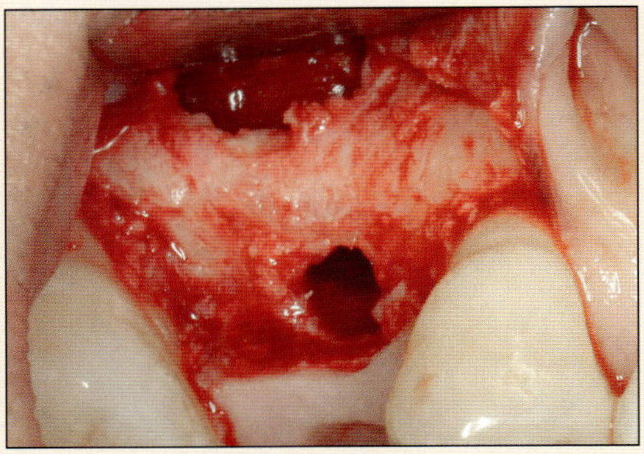

Fig 3-3i Surgical access is created for sinus elevation and implant placement on the right side.

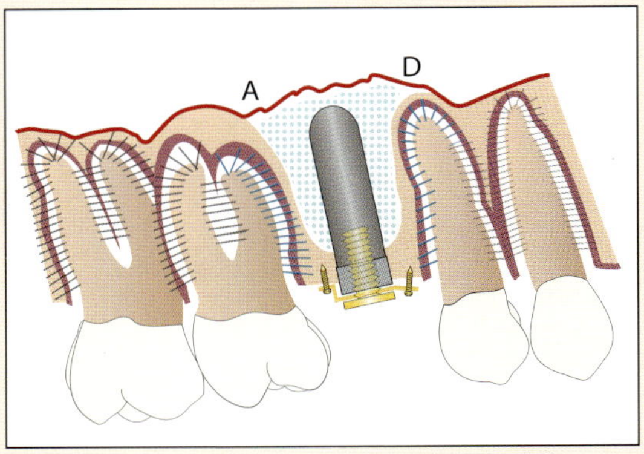

Fig 3-3j Surgical plan for implant placement and stabilization. No mechanical stability is achieved by contact between the implant and the native bone. A supporting bone plate will establish primary stability.

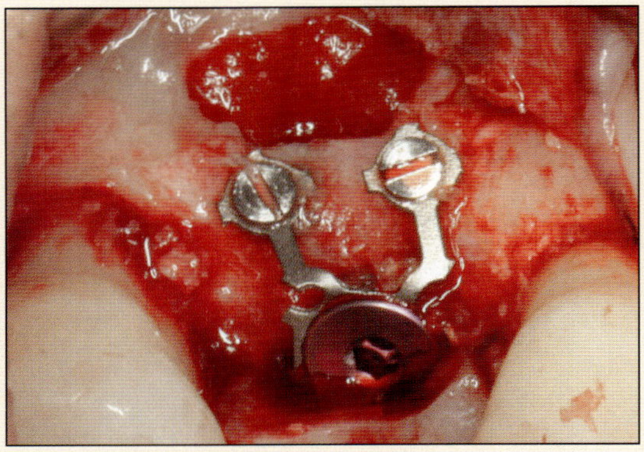

Fig 3-3k The implant and stabilizing bone plate are placed. A sinus elevation graft of rhBMP-2/ACS fills the regeneration chamber.

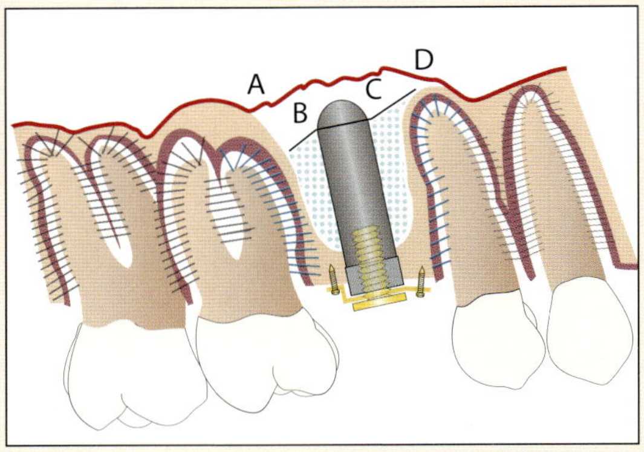

Fig 3-3l The constructed environment on the right side includes the centrally positioned implant with supporting bone plate, stable native bone at points A and D, constructed stable points at B and C, and an rhBMP-2/ACS graft.

→

The objective was to place implants at the sites of the maxillary left canine and first premolar. Surgical planning begins not with the defect itself but with analysis and comprehensive diagnosis of the adjacent structures. In the alveolar process, the adjacent teeth are the most important source of neuromuscular signaling. In this patient, the alveolar bone at point A was formed and maintained primarily under the regulation of the left lateral incisor and its periodontal system. This region was also under the influence of the muscles that control and exert force on the midfacial structures. Bone grows immediately distal to the lateral incisor because this region is part of the piriform buttress. Even in the completely edentulous maxilla, neuromuscular function will maintain some bone in the canine regions because the piriform buttress remains under function. Although the bone volume in this patient was minimal at the potential site for the canine implant, successful osseointegration was likely because the environment was regulated by neuromuscular signaling from two sources. At the posterior extent of the defect, bone was maintained by the periodontal system at the labial roots of the first molar (point F).

Two dental implants were planned because two were needed to meet the prosthodontic objective. The implants would fulfill multiple roles within the bone-forming construct design. The stabilized implant cylinders would interact with the forces imparted by the periodontal ligament systems, existing periosteal Sharpey fiber systems, and elevated sinus membrane. Engineering analysis of the planned bone-forming construct showed that the potential bone-forming environment would extend from points A to B to C to D to E to F. Each of these landmarks would determine how the environment would support bone growth. Extending the graft beyond this boundary would not have been useful. The remaining, minimal chamber volume was the only place that needed bone-forming cells.

The engineering problem posed by the left side was the graft volume between the two implant cylinders. This volume was at risk for consolidation to fail because it was distant from the primary neuromuscular regulation sources of the periodontal ligament systems. Moreover, the posterior implant cylinder actually would obstruct the potential signaling from the molar periodontal system, and the first molar position within the skeleton lacks indirect regulation from the major facial muscle systems.

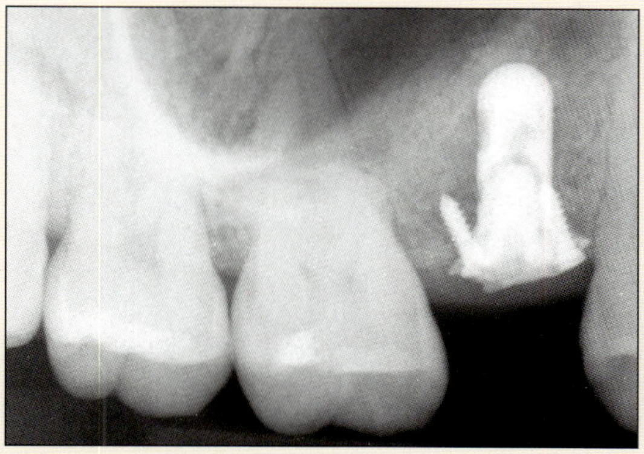

Fig 3-3m Radiograph of the maxillary right implant 16 weeks after placement and grafting.

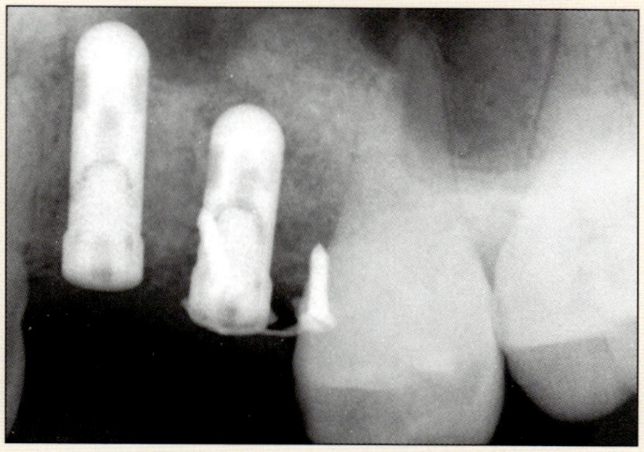

Fig 3-3n Radiograph of the maxillary left implants 16 weeks after placement and grafting.

→

In this case, placement of rhBMP-2 carried on a collagen sponge might not be effective because of its limited duration of action. An ACS is likely to resorb within 14 days. When necessary, the surgical designer may choose an alternative carrier that will prolong the remodeling time. In this case, the choice was made to carry rhBMP-2 to the chamber on solvent-dehydrated cancellous bone particles (Puros, Zimmer Dental). The reasons for the use of solvent-dehydrated bone rather than freeze-dried bone are discussed in chapter 4.

Clinical procedure

On the right side, a sinus elevation procedure was performed through a lateral window (Fig 3-3i). With the membrane retracted, an implant osteotomy was placed through the alveolar crest. Only 2 mm of bone was drilled through before the sinus floor was penetrated.

With this surgical plan, an implant cylinder (Camlog) is positioned through the osteotomy (Fig 3-3j). The polished collar of the implant is thicker than the bone and is not expected to osseointegrate. The titanium plasma-sprayed zone of the implant surface is the only portion on which osseointegration is likely to occur, and in this site the entire plasma-sprayed portion projects into the sinus elevation chamber. No native bone is in contact with the plasma-sprayed surface. No mechanical stability is achieved by contact between the implant and the native bone. If primary stability is to be established, an auxiliary method is required.

A dental implant was placed through the osteotomy, and the main body of the implant extended beyond the sinus floor (Fig 3-3k). A titanium plate was attached to the cover screw, and 1.2-mm microscrews were used to secure the plate to adjacent bone. A graft consisting of rhBMP-2 (Medtronic) carried on a collagen sponge (Integra Life Sciences) was placed. The dose was 0.25 mg of rhBMP-2 in 1 mL of water.

The resulting engineered environment (Fig 3-3l) included the centrally positioned implant with supporting bone plate, stable native bone at points A and D, constructed stable points B and C, and an rhBMP-2 graft carried on an ACS. According to the engineering parameters, bone will form and be maintained in the chamber below the black line.

In this regenerative approach, the dental implant assumed multiple roles. The first purpose of the dental implant was to stabilize the central portion of the regeneration chamber so that newly arriving osteogenic cells would have the best mechanical environment in which to mature and consolidate. Long-term follow-up of many implants placed with this technique suggests that the influence of the parallel walls of the implant cylinder is different from the effect of the hemispherical dome. Viable bone forms around the implant cylinder and extends to the level where the dome radius begins. Bone may initially form to cover the dome but will eventually resorb until only the vertical walls remain osseointegrated. The mechanism that governs this process is unknown. Furthermore, bone will not form and remain above the level of the stable native sites, point A and point D. Extending the graft beyond these boundaries would not have been effective or necessary.

The second purpose of the dental implant was to provide for anchorage of the prosthesis. Successful osseointegration is a prerequisite to establishing a functional prosthesis. In this situation, all of the bone involved in osseointegration was derived from the construction process.

Sixteen-week postsurgery follow-up

The bone-forming construct, including the dental implant and supporting bone plate, was examined 16 weeks after surgery (Fig 3-3m). Initially, the graft material extended beyond the confines of the regeneration chamber. In this state of incomplete organization, there was no distinct cortical outline at the sinus floor. This indicated that functional consolidation of the graft was not yet complete.

A radiograph of the left side, taken 16 weeks after placement of the rhBMP-2 and solvent-dehydrated bone graft, revealed that the graft opacity extended well apical, to the apex of the distal implant (Fig 3-3n).

Sixteen weeks after placement of the implants and grafts, both right and left maxillary sites were reentered to remove

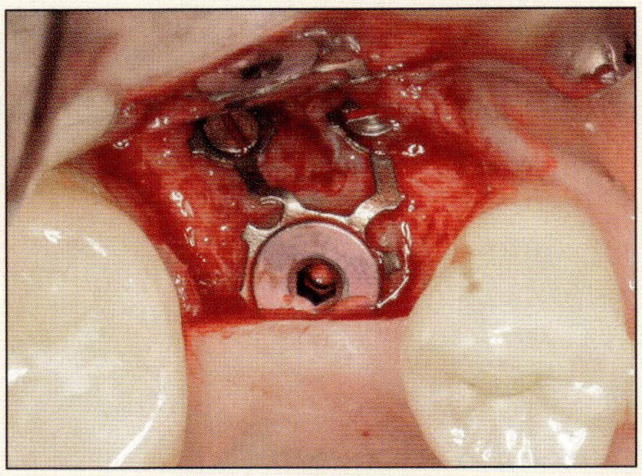

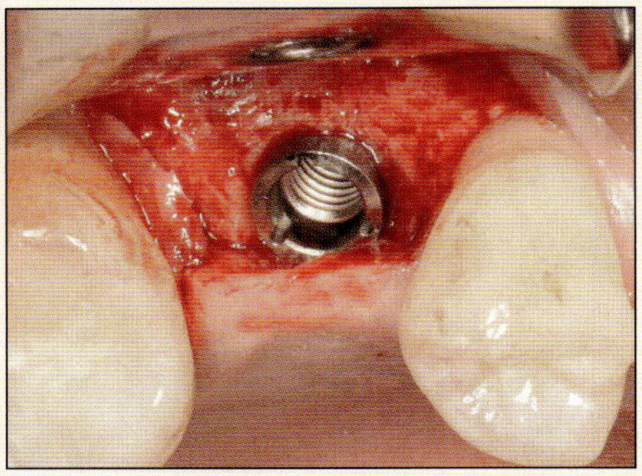

Fig 3-3o *(far left)* Appearance of the bone plate at the right implant 16 weeks after surgery.

Fig 3-3p *(left)* Alveolar ridge remodeling exposes the polished collar of the right implant.

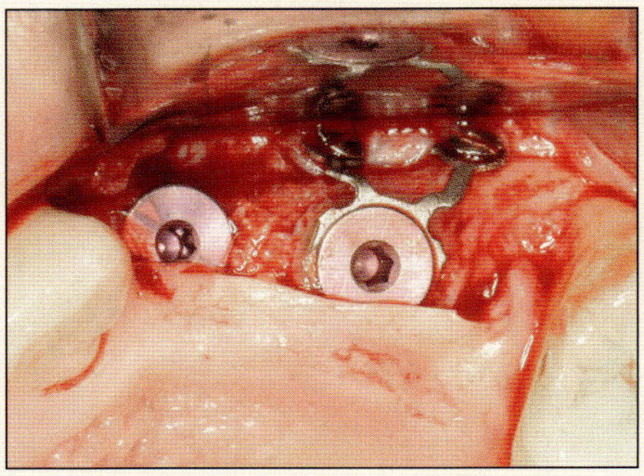

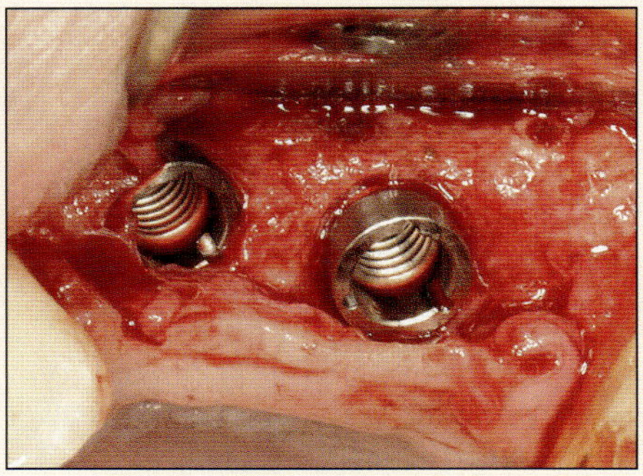

Fig 3-3q *(far left)* Appearance of the bone plate at the left implant 16 weeks after surgery.

Fig 3-3r *(left)* After the bone plate is removed, the ridge crest is visible at the level of the polished collars.

→

the bone plates and to place abutments. The bone plate on the right side remained stable (Fig 3-3o). Removal of the bone plate revealed that the implant was clinically stable. The polished collar was not covered by bone, but the titanium plasma-sprayed surface was fully invested in normal-appearing bone (Fig 3-3p).

Findings at the left-side implants were similar. The bone plate on the left posterior implant remained stable (Fig 3-3q). Removal of the bone plate revealed that the bone had healed at the level of the titanium plasma-sprayed surface of the implant. The typical finding was that the bone had remodeled to leave the polished implant collar exposed (Fig 3-3r).

All three implants were restored with single crowns.

Seven-year post-restoration follow-up, right side

Seven years after the crowns were placed, the patient was recalled for follow-up evaluation (Fig 3-3s). The single crown on the right side had been in function without complications (Fig 3-3t). A radiograph of the right implant revealed the result of 7 years of remodeling (Fig 3u). There was a clear cortical outline representing the floor of the maxillary sinus.

The steady state established among the existing bone, implant, and constructed bone on the right side was determined by the predicted engineering parameters. The bone level at point A was under the control of the periodontal system of the mesiolabial molar root. The bone level rose to meet the cylinder at the junctions between the parallel body and the hemispherical apex. The bone level was then continuous with the bone that was adjacent to the apex of the premolar root at point D. Over time, the bone that was formed by the construction process became continuous with the native bone. To be a completely integrated construct, the new bone and implant had to be seamlessly integrated into the anatomical and physiologic processes of the native skeleton.

Seven-year post-restoration follow-up, left side

The performance of the maxillary left reconstruction followed a similar course. The two crowns on the left side had also been in function without complications (Fig 3-3v). A radiograph at the 7-year follow-up revealed that remodeling of the bone construct followed the form predicted by the surgical engineering and design (Fig 3-3w). The bone construct was radiographically continuous with the native bone and had become fully integrated with its physiology.

The functional and mechanical parameters of the surgical design regulated the steady-state morphology of the bone construct as intended. A well-defined cortical outline represented the sinus floor in the remodeled steady state. The bone volume began on the mesial aspect at point A, which was under the regulation of the lateral incisor periodontal system. The bone level descended to meet the implant cylinders at the junctions of their parallel walls and their hemispherical apices. The distal-most extent of the bone construct was continuous with the bone covering the apex of the labial molar root.

Discussion

In this patient, the specific conditions that challenged successful healing were different on the right and left sides; however, the basic strategy for design of bone-forming constructs containing dental implants was the same. The implants were used to provide mechanical stability to the center of the bone-forming environment. The bone-forming chambers were isolated from oral

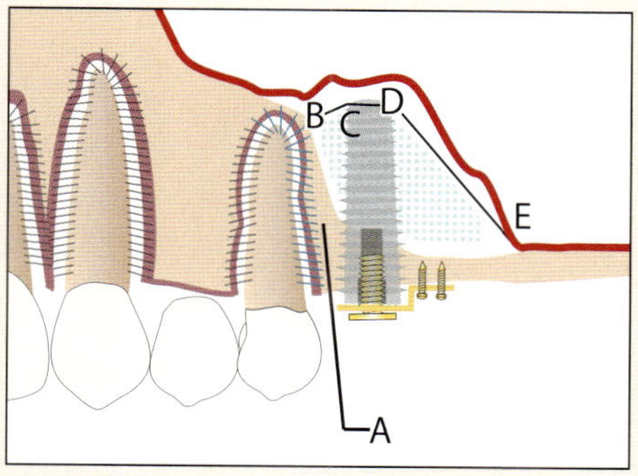

Fig 3-4j Important landmarks of the assembled bone-forming construct: A, bone that houses the Sharpey fibers of the periodontal ligament system, which is the primary source of neuromuscular signaling into the regeneration site; B, the apical limit of the existing bone volume; C and D, the constructed limits of the stabilized environment; E, a stable point on the existing sinus floor. The implant serves as the central mechanical element of the constructed environment.

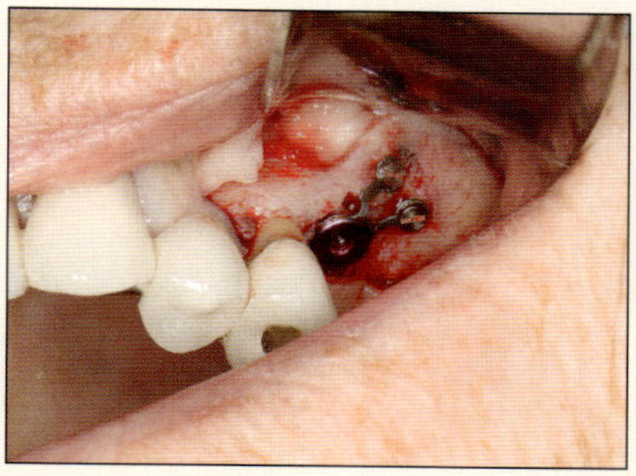

Fig 3-4k A collagen sponge containing rhBMP-2 surrounds the implant and fills the sinus elevation volume.

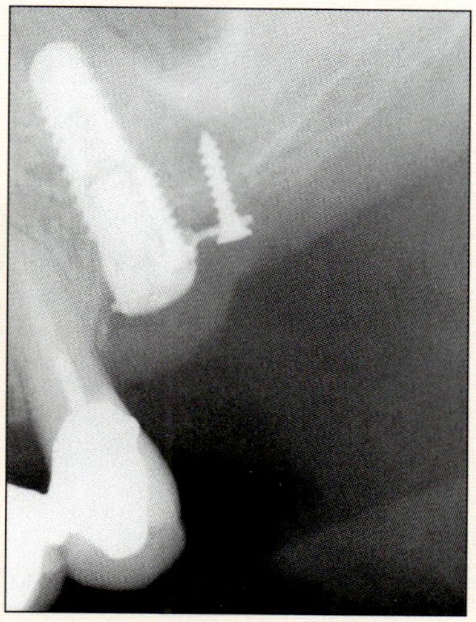

Fig 3-4l A postoperative radiograph shows the implant rising above the sinus floor, the bone plate, and one of the two microscrews. The implant is positioned close to the dental root to take advantage of the stimulating potential of its periodontal ligament–Sharpey fiber system.

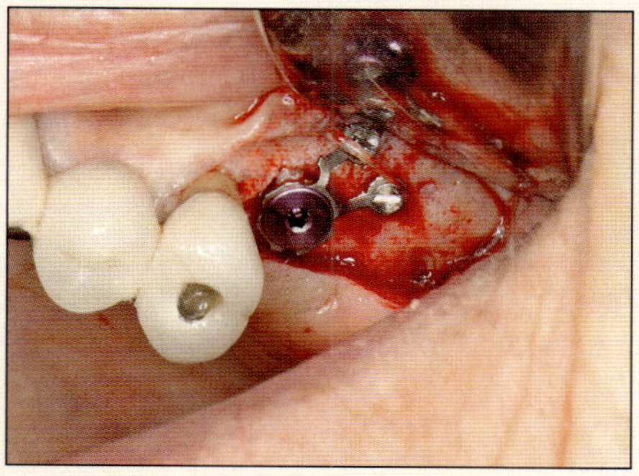

Fig 3-4m At reentry 4 months postoperatively, typical limited resorption is observed around the coronal 2 mm of the implant head.

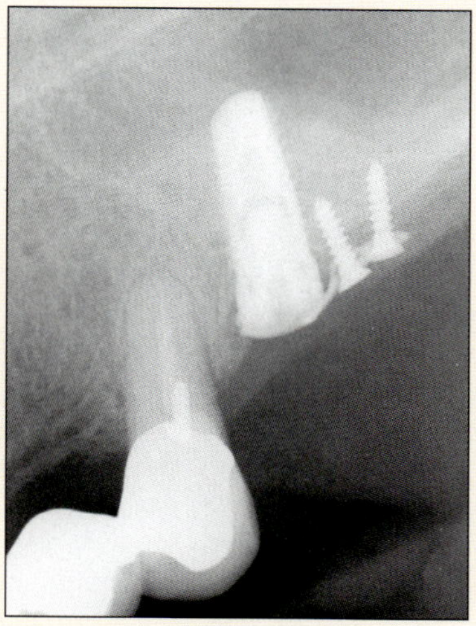

Fig 3-4n A radiograph taken 4 months postoperatively reveals bone consolidation around the implant and remodeling that has resorbed all of the graft volume extending beyond the implant and the mechanically sheltered zone.

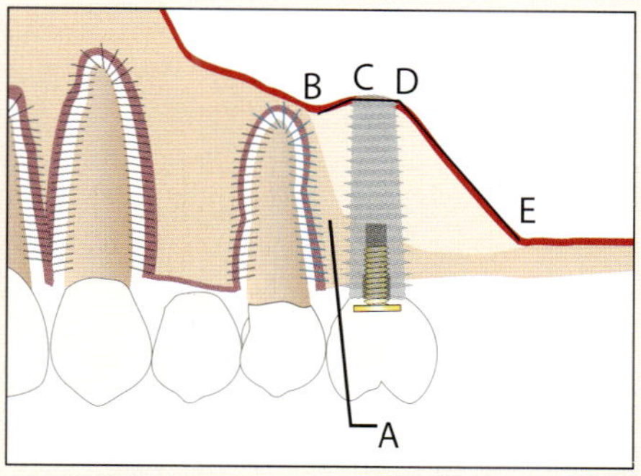

Fig 3-4o The rhBMP-2–containing collagen sponge has produced an ossified mass that extends to, but not beyond, the functional landmarks of the constructed environment. The collagen sponge has resorbed rapidly, leaving no particulate matter.

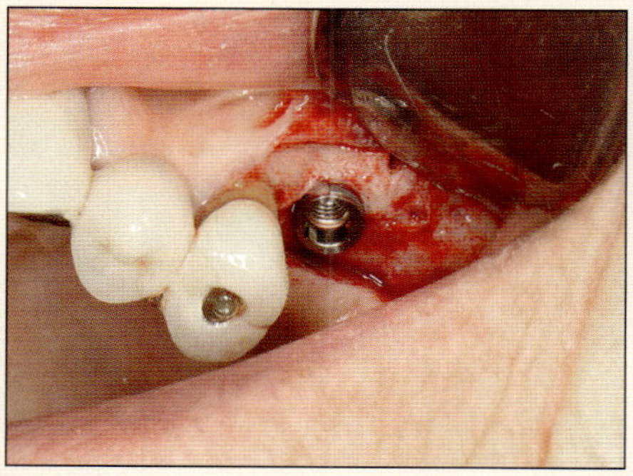

Fig 3-4p When the bone plate is removed, the implant projects 2 mm beyond the new ridge crest.

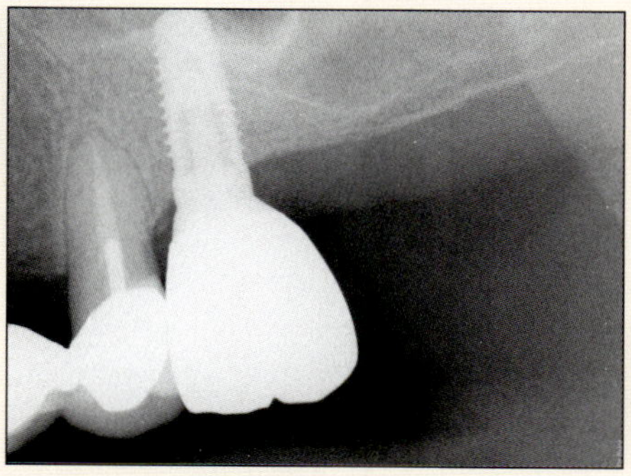

Fig 3-4q A radiograph taken 10 months postoperatively shows maturation of the constructed bone volume, reflecting progressive functional integration.

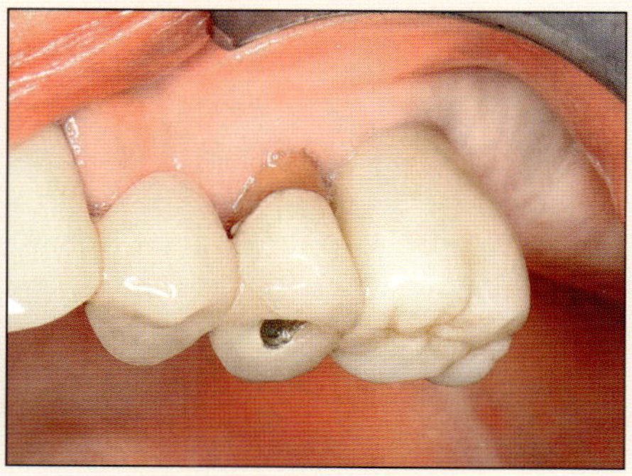

Fig 3-4r Crown in place.

Functional Analysis of Graft Positioning and Volume Requirements

An understanding of which parameters determine the optimal volume of the graft needed during a sinus elevation procedure is important for the efficient and safe use of these materials. There is a tendency to overbuild sinus elevation grafts. Surgeons place much more graft material than is needed because their experience is that the graft often collapses and resorbs before implants can be placed. Excessive graft volumes introduce additional risks, increase costs, and do not substantially benefit the reconstruction.

If the reconstruction is successful, it will result in a stable implant in a steady-state relationship with surrounding structural bone. Bone that might initially extend outside the boundaries of functional stimulation or direct mechanical support from the implant will eventually be lost through resorption and remodeling. Sinus grafts that contain unresorbable or slowly resorbable materials may extend the volume beyond that required to support the implant. The extra volume does not contribute to the function or predictability of the implant.

Placement of an excessive volume of graft materials during sinus elevation procedures may increase the risk of membrane perforation because of unnecessary dissection. If there is a breach of the sinus membrane during dissection or a perforation occurs due to sinus infection, graft material can escape into the antrum. This material may become a surgical salvage problem or may challenge the patient's natural process for clearing foreign bodies from the sinus. Minimizing the volume of graft material limits this risk.

Placing implants at the time of sinus elevation grafting decreases the graft volume in two ways. First, the volume displaced by the implant cylinder does not require grafting. Second, the position of the implant is known, so graft material can be positioned specifically to surround the cylinder and fill the anticipated structural volume. In most cases, the total volume of rhBMP-2 applied can be limited to a fraction of what is needed if the sinus is grafted first and the implant is placed in a delayed procedure.

Limiting the total volume of graft needed provides several additional benefits. Modern graft materials may be expensive or difficult to obtain. Minimizing their use will reduce costs. If autogenous bone is used, the morbidity of graft harvesting can be reduced by limiting the amount of bone needed. In addition, all graft materials elicit an inflammatory response because it is integral to the healing process. Pronounced swelling has been attributed to rhBMP-2 carried on ACSs.[16] Increasing the volume of the rhBMP-2 device and the total dose of rhBMP-2 beyond the necessary amount increases the risk of swelling-related complications.

The following case demonstrates a strategy to place a dental implant and to grow structural bone in a single stage. Analysis of the volume of bone necessary for a functional result allowed use of minimal volumes of graft materials.

Case description

A 65-year-old man presented with a failing maxillary left first molar. Despite frequent periodontal care, the tooth experienced progressive bone loss. The patient requested that the tooth be removed and a dental implant be placed. At the time of his initial presentation, a radiograph showed bone loss involving all three roots of the first molar (Fig 3-5a). The sinus floor was in close proximity to the root apices.

The tooth was removed, and the extraction site was treated with rhBMP-2/ACS. The socket lacked confining walls, and the root surfaces of adjacent teeth made up the anterior and posterior walls of the defect. Very little vertical bone developed in response to the placement of rhBMP-2 (Fig 3-5b).

Design of a bone-forming construct for this defect began with an analysis of how the remaining bone was being maintained (Fig 3-5c). This is always a critical step in defining a comprehensive diagnosis. Diagnosis is part of the engineering phase of the treatment process and provides the basis for creating alternative surgical designs.

The anterior wall (A) of the prospective graft site was maintained by the periodontal ligaments that insert into the lamina dura at this location. Point B was maintained by the structural support from the premolar root and the periodontal ligament insertions at the root apex. Bone was similarly maintained posteriorly at points C and D. The neuromuscular stimulating effects extending from the periodontal systems of the teeth adjacent to the defect diminished with distance from these structures. The effect was weakest at the midpoint between the two roots.

As part of the bone-forming construct, a dental implant was to be placed in the center of the defect (Fig 3-5d). The sinus membrane was elevated, and the cylinder was positioned. A bone plate was required to support the implant because of the lack of native bone. The presence of the implant introduced two new points, E and F. These are mechanically sheltered points in this bone-forming environment. A cell positioned next to the cylinder at point E or F would experience less mechanical stress than a cell in the center of the chamber.

Cells occupying the volume under the line extending from points B to E to F to C would experience a sheltered environment and would be protected from major forces (Fig 3-5e). Bone within this limited volume has the potential to become a viable skeletal unit and exist in a steady state long term. Bone that is viable and has remodeling capability could not exist long term beyond these boundaries. Nevertheless, collagen sponges with rhBMP-2 were placed between the implant apex and the sinus membrane. This was done to avoid having the sinus membrane drape directly over the hemispherical implant dome. The graft material therefore extended beyond the confines of the bone-forming chamber (Fig 3-5f).

Four months after placement of the implant, cover screw, and bone plate, bone had formed to cover the anterior arm of the bone plate (Fig 3-5g). The 4-month radiograph revealed radiopaque material surrounding the implant (Fig 3-5h). The neuromuscular and mechanical stabilization effect was best between the premolar root and the anterior face of the implant cylinder. Bone rose on each side toward the junctions of the parallel cyl-

Fig 3-5 Functional analysis of graft positioning and volume requirements in a 65-year-old man with a failed maxillary left first molar.

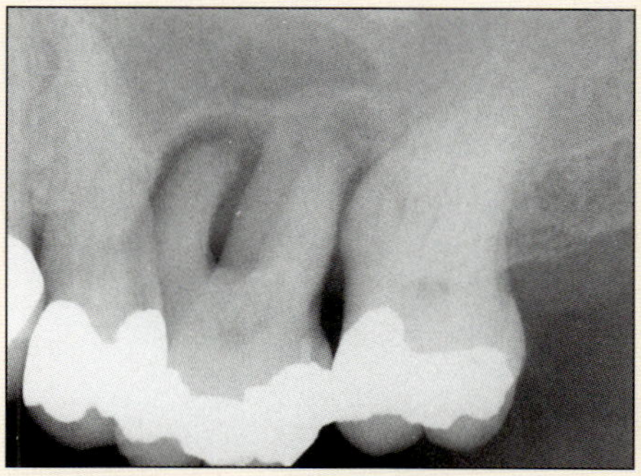

Fig 3-5a The initial radiograph of the first molar reveals bone loss involving all three roots.

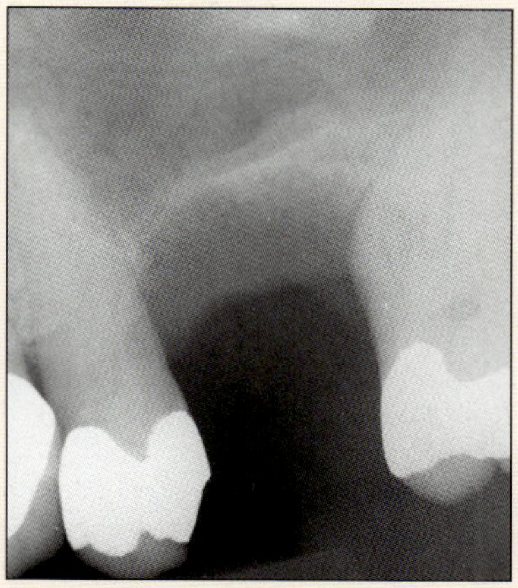

Fig 3-5b A radiograph of the site taken 2 months after tooth extraction and rhBMP-2/ACS grafting reveals that little vertical bone has developed.

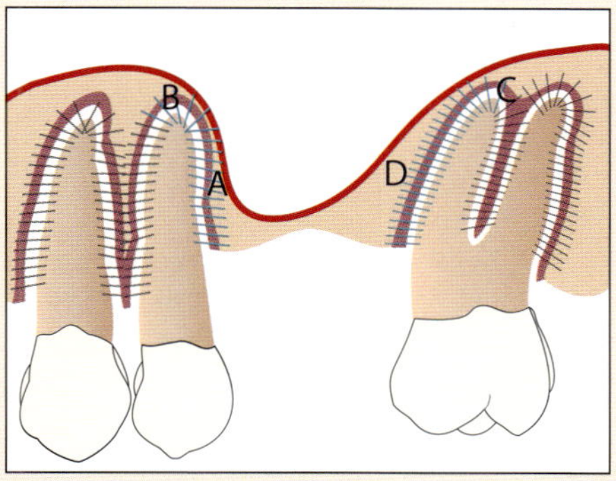

Fig 3-5c Analysis of the existing physiologic elements of the site. The anterior wall (A) of the prospective graft site is maintained by the periodontal ligaments that insert into the lamina dura at this location. Point B is maintained by the structural support from the premolar root and the periodontal ligament insertions at the root apex. Bone is similarly maintained posteriorly at points C and D. The neuromuscular stimulating effects extending from the periodontal systems of the teeth adjacent to the defect diminish as the distance from these structures increases. The effect is weakest at the midpoint between the two roots.

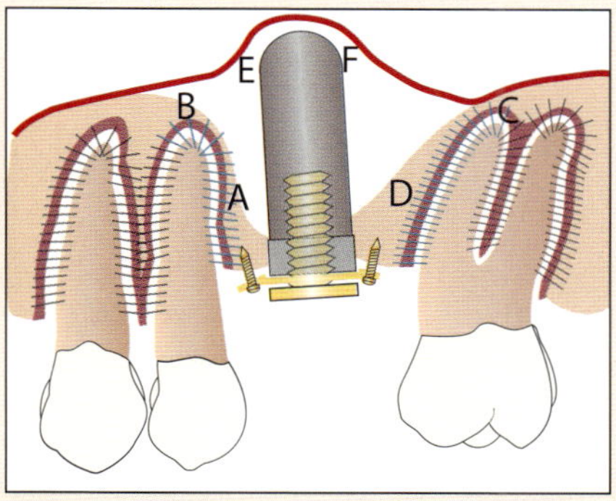

Fig 3-5d The stabilized implant introduces two new points, E and F. These are mechanically sheltered points in this bone-forming environment.

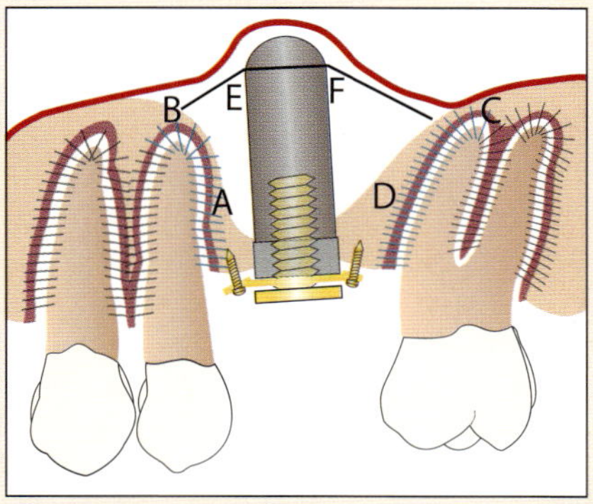

Fig 3-5e Defining the potential occupying volume of the graft. Cells that come to occupy the volume under the B-E-F-C line will experience a sheltered environment and be protected from major forces.

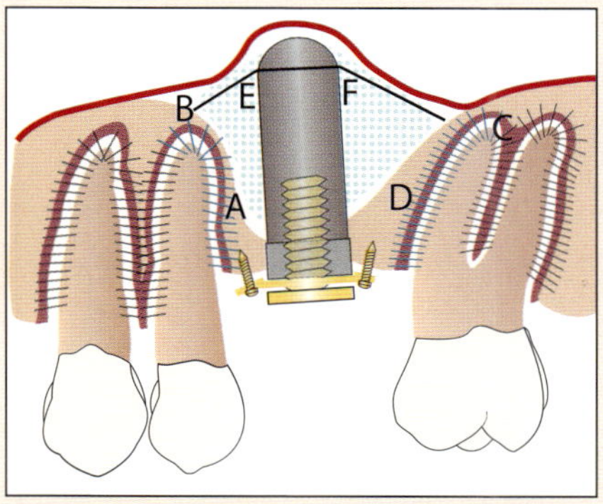

Fig 3-5f The initial sinus elevation volume extends beyond the graft boundaries.

→

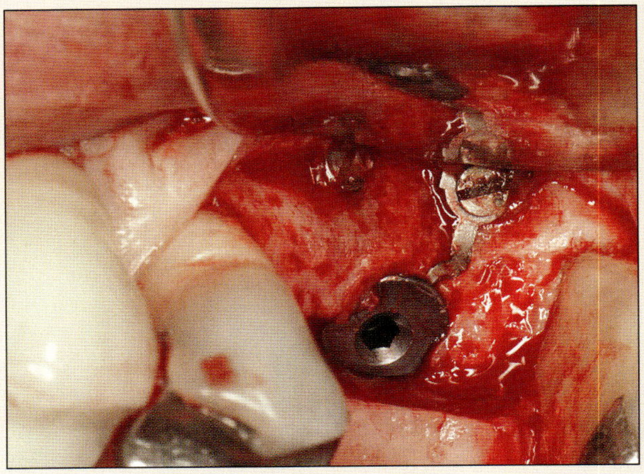

Fig 3-5g Clinical appearance 4 months after placement of the implant and rhBMP-2 graft.

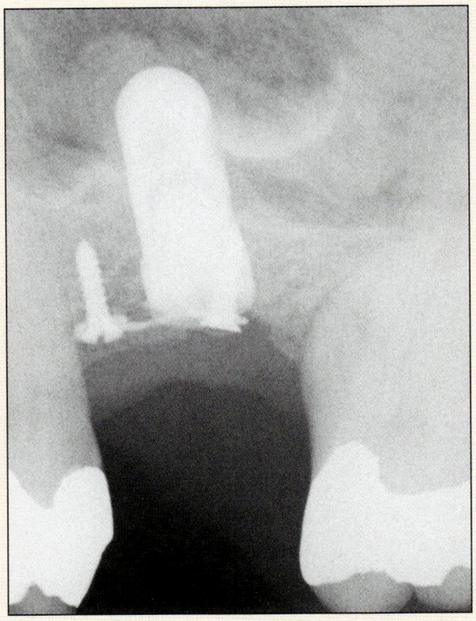

Fig 3-5h Four-month postoperative radiograph shows radiopaque material surrounding the implant.

→

inder and the hemispherical dome. Bone also extended to the posterior side of the bone-forming chamber. Less stimulation and support were derived from the second molar because it was located farther from the implant.

After the bone plate was removed, the implant was noted to be slightly below the crestal bone level (Fig 3-5i). This was an unusual finding because, in general, 2 mm of the implant is exposed by crestal bone resorption. This result was observed in one other patient treated by the author. The two cases had a treatment step in common: Both patients had a history of initial rhBMP-2 treatment involving the crestal bone. How rhBMP-2–derived engineered bone responds to subsequent surgery is incompletely understood.[17]

A radiograph taken after removal of the bone plate revealed a cortical plate forming at the new sinus floor (Fig 3-5j). The cortex followed the boundaries of the bone-forming chamber. Remodeling and organization of the sinus graft created a skeletal unit that could exist within the regulatory limits of the adjacent teeth and implant (Fig 3-5k).

When the graft material results in bone that has the capability of both consolidation and organization, the new ossicle will consistently remodel into the shape predicted in the design process. Functional parameters working on the maturing bone segment direct it to conform to a shape that follows the rules of bone formation. Nonresorbable graft particles act as implants themselves and can maintain newly formed bone beyond the boundaries of the dental implant environment.

After 4 years in function, the implant was found to be stable, and the morphology of the bone generated had been maintained (Fig 3-5l). The clear cortical outlines and normal trabecular patterns confirmed that bone remodeling and organization were occurring under the influence of signals common to the original, natural skeleton. The bone synthesized was seamlessly integrated into the structural and physiologic systems of the patient's existing skeleton, allowing placement of a functional single-tooth restoration (Fig 3-5m).

Discussion

Replacement of a missing maxillary first molar is one of the most common problems that present to a surgical practice. The 6-year molar enters service when the patient is most caries prone. Restorative treatment is often initiated at a young age and continues for many years. Failure of the tooth may be related to structural compromise that accumulates over increasingly extensive restorative treatments. This tooth also has a propensity for bone loss related to periodontal failure. In this patient, the maxillary first molar on the contralateral side failed in the same manner 4 years later.

Placement of dental implants to replace maxillary first molars is challenging because of the anatomical features of the site. The maxillary first molar is the largest tooth in the maxillary arch but often exists in limited alveolar bone volume. Following loss of a maxillary first molar, the alveolar process atrophies and the sinus floor descends. The result is minimal available bone volume in which to place an implant.

By understanding the limits of the mechanisms that regulate bone physiology at the site, the surgeon can create an efficient and effective surgical design that meets all of the essential elements for bone formation and long-term maintenance while minimizing the volume of graft materials that will be applied. The latter is important to control the cost of the procedure as well as the exposure of the patient to the side effects and risks inherent to these materials.

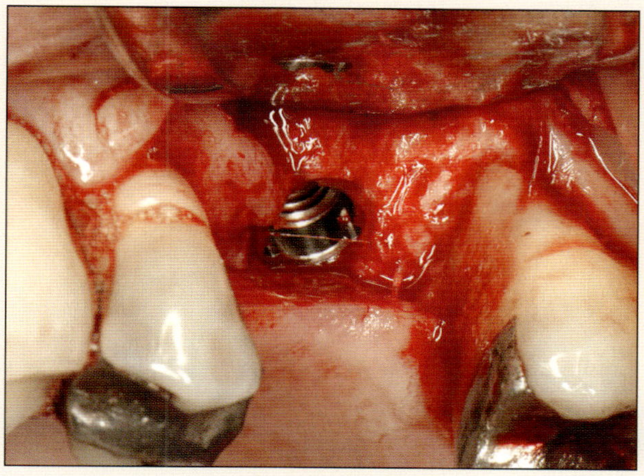

Fig 3-5i Bone growth over the polished titanium collar of the implant is an unusual finding because 2 mm of the implant is usually exposed by resorption.

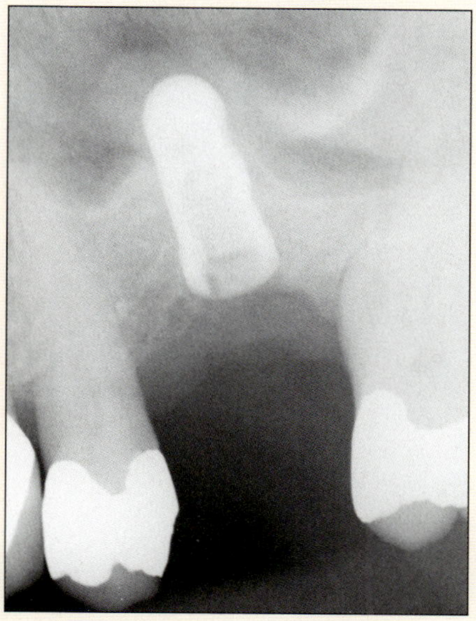

Fig 3-5j Follow-up radiograph taken after removal of the bone plate at 4 months shows the implant slightly below the crestal bone level.

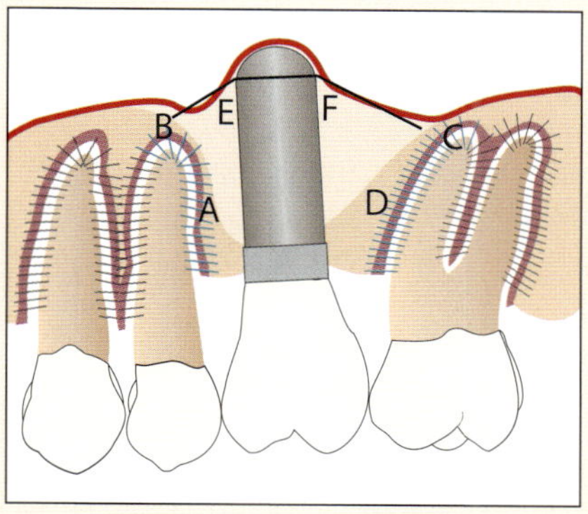

Fig 3-5k *(right)* The remodeled sinus graft follows the limits of the site physiology.

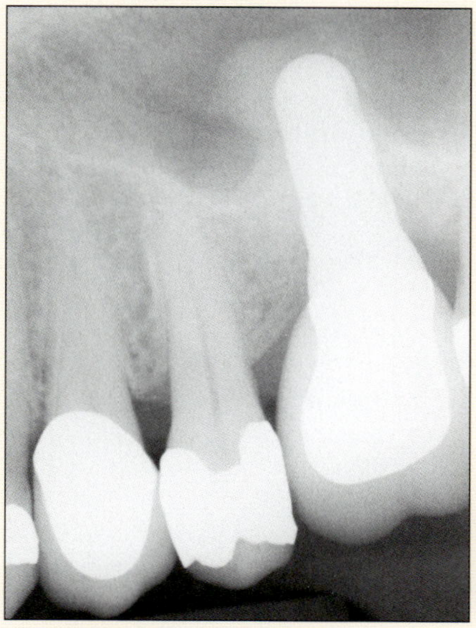

Fig 3-5l After 4 years in function, the implant occupies a volume of constructed bone that can be maintained in a steady state for many years. Formation of normal cortical layers and appropriate trabecular architecture demonstrates that the new bone is interacting at a functional level with the host.

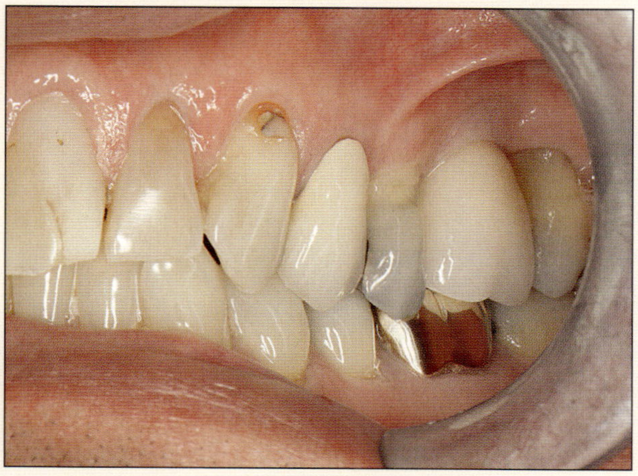

Fig 3-5m Clinical view of the prosthesis after 4 years.

Management of a Deficiency in Neuromuscular Input

One of the essential components of the bone-forming construct is the source of neuromuscular input. Stimulation and control of the bone growth within the regeneration chamber are dependent on these signals. Muscle attachments are the primary source of these signals. Healthy teeth with intact periodontal ligament systems also can furnish these signals, particularly within the alveolar process.

One common challenge to successful surgical design is multiple missing adjacent teeth in the posterior maxilla. This area is normally weakly regulated by muscle function. The primary source of stimulation and regulation of the posterior maxillary alveolus is healthy teeth.

When placing multiple implants in the posterior maxilla, the clinician must determine where regulatory signals arise from and recognize that their effect is distance dependent. Although dental implants may stabilize the adjacent area, they do impede the mechanical signals traveling through the chamber. The locations within the regeneration chamber that have deficient signaling are predisposed to poor graft organization. During the surgical design process, it may be possible to compensate for the deficiency by choosing the proper graft material or increasing the availability of bone morphogenetic proteins. The following case demonstrates careful planning of a bone-forming construct to meet the challenge of a large regeneration site.

Case description

A 79-year-old woman presented with a failing fixed partial denture extending from the maxillary right second molar to second premolar. The posterior abutment tooth had failed. The objective was to remove the failed abutment tooth and place implants at the first and second molar sites for an implant-supported fixed prosthesis.

Minimal bone was present at the sinus floor (Fig 3-6a). A vertical septum divided the maxillary sinus into a main anterior section and a smaller posterior section. The presenting skeletal architecture had been in a steady state for many years (Fig 3-6b). The alveolar process housing the second premolar maintained stable bone at points A and B. The septum at point C partially partitioned the sinus chamber. The functional dynamics that create and maintain sinus septa are unknown. The presence of the structure implies that some source of stimulation and regulation must be operating. Bone at the posterior sinus is under the regulation of the pterygomaxillary junction.

To meet the requirements of the restorative objective, the surgical design included two implants (Fig 3-6c). The posterior implant would be placed anterior to the sinus septum, avoiding the need to elevate both sinus chambers. Placement of two adjacent implants would introduce four areas that would interact with the bone-forming chamber. The landmarks for surgical planning were at points E, F, G, and H. These landmarks represented the junctions between the cylindric body of the implant and its hemispherical apex.

The fixed partial denture was divided, preserving the anterior premolar abutment. The distal abutment was removed. After 4 weeks of healing, a sinus elevation graft procedure with rhBMP-2 was performed, and two implants were placed (Fig 3-6d). The sinus floor was not thick enough to achieve primary stability. Bone plates allowed stabilization of the two implants to the adjacent alveolar bone. A radiograph showed graft consolidation at 4 months.

Initially the graft material extended somewhat apical to the implant cylinders (Fig 3-6e). During surgery, collagen sponges carried rhBMP-2 above the apices of the implant cylinders. The rhBMP-2/ACS device was interposed between the implant apices and the elevated sinus membrane. In this bone-forming construct, the graft material adjacent to points A, B, and C would consolidate most readily. These regions were closest to the existing native bone with its established regulatory mechanisms.

The challenge in this configuration was the volume between the two cylinders. The center of the regeneration volume was the greatest distance from regulating signals and a native source of cells. The rhBMP-2 material was prepared at 0.5 mg/mL. One collagen sponge, 2 × 20 × 40 mm, received 1 mL of rhBMP-2. Banked bone, in the form of 1 mL of cancellous particles, also received 1 mL of rhBMP-2 for reconstitution. The total dose of rhBMP-2 was therefore 1.0 mg. The collagen sponge filled the periphery of the chamber. The bone graft carrying rhBMP-2 was placed in the center of the chamber, between the two implant cylinders.

The stabilizing bone plates and anchoring screws were evaluated 4 months after simultaneous implant and graft placement (Fig 3-6f). The bone plates were stable. After the bone plates were removed, 1 to 2 mm of the polished collar was found to be surrounded by soft tissue (Fig 3-6g).

On a radiograph taken 6 months after placement of the implants and rhBMP-2 graft, the graft adjacent to the native sinus floor showed organization and formation of trabeculae (Fig 3-6h). The portion of the graft near the implant apices was diffuse and lacked organization. There were no clear trabeculae. There was no cortical outline between the graft mass and the sinus membrane. Mineralization of the graft extended just beyond the implant apices. The implants were clinically stable and responded normally to percussion.

As the graft matured, the newly formed ossicle organized (Fig 3-6i). Resorption of the graft mass removed bone that was outside the functional environment. The mineralized volume collapsed, exposing the hemispherical domes and the implant apices.

Five years after implant and graft placement, there were signs of consolidation and maturation (Fig 3-6j). Trabeculae extended to the apical region of the graft. A cortical layer had formed at the interface between the graft and the sinus membrane. Bone consolidation on each side of the implant extended to the junctions of the implant cylinder and the apical dome. The dome portion was not covered by bone. The cortical formation extended between the cylindric aspects of the adjacent implants, even if they were at different levels. The implant crowns had functioned successfully for 5 years (Fig 3-6k).

Fig 3-6 Management of deficient neuromuscular input after removal of a mobile, failed abutment tooth resulted in a large edentulous span.

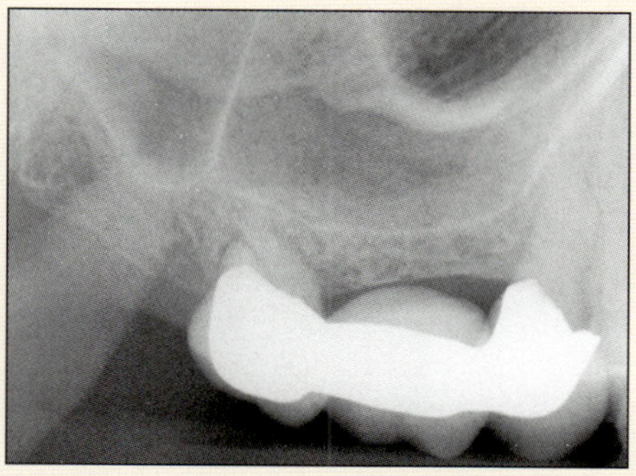

Fig 3-6a A radiograph of the site shows compromised abutment teeth and a thin maxillary sinus floor.

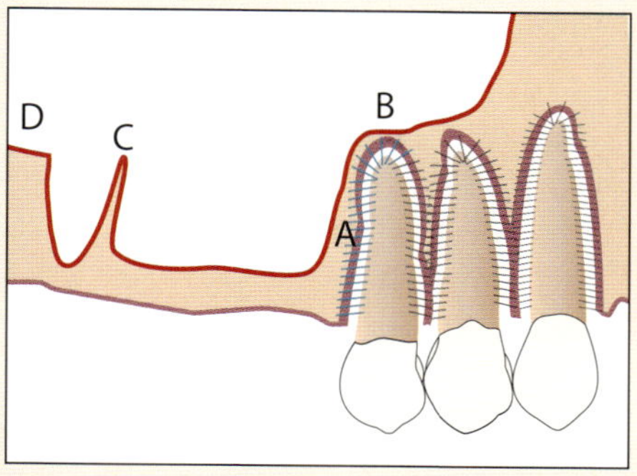

Fig 3-6b Analysis of the functional skeletal elements that maintain the existing site morphology. The alveolar process housing the second premolar maintains stable bone (A and B). The septum (C) partially partitions the sinus chamber. Bone at the posterior sinus (D) is under the regulation of the pterygomaxillary junction.

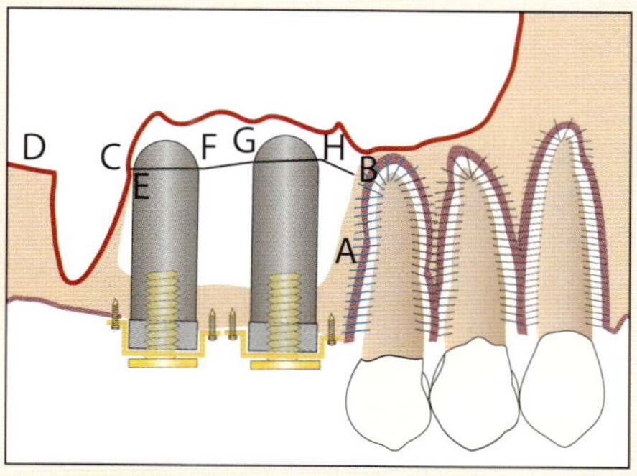

Fig 3-6c Strategy for a possible bone-forming construct including two implants. Introduction of two stabilized implants to the proposed reconstruction site has the potential to establish a volume that has relative mechanical stability. Placement of adjacent implants introduces four areas that will interact with the bone-forming chamber; these landmarks represent the junctions between the cylindric body of the implants and their hemispherical apex (E, F, G, and H).

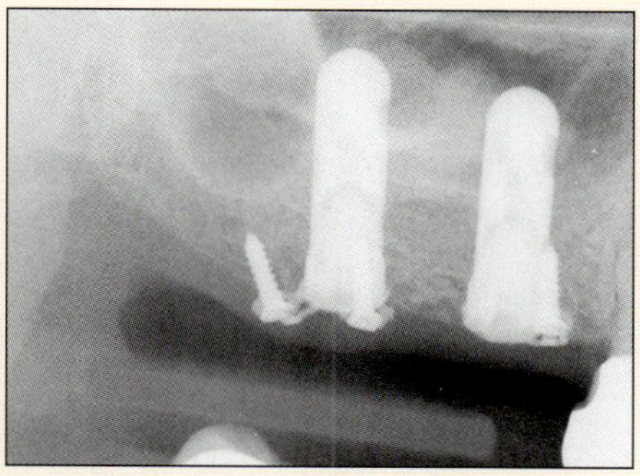

Fig 3-6d Two implants, each with a stabilizing bone plate, are placed.

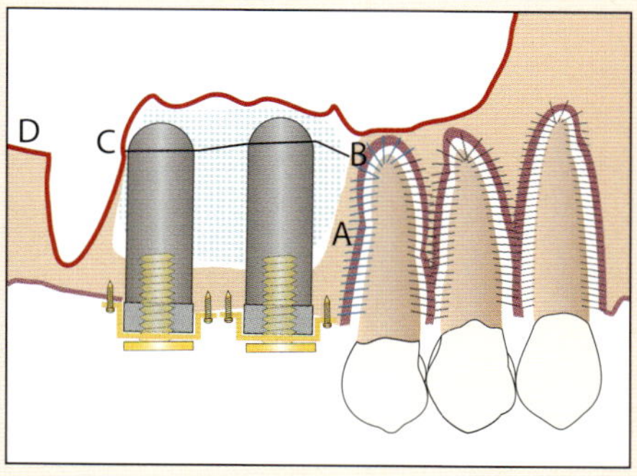

Fig 3-6e The graft will extend initially beyond the apices of the two implants. A viable graft will not be maintained beyond the volume *(area under black line)* that obtains its relative mechanical stability from the implants and surrounding bone.

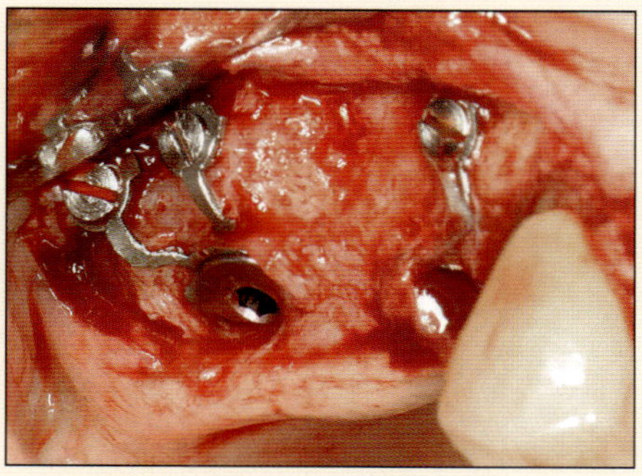

Fig 3-6f Bone plates securing the implants are stable after 4 months.

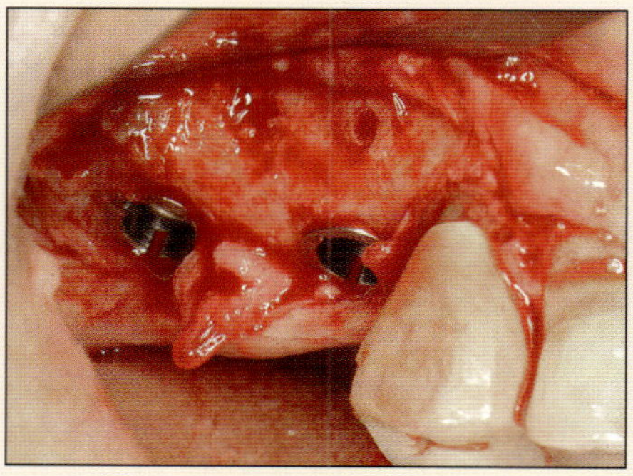

Fig 3-6g Following removal of the bone plates, the implants are stable. About 1 to 2 mm of the polished collars is surrounded by soft tissue.

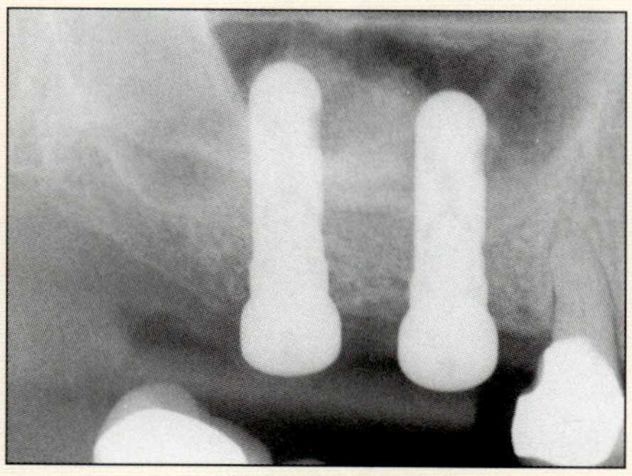

Fig 3-6h Radiograph taken 6 months postoperatively shows trabeculae in the area of the graft adjacent to the native sinus floor but not near the apices of the implants.

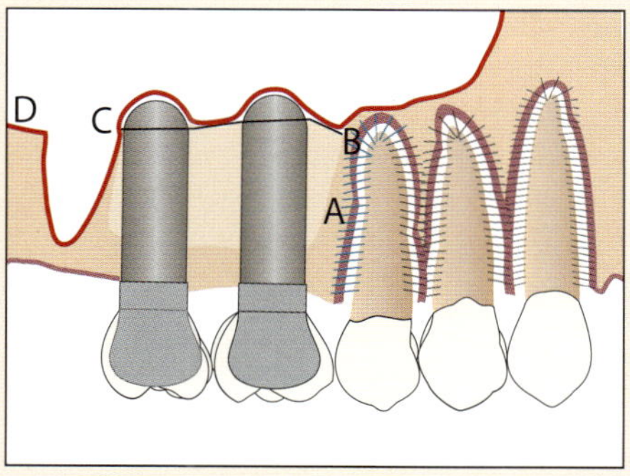

Fig 3-6i Remodeling removes the part of the graft that extended beyond the volume of the mechanically stable environment.

→

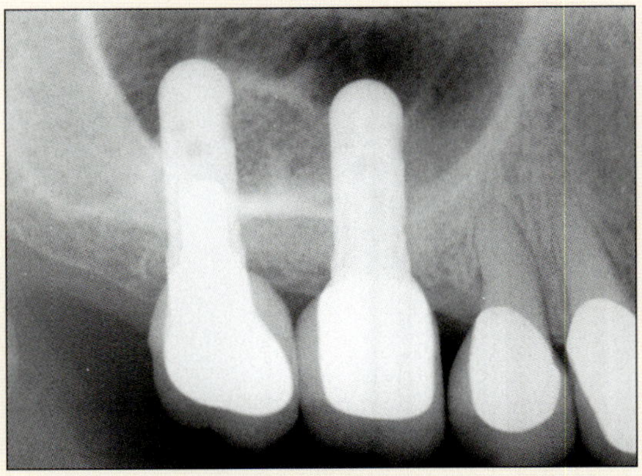

Fig 3-6j A 5-year follow-up radiograph shows the maturation of the graft with establishment of normal cortical layers and appropriate trabecular architecture.

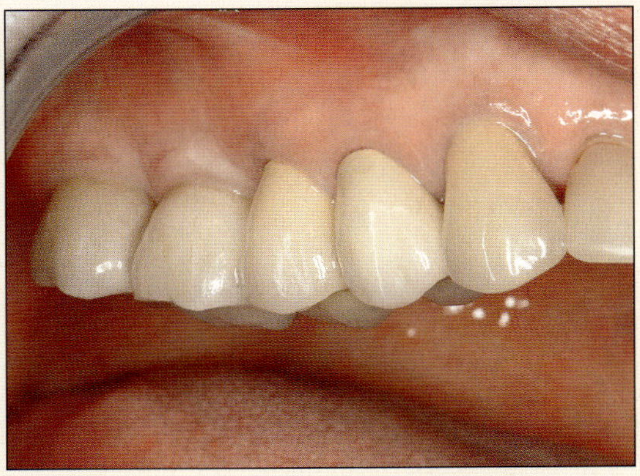

Fig 3-6k Implant crowns in function after 5 years.

Discussion

Graft selection requires an understanding of how the material functions within the bone-forming construct. Optimal performance and minimal risk are the objectives. In this case, a combination of rhBMP-2, banked bone, and collagen sponge was designed into the construct. Placement of two implants at the time of sinus elevation grafting created an environment that supported bone growth with low doses of rhBMP-2. With the implants in place, it was clear where bone was deficient and needed. The volume displaced by the implants decreased the volume of graft material needed. The apices of the implants established a boundary within which bone would be structurally useful. They also defined a boundary beyond which bone would not be maintained and should not be extended.

The proposed surgical design anticipated a challenge to bone formation in the central region. To improve the probability of successful bone formation in the compromised site, cancellous banked bone treated with rhBMP-2 was chosen to fill the central region between the implants. The collagen sponges were expected to resorb in about 15 days. The cancellous banked bone would remain in place for at least 8 weeks. This prolonged the time available for development of new bone in the central zone.

Banked bone was not considered for filling the entire chamber because it would have required resorption to free the volume to fill with new bone. The small portion of particulate bone is less hazardous than a large volume should the sinus membrane develop a perforation, allowing the escape of particles into the maxillary sinus.

Alveolar Construction in a Site of Extreme Alveolar Atrophy

Construction of a bone segment and osseointegration of implants are most challenging when there is no adjacent native bone as well as no preexisting bone. The bone is being constructed in an environment that lacks support from a neuromuscular source. When this bone is constructed and implants are placed in the maxillary sinus, there is also risk of confronting sinus pathosis. Mucous clearance disorders or sinus membrane perforation may complicate the healing process. However, successful treatment can be achieved if all of the elements required for construction are met. In the following case of severe atrophy, a functional and stable result was achieved even though no adjacent bone was available to stabilize the implant or to provide osteogenic cells.

Case description

A patient presented with a failing maxillary reconstruction that had served her for many years (Fig 3-7a). Despite exceptional personal and professional maintenance, the teeth supporting the complete-arch fixed prosthesis failed and were not restorable. The remaining teeth were extracted, and an immediate denture was placed. After the complete maxillary denture had been placed, the patient requested placement of dental implants for a fixed prosthesis.

When the maxillary teeth were removed, the extraction sites had been treated with rhBMP-2/ACS. The anterior maxilla re-

Fig 3-7 Immediate placement of implants at a site of sinus floor discontinuity.

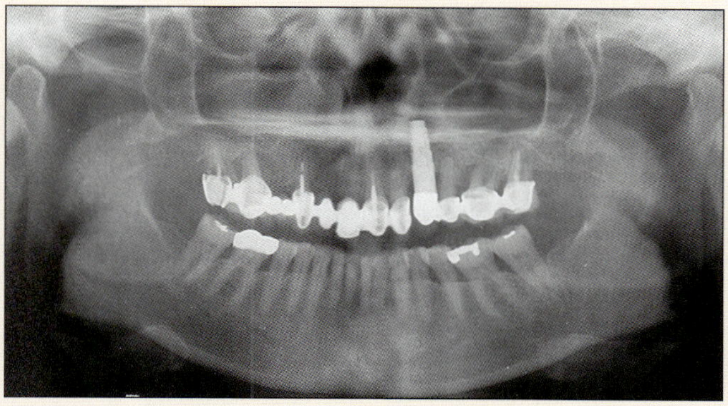

Fig 3-7a The pretreatment panoramic radiograph shows advanced bone loss at multiple sites.

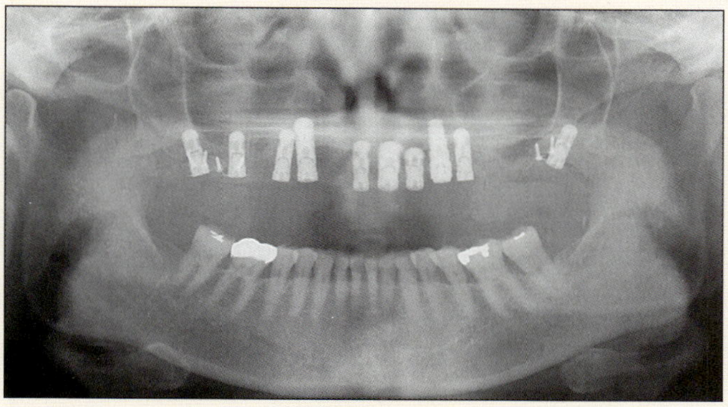

Fig 3-7b Following removal of the maxillary teeth and rhBMP-2 ridge preservation, implants are placed at the sites exhibiting adequate bone regeneration.

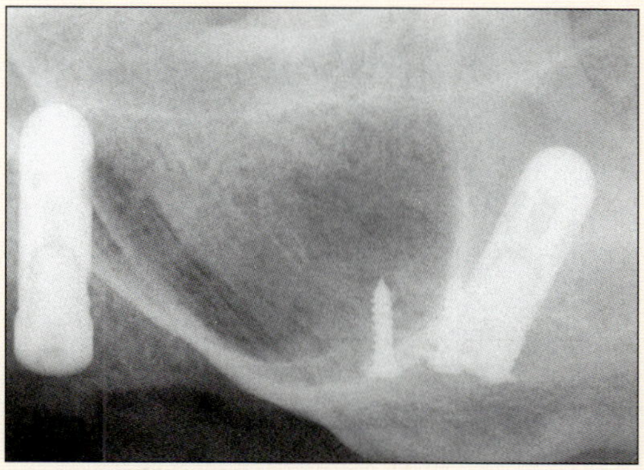

Fig 3-7c The maxillary left first molar site has not formed bone in response to placement of rhBMP-2 at the time of extraction. The sinus floor descends to the ridge crest.

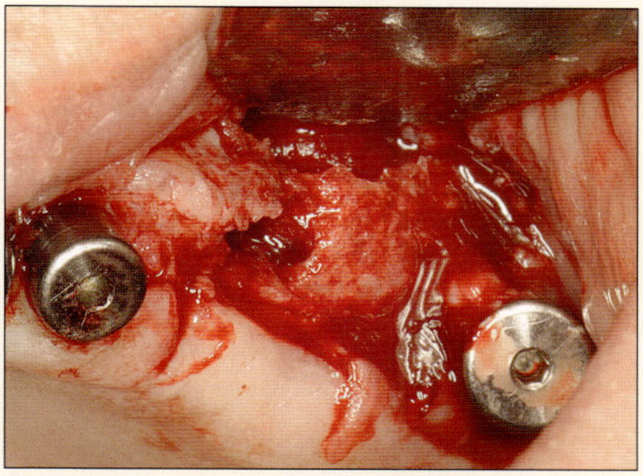

Fig 3-7d Four months following the placement of anterior and third molar implants. The thin bone between the sinus elevation window and the implant osteotomy site is lost.

→

sponded well to the rhBMP-2, and sufficient bone developed to place dental implants. Bone loss around the maxillary right and left first molars, however, was extensive. Despite use of rhBMP-2 at the time of extraction, only the thin sinus floor remained at these sites. The patient wished the restoration to include the first and second molars, so placement of posterior implants was indicated.

After initial healing of the extraction sites, dental implants were placed. Six implants (Camlog) were placed in the anterior region, and the existing implant (Frialit-2, Dentsply) in the site of the left canine was retained. On the right side of the maxilla, a sinus elevation graft was performed using rhBMP-2. Dental implants were placed immediately in the rhBMP-2 graft. The thickness of native bone at the sites of the right first and second molars and left third molar was not enough to achieve primary stability. Titanium plates were used to stabilize the implants in those positions. The bone comprising the sinus floor of the left side of the posterior maxilla was extremely thin, and there was a perforation of the sinus membrane during the dissection. Because of the extensive disruption of the sinus membrane, implants were not placed in the left-side first and second molar sites (Fig 3-7b).

The left-side third molar implant was placed in the maxillary tuberosity, where the bone was primarily cancellous. A bone plate was placed for added stability and to prevent displacement should it fail to osseointegrate. The remaining challenge was to place an implant into the site of the first molar, where the bone was extremely thin (Fig 3-7c).

Four months after initial placement of implants, the patient returned for a second attempt at sinus elevation of the left side of the maxilla and placement of an implant in the left first molar site. A flap was raised and a lateral window created to elevate the sinus membrane. The bone was thin and very soft, but the sinus membrane was successfully elevated without perforation. An osteotomy was started through the ridge crest, but the integrity of the sinus floor could not be maintained. This resulted in a large discontinuity defect in the alveolus where the implant osteotomy was continuous with the lateral sinus window (Fig 3-7d). The surrounding bone was thin and of a soft consistency. Although the large bone defect and poor bone quality made stabilizing an implant challenging, the intact sinus membrane offered the opportunity to construct an environment that could act as a bone-forming chamber.

While implants had been successfully placed at the sites of the left second premolar and third molar, an implant at the first molar site would improve the response to functional load challenges and offer more restorative options. However, there were obvious anatomical challenges. The bone adjacent to the bone gap was thin and structurally compromised (Fig 3-7e). Although successful implants had healed at the mesial and distal boundaries of the defect, they were too far from the center to offer much stabilizing effect on a graft.

One option was to place a sinus elevation graft as a first stage (Fig 3-7f). After some months of healing and maturation, an implant could be placed if the graft were successful. In this type of defect, a large volume of graft material would be necessary because the volume deficiency was large and the boundaries were wide. The surrounding anatomy did not lend any mechanical support to maintenance of the graft volume. This was essentially a one-wall defect. The collagen sponge that carries rhBMP-2 to the sinus grafts resorbs within about 2 weeks (Fig 3-7g). Although rhBMP-2 recruits cells that have osteogenic potential, there is no physical or physiologic space for structural, living bone to form. After 4 months, little or no bone is available for implant placement.

Placement of autogenous or allogeneic human bone was another option. In many environments, successful bone construction can be realized with this method. However, autogenous bone of this volume would likely have required harvesting from the patient's iliac crest or tibia, involving substantial risk and expense. Banked bone also must undergo a sequence of maturation steps before it can be considered suitable for implant anchorage. First, the banked bone graft must be tolerated by the soft tissue envelope and successfully heal. Second, the material must be resorbed and replaced by living bone. In general, in sites with large defects and greater limitation to access existing viable bone cells, the predictability of allogeneic grafts is compromised.

Because of the disadvantages associated with the other management options, an implant was positioned within the sinus elevation regeneration chamber (Figs 3-7h and 3-7i). The implant was secured by a malleable titanium bone plate anchored to the distal alveolar ridge with two 1.2-mm screws and attached to the implant with the cover screw. The plate was oriented on the distal aspect because the labial bone was absent. Anchorage of the implant was not dependent on the integrity of the osteotomy site. The small screws that anchored the plate required minimal bone.

The lateral aspect of the implant cylinder was visible through the discontinuity of the lateral sinus wall. Small-particle (0.5- to 1.0-mm), solvent-dehydrated, cancellous allogeneic bone (Puros) was reconstituted in bone morphogenetic protein (Infuse, Medtronic) at a concentration of 0.5 mg/mL. ACSs (Integra Life Sciences) were soaked in rhBMP-2 at a concentration of 0.5 mg/mL. The total dose of rhBMP-2 was 1.0 mg in 2.0 mL of sterile water. One rhBMP-2 sponge was positioned between the sinus membrane and the apex of the implant. The bone graft particles were placed to surround the implant cylinder. A second rhBMP-2–soaked sponge was used to cover the lateral aspect of the graft and to fill the sinus elevation window (Fig 3-7j). At this stage, the graft volume extended somewhat beyond the confines of the anticipated bone-formation chamber.

To be successful, all of the critical components for bone construction must be present (Fig 3-7k). The secured implant device provided mechanical stabilization of the regeneration chamber. The malleable bone plate and microscrews established a semirigid structure in the center of the engineering environment. As noted earlier, the vertical walls of the cylinder and the hemispherical apex interact differently with the bone-forming environment. The junctions between each side of the cylinder and the apex are important engineering landmarks. Bone important to the long-term stability of the implant will not form apical to these landmarks. Extending the graft beyond these landmarks is therefore not clinically useful.

Because there were no adjacent teeth in this site, the nearest segments of stable bone were under the influence of the existing implants. Bone adjacent to the two existing implants was relatively stable. The graft would not heal beyond the level of the bone stabilized by the implants. The new implant was closer to the first premolar implant than it was to the third molar implant. The most supportive environment extended mesially from the new implant cylinder to the bone housing the first premolar implant. Bone formed by this process would not consolidate apical to the cylinder-apex junctions of the existing implant. On the distal aspect of the new implant, the environment was mostly developed by the implant itself. Placement of grafting material beyond the boundary that was under the stabilizing influence of the construct (see Fig 3-7k) would not have been useful because it was unlikely to develop into structural bone.

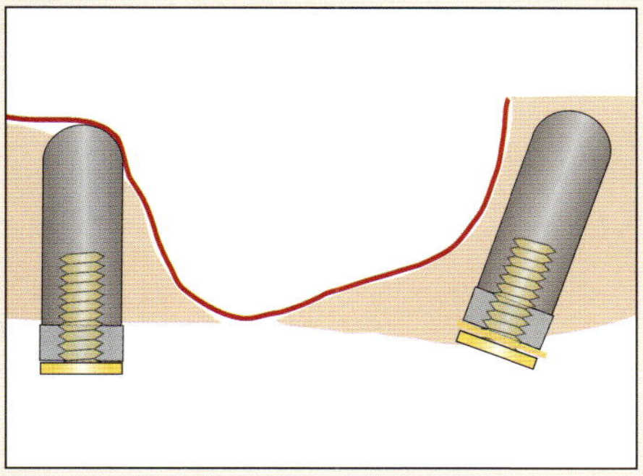

Fig 3-7e The implant site represents a discontinuity of the alveolar crest. The bone adjacent to the bone gap is thin and structurally compromised.

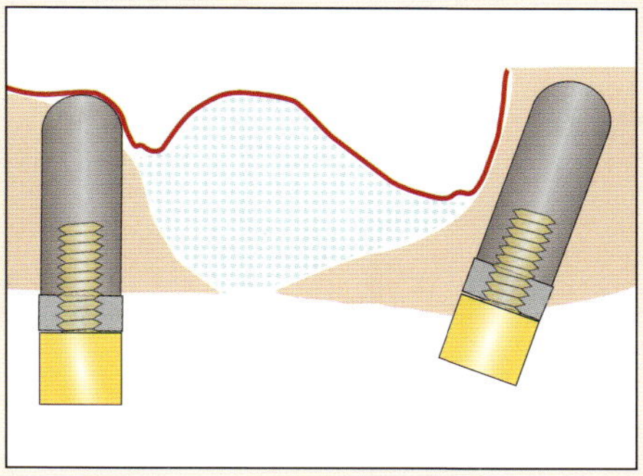

Fig 3-7f One option is to place a sinus elevation graft and allow it to heal before the dental implant is placed.

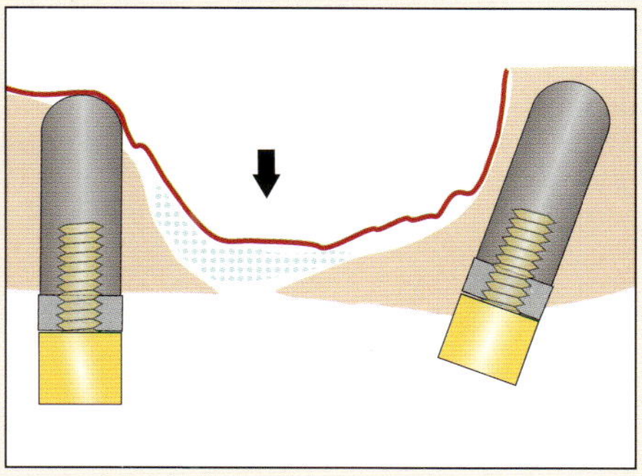

Fig 3-7g Sinus elevation grafts that use rhBMP-2 on collagen sponges tend to fail because they lack the ability to maintain volume as the sponge resorbs. (The *arrow* indicates collapse of the graft.)

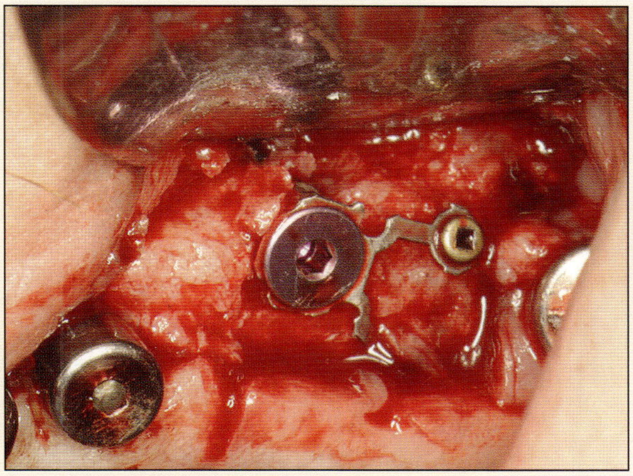

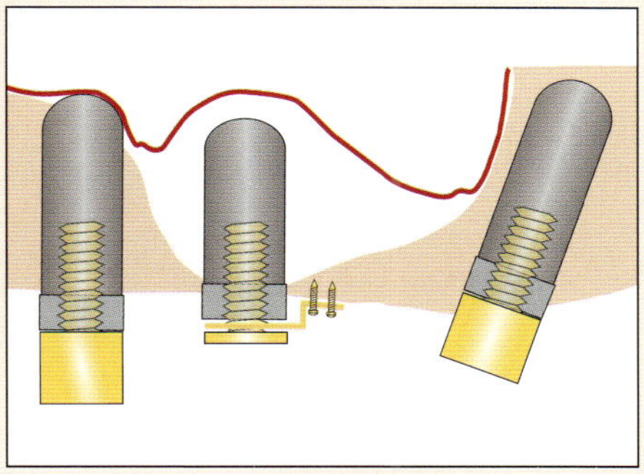

Fig 3-7h *(left)* An implant is positioned and secured with a bone plate as part of the bone-forming construct. The lateral sinus wall is absent, exposing the entire lateral surface of the implant. The bone plate is attached to the implant using the cover screw.

Fig 3-7i *(right)* An outline of the surgical design shows the implant suspended in the sinus elevation chamber and secured by the bone plate and microscrews.

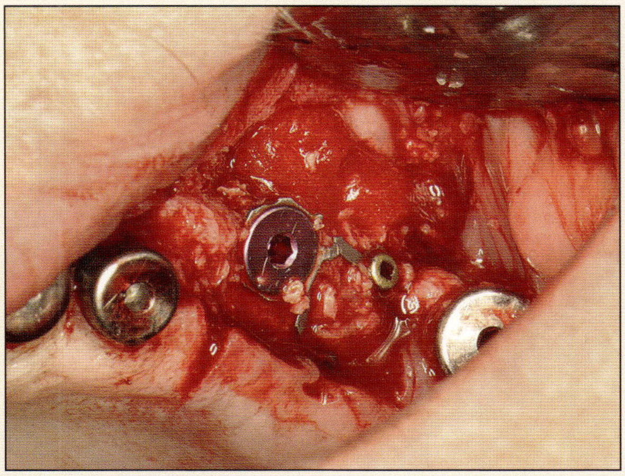

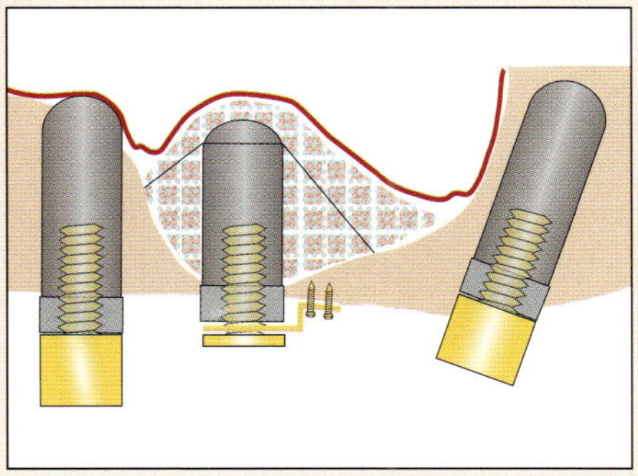

Fig 3-7j *(left)* The sinus elevation volume is filled with a combination of rhBMP-2 on collagen sponges and solvent-dehydrated cancellous bone particles reconstituted in rhBMP-2.

Fig 3-7k *(right)* The potential bone-forming environment *(area under black line)* is defined by the existing skeletal anatomy and the cylindric portion of the implant. Cells will be needed to fill this engineered volume. Extending the sinus elevation graft beyond the boundary of the bone-forming environment will not improve healing. Excessive graft volumes may increase the risk of membrane perforation. If particulate graft material escapes into the maxillary sinus, infection or obstruction of the ostium may occur.

→

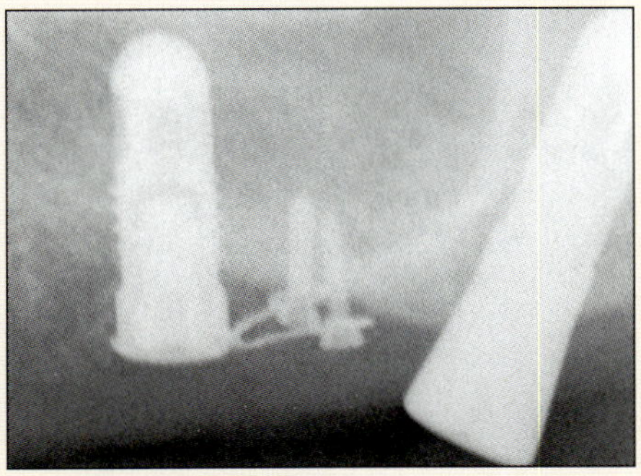

Fig 3-7l The bone plate arms are extended posteriorly because this is the site of stable, existing bone. The graft particles extend well above the apex of the implant.

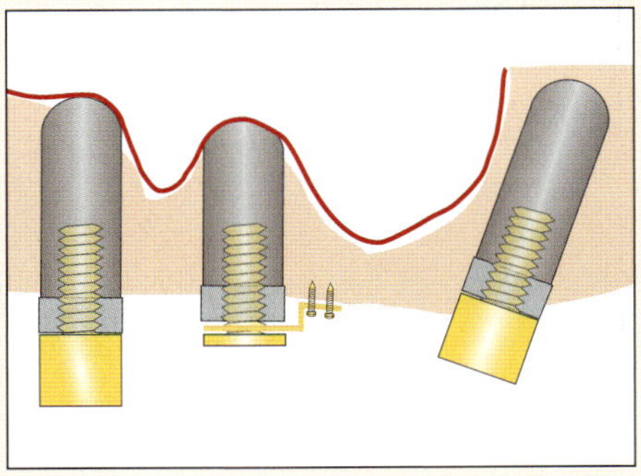

Fig 3-7m As the graft consolidates and remodels, the volume will be determined by the structural and physiologic parameters of the bone-forming construct. The remainder of the graft volume will be removed by resorption.

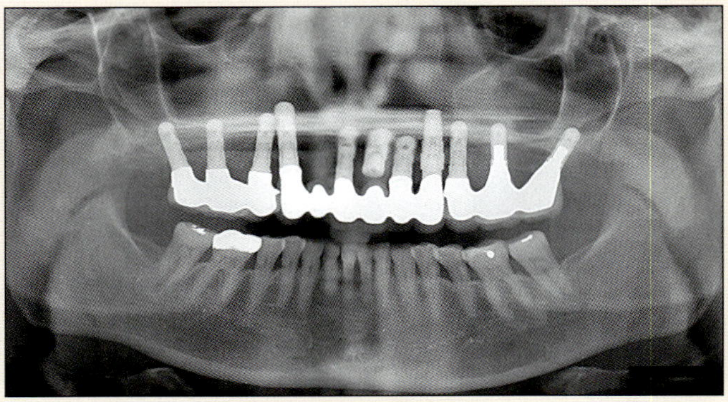

Fig 3-7n Four years after surgery, a panoramic radiograph shows the definitive prosthesis in place.

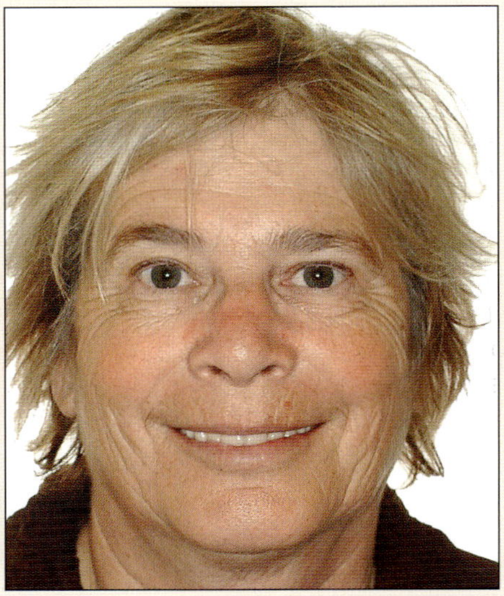

Fig 3-7o Patient's appearance after implants have achieved 5 years in function.

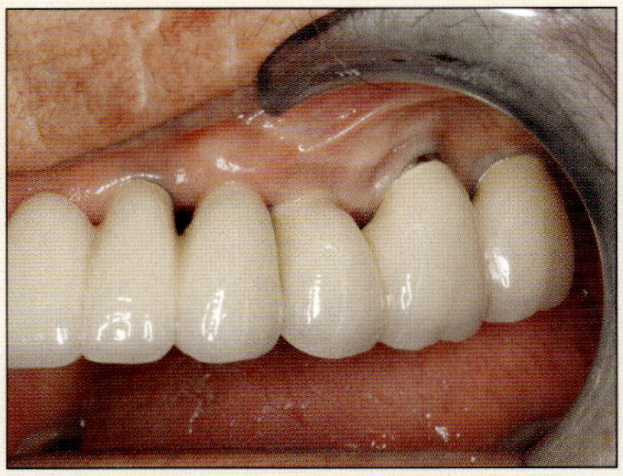

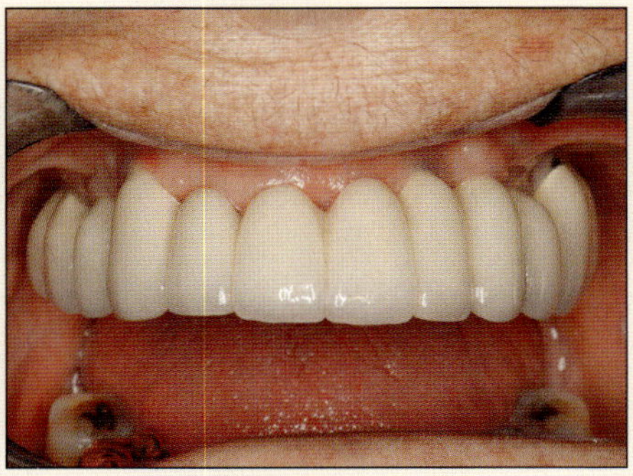

Figs 3-7p and 3-7q Definitive prosthesis after 5 years in function.

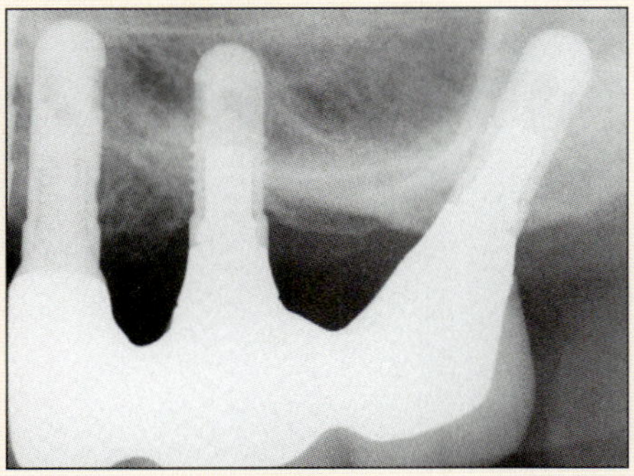

Fig 3-7r The maxillary left first molar implant is surrounded by bone that has remodeled into the form predicted by the engineering and design principles. The bone volume invests the cylindric portion of the implant but not the hemispherical dome. The local environment adjacent to the apical dome does not support bone formation.

A 5-month postsurgical radiograph of the implant and bone-forming construct in place revealed that the graft material was not fully organized and extended beyond the stabilized area (Fig 3-7l). As the graft matured, the sinus floor would be expected to descend to the level dictated by the newly formed bone (Fig 3-7m). The radiographic appearance 4 years after surgery shows that the graft has remodeled with bone surrounding the implant. The graft material that was placed beyond the constructed environment has been resorbed (Fig 3-7n).

The patient was reexamined 5 years after surgery, and the reconstruction was found to be functional and stable (Figs 3-7o to 3-7q). A radiograph taken at that time revealed that the constructed bone segment had consolidated with the existing sinus floor (Fig 3-7r). Development of a cortical outline and normal trabeculae indicated that the bone had matured into a functioning structural element. The cortical outline of the new sinus floor extended apically to just below the hemispherical implant apex and descended coronally to meet the bone stabilizing the existing implants.

Discussion

This case illustrates the potential of properly engineered and constructed regeneration environments. Although there was no adjacent natural bone to provide implant stability or a source of cells for osseointegration, a new maxillary bone segment was developed. The newly formed bone surrounded the implant that was suspended within the chamber environment. The newly generated bone provided stable anchorage for the implant and the fixed dental restoration. Five-year follow-up demonstrated that the bone segment had been physiologically integrated as a functional skeletal unit.

Conclusion

This chapter has presented cases encompassing a variety of clinical challenges in patients of different ages to demonstrate successful application of the theory of bone formation to management of real-world problems. The keys to producing a successful outcome in a compromised site are careful analysis and comprehensive diagnosis of the regeneration site and adjacent structures to ensure that all necessary elements of the bone-forming construct are in place.

References

1. Harvold EP. The theoretical basis for the treatment of hemifacial microsomia. In: Harvold EP, Vargervik K, Chierici G (eds). Treatment of Hemifacial Microsomia. New York: Alan R. Liss, 1983.
2. Brånemark PI. Osseointegration and its experimental background. J Prosthet Dent 1983;50:399–410.
3. Kasemo B. Biocompatibility of titanium implants: Surface science aspects. J Prosthet Dent 1983;49:832–837.
4. Albrektsson T. Surface roughness of intraoral dental implant fixtures. Dent Implantol Update 1998;9:73–77.
5. Oates TW, Valderrama P, Bischof M, et al. Enhanced implant stability with a chemically modified SLA surface: A randomized pilot study. Int J Oral Maxillofac Implants 2007;22:755–760.
6. Degidi M, Nardi D, Piattelli A. 10-year follow-up of immediately loaded implants with TiUnite porous anodized surface. Clin Implant Dent Relat Res 2012;14:828–838.
7. Jungner M, Lundqvist P, Lundgren S. Oxidized titanium implants (Nobel Biocare TiUnite) compared with turned titanium implants (Nobel Biocare Mark III) with respect to implant failure in a group of consecutive patients treated with early functional loading and two-stage protocol. Clin Oral Implants Res 2005;16:308–312.
8. Huang YH, Xiropaidis AV, Sorensen RG, Albandar JM, Hall J, Wikesjö UM. Bone formation at titanium porous oxide (TiUnite) oral implants in type IV bone. Clin Oral Implants Res 2005;16:105–111.
9. Sul YT, Johansson C, Albrektsson T. Which surface properties enhance bone response to implants? Comparison of oxidized magnesium, TiUnite, and Osseotite implant surfaces. Int J Prosthodont 2006;19:319–328.
10. Brattstrom V, McWilliam J. The influence of bone grafting age on dental abnormalities and alveolar bone height in patients with unilateral cleft lip and palate. Eur J Orthod 1989;11:351–358.
11. Calvo AM, Trindade-Suedam IK, da Silva Filho OG, et al. Increase in age is associated with worse outcomes in alveolar bone grafting in patients with bilateral complete cleft palate. J Craniofac Surg 2014;25:380–382. Amler MH. The age factor in human extraction wound healing. J Oral Surg 1977;35:193–197.
12. Engeland CG, Bosch JA, Cacioppo JT, Marucha PT. Mucosal wound healing: The roles of age and sex. Arch Surg 2006;141:1193–1197; discussion 1198.
13. Garvin K, Feschuk C, Sharp JG, Berger A. Does the number or quality of pluripotent bone marrow stem cells decrease with age? Clin Orthop Relat Res 2007;465:202–207.
14. Izumi-Hisha H, Ito Y, Sugimoto K, Oshima H, Mori KJ. Age-related decrease in the number of hemopoietic stem cells and progenitors in senescence accelerated mice. Mech Ageing Dev 1990;56:89–97.
15. US Department of Health and Human Services. FDA Public Health Notification: Life-threatening Complications Associated with Recombinant Human Bone Morphogenetic Protein in Cervical Spine Fusion. Issued 1 July 2008. http://www.fda.gov/MedicalDevices/Safety/AlertsandNotices/PublicHealthNotifications/ucm062000.htm. Accessed 17 November 2014.
16. Tom WK, Chin, M, Ng T, Carstens M. Distraction of rhBMP-2 Generated Mandible: How Good Is Engineered Bone Response to Subsequent Surgeries? Presented at the 5th International Congress of Maxillofacial and Craniofacial Distraction, Paris, France, 2006.

4 Using Bone Morphogenetic Protein to Generate Bone

Successful, safe, and efficient use of emerging biologic agents such as recombinant human bone morphogenetic protein 2 (rhBMP-2) is one of the most important challenges for the modern surgeon. To be effective and predictable, these new materials must be thoughtfully engineered into tissue-forming systems. Growth factors and bone morphogenetic proteins (BMPs) should not be viewed as stand-alone products. Used on their own, they will not form skeletal units or organs.[1] To function properly, these biologic agents must interact with multiple components of tissue-forming and organ-maintaining environments. The biologic engineer must understand the capabilities and limitations of these agents before designing them into a surgical construct. When these agents are properly integrated into a bone-forming construct, an otherwise deficient system can be made to perform and produce structures that are biologically stable.

Basic scientists have identified these agents as important players in normal embryologic development.[2] Modern scientists now recognize that many mechanisms of embryologic development that were believed lost in the adult actually remain intact.[3] Instead of abandoning embryologic processes, the developing organism recruits the pathway to another related use.[4] BMPs are important in the development of the skeleton in the embryo. The processes are retained in the adult and used during the healing of bone fractures. In these cases, endogenous BMPs sequestered within the mineralized matrix of vital bone enter the fracture site to initiate and promote healing.

Deliberate design of procedures to exploit the healing mechanism of BMPs can improve the outcome of treatment. This potential is expanded by the option to introduce exogenous BMPs synthesized through recombinant technology.[5] In 2002, the US Food and Drug Administration (FDA) cleared rhBMP-2 (Infuse, Medtronic) for clinical use.[6] The on-label use was limited to fusion of the lumbar spine following a very specific surgical technique. Clearance for use in maxillofacial surgery came in 2008.

At that time, practical experience with this novel material was limited. Following the use of rhBMP-2 documented in clinical trials, maxillofacial application focused on enhancement of dental extraction site healing and sinus floor augmentation for dental implants. Although reported outcomes with these materials showed consistent bone growth, the results were difficult to reproduce in the clinical setting. Clinical practice challenged rhBMP-2 performance with a wider range of anatomical deformities, patient health conditions, and surgeon-specific techniques than did the rigidly controlled FDA trials. Although the recommended instructions for use were followed, bone formation was inconsistent.

It became clear that successful use of these materials required more than simple application. To fully exploit the potential of morphogenetic proteins, clinicians must understand how BMPs participate in the complex process of bone growth and organization. The cases presented in this chapter are intended to demonstrate that successful use of these agents depends on their proper engineering into bone-forming systems.

When bone-forming constructs are engineered, a source of cells is an essential component. Cells are the basic substrate from which skeletal systems develop. In some situations, cells are drawn into the bone-forming chamber from the adjacent tissue.[7] Local recruitment of cells may not be possible if the surrounding tissue is compromised or if the size of the bone defect exceeds a critical dimension. In these cases, introduction of cells from an alternative source is necessary. Providing a source of cells is part of the engineering and design of the bone-forming construct. In the past, autogenous bone grafting was the principle method for supplying cells to a deficient site. Use of BMPs is a new and powerful method of supplying cells to a site undergoing regeneration or de novo construction.

Before BMPs can be efficiently designed into the construction plan, the engineer must have a general understanding as to how these agents operate in a clinical setting. When BMPs are placed in a surgical site, the result is an increase in the number of available bone-forming cells. It is believed that BMPs draw bone precursor cells to the location and then effect a morphologic transformation of these cells to a bone-forming phenotype.[4,7]

While an important part of the bone-forming process, BMPs will not form organized bone or skeletal units without external regulation. Cells are only potential building material, not a functioning organ. The environment of the bone-forming chamber must provide signals that direct these bone-forming cells to create and organize a skeletal system.

For a specific bone-forming construct design to perform successfully, its essential parameters must follow the previously discussed working theory (see chapter 1). The essential elements are a mechanically stabilized environment, a source of cells, neuromuscular input, and an absence of pathology. These are co-dependent parameters. The requirement that cells be introduced to the construct depends on the contribution of the other parameters.

Delivery of rhBMP-2

All use of rhBMP-2 involves combining it with a carrier or graft material. The material comes from the manufacturer as a lyophilized protein powder that is reconstituted with sterile water. The solution by itself is impossible to retain at a surgical site. Loss of the protein from the regeneration site decreases its effectiveness and exposes adjacent structures to undesirable bone growth and inflammation. The protocol cleared by the FDA involves use of rhBMP-2 with an absorbable collagen sponge (ACS) carrier. Following FDA clearance of rhBMP-2 for spinal fusion in 2002, clinicians have modified the delivery method for rhBMP-2 in every possible way,[8] despite the fact that the FDA has not cleared any carrier other than the ACS.[6]

When surgeons began using rhBMP-2 with the ACS as a carrier in procedures involving facial bone, the results were often disappointing. Although substantial doses of rhBMP-2 were placed, the resulting volume of bone produced was not substantially more than would be produced with more familiar materials. Because the ACS carrier is mechanically weak, it may not provide a stable volume in which bone can form. The typical resorption time for the collagen sponge is about 2 weeks. Collapse of the soft tissue envelope that comprises the bone-forming chamber within 3 weeks prevents formation of the desired volume of bone.

To address this problem, surgeons combined collagen sponges carrying rhBMP-2 with particulate graft materials or used rhBMP-2 to reconstitute dry graft materials. The strategy was to use rhBMP-2 to deliver a population of bone-forming cells to the regeneration site and then to have the particulate graft material maintain the physical volume of the chamber while the maturing bone established structural integrity. Another strategy was to compress multiple rhBMP-2–containing collagen sponges into a dense mass to prolong the resorption time.[9] While potentially effective, this approach substantially increases the dose of rhBMP-2. High doses of rhBMP-2 have been associated with inflammation, swelling, and their associated complications.[10,11] The associated increase in the cost also made the approach of using large doses of rhBMP-2 impractical for many dental procedures.

The FDA-cleared protocol for spinal fusion followed a method of use demonstrated as effective during clinical trials. Delivery of collagen sponges carrying rhBMP-2 to the spinal fusion site involved housing the material in a titanium cage.[12] The cage provided continuous mechanical support and space maintenance. This protocol confirmed the principle that a titanium implant could be placed together with the rhBMP-2/ACS to provide a source of bone-forming cells and maintain mechanical support of the site.

Delivery on absorbable collagen sponges

In clinical situations in which the mechanical support of the bone-forming environment has been achieved by some other means, it is best to use rhBMP-2 carried on ACSs alone, without any particulate graft material. Well-formed distraction osteogenesis chambers are an example in which rhBMP-2/ACS is used alone to increase the population of cells with bone-forming capability.[13–15]

A second indication for using rhBMP-2/ACS alone is when introduction of particulate graft material poses an increased risk of infection. If a sinus elevation graft is being placed in a patient with a history of sinus infection, particulate graft material may complicate management should the sinus membrane be compromised. Although sinus infections can occur with the use of rhBMP-2 carried on collagen sponges, the carrier is rapidly resorbed, unlike particulate graft material; placing rhBMP-2/ACS without a graft avoids the need to surgically remove migrating bone graft particles in the event of infection.

Another indication for using rhBMP-2/ACS alone is when a patient cannot tolerate antibiotic treatment for medical reasons. Multiple antibiotic allergies or moderate organ compromise may pose a clinical dilemma if an infection occurs. The rhBMP-2/ACS system is less likely to be colonized by pathogenic bacteria than is a graft that includes particulate cadaveric bone or synthetic material. If infection occurs with a particulate graft in place, debridement of the material may present a challenge to the surgeon. In these cases, the inherent resorptive feature of the collagen sponge is again a substantial advantage.

Delivery in combination with particulate graft materials

The rhBMP-2/ACS system should be combined with particulate graft materials when the likely benefits exceed the potential risks. The most common reason to combine rhBMP-2 with a material other than the collagen sponge is to maintain the volume of the regeneration site until viable bone has had the opportunity to consolidate and organize.

Freeze-dried cadaveric bone

The use of rhBMP-2 in combination with freeze-dried cadaveric bone has been reported by a limited number of surgeons with some success. Concerns about freeze-dried cadaveric bone include its theoretical safety profile, variations in the preparation process, and compromise of the mechanical integrity from the freeze-drying process.

Solvent-dehydrated donor bone

An alternative to freeze-dried cadaveric bone is solvent-dehydrated cadaveric bone. Although these products are used interchangeably in oral surgery, there are important differences between the materials. Solvent-dehydrated cadaveric bone is available in the United States as Puros (Zimmer Dental). The proprietary process (Tutoplast, Tutogen) that produces Puros includes solvent dehydration. This spares the bone the freeze-drying process that may compromise the structural integrity of the material. This is important because structural support is the primary reason to add grafting material to the bone-forming construct.

Safety profile. Puros bone allogeneic bone graft is a product of RTI Biologics. This material is used when the requirements of the bone-forming construct require prolonged mechanical stability beyond the capability of the rhBMP-2/ACS device. Puros was chosen as the material to carry rhBMP-2 because of its favorable mechanical properties and excellent safety profile. Puros is produced by the Tutoplast process that was developed by Tutogen Medical GmbH. In this process, cadaveric bone is subjected to a series of chemical treatments comprising solvent dehydration followed by gamma radiation. Unlike most banked human bone, this product is not freeze-dried because, according to the manufacturer, sparing the bone from freezing preserves important mechanical properties. The combination of chemical treatment and gamma radiation achieves a sterility assurance level of 10^{-6} in compliance with the FDA.

The Tutoplast process is proprietary, and the specific method is protected as a trade secret. Studies supporting the efficacy of the method were commissioned by Tutogen and remain confidential. The FDA is mandated only to assure the safety and efficacy of the product to the standards they set to evaluate other similar products. Tutogen and RTI Biologics have an excellent record of consistent compliance.

Donor screening is the first step in preventing pathogens from entering the pool of banked tissue, but it has limitations. Laboratory testing may produce a false-negative finding if the timing of infection is unfavorable. If the tissue is harvested after the donor has been infected but before antibodies have developed, the tests will be seronegative.[16] Therefore, it is advantageous to have a system that offers the redundancy of pathogen inactivation through processing.[17]

The recognition of prions as potential infective agents poses new challenges to protocols to prevent disease transmission.[18–22] Prions represent a new class of hazardous substance. Because they lack nucleic acids common to bacteria, viruses, and fungi, prions are not disabled by conventional sterilizing methods.[23] These unconventional pathogens replicate in the host and are particularly difficult to inactivate.[24–27] Prions may retain their infective capability after being subjected to steam autoclaving.[26] They have been known to survive in the environment, outside the living host, for 16 years or more and still retain the ability to infect and kill.[28] There is no known treatment for infection by prions. Donors are not routinely examined by autopsy to rule out Creutzfeldt-Jakob disease (CJD), which is caused by prions. Transmission of CJD through donor bone not harvested adjacent to the central nervous system is considered low risk.[29,30] Nevertheless, a method to inactivate prions though processing would be attractive if it did not adversely affect the efficacy of the tissue.

Both the manufacturer and the distributor of Puros have stated that the Tutoplast process may have a redundant or extended capability to inactivate pathogens.[31–34] Yet full evaluation of the potential safety advantage of this material is limited by an inability to analyze the details of the Tutoplast process, since it is protected as a trade secret. Other manufacturers have developed proprietary tissue-processing methods as well. Until the

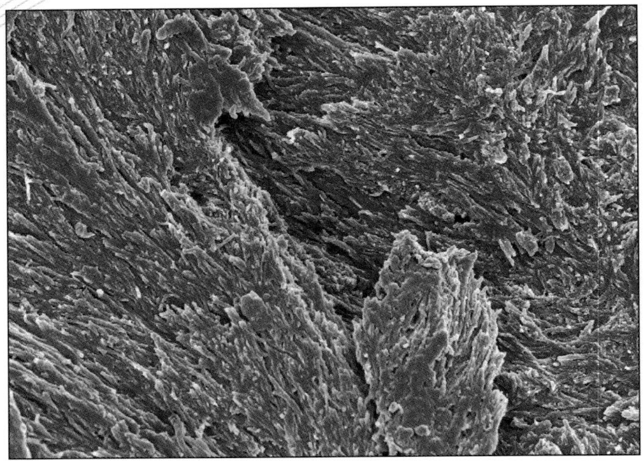

Fig 4-1a Scanning electron micrograph of freeze-dried cancellous human bone for transplantation. The width of the image is 15.4 µm.

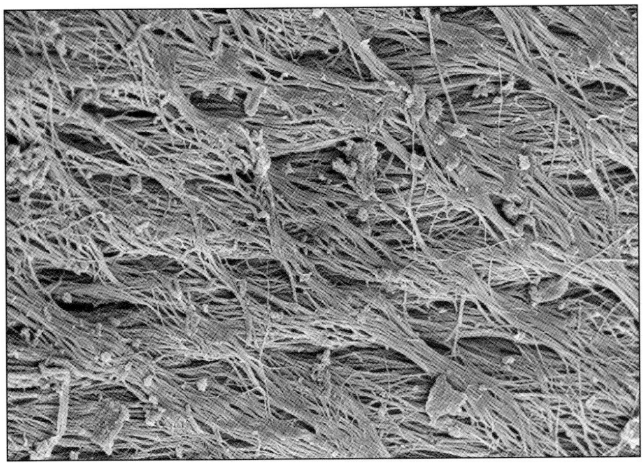

Fig 4-1b Scanning electron micrograph of solvent-dehydrated cancellous human bone (Puros) for transplantation. The width of the image is 15.4 µm.

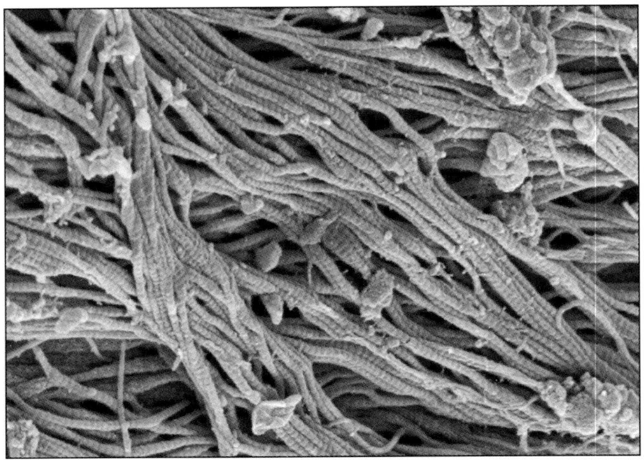

Fig 4-1c Higher magnification of Fig 4-1b. The width of the image is 200 nm.

details of these techniques are revealed, independent validation cannot be undertaken. Examining reports of adverse outcomes is one method to grossly estimate the safety of these products. Science and patient care would benefit from an accurate understanding and assessment of the secret processing methods. Independent, reproducible testing of the exact processing technique would be the best method to assure optimal patient safety and extend the potential of this technology.

Comparison of the physical features of freeze-dried and solvent-dehydrated cadaveric bone

When rhBMP-2 is mixed with freeze-dried cancellous human bone, the manner in which the components combine depends on how the graft has been processed by the manufacturer. Considerable variation in the consistency of graft material occurs among different sources.

The lyophilized rhBMP-2 powder is reconstituted with sterile water. The liquid is then mixed with the bone particles. Unlike the collagen sponge, freeze-dried particles do not readily absorb the liquid rhBMP-2, and the two ingredients tend to remain separate. This presents a challenge when the material is delivered to the surgical site. Delivery of the rhBMP-2 to the site on sheets or pieces of collagen sponge material is an option. If this is done, the sponge pieces are compressed between bone particles. As the sponges exert a tendency to expand, the graft particles are displaced. From a clinical standpoint, the combination of rhBMP-2 and freeze-dried human bone produces a moderate positive healing result.

When reconstituted rhBMP-2 is mixed with solvent-dehydrated human bone, the liquid volume absorbs into the particles of graft material. The difference in handling compared to freeze-dried bone has been explored by Dr Sean Meitner (personal communication, 2012), who studied different graft materials under the scanning electron microscope.[30] There was a clear difference in architecture between the two graft materials (Fig 4-1). The solvent dehydration process produces a material that is porous and preserves the continuity of the collagen fibers. The solvent dehydration process also preserves the mechanical strength of the graft by limiting structural damage normally caused by the freeze-drying process. When rhBMP-2 and solvent-dehydrated bone are combined, it is possible that the morphogenetic protein liquid is simply trapped within the pores of the material. There is a possibility that the protein becomes bound by the collagen fibers by the same mechanism that occurs when the material is allowed to soak in the ACSs.

With rhBMP-2 and solvent-dehydrated bone combined as a single mass, the material can be delivered to the bone construc-

Fig 4-2 Use of rhBMP-2 carried on an ACS.

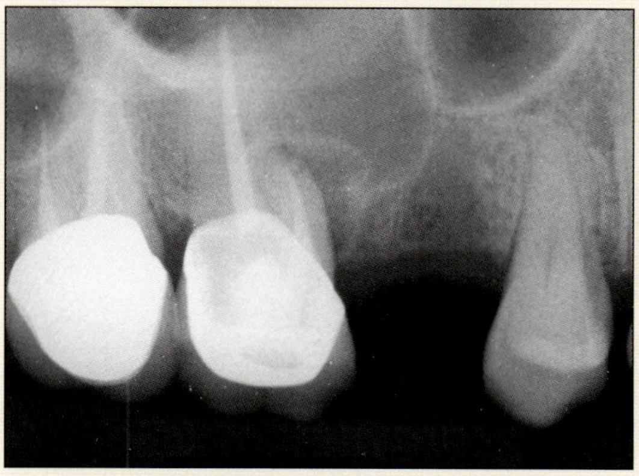

Fig 4-2a A radiograph of the healed maxillary second premolar extraction site shows a bone septum dividing the sinus cavity.

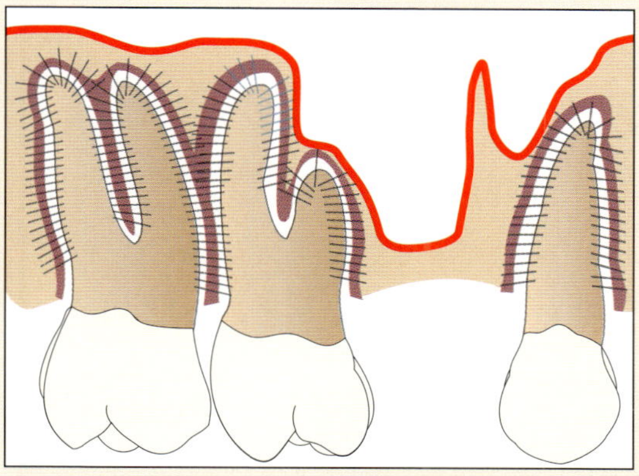

Fig 4-2b The existing skeletal morphology is maintained by the periodontal ligament systems of the adjacent teeth. The sinus membrane and natural physiology create and maintain the septum.

→

tion site. Collagen sponges carrying rhBMP-2 can be used to cover the particulate graft mass. This confines the graft particles and reinforces the integrity of mucosal suture lines that may overlie the graft site.

The combination of rhBMP-2 and solvent-dehydrated cancellous bone has produced uncomplicated healing and bone formation in many cases. Nevertheless, the material is only one component of the bone-forming construct. Successful outcomes depend on design and assembly of a bone-forming construct that meets all of the essential requirements for skeletal regeneration. This will be demonstrated in a case report later in this chapter.

Clinical Applications

The case reports presented in this chapter demonstrate use of rhBMP-2 in a range of clinical applications. Follow-up results range from 2 to 12 years. In this series of patients, rhBMP-2 was considered as the principal method for introducing cells into bone-forming constructs. Experience has shown that the performance of the construct is dependent on the integrity of the design and the construction of the system.

rhBMP-2 Carried on an ACS

In a healthy site with a four-wall defect and intact neuromuscular input, no cells may be needed other than those introduced from the adjacent tissue. In contrast, if the environment is not mechanically sheltered and lacks neuromuscular input, even high doses of rhBMP-2 will not produce growth of a skeletal unit.

The dose of rhBMP-2 designed as part of the bone-forming construct depends on the analysis and understanding of the other governing components. Placing the implant in the chamber at the time of grafting indicates where bone formation is needed. This approach enables very efficient use of rhBMP-2. Overbuilding the volume of bone serves no long-term useful purpose. If the new bone unit is viable and functional, excess bone will be removed by remodeling until it meets a steady state with the local environment.

Case description

A 37-year-old patient was missing the maxillary right second premolar. A radiograph revealed that the sinus floor had descended into the alveolus and endodontic lesions were resolving as well as the presence of a septum dividing the antrum (Fig 4-2a). This was a narrow, confined alveolar defect. The projection of the alveolar process apically into the sinus was maintained by the first molar roots and periodontal ligament attachments (Fig 4-2b).

The engineering and design processes yielded a plan to elevate the sinus membrane to create a space isolated from respiratory and oral bacteria (Fig 4-2c). A dental implant was to be placed and stabilized by a bone plate. The purpose of the implant was to provide mechanical stability of the bone-forming chamber, displace volume of the construct that would require bone synthesis, and provide the anchorage for a dental prosthesis. The titanium bone plate, which could accommodate various sizes of implants, was to be fixed to the implant by the cover screw (Fig 4-2d). The stabilizing arms of the plate were malleable and could be bent to meet the bone contour with the implant in place.

The sinus elevation was performed through a lateral window. The membrane lining the posterior compartment of the partitioned sinus was elevated, and rhBMP-2 on an ACS was placed in the space created (Fig 4-2e). In this case, a piece of ACS (Integra Life Sciences) was used to carry the rhBMP-2 to the sinus elevation cavity (Fig 4-2f). The 20 × 40 × 3–mm collagen sponge was cut in half to a dimension of 20 × 20 × 3 mm and contained 0.25 mg of rhBMP-2 in 0.50 mL of water.

Clearly defining where bone growth is required to establish osseointegration allows reduction of the graft volume and ef-

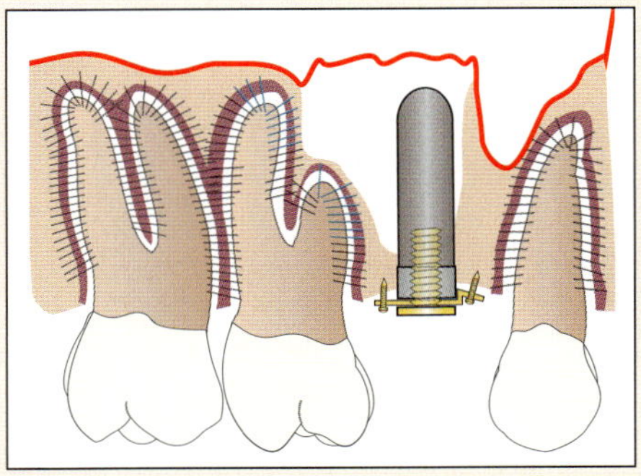

Fig 4-2c The surgical strategy is to assemble a bone-forming construct in the posterior chamber of the divided sinus. The anterior surface of the implant is positioned against the existing bone, leaving a posterior chamber that will require grafting. The graft will derive its regulatory signaling from the first molar periodontal ligament system. Additional input may be recruited from the sinus membrane and exposed sinus floor.

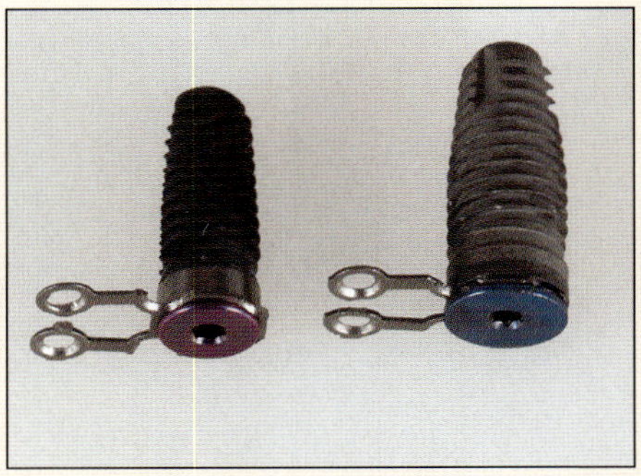

Fig 4-2d A bone plate will stabilize the implant. A variety of implant types and sizes can be used with bone plates.

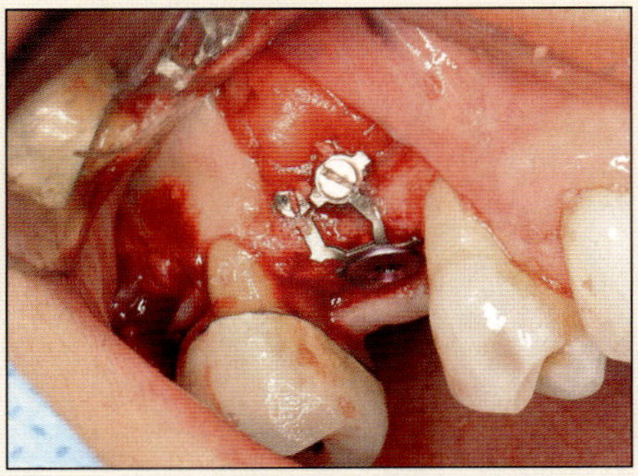

Fig 4-2e The implant (Camlog) is positioned and secured. A collagen sponge containing rhBMP-2 is placed to surround the implant and fill the sinus elevation chamber.

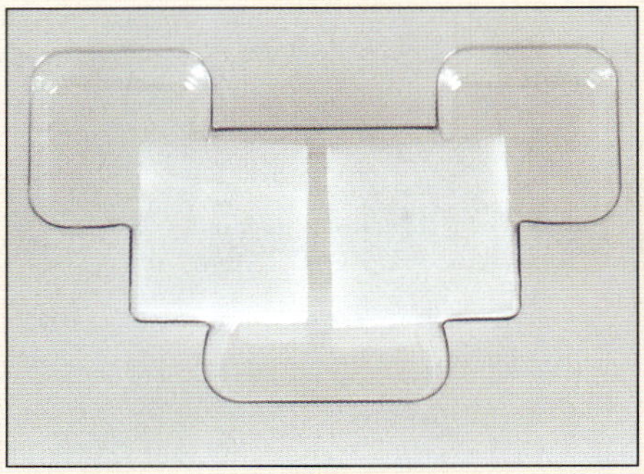

Fig 4-2f The graft consists of a 20 × 40–mm collagen sponge containing 0.25 mg of rhBMP-2 (Medtronic). No particulate graft material will be used in this patient.

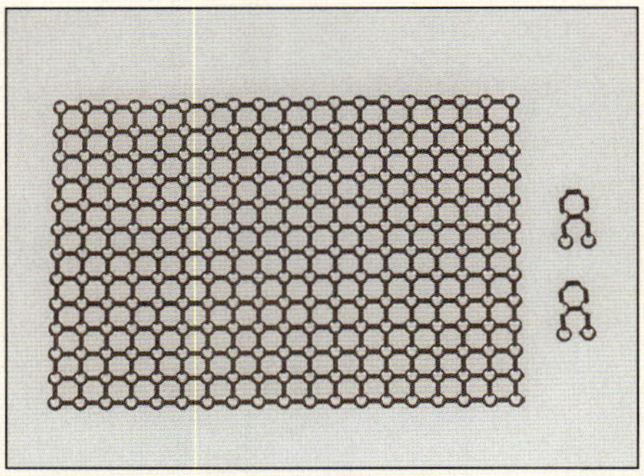

Fig 4-2g The bone plate is cut from a stock piece of surgical mesh.

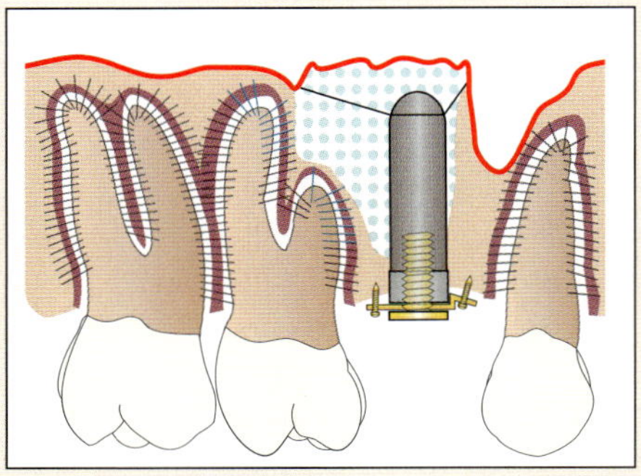

Fig 4-2h A diagram shows the assembled bone-forming construct incorporating the dental implant. The *black line* indicates the superior boundary of the bone-forming chamber.

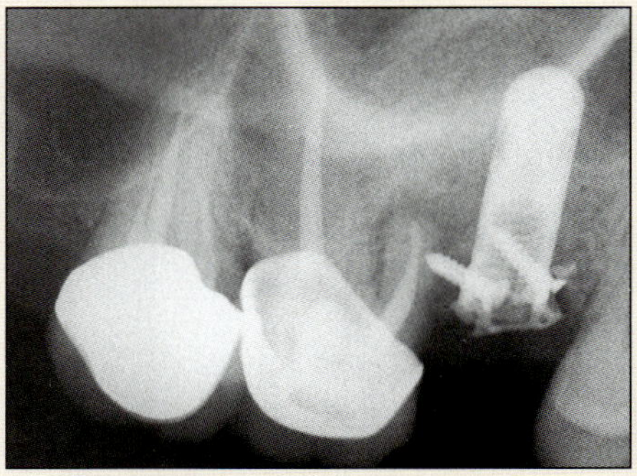

Fig 4-2i The implant in place.

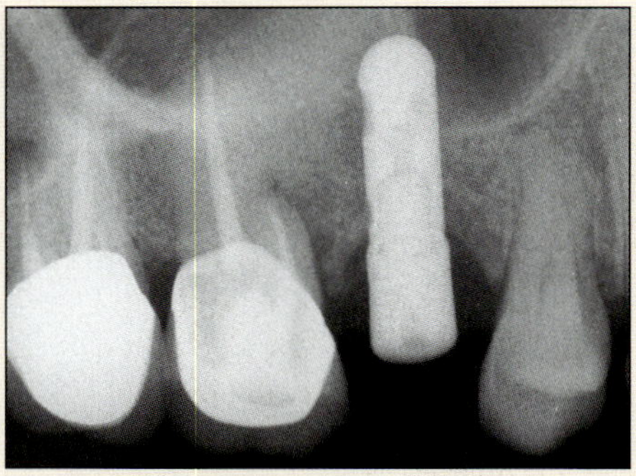

Fig 4-2j Four months after the initial surgery, the site is opened for removal of the bone plate and placement of a gingival former.

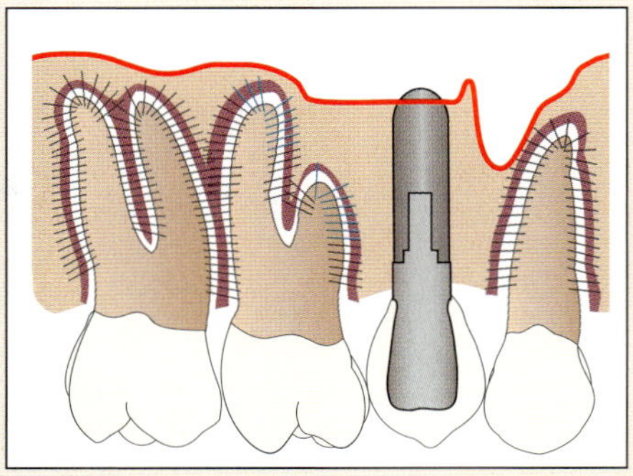

Fig 4-2k The sinus elevation chamber fills with bone under the mechanical shelter of the implant and sinus floor.

→

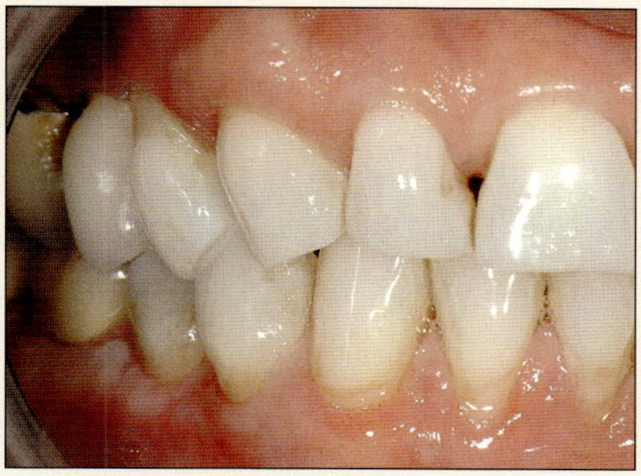

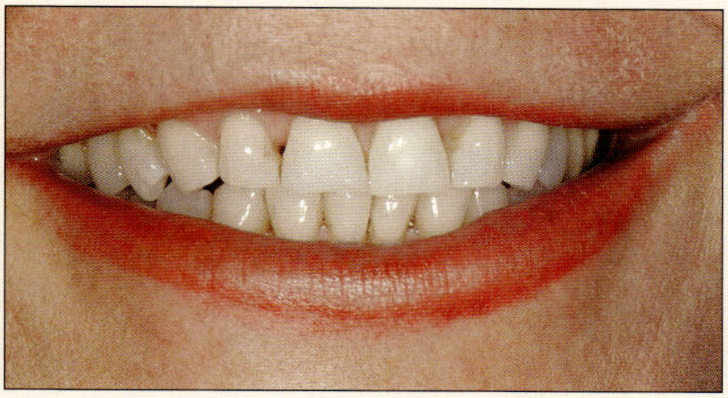

Figs 4-2l and 4-2m Prosthesis in function at the 7-year follow-up.

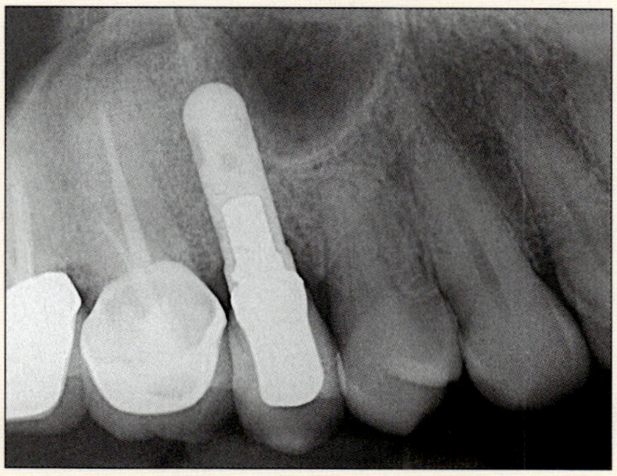

Fig 4-2n The radiographic appearance after 7 years of implant function reveals maturation of the graft and a stable bone level at the crest.

ficient use of rhBMP-2. It is most important to provide enough cells in the central portion of the regeneration chamber. The walls of the defect comprise viable bone under the direct stimulation of roots and periodontal ligaments. The periphery of the defect has the potential to recruit bone-forming cells locally and needs only minimal enhancement from exogenous BMP.

Implant-supporting bone plates were cut from standard maxillofacial reconstruction mesh (KLS Martin) of 0.3-mm-thick commercially pure titanium (Fig 4-2g). The small holes could accommodate 1.0- to 1.2-mm-diameter screws. Because the site of reconstruction was thin (as is usually the case), pilot holes were placed with 0.7-mm drills.

The design of the construct satisfied all of the principal requirements for successful bone formation (Fig 4-2h). The space was physically confined and moderately stable. The bone plate was not intended to provide rigid immobilization of the dental implant, which is not necessary or desirable. The adjacent periodontal systems provided neuromuscular regulation. The intact, elevated sinus membrane isolated the chamber from sinus secretions and bacteria. In this circumstance, the demand to introduce additional cells in large numbers was limited. Placing the dental implant at the time of grafting decreased the amount of rhBMP-2 needed, because the volume of bone that needed to be generated was decreased. In the supportive environment of this well-designed construct, only a few cells were necessary to initiate the process of bone growth and organization.

A radiograph taken at the time of implant placement and rhBMP-2 grafting revealed the assembled components of the bone-forming construct within the anatomical environment (Fig 4-2i). Four months after grafting, bone initially had formed beyond the confines of the planned construct (Fig 4-2j). After initial bone formation, the new skeletal unit remodeled and resorbed until it collapsed into the volume dictated by the stabilizing structures (Fig 4-2k). The apical portion of the implant was one important stabilizing structure. The newly formed bone descended until it encountered the implant cylinder.

Follow-up after the implant had been in function for 7 years revealed the maturation of the graft and a stable bone level (Figs 4-2l to 4-2n).

Discussion

Treatment was successful and stable because all the requirements for bone formation were met. The implant achieved osseointegration because it was suspended in a semirigid manner within the bone-forming chamber. New bone surrounded the bare implant cylinder and established osseointegration. Very little rhBMP-2 was necessary because of the quality of the bone-forming construct and the minimal volume of bone needed to fully cover the implant.

Fig 4-3 Use of rhBMP-2 in combination with other materials.

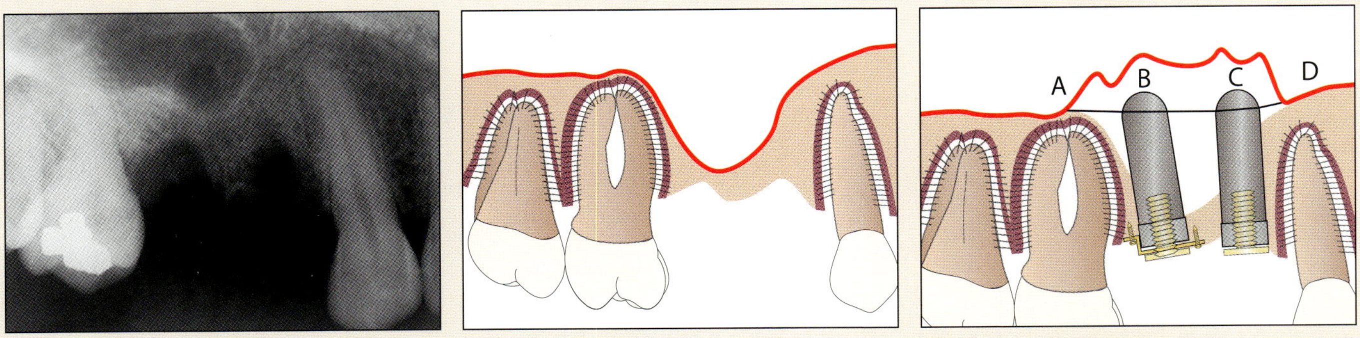

Fig 4-3a The initial radiograph of the site of the lost maxillary right premolars shows minimal bone at the sinus floor to allow placement of implants.

Fig 4-3b Analysis of the functional elements that regulate the existing site morphology.

Fig 4-3c Surgical design strategy for assembly of a bone-forming construct incorporating two implants.

→

rhBMP-2 in Combination with Other Materials

Some clinical situations are best managed with a combination of rhBMP-2 and other materials. However, the clinician who randomly combines rhBMP-2 and other materials without understanding the underlying mechanisms will obtain unpredictable and often disappointing results. Each clinical situation poses specific engineering demands. Before introducing another material to the surgical design, the surgical engineer must understand how the added component might promote healing. The potential to improve bone development must be balanced against the hazard introduced by the addition of another component to the construct design.

In many clinical situations, design and construction of an ideal bone-forming environment is not possible. When the construct has more than one deficient parameter, one engineering strategy is to increase the cell population. There are several design options to increase the number of cells and to prolong their presence: *(1)* increase the dose of rhBMP-2 used in one application, *(2)* administer rhBMP-2 to the site in repeated doses, or *(3)* combine rhBMP-2 with a material that will prolong the remodeling phase. The following case is an example of using a minimal dose of rhBMP-2 in an imperfect construct. The action of a small dose of rhBMP-2 was enhanced by combining it in a specific manner with human allogeneic bone graft.

Case description

A 40-year-old patient presented with recent loss of the maxillary right premolars and defects in the two adjacent extraction sites (Fig 4-3a). The sinus floor descended into the second premolar position, resulting in residual bone of 3 to 4 mm.

The diagnostic process began with an analysis of how the current bone architecture was maintained in the existing morphology. Posterior to the edentulous site, the volume of the alveolus was maintained by the first molar root and its periodontal attachment to the lamina dura (Fig 4-3b). The anterior aspect of this potential bone-forming environment was bounded by the canine root and its periodontal system. In this environment, the neuromuscular input generated by the periodontal systems diminished in effect toward the center of the defect.

Two dental implants were needed to meet the restorative goals (Fig 4-3c). If rhBMP-2 were used at a typical dose carried on an ACS, it might not result in bone consolidation in the center of the construct. Because the neuromuscular input delivered to the site was weakest in the center, bone formation and organization would propagate from the mesial and distal walls of the chamber. The collagen sponge containing rhBMP-2 would resorb by the 14th day, and the cell population would diminish before the bone filled the central site.

One strategy to alleviate this problem was to use a hybrid graft. The ideal hybrid graft material would bind rhBMP-2 and hold it at the reconstruction site for precisely the time needed to initiate the bone-consolidation process. After its role of cell introduction was completed, the material would ideally resorb to allow the chamber to fill completely with viable bone. Grafting material that resorbs too slowly is a liability if it is displaced in the sinus. Perforation of the sinus membrane during the surgical elevation procedure or breach of the membrane by postoperative sinus infection is always a risk. If a portion of the graft is displaced into the sinus, it is an advantage for the graft to be a material that is readily absorbed or small enough to be cleared by the ciliary system.

If, during elevation of the sinus membrane, the integrity and quality of the membrane are found to be good, a graft combining rhBMP-2 and small-particle bone can be used. If the membrane appears intact but friable, consideration might be made to place rhBMP-2/ACS without a bone graft but to increase the dose from 0.5 mg to 4.0 mg.

In this patient, two implants were placed within a sinus elevation graft combining rhBMP-2 and allogeneic bone (Fig 4-3d). The

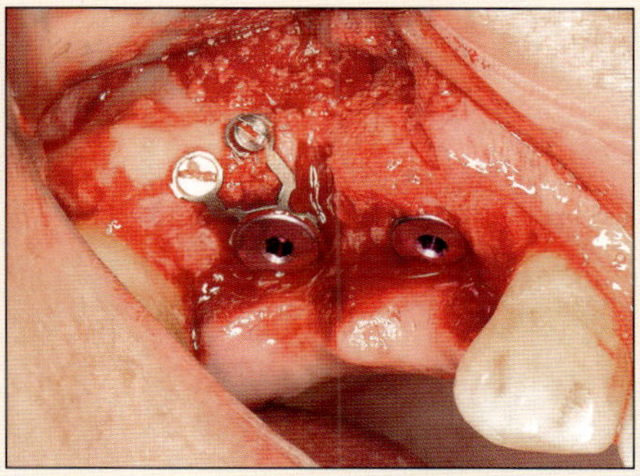

Fig 4-3d Two implants and a hybrid graft have been placed. The sinus elevation chamber has been lined with collagen sponges carrying rhBMP-2 (Medtronic). Solvent-dehydrated allogeneic human bone (Puros) reconstituted in rhBMP-2 fills the remainder of the chamber.

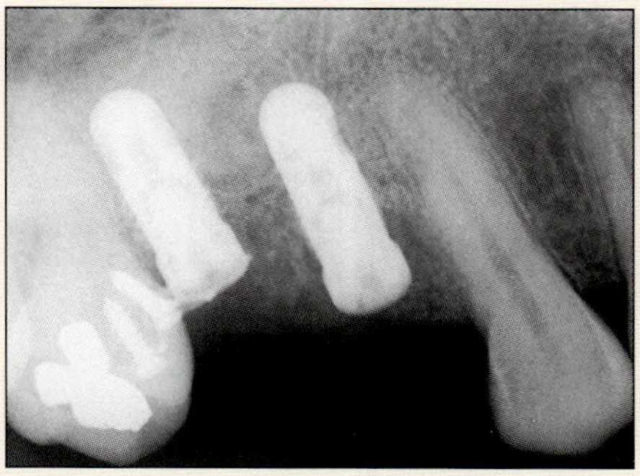

Fig 4-3e The mineralized bone graft can be seen on the radiograph at the time of initial placement. The material extends well beyond the boundary of the bone-forming environment.

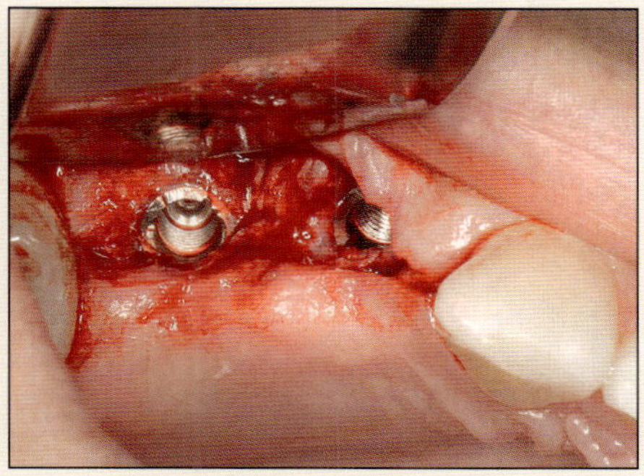

Fig 4-3f Surgical findings 4 months after the initial surgery reveal stable implants and typical granulation tissue around the polished collar of the proximal implant.

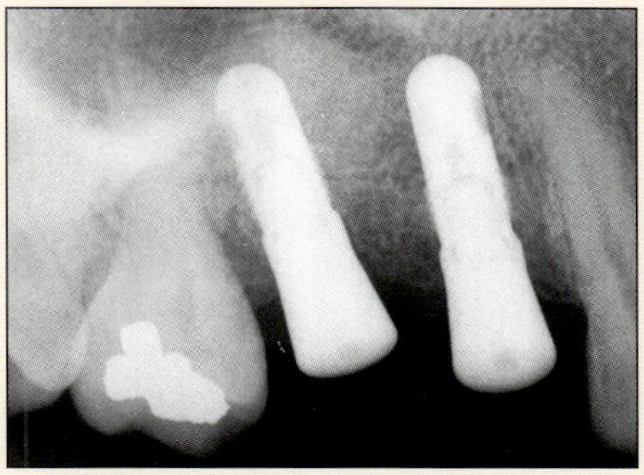

Fig 4-3g Four months after implant and graft placement, the radiograph shows that the graft has remodeled and descended to the level of the implant apices.

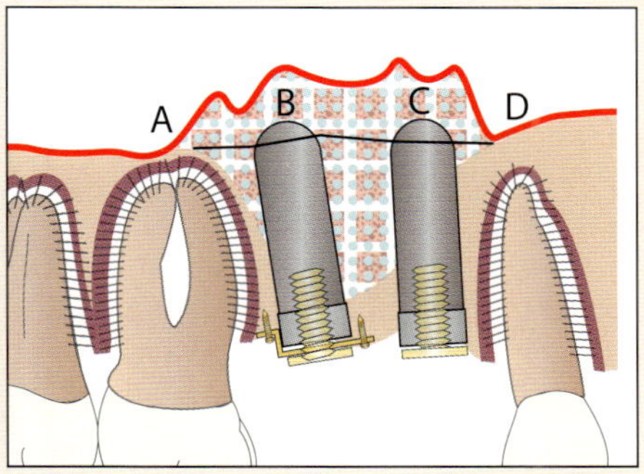

Fig 4-3h The diagram illustrates that the graft volume between the implant cylinders lacks an adjacent source of neuromuscular regulation. The sinus floor and sinus membrane may introduce some direction to the immature cell population, but the center of the graft is still vulnerable to incomplete consolidation. Filling the center with cancellous bone particles carrying rhBMP-2 prolongs the remodeling phase beyond that associated with the standard rhBMP-2/ACS device alone.

distal implant was supported by a bone plate. Bone graft preparations vary widely among sources. The behavior of rhBMP-2 and allogeneic bone graft hybrids depends heavily on how the bone component has been prepared. In this case, 1.0 mL of cancellous Puros (0.25- to 1.00-mm particle size) was used. The Puros was mixed with 0.50 mg of rhBMP-2 in 0.50 mL of sterile water.

Hybrid grafts that included particulate material showed immediately on the radiograph and could be seen to extend beyond the borders of the planned bone-forming construct (Fig 4-3e). After 4 months, the bone plate was removed and healing abutments were placed. On removal of the bone plate, the implants were confirmed to be stable (Fig 4-3f). In response to the bone plate, the coronal 2 mm of the implant was not osseointegrated. The graft had partially remodeled (Fig 4-3g). The emerging trabecular pattern indicated that structural organization of the graft was proceeding.

The rate of remodeling was moderate, reflecting the resorption kinetics of small-particle cancellous Puros. As Puros resorbs, the sinus floor descends until it meets the apical domes of the implants (Fig 4-3h). At the mesial and distal aspects, resorption continues until the bone construct comes under the influence of the root tips. The Puros particles in this construct prolong the remodeling period. This allows bone to fill the central part of the construct between the implants.

The implant crowns were assessed after 6 years in function (Fig 4-3i). At that time, the remodeling of the hybrid graft was complete, and a steady state had been established (Fig 4-3j). The graft descended until it encountered the junction of the implant tip and the cylinder wall. This was a point of mechanical stability. At the distal aspect of the graft, the existing sinus floor above the molar tooth roots was the stable point. A well-defined cortical outline was present at the new sinus floor, demonstrat-

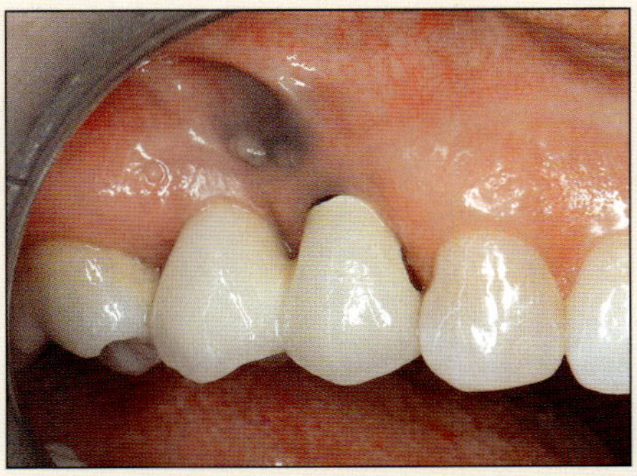

Fig 4-3i The implant crowns have been in function for 6 years. The irregularity of the vestibular mucosa and pigmented area is the result of a prior apical endodontic procedure.

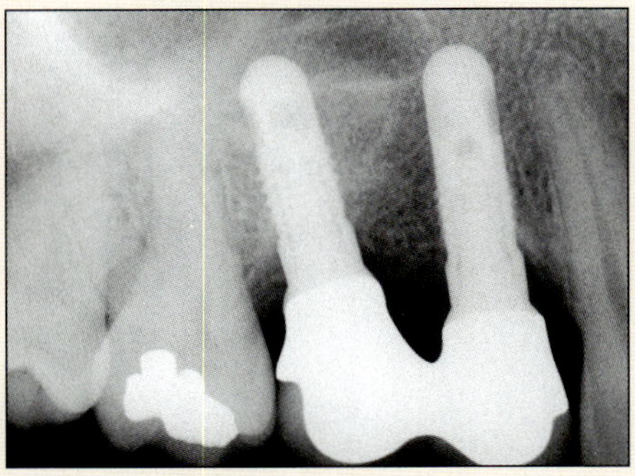

Fig 4-3j A radiograph taken after 6 years shows the steady state of graft remodeling. A well-defined sinus floor cortex has been established.

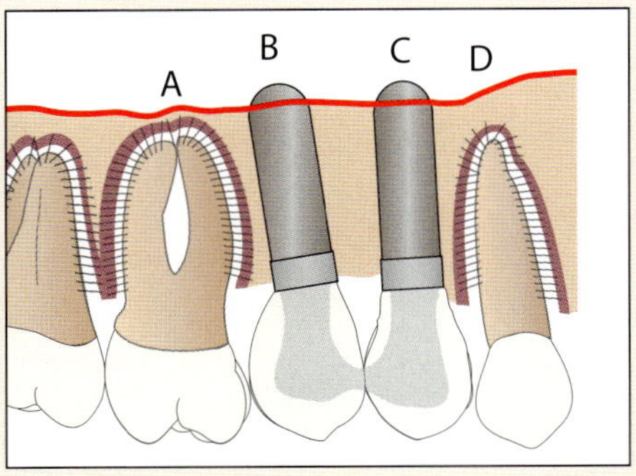

Fig 4-3k The morphology of the mature reconstruction is maintained by the periodontal ligament systems (A and D); the central control is introduced by the implants (B and C).

ing that the constructed bone volume had reached a steady state of resorption and deposition.

A diagram illustrates how the graft remodeled until it conformed to the projected volume predicted by engineering and design principles (Fig 4-3k). Points A and D were stabilized by the dental roots and periodontal ligament attachments. Points B and C were stabilized by the implant cylinder walls. The hemispherical implant apices did not support the bone volume.

Discussion

When this skeletal construct was engineered, the decision was made to use a hybrid graft consisting of rhBMP-2 and small-particle cancellous Puros. There are many possible choices of graft material. One choice would have been to use rhBMP-2/ACS alone. The challenge with this combination would have been to generate enough bone in the central area of the construct. At the mesial and distal aspects of the reconstruction site, the rhBMP-2/ACS combination would likely have performed well because those zones were physically stable, had local neuromuscular input from the periodontal systems, and had a source of local cells. The central portion of the reconstruction site, however, required more support. The combination of rhBMP-2 and Puros prolonged the direct bone-forming stimulation because the Puros particles resorb more slowly than the collagen sponge and may prolong the release of rhBMP-2 from its fibrillar architecture.

Another strategy would have been to increase the concentration and total dose of rhBMP-2. In the case presented, the total dose was 0.5 mg and the concentration was 0.5 mg/mL. Used alone, the rhBMP-2 could have been placed at 1.5 mg/mL in a device volume of 3.0 mL. This would have provided a total dose of 4.50 mg of rhBMP-2, which would have increased the bone-forming potential.

Another option would have been to place rhBMP-2/ACS without simultaneous implants. If this approach had been chosen, the implant volume would have had to be occupied by rhBMP-2. Also, because the central portion of the chamber lacked mechanical stability, it would have been necessary to increase the total dose of rhBMP-2. If a 4-mL sinus elevation volume were to be placed in anticipation of graft settling, the total dose of rhBMP-2 would have to be 6 mg. An increased dose of rhBMP-2 may produce a clinical result, but the benefits of higher doses must be weighed against the increase in local inflammatory reactions and expense.

There are alternative grafting materials that can be considered for combination with rhBMP-2. When any grafting material is considered for the sinus area, the potential risks must be weighed against the benefits. In this case, small-particle Puros was chosen after the quality of the sinus membrane was examined.

Large Doses of rhBMP-2 Without Bone Grafting

In some patients, placement of particulate bone grafts poses a potential hazard. In these cases, an increase in the dose and volume of the rhBMP-2 graft is a good option. Patients with a history of infection after oral surgery or who are unable to take antibiotics may not be good candidates for placing banked bone particulate. Infections of the maxillary sinus or oral site may be difficult to manage if free cadaveric bone particles are present within the wound. Collagen sponges with rhBMP-2 have a degree of safety because the collagen resorbs within about 2 weeks and does not provide a long-term site that will harbor bacteria.

Case description

A 65-year-old woman had a history of multiple sinus, facial bone, and facial space infections after oral surgery. She developed allergies to many antibiotics following treatment for osteomyelitis

Fig 4-4 Use of large doses of rhBMP-2 without bone grafting.

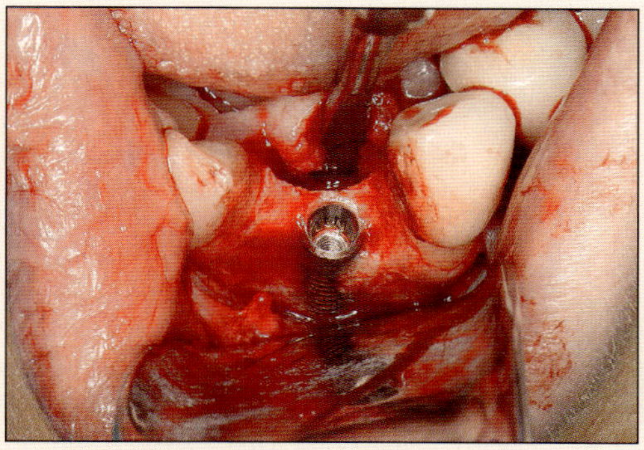

Fig 4-4a This failed implant has become infected repeatedly.

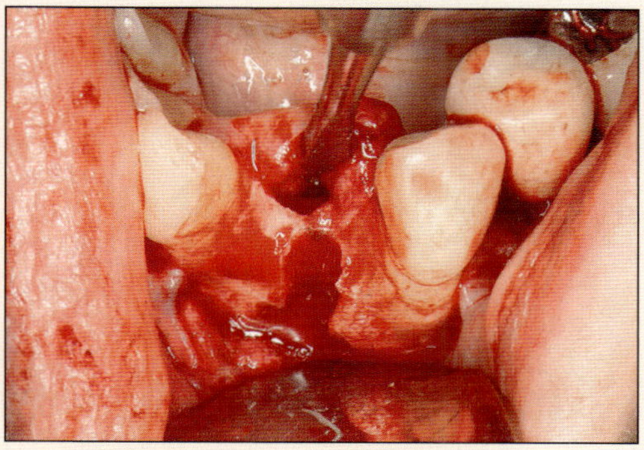

Fig 4-4b The implant has been removed, leaving a substantial defect.

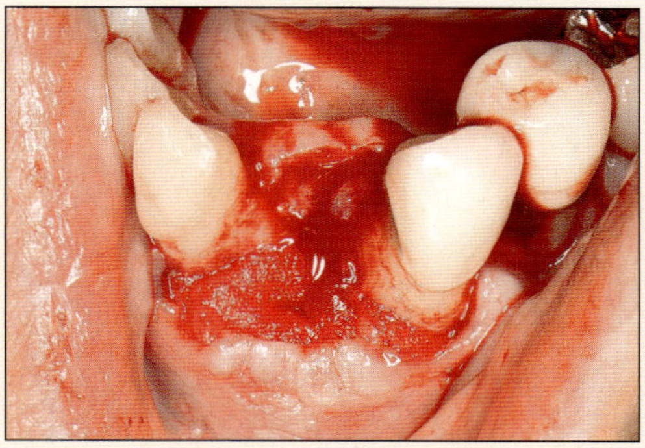

Fig 4-4c The site is repaired with rhBMP-2 carried on collagen sponges. No particulate graft material is used.

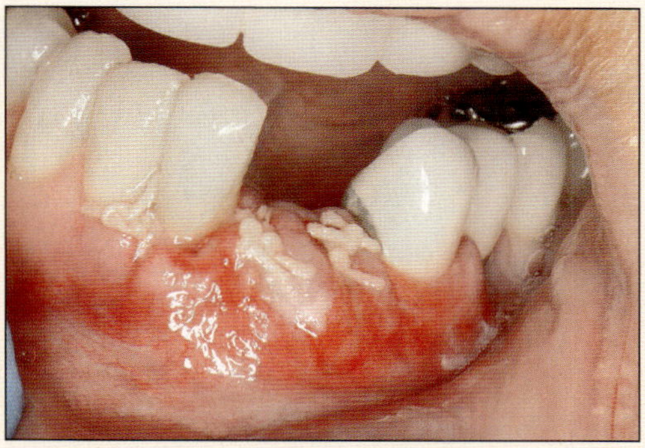

Fig 4-4d Two weeks after implant removal and site repair, the site exhibits normal accentuated edema and erythema. This is the normal healing process for the rhBMP-2/ACS device.

of the maxilla and mandible. After she had spent many years in a stable dental condition, a mandibular incisor failed and was removed. An implant was placed, but bone loss and pain developed at the site. Removal of the implant was recommended, but the anticipated bone defect from the implant and the existing local bone loss would require repair of the lost volume. Use of a moderate to high dose of rhBMP-2 on a collagen sponge carrier was indicated.

The original implant had been placed in an inadequate volume of bone. The exposed threads on the labial aspect developed an infection that did not resolve (Fig 4-4a). Removal of the implant resulted in a large bone defect (Fig 4-4b). This patient had adverse reactions to multiple antibiotics, and a previous sinus elevation procedure using autogenous bone grafting from the iliac crest had failed. Because regeneration of the site was a goal, use of an rhBMP-2/ACS device had advantages. However, because the environment was poorly contained and the adjacent teeth exhibited periodontal compromise, treatment with a minimal dose of rhBMP-2 was not likely to produce the desired result.

An rhBMP-2/ACS graft was prepared to deliver a moderate dose of BMP (Fig 4-4c). The rhBMP-2 device (Infuse) was prepared using 4 mg of rhBMP-2 in 2 mL of sterile water. The 2-mg/mL preparation was carried on a 40 × 40–mm collagen sponge.

Two weeks after surgery, typical intense erythema developed on the overlying mucosa (Fig 4-4d). The patient's recovery and healing were uneventful, despite minimal use of antibiotics. The healing of this patient was uncomplicated, and the missing teeth were replaced with a conventional fixed partial denture.

Discussion

In this case, rhBMP-2 at a relatively high dose and carried on an ACS was used to promote regeneration of the bone defect. The advantage of this material is that it contains no particulate matter, has a high bone-inductive potential, and is rapidly resorbed. Because infection was the result of multiple prior oral surgeries, there was an increased risk of a similar outcome with subsequent grafting procedures. If an infection had occurred, the absence of nonvital, slowly resorbing graft particles at the

Fig 4-5 Use of rhBMP-2 and solvent-dehydrated bone for the repair of an alveolar cleft.

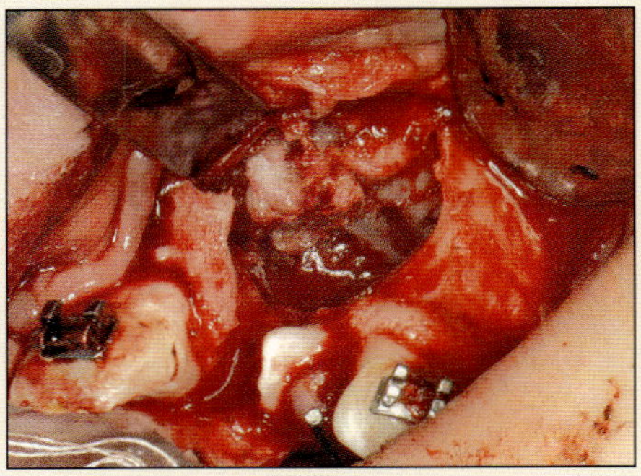

Fig 4-5a An alveolar cleft is present in a 10-year-old patient.

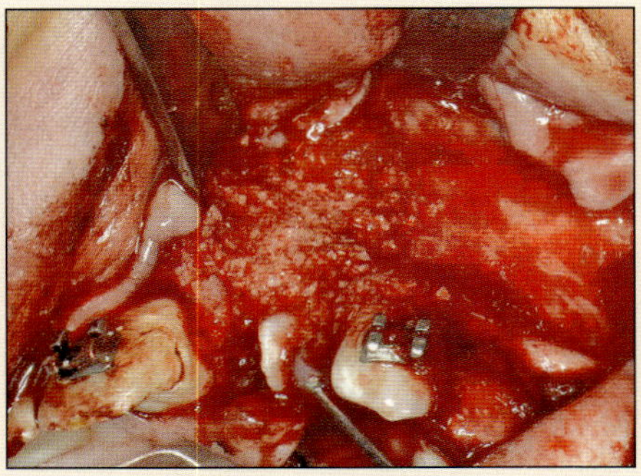

Fig 4-5b The alveolar cleft defect is filled with rhBMP-2 carried on solvent-dehydrated cancellous bone particles.

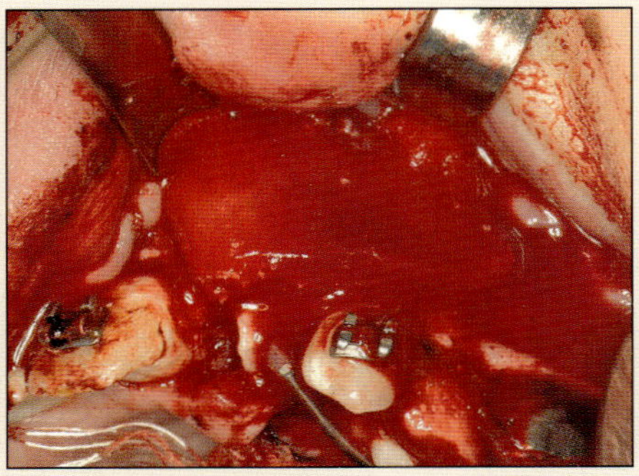

Fig 4-5c The mass of bone particles is covered with a collagen sponge containing rhBMP-2.

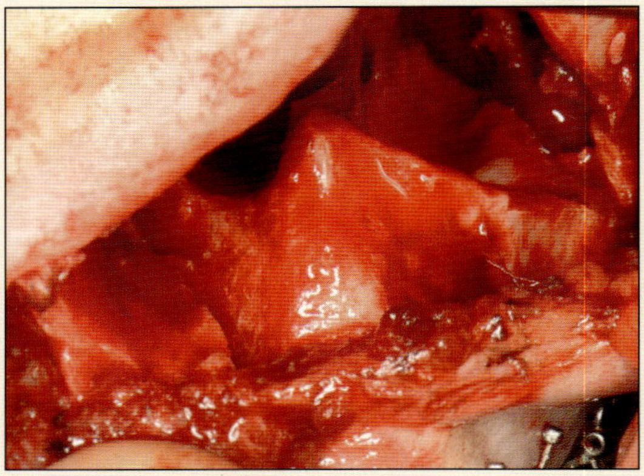

Fig 4-5d The alveolar cleft repair site in the same patient at age 19 years. An osteotomy has been placed through the graft site during a segmental Le Fort I osteotomy to advance the maxilla.

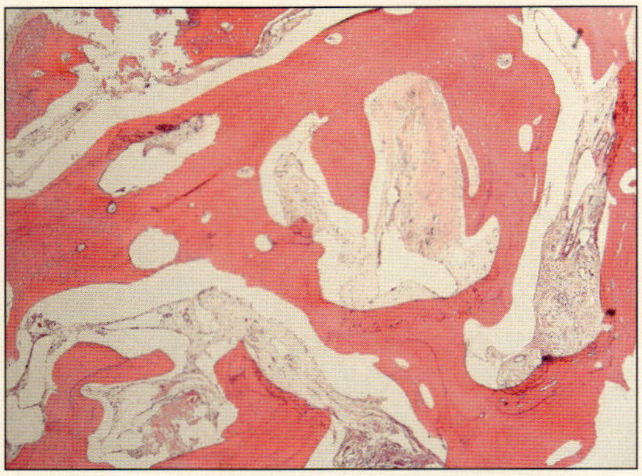

Fig 4-5e Histologic analysis of the graft 9 years after initial placement reveals normal, vital bone. (Hematoxylin and eosin, original magnification ×40.)

site would have been an advantage. Collagen sponges carrying rhBMP-2 introduce bone-forming enrichment while limiting the risk of complicating an infection with graft particles.

rhBMP-2 and Solvent-Dehydrated Bone for the Repair of an Alveolar Cleft

The combination of rhBMP-2 and solvent-dehydrated cancellous bone is useful and effective for the repair of alveolar clefts. The material can be used for patients with a wide range of ages and spares patients the need for harvesting of autogenous bone from the iliac crest. The volume-maintaining ability of the cancellous bone particles is necessary because the osseous walls of the cleft will not prevent the mucosal flaps from collapsing before the graft has healed. This is particularly true when the secondary dentition has already erupted in the dental arch.

When a missing skeletal segment is constructed in a child in the primary dentition, rhBMP-2 can be delivered on a collagen sponge alone, because the child only requires enough bone mass to allow secondary teeth an environment to erupt. The eruption process itself will result in enlargement and organization of the alveolar process.

Case description

In this 10-year-old, the permanent central incisor was already in place. The volume of the alveolar deficiency was substantial (Fig 4-5a). The positions of the primary teeth roots were unfavorable to recruit their periodontal systems to promote bone growth at the cleft defect.

To establish and maintain a substantial volume to form bone, solvent-dehydrated cancellous bone was treated with rhBMP-2 and then placed to fill the entire cleft defect (Fig 4-5b).

After the bone particles carrying rhBMP-2 were placed, a collagen sponge carrying rhBMP-2 was placed to cover the graft mass (Fig 4-5c). The collagen sponge was used to deliver additional rhBMP-2 to the site, prevent migration of the bone particles, and create a collagen–rhBMP-2 bed over which the mucosa suture line would rest.

The alveolar cleft reconstruction site was reentered after 9 years to perform a Le Fort I osteotomy to advance the maxilla (Fig 4-5d).

A solid mass of normal-appearing bone occupied the prior cleft defect. A vertical osteotomy was made through the repair site as part of the multiple-segment maxillary osteotomy. Histologic assessment of the bone from the repair site showed normal structural bone (Fig 4-5e).

Discussion

The combination of rhBMP-2 and solvent-dehydrated cancellous bone particles is an effective and predictable component of a successful bone-forming construct. The process of solvent dehydration results in a material that has consistent mechanical properties. The apparent preservation of the collagen architecture may be an advantage when the material is used as a vehicle to deliver rhBMP-2 to the bone-forming site. Treating the donor bone with solvent dehydration may afford additional safety against transmission of currently known and yet to be discovered pathogenic agents.

Conclusion

Procedures that exploit the healing potential of BMPs, via the application of exogenous BMPs synthesized through recombinant technology, can improve the outcome of treatment. Clinical application of these materials demands a thoughtful and deliberate strategy. If these biologic agents are properly integrated into a bone-forming construct that includes all of the essential elements for success, an otherwise deficient system can produce structures that are biologically stable.

References

1. Razzouk S. BMP-2: Biological challenges to its clinical use. N Y State Dent J 2012;78(5):37–39.
2. Carlson BM. Human Embryology and Developmental Biology, ed 5. Philadelphia: Elsevier Saunders, 2013:156–472.
3. Urist MR. Bone: Formation by autoinduction. Science 1965;150: 893–899.
4. Wozney JM, Rosen V, Celeste AJ, et al. Novel regulators of bone formation: Molecular clones and activities. Science 1988;242: 1528–1534.
5. Chin M, Ng T, Tom WK, Carstens M. Repair of alveolar clefts with recombinant human bone morphogenetic protein (rhBMP-2) in patients with clefts. J Craniofac Surg 2005;16:778–789.
6. US Food and Drug Administration, Center for Devices and Radiologic Health. Premarket Application Approval No. P000058, InFUSE™ Bone Graft/LT-CAGE™ Lumbar Tapered Fusion Device. http://www.accessdata.fda.gov/cdrh_docs/pdf/P000058a.pdf. Issued 2 July 2002. Accessed 17 September 2014.
7. Wozney JM, Wikesjö UME. rhBMP-2: Biology and applications in oral and maxillofacial surgery and periodontics. In: Lynch SE, Marx RE, Nevins M, Wisner-Lynch LA (eds). Tissue Engineering: Applications in Oral and Maxillofacial Surgery and Periodontics. Chicago: Quintessence, 2008:159–177.
8. Schwartz Z, Somers A, Mellonig JT, et al. Addition of human recombinant bone morphogenetic protein-2 to inactive commercial human demineralized freeze-dried bone allograft makes an effective composite bone inductive implant material. J Periodontol 1998;69:1337–1345.
9. Triplett R. Bone augmentation of the maxillary sinus floor with rhBMP-2. In: Lynch SE, Marx RE, Nevins M, Wisner-Lynch LA (eds). Tissue Engineering: Applications in Oral and Maxillofacial Surgery and Periodontics. Chicago: Quintessence, 2008:186–202.
10. Deutsch H. High-dose bone morphogenetic protein-induced ectopic abdomen bone growth. Spine J 2010;10(2):e1–e4.
11. US Department of Health and Human Services. FDA Public Health Notification: Life-threatening Complications Associated with Recombinant Human Bone Morphogenetic Protein in Cervical Spine Fusion. http://www.fda.gov/MedicalDevices/Safety/AlertsandNotices/PublicHealthNotifications/ucm062000.htm. Issued 1 July 2008. Accessed 17 September 2014.
12. Burkus JK, Heim SE, Gornet MF, Zdeblick TA. Is INFUSE bone graft superior to autograft bone? An integrated analysis of clinical trials using the LT-CAGE lumbar tapered fusion device. J Spinal Disord Tech 2003;16:113–122.
13. Chin M. Bone morphogenetic protein enhancement of alveolar distraction in humans. Presented at the 4th International Congress of Maxillofacial and Craniofacial Distraction, Paris, 2–5 July 2003.
14. Chin M, Ng T, Tom WK, Carstens M. Tissue engineering with rhBMP-2: Human in situ skeletal construction in 250 cases. Presented at the 5th International Congress of Maxillofacial and Craniofacial Distraction, Paris, 21–24 June 2006.
15. Chin M, Ng T, Tom WK. New protocol of alveolar distraction: Review of 50 cases. Presented at the 5th International Congress of Maxillofacial and Craniofacial Distraction, Paris, 21–24 June 2006.
16. Simonds RJ, Holmberg SD, Hurwitz RL, et al. Transmission of human immunodeficiency virus type 1 from a seronegative organ and tissue donor. N Engl J Med 1992;326:726–732.
17. Marthy S, Richter M. Human immunodeficiency virus activity in rib allografts. J Oral Maxillofac Surg 1998;56:474–476.
18. Prusiner SB. Novel structure and genetics of prions causing neurodegeneration in humans and animals. Biologicals 1990;18:247–262.
19. Prusiner SB. Neurodegeneration in humans caused by prions. West J Med 1994;161:264–272.
20. Prusiner SB. Human prion diseases and neurodegeneration. Curr Top Microbiol Immunol 1996;207:1–17.
21. Prusiner SB. Biology and genetics of prions causing neurodegeneration. Ann Rev Genetics 2013;47:601–623.
22. Noumbissi SS, Lozada JL, Boyne PJ, et al. Clinical, histologic, and histomorphometric evaluation of mineralized solvent-dehydrated bone allograft (Puros) in human maxillary sinus grafts. J Oral Implantol 2005;31:171–179.
23. Alper T, Cramp WA, Haig DA, Clarke MC. Does the agent of scrapie replicate without nucleic acid? Nature 1967;214:764–766.
24. Bellinger-Kawahara C, Cleaver JE, Diener TO, Prusiner SB. Purified scrapie prions resist inactivation by UV irradiation. J Virol 1987; 61:159–166.
25. Bellinger-Kawahara C, Diener TO, McKinley MP, Groth DF, Smith DR, Prusiner SB. Purified scrapie prions resist inactivation by procedures that hydrolyze, modify, or shear nucleic acids. Virology 1987;160:271–274.
26. Brown P, Liberski PP, Wolff A, Gajdusek DC. Resistance of scrapie infectivity to steam autoclaving after formaldehyde fixation and limited survival after ashing at 360°C: Practical and theoretical implications. J Infect Dis 1990;161:467–472.

27. Brown P, Liberski PP, Wolff A, Gajdusek DC. Conservation of infectivity in purified fibrillary extracts of scrapie-infected hamster brain after sequential enzymatic digestion or polyacrylamide gel electrophoresis. Proc Natl Acad Sci U S A 1990;87:7240–7244.
28. Georgsson G, Sigurdarson S, Brown P. Infectious agent of sheep scrapie may persist in the environment for at least 16 years. J Gen Virol 2006;87:3737–3740.
29. US Food and Drug Administration. Processing of Orthopedic, Cardiovascular, and Skin Allografts Workshop. Bethesda, MD: National Institutes of Health, 2007.
30. Günther KP, Scharf HP, Pesch HJ, Puhl W. Osteointegration of solvent-preserved bone transplants in an animal model. Osteologie 1996;5(1):4–12.
31. US Securities and Exchange Commission. Form 10-K. Washington, DC: US Securities and Exchange Commission, 2011.
32. Zimmer Dental. Regenerative Product Catalog. Carlsbad, CA: Zimmer Dental, 2008.
33. Schoepf C. Allograft safety: The efficacy of the Tutoplast Process. Int Magazine Oral Implant 2006;1:10–15.
34. Kim Y, Nowzari H, Rich SK. Risk of prion disease transmission through bovine-derived bone substitutes. A systematic review. Clin Implant Dent Relat Res 2013;15:645–653.

5 Using Developing Teeth to Generate Bone

The relationship between alveolar bone growth and dental eruption has been observed for many years. The underlying mechanisms by which this occurs are still obscure. Nevertheless, integration of tooth development into long-term management of dental and jaw deformities can improve the treatment outcome and decrease the need for complicated surgery. This approach to correcting alveolar defects combines dental development, recombinant human bone morphogenetic protein 2 (rhBMP-2), and surgical design modifications.

Role of Periodontal Ligaments in Regulation of Bone Growth

Teeth and their periodontal ligament systems are important elements in the engineering and design of bone-forming constructs. The system is used to deliver critical mechanical signals to the environment in which bone is forming. A source of neuromuscular input is a basic and essential component of an effective bone-forming environment. The anatomical path along which these signals travel is poorly understood. Because this is a critical element of successful bone-forming environments, it is important to understand what is known about the anatomy and physiology of the system.

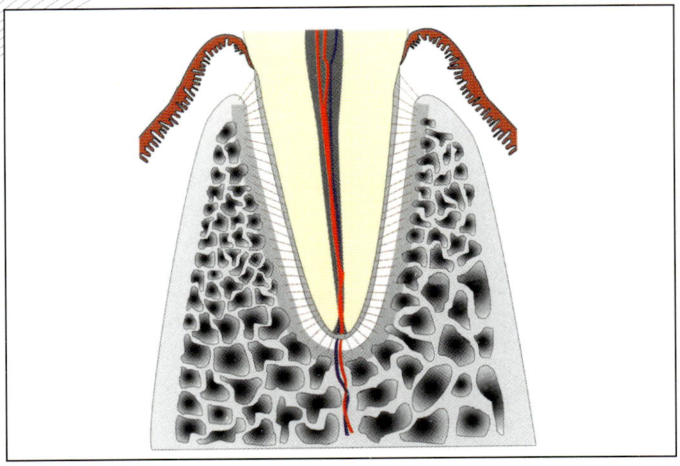

Fig 5-1 Standard depiction of the periodontal ligament. (Reprinted from Holmstrup[1] with permission.)

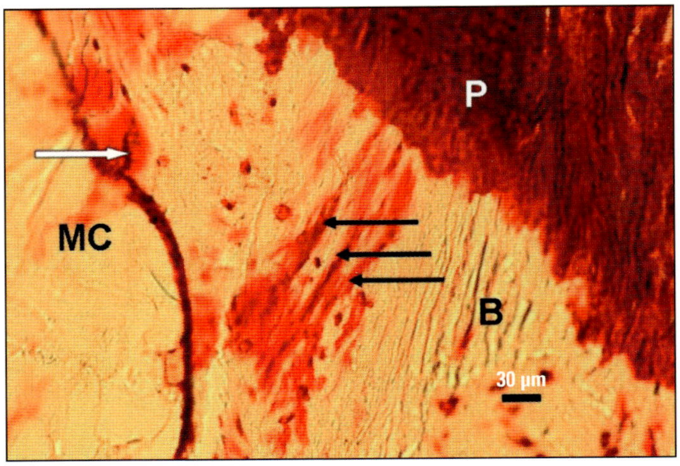

Fig 5-2 Photomicrograph of a typical representative array of three periosteal Sharpey fibers *(black arrows)*, each about 15 µm thick, extending from the periosteum (P), through the bone (B), toward the endosteum outside, which is the marrow cavity (MC). In addition, nearby are stress-induced microcracks; for example, one *(white arrow)* is surrounded by bone matrix that has become "leaky" to the stain (normally impervious), apparently due to submicroscopic fatigue fissures increasing accessibility of the dye. Human proximal femur. En bloc gentian violet stain. (Reprinted from Aaron[3] with permission.)

Within the maxillofacial skeletal system, the primary muscle attachments that deliver neuromuscular signals are confined to the basilar bone structures. The action of the muscles of mastication maintains the morphology of the mandible even when challenged by extensive alveolar atrophy. The alveolar process lacks major muscle attachments and depends on teeth to develop and maintain its structural integrity. Within the alveolar process, the system of teeth, periodontal ligaments, and Sharpey fibers function in a role similar to that of a muscle attachment.

Both muscle attachments and periodontal ligament insertion into the alveolar process deliver regulatory signaling. The common anatomical structure shared between the dental and skeletal systems is the Sharpey fiber. Although Sharpey fibers have been recognized for many years as the interface between bone and skeletal muscle, their full role and mechanism of action have been underappreciated. The mechanism by which teeth act to deliver regulatory signaling to alveolar bone is also not well understood. The current state of understanding of this process represents a synthesis of years of clinical observation and modern innovations in immunohistochemistry. The following is a discussion of the possible underlying mechanisms by which this system operates.

Basic descriptions of periodontal ligaments are limited to their role connecting the root surface to the lamina dura of the alveolar process (Fig 5-1). The ligaments are described as a method to suspend the tooth within the socket in a manner that allows a degree of movement. The ligaments themselves are described as fibers that are embedded in the cementum, cross the narrow gap between the root and the socket, and are inserted in the surface of the lamina dura. Typical diagrams depict the ligaments as simple, single fibers that are aligned to stabilize the tooth against vertical loading forces. Few details are given as to the manner in which or extent to which the fibers penetrate the alveolar bone.

In 1954, Sicher[2] offered a more detailed description of the organization of the ligaments. He revealed that the fibers were not continuous single fibers across the periodontal ligament space. Instead, fibers from the cementum side and the lamina dura side converge in the middle to join in a plexus. Although the functional nature of the ligament plexus remains obscure, its complex architecture suggests that the system is involved in processes beyond simple anchorage.

Modern investigators[3] have used new methods to reveal how these fibers are embedded in bone. Advancements in immunohistochemistry have provided a better understanding of the extent to which these fibers penetrate bone (Fig 5-2). Aaron and Skerry[4] demonstrated that Sharpey fibers extend through the cortex of the proximal femur toward the medullary space (Fig 5-3). Immunohistochemical studies show evidence of these fibers within the marrow space. The presence of these fibers in locations not associated with muscle attachment is compelling evidence that their function extends further than anchorage.

The concept that Sharpey fibers affect bone activity beyond the surface at which they insert is consistent with clinical events in the alveolar process. It is clear that normal bone within the alveolar housing that surrounds teeth establishes a trabecular architecture that reflects the functional demands of tooth loading. The phenomenon is attributed to Wolff's law. Wolff's law is commonly interpreted to describe the tendency of bone to form and adapt in a manner to accommodate the net functional stress placed upon it.

The underlying mechanism that directs and maintains the anatomical architecture remains obscure. One explanation is that forces absorbed by teeth are transmitted via the periodontal ligaments to the lamina dura, and those forces are mechanically transmitted to the underlying trabeculae of the cancellous bone. The medullary bone remodels in response to the mechanical load placed on it through the cortex. This follows the Frost prin-

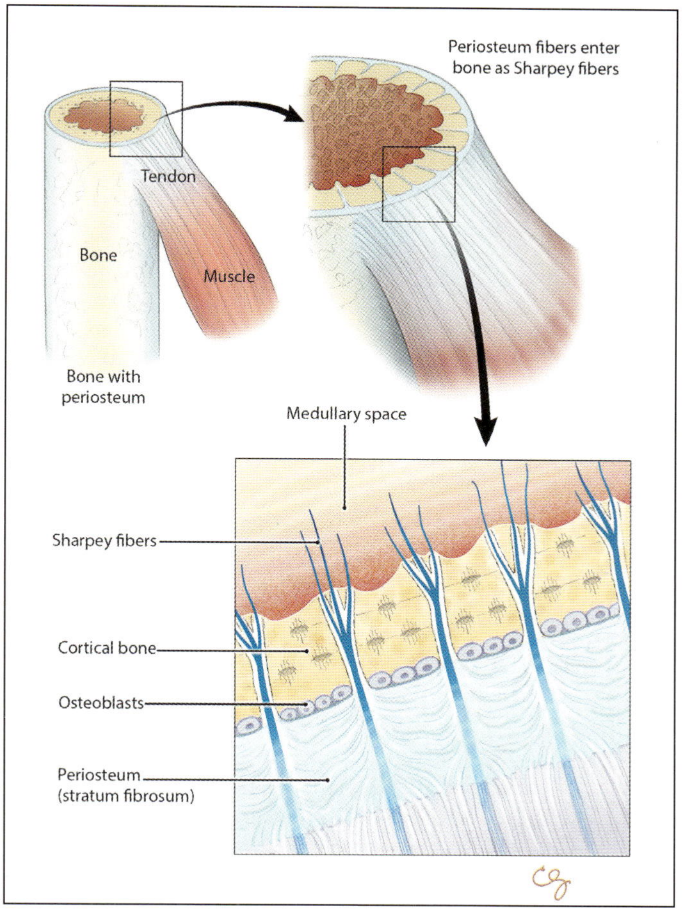

Fig 5-3 Sharpey fibers arise from tendon insertions, periodontal ligaments, and normal periosteum. *First inset*: Sharpey fibers penetrate through the width of the cortical bone. *Second inset*: Extensions of Sharpey fibers continue into the medullary space.

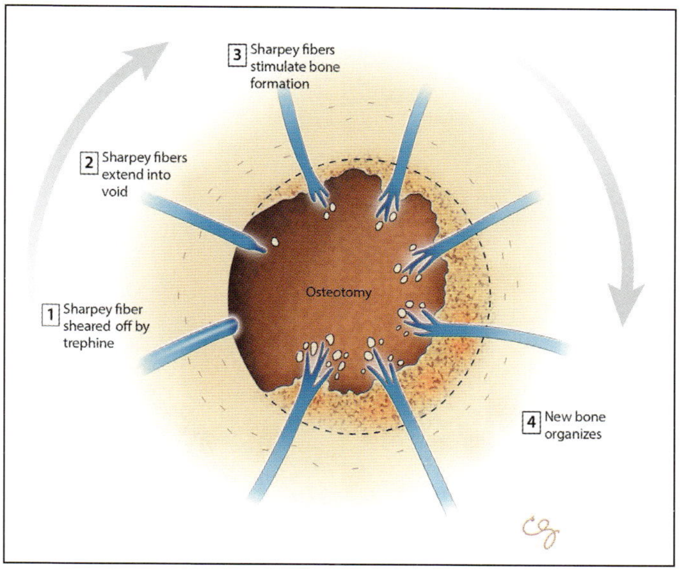

Fig 5-4 Membranous healing stages of an osteotomy defect. Sharpey fibers grow into the defect before trabecular bone formation occurs.

ciple of remodeling in response to microstrains. Compromised structural bone is replaced and renewed through resorption and deposition. The structure itself transmits load, and microstrains are absorbed following known mechanical laws. Even if the Frost principle is operating, additional processes must be in place that regulate and direct the maintenance of the structural morphology, or a steady state could not be maintained.

An alternative or additional explanation is that penetrating Sharpey fibers transmit signals from the periodontal ligament to the lamina dura and beyond to the medullary space. This is an attractive model because it explains how ligaments and their penetrating Sharpey fiber ends might regulate the growth and architecture of developing or mature bone. In embryologic skeletal development and in a surgical bone-forming construct, Sharpey fibers from existing muscles occupy their insertion sites before structural bone has formed. This process occurs without transfer of microstrains because there is no existing mechanical environment to transmit and focus forces. For either of these systems to yield a skeletal unit, another regulatory mechanism must be in place. Extension of Sharpey fibers into the environment adjacent to developing teeth is a likely mechanism that promotes the growth of the alveolar process. In the adult, the persistence of Sharpey fibers through the lamina dura and in the medullary bone is very likely involved in maintenance and repair of these structures. The role of Sharpey fibers in the repair of surgical defects has been demonstrated in an experimental lamb model.[5] A cylindric void heals and fills with vital bone following a specific sequence (Fig 5-4). First, Sharpey fibers severed by the trephine drill grow into the osteotomy void. Second, trabecular bone forms around the Sharpey fiber extensions. Trabecular bone does not form without the restoration of the embedded fiber system. Histology of the repair site is identical to that of fetal lamb membranous bone development. Even though the lamb experimental site is endochondral in origin, it still heals by a mechanism that follows membranous bone development. This confirms Harvold's theory that fetal bone development processes are preserved in the adult.[6] The embedded fiber system joins muscle attachment, periosteum, and periodontal ligaments into a network that is the likely conduit for regulatory control signals to form and maintain the skeleton. Use of teeth and their periodontal systems to promote healing of reconstructive procedures is intended to exploit these regulatory processes to the advantage of successful healing.

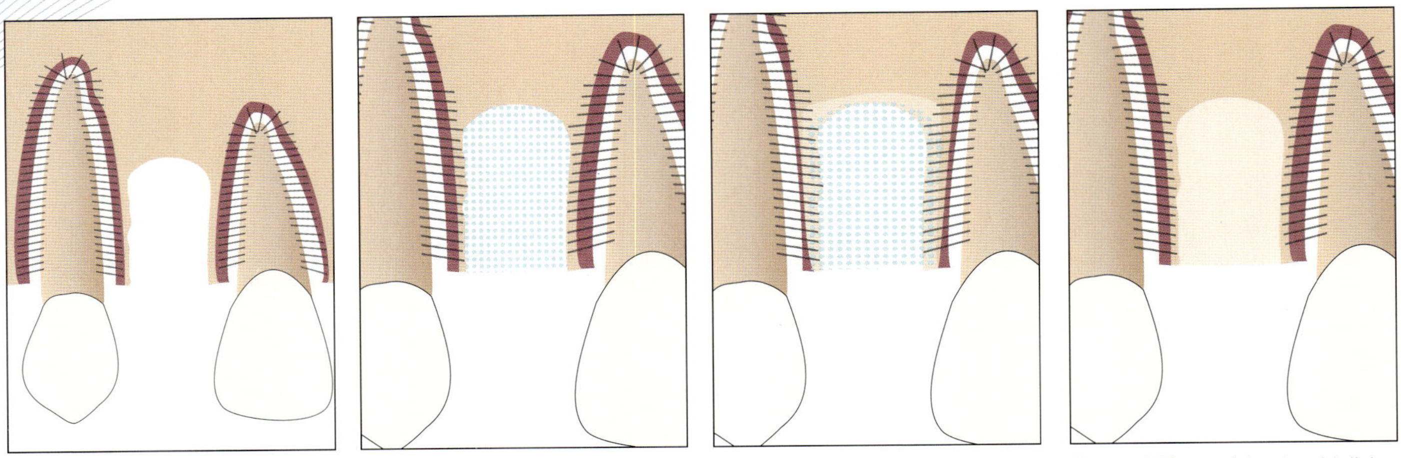

Fig 5-5a An extraction site has healed with a large defect.

Fig 5-5b A collagen sponge impregnated with rhBMP-2 is placed.

Fig 5-5c Sharpey fibers become continuous with the graft and immature cells.

Fig 5-5d The graft heals with living and organized bone.

Surgical Design and Procedures

Periodontal ligament systems can be exploited to regulate bone growth in many common clinical situations.

I. Sharpey fibers and bone grafting of adjacent defects

Theoretical basis of surgical design

A challenging, common alveolar problem is when two intact teeth are adjacent to a large defect (Fig 5-5a). The teeth adjacent to the defect have good periodontal attachment levels. The thin layer of bone that covers the root surfaces facing the defect houses the attachment sites for the periodontal ligament fibers. The Sharpey fibers that extend from the periodontal ligament into the lamina dura are inherently resistant to demineralization. Following placement of a collagen sponge with rhBMP-2 (Fig 5-5b), the walls of the defect respond by demineralization. This process exposes the Sharpey fibers that are embedded in the socket wall.

As new bone grows and begins to remineralize, the Sharpey fibers of the periodontal ligament become invested in the graft mass (Fig 5-5c). The rhBMP-2 graft concentrates a cell population with bone-growing potential at the regeneration site. The regulatory process that the fibers originally used to create and maintain the thin socket wall is now distributed to the graft mass. This effect is distance dependent, so the primary influence of the fibers is at the periphery. The defect fills as the graft-derived tissue merges seamlessly with the adjacent alveolar bone (Fig 5-5d).

Discussion

Successful healing requires concentration of a sufficient number of bone-forming cells at the site. The rhBMP-2 graft satisfies this condition. Although the cells have bone-forming potential, however, they will not necessarily perform this function with optimal efficiency in the absence of direction. Organization of the amorphous tissue mass into an organized structural system requires regulation of the construction and assembly process.

Although bone morphogenetic proteins can effect de novo bone formation in an ectopic site, the resulting bone will not mature into a functional skeletal unless transferred to a supportive environment.[7] Neuromuscular input provides direction to grow bone. Physiologic coordination of the new, living bone segment requires integration into the neuromuscular system to establish morphology on the cellular and tissue architecture levels for both construction and maintenance of the skeletal organ system.

II. Sharpey fibers and bone growth in osteotomy sites

Theoretical basis of surgical design

Osteotomies between adjacent roots can be performed to transport dentoalveolar segments. The two adjacent teeth share support from the interproximal bone (Fig 5-6a). Within the volume of bone between the roots, their periodontal systems overlap (Fig 5-6b). The interproximal bone was formed and is maintained by a process that must be coordinated and shared by the periodontal systems of both teeth. Regulation of this process requires a path by which signals can pass. The Sharpey fiber network is the likely route through which communication propagates.

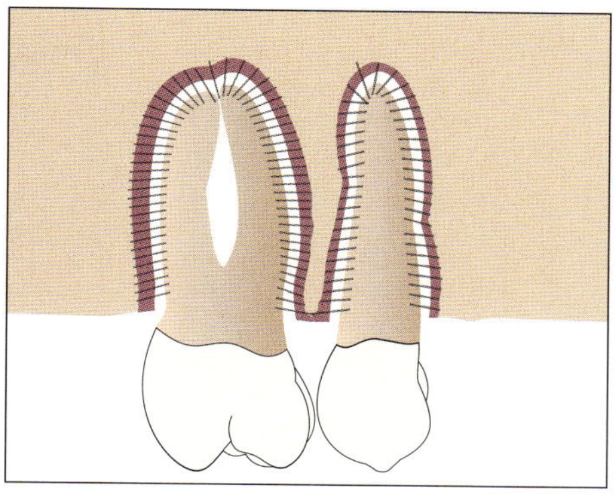

Fig 5-6a Two typical teeth share support from the interproximal bone.

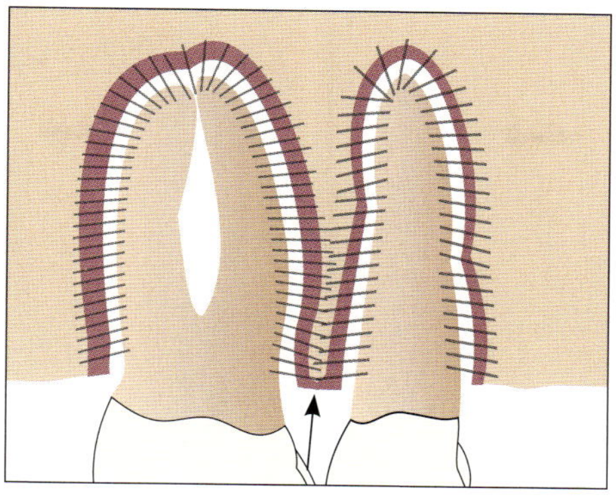

Fig 5-6b New evidence shows that periodontal systems overlap within the interproximal bone. The interproximal bone *(arrow)* was formed and is maintained by a process that must be coordinated and shared by the periodontal systems of both teeth. Regulation requires a path by which signals can pass.

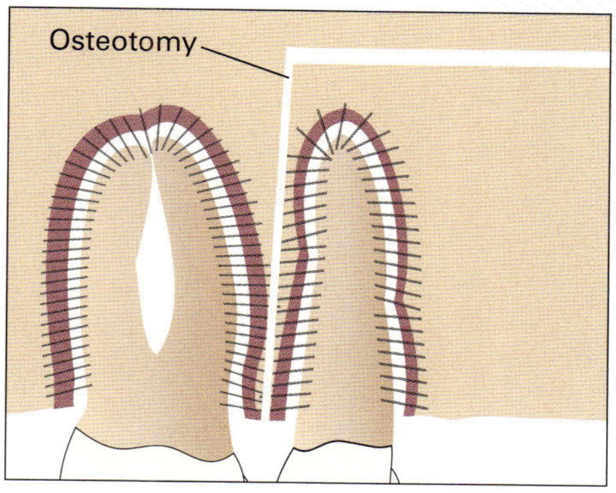

Fig 5-6c This type of osteotomy would be used to mobilize an alveolar segment for orthognathic surgery or distraction osteogenesis. The bone cut divides the two periodontal systems but also transects some of the Sharpey fibers.

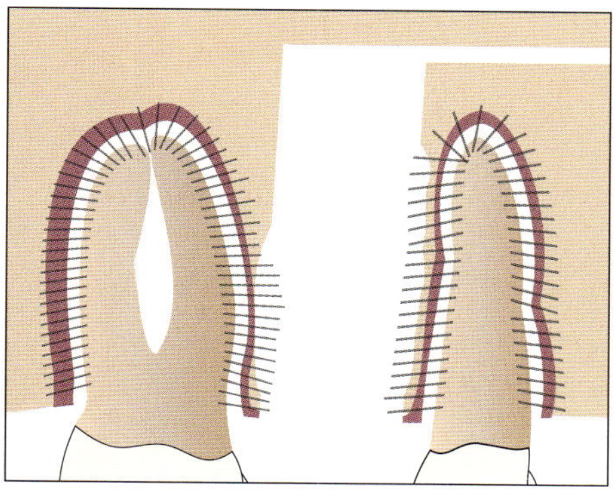

Fig 5-6d Segment transport separates the anatomical units and the regulatory network.

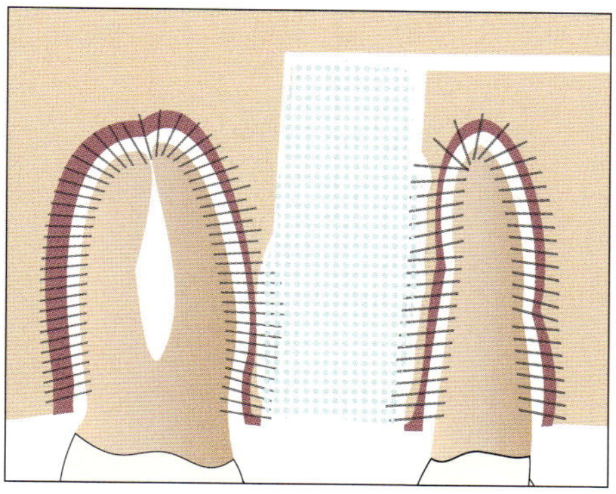

Fig 5-6e The cut surfaces of the osteotomy site undergo demineralization. Absorbable collagen sponges containing rhBMP-2 are placed in the discontinuity gap.

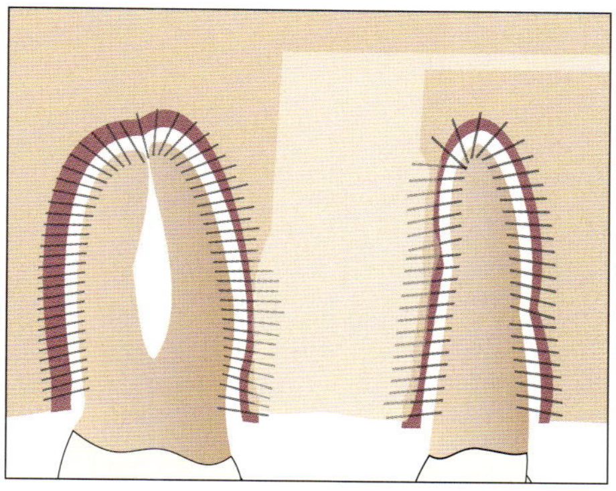

Fig 5-6f The Sharpey fibers of the periodontal ligament system become invested in the new bone mass.

An interproximal osteotomy is performed to divide the bone and the Sharpey fiber network in order to mobilize an alveolar segment for orthognathic surgery or distraction osteogenesis (Fig 5-6c). The bone cut divides the two periodontal systems but also transects some of the Sharpey fibers. Segment transport separates the anatomical units and the regulatory network (Fig 5-6d).

The surgical cut through the site divides the anatomical structure but also the physiologic system contained within. Some Sharpey fibers are transected, and their distal ends remain embedded in the opposite side of the segment. The existing network is disrupted. Normal bone physiology involves resorption and deposition of the mineralized, structural component. The Sharpey fibers embedded in the bone remain intact throughout the remodeling process because they are resistant to demineralization.

Absorbable collagen sponges (ACSs) containing rhBMP-2 are placed in the discontinuity gap. The bone underlying the line of osteotomy demineralizes in response to the bone cut and the presence of the rhBMP-2 graft. As the bone resorbs, more of the Sharpey fiber network is exposed (Fig 5-6e).

During the process of healing, the existing bone that was the interproximal bone demineralizes and becomes continuous with the mass of immature cells drawn to the site by the rhBMP-2. A new relationship is established between the periodontal ligament system, its Sharpey fiber extensions, and the new mass of bone (Fig 5-6f).

Discussion

The conventional assumption is that the primary role of the periodontal ligament is to suspend the tooth within the socket. Evidence demonstrating the deep penetration of these fibers into the lamina dura and their likely presence in the medullary space supports the concept that their role is more complicated. The structural stability and resistance to demineralization of Sharpey fibers make them an attractive explanation for morphologic stability within an environment of constant remodeling. If this fiber network is involved in the maintenance of bone through a process similar to that provided by a skeletal muscle attachment, recruiting its effect by deliberate surgical design has the potential to improve healing and the treatment outcome.

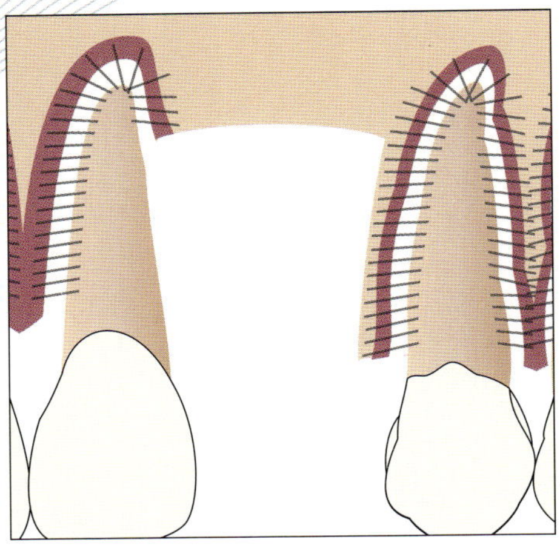

Fig 5-7a A lateral incisor with a periodontal defect is adjacent to an alveolar bone defect.

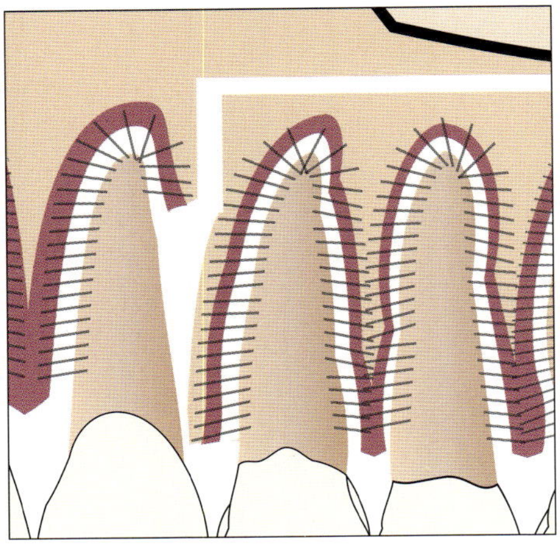

Fig 5-7b A segmental osteotomy transports the posterior teeth anteriorly, establishing a narrow, sheltered bone-forming chamber.

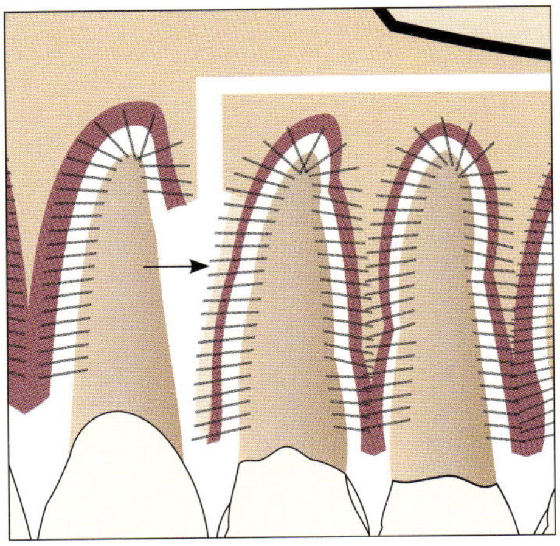

Fig 5-7c Demineralization of the bone covering the premolar root leaves Sharpey fibers projecting into the regeneration site *(arrow)*.

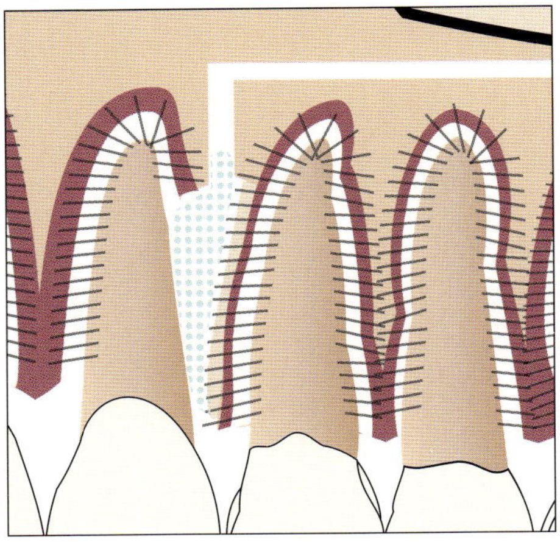

Fig 5-7d A collagen sponge containing rhBMP-2 is placed as a graft.

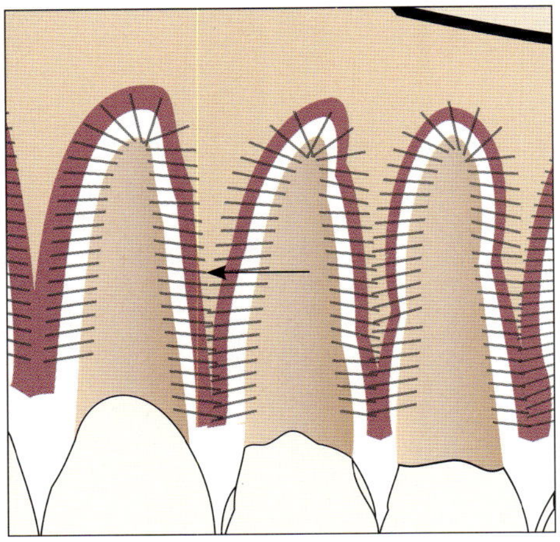

Fig 5-7e Bone fills the interproximal space and matures into normal structural bone. The site shows possible growth of a new periodontal ligament and attachment system *(arrow)*.

III. Asymmetric regeneration using the periodontal ligament–Sharpey fiber network

Theoretical basis of surgical design

A periodontal defect on the lateral incisor is sometimes the result of a failed attempt to manage an impacted canine tooth. In this familiar scenario, the canine is eventually extracted but the treatment leaves a large defect in the alveolus and damages the root and periodontal ligament system of the lateral incisor (Fig 5-7a). Simple grafting will not restore the attachment level defect. In the example shown here, the premolar tooth also has sustained damage after multiple prior grafting attempts. This situation can be treated through a strategy that uses the periodontal ligament and Sharpey fiber system to promote regeneration of the lateral incisor attachment.

The objective is to construct a bone-forming environment that has optimal regeneration capability. The first step is to mobilize an osteotomy segment and transport the teeth, bone, and periodontal ligament systems anteriorly to eliminate most of the volume of the alveolar bone defect (Fig 5-7b). What remains is the distal and facial root surface defect on the lateral incisor where the periodontal ligament attachment has been damaged.

Transportation of the osteotomy segment through the alveolar bone defect places the premolar root in close proximity to the damaged surface of the lateral incisor. The effect is to move a working periodontal ligament–Sharpey fiber system into the repair site (Fig 5-7c). The Sharpey fibers of the premolar maintain the bone that covers its mesial side. The defect repair is asymmetric because the damaged lateral incisor root lacks a periodontal system to contribute to the regeneration process.

A collagen sponge containing rhBMP-2 is positioned in the interproximal space and over the labial root surface of the lateral incisor (Fig 5-7d). The bone that is between the roots demineralizes in response to both elevation of the mucoperiosteum and the rhBMP-2/ACS graft. Immature cells are concentrated in the space by the action of rhBMP-2. These cells occupy an environ-

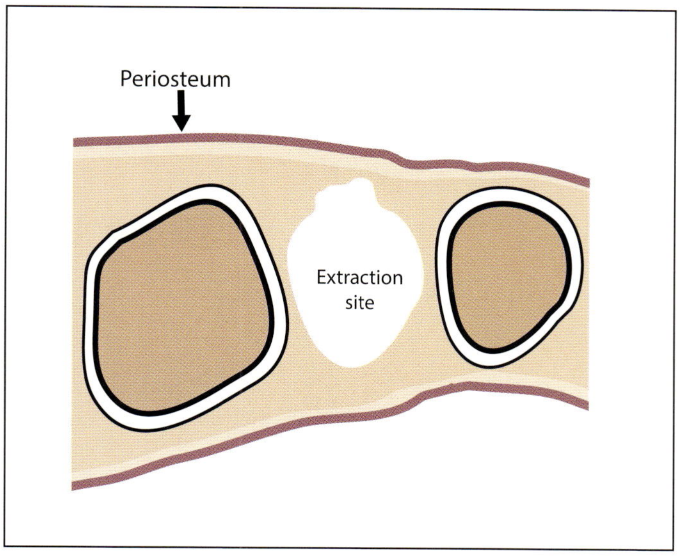

Fig 5-8a Occlusal view of an extraction site of a premolar.

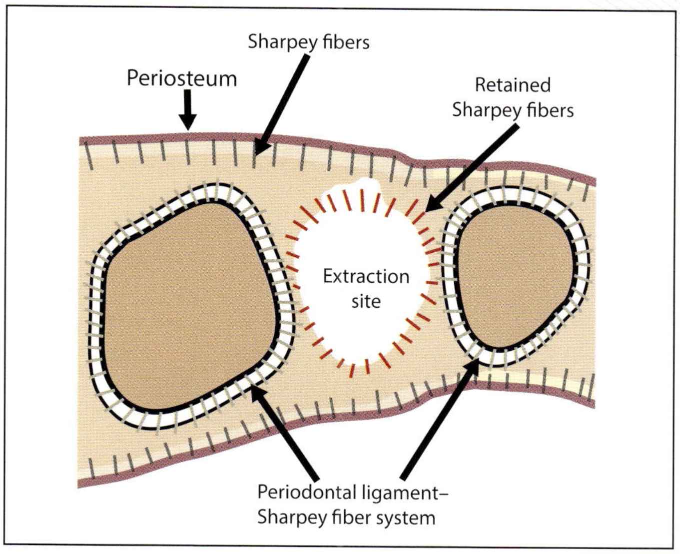

Fig 5-8b Sharpey fiber systems associated with the teeth and periosteum.

ment that is now shared by the exposed Sharpey fiber system from the premolar periodontal ligament system.

Within the constructed environment, bone fills the interproximal space (Fig 5-7e). Over many months, the site remodels and takes on the fine structural architecture of a normal, healthy interproximal bone unit. A well-defined lamina dura forms opposite the damaged lateral incisor root. The hypermobility and gingival recession of the tooth are reduced.

Discussion

The objective is to restore the lost periodontal ligament and attachment system on the lateral incisor. Although histology of the reconstructed site would be necessary to confirm if a new attachment has been synthesized, radiographic and clinical evaluations could suggest whether the site has been restored to normal anatomy. The development of a normal lamina dura would suggest that a functional load is being transferred from the tooth root to the alveolar bone.

IV. Combination of the periodontal and periosteal Sharpey fiber networks to promote bone growth

The periodontal ligament system and its Sharpey fiber extensions operate in an environment that is also under the influence of the periosteal system, which has its own Sharpey fiber extensions. Figure 5-8a depicts the extraction site of a premolar that has a labial bone defect. The gross presentation is of an extraction site void in the alveolar bone located adjacent to the roots of intact teeth.

Hidden within the volume of calcified bone are the embedded Sharpey fibers (Fig 5-8b). These fibers extend from the cementum of the remaining roots to cross the periodontal ligament space. They penetrate the lamina dura of the socket wall to enter the medullary space of the alveolar process. When roots are in close proximity, the fibers of one tooth reach the fibers of the adjacent tooth. When a tooth is extracted, its anchoring Sharpey fibers are disrupted, leaving severed pieces of fibers in the socket wall. If the periosteum of the alveolar process follows the structure demonstrated for the femur, Sharpey fibers penetrate the cortical bone to reach the medullary space.[8]

Sharpey fibers form a hidden web of interconnecting structures that provide a route for mechanical regulatory signaling within the bone (see Fig 5-8b). They have the important ability to transmit forces from stimuli outside the bone to structures and cells within the solid skeletal mass.

Discussion

Growth of alveolar bone around erupting teeth has been observed for many years. The mechanism of how the tooth promotes bone growth and how the alveolar process maintains its morphology is poorly understood. There is substantial evidence that the periodontal ligament–Sharpey fiber system is an important mechanism for growth and maintenance of alveolar bone. It is now clear that the periodontal ligament system extends from the root, across the periodontal ligament space, and penetrates deeply into the alveolar bone. Invested in the alveolar bone as Sharpey fibers, this system is well suited to transmit force and regulatory signals into the environment that will form bone and maintain its morphology.

Unlike the surrounding calcified structural bone, the periodontal ligament–Sharpey fiber system is resistant to demineralization. These fibers are not calcified and are not affected by bone's necessary remodeling process. This means that as bone undergoes its natural process of resorption and deposition to maintain its structural integrity and health, the embedded Sharpey fiber system remains stable and continuously operating.

If the gross morphology of any facial bone segment is to remain in a steady state through multiple cycles of bone renewal, there must be anatomical and physiologic systems that remain constant. The features of the Sharpey fiber network can deliver anatomical stability when considered in their relationship with skeletal muscle, periosteum, periodontal ligaments, and cranial sutures.

If the skeletal unit is to form initially and maintain its morphology over years, it must have the ability to receive and process neuromuscular signals. The Sharpey fiber system is also well suited to transmitting mechanical signals. In the musculoskeletal system, nerves deliver signals from the central nervous system to the muscle body. The muscle delivers the forces to the tendon and then to the muscle attachment through Sharpey fibers. By this path, the brain has communication with the bone and the cells within. In the alveolar process, regulatory signals are transmitted from the oral environment to the teeth. The teeth transmit mechanical forces to the periodontal ligaments and beyond the Sharpey fibers. The Sharpey fibers embedded in the bone transmit regulatory forces deep into the bone and to the cells within. Cellular sensitivity to mechanical forces has the potential to receive regulatory signals.[9–14]

Understanding of the anatomical extent and complexity of these fiber systems has been greatly improved by modern investigators. A working model can be established when the anatomical findings are combined with the behavior of these structures in the clinical setting.

Harvold[14] formulated a working theory on how bone forms in the embryologic environment. He believed that skeletal formation was the result of the combined factors of a stabilized physical environment, a source of cells, and neuromuscular input. He recognized that major facial bones developed consistently within a tissue volume that was adjacent to an existing muscle. He postulated that muscle activity resulted in specific and deliberate distortion of the adjacent soft tissue volume. The concept held that mechanical distortion of their surroundings caused the cells to modify their activity and morphology in favor of bone formation. No explanation was offered at that time as to how a cell might interpret mechanical signaling, and the concept of tensegrity had not yet been described.

Harvold[14] speculated that if the mechanisms that promoted skeletal formation in the embryo persist after birth, it may be possible to recruit the processes to aid in healing of reconstructive surgeries. The interaction of muscle attachments and bone formation was a primary focus of his research. He also recognized that developing teeth were associated with bone growth and seemed to satisfy the requirement for neuromuscular input. However, the mechanism that allowed teeth to fulfill this function was unknown.

Clinical experience and histologic studies show that developing teeth are associated with bone formation even though they are not directly associated with muscle attachments. The likely explanation for this shared ability of muscle attachments and periodontal ligaments to regulate bone formation is the Sharpey fibers that anchor both teeth and tendons to bone. Although teeth and muscles present as very different anatomical structures, they both use Sharpey fibers to establish bone anchorage. The role of Sharpey fibers in the development, growth, maintenance, and repair of bone is slowly becoming clearer as the result of new analysis techniques. Thus, when surgical procedures that involve bone growth of alveolar structures are designed, teeth are the most obvious source of neuromuscular input.

Exploitation of Tooth Development and Eruption to Create Bone-Forming Constructs

Bone formation associated with tooth development is an essential mechanism for the natural development of the maxilla and mandible. The alveolar processes of the jaws depend on the formation and eruption of teeth to achieve normal morphology. As teeth form and erupt, supporting bone develops simultaneously. The morphology of the resultant skeletal systems conforms to the presence of the periodontal ligament systems that connect the dental roots to the adjacent bone.

The growth and development of the alveolar processes of the jaws appear to be related more to the presence of teeth than to the influence of the muscle attachments inserting on the adjacent bone. This observation leads to the conclusion that development of the teeth and their functional attachment via ligaments to the surrounding bone imparts a stimulating and regulating effect on the bone itself. In this manner, teeth and their functioning periodontal apparatus function as neuromuscular regulating mechanisms analogous to muscle attachments.

If teeth do not develop or erupt successfully, hypoplasia of the involved skeletal unit is the result. The mechanism by which teeth stimulate bone to grow is incompletely understood. The periodontal ligaments form an anatomical connection between the tooth and the surrounding bone. This establishes a mechanical route by which regulatory signals can pass between the functioning tooth and the adjacent bone. The pattern, nature, and physiology of the specific signaling are unknown. The mechanism that directs the path of movement in both normal and abnormal tooth eruption is also unidentified. Current understanding is mostly derived from clinical observation of normal and abnormal tooth development and its apparent effect on the development of bone. Because alveolar development depends on dental development, all of the mechanisms that direct tooth formation regulate bone formation.

The development and eruption of teeth are important processes in children to generate bone and form normal jaws. The alveolar process forms in unison with tooth development. Clinical observation shows that bone forms around the anatomical system that includes the tooth and the periodontal support apparatus. As the root forms, an alveolar process grows to encase it. As a tooth moves along a natural eruption path, bone forms to maintain structural support of the root. If orthodontic traction is placed on a tooth, the alveolar housing adapts to maintain support of the displaced root. In contrast, a tooth without an intact periodontal support system will not form bone if moved by natural eruption or orthodontic traction.

For a skeletal unit to be formed in relation to teeth, an intact periodontal apparatus must be present. Periodontal ligaments connect semimobile teeth to the lamina dura of the alveolar housing. The periodontal ligaments act on alveolar bone in a fashion similar to the way that muscle attachments act on other bones. Physiologic movement of the teeth results in forces transmitted through the periodontal ligaments to the lamina dura. This is a source of neuromuscular signaling that participates in the regulation of bone physiology within the alveolar process.

It is possible to engineer bone-forming constructs that exploit the stimulating abilities of teeth to generate skeletal structures. However, designing bone-forming constructs that exploit tooth development and eruption is challenging for multiple reasons. Tooth eruption follows a specific timeline in growth and development. It is currently not possible for the clinician to control the time of initiation or completion of tooth eruption. For this reason, these treatments must be initiated at an age when dental development is occurring naturally.

Both primary and secondary teeth have bone-forming potential. The potential age to take advantage of this process begins as the first primary teeth are developing. Surgical incursion into the immature site must be designed to avoid damage to the developing adjacent structures. Impairment of jaw growth has been a concern if early surgery damages the site. Preserving the potential for future growth of the repaired site is a critical aspect of the surgical design.

Surgeons in the past recognized that the procedures they performed on children resulted in growth impairment. The mechanisms by which this occurred were mostly a matter of speculation. Studies to define the mechanism of growth impairment lacked validity because most were conducted on surgically created cleftlike defects. These experimental animals lacked the more complex field deficiency of a naturally occurring developmental cleft.[15,16]

The availability of recombinant growth factors and morphogenetic agents offers surgeons the potential to design new surgical treatments. However, to fully realize the potential of children to grow and maintain bone within a developmentally challenged anatomical field, all aspects of bone physiology must be understood. Emerging knowledge in the fields of biotechnology and neuroscience will increasingly direct the types of treatment that can be offered to these children.

Clinical Applications

Discontinuity defects of the maxilla related to cleft lip and palate are among the most common bone deficiency disorders treated by craniofacial surgery centers. In the past, rehabilitation of alveolar clefts was performed when patients were between the ages of 9 and 11 years. This staging protocol depended on multiple factors, including the stage of dental eruption, the presence of an adequate volume of bone at the iliac crest donor site, and the patient's ability to cooperate in orthodontic preparation. The use of rhBMP-2 in children necessitates redesign of the surgical process.

Engineering Bone-Forming Constructs in the Primary Dentition

The mechanism that directs the path of tooth eruption is poorly understood. Alveolar development is controlled by the process of tooth development. Regardless of how the path and rate of tooth eruption are controlled, the process results in a net anabolic state adjacent to the tooth, allowing the volume of the alveolar process to increase. The alveolar process of the posterior maxillary segments form under the same mechanism. In the patient with an alveolar cleft, the bone adjacent to the cleft forms and is maintained under the influence of the developing teeth.

Initially, the process of eruption results in growth of the alveolar housing. After the tooth has erupted, the functioning periodontal ligaments act on the bone to provide stimulation and regulation of remodeling. The mechanisms that successfully formed the bone adjacent to the clefts can be recruited to improve the healing response to bone grafting.

Engineering parameters that direct the design of the bone-forming construct must be understood and applied for the best response. Manipulation of the tissue and graft material requires care and technical ability. The success of the treatment depends on the optimal combination of *(1)* engineering—the best understanding of the underlying physical and biologic mechanisms governing the creation of the defect and the patient's response to surgery; *(2)* design—application of basic science to determine what type of environment and arrangement of materials will heal toward the desired result; and *(3)* construction—surgical manipulation of tissues and graft materials in a manner that will minimize short-term healing problems and long-term growth impairment.

Case description

A 4-year-old girl with bilateral cleft lip and palate presented for management (Fig 5-9a). Other than the lip closure, which had been performed when the child was 12 weeks of age, no other treatment had been provided. There was no osseous continuity between the incisive bone and the maxilla (Fig 5-9b). The oronasal fistula extended to the right and left vestibules and across the palate.

A diagram shows how the developing teeth were responsible for the development of the existing alveolar bone volume (Fig 5-9c). The incisive bone was connected to the face by the labial gingiva and the nasal septum. Radiographs revealed cleft discontinuities (Figs 5-9d and 5-9e). The developing permanent teeth were still completely covered with bone.

Design of any bone-forming construct begins with an appreciation of the defect itself. Rather than focusing on the obvious cleft gaps, it is more valuable to study the surroundings (Fig 5-9f). The incisive bone formed because it had all of the essential elements to develop and maintain a morphologic steady state. Muscle-related neuromuscular input was lacking, but the developing teeth served as the signaling mechanism.

Fig 5-9 Engineering bone-forming constructs in the primary dentition.

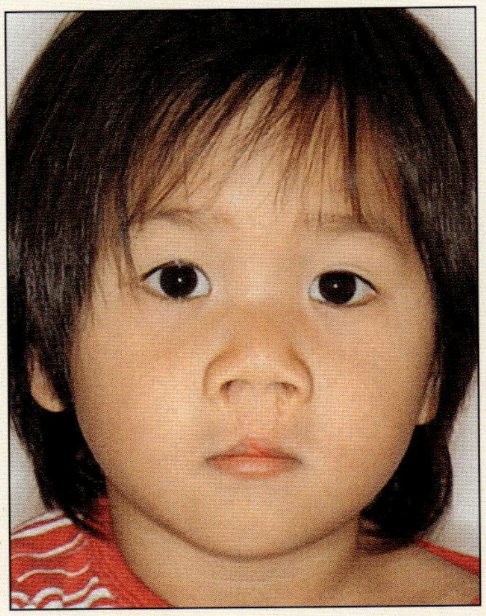

Fig 5-9a A 4-year-old girl with bilateral cleft lip and palate presents for long-term management of maxillary clefts, oronasal fistula, and dental development.

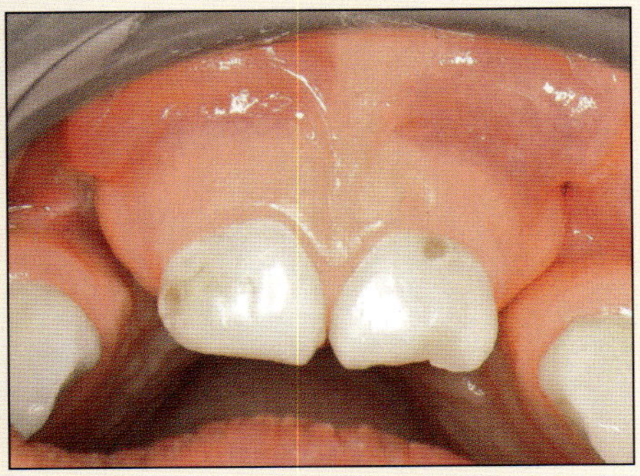

Fig 5-9b The patient exhibits typical oral features of bilateral maxillary clefts, including a mobile premaxilla and missing primary lateral incisors.

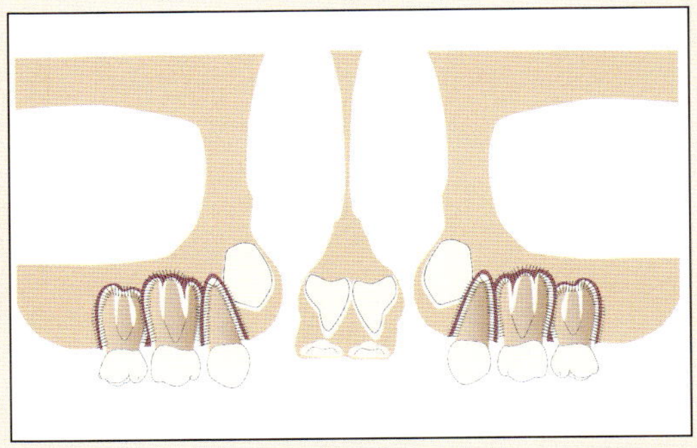

Fig 5-9c Analysis of the functional skeletal anatomy that regulates this defect shows that the bone has developed in response to dental eruption.

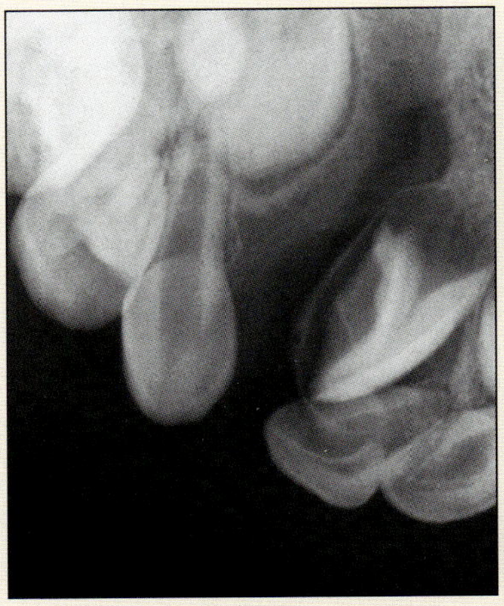

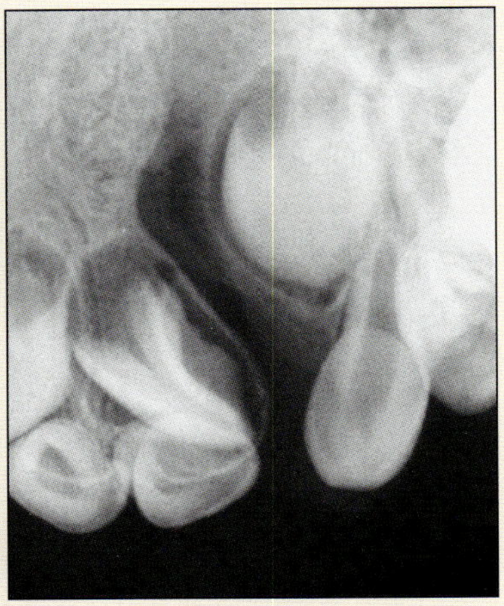

Fig 5-9d *(far left)* A radiograph of the right cleft reveals that the alveolar process has developed vertically in response to eruption of the primary teeth. The permanent central incisor and permanent canine are positioned to continue alveolar bone development following the exfoliation of the primary teeth. The discontinuity defect at the cleft fails to grow bone because there is no tooth to provide neuromuscular signal through its periodontal ligament–Sharpey fiber network.

Fig 5-9e *(left)* A radiograph of the left cleft shows a development process parallel to that of the right side.

→

Surgical exposure of the left cleft revealed the extent of the osseous deficiency. Mucosal flaps were elevated, advanced, and sutured to close the oronasal fistula (Fig 5-9g). Creation of a physical barrier between the nasal cavity and the potential site of new bone formation was part of the design of the bone-forming construct. Nasal flora and secretions must be isolated from the regeneration chamber to prevent contamination and infection.

Elevation of the nasal and oral mucosa exposed a portion of the gap in the maxillary bone. The bone that faced the discontinuity had been formed by the development and eruption of the primary central incisors and canine teeth. The interaction of these teeth and the alveolar bone was critical to bone formation, maintenance, and remodeling of the skeleton as it presented.

Before the surgeon considers how to fill the cleft void, he or she must understand what forces can be recruited from the surroundings. When a bone-forming construct is designed to grow a skeletal unit across a cleft, the stimulating input from teeth is critical. In this patient, immediately after surgery, the primary teeth would be most important. As the patient and maxilla developed over several years, the permanent teeth would be the important stimulating force.

To create the roof and palatal wall of the regeneration chamber, mucosa was elevated from the cleft margins, rotated as flaps, and sutured (see Fig 5-9g). The rhBMP-2 graft was extended to fill the entire defect, including the piriform rim and extension of the cleft at the hard palate. The remaining labial aspect was used for access to place rhBMP-2 carried on ACSs to fill the chamber volume (Figs 5-9h and 5-9i).

The palatal mucosa cleft was closed in two layers. The deep aspect of the palatal flap was approximated with buried 4-0 polyglactin 910 sutures. The mucosa was then closed with interrupt-

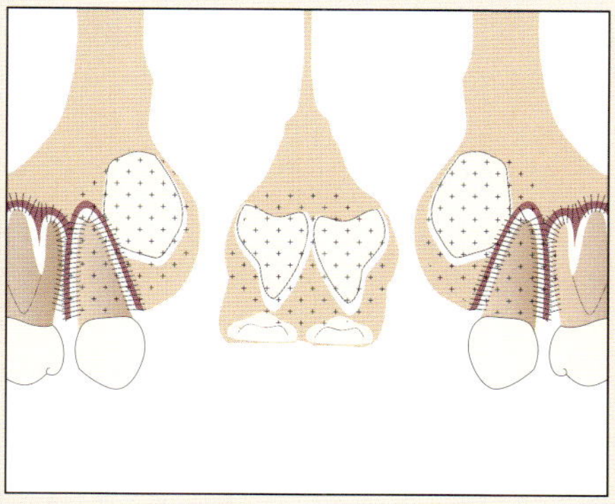

Fig 5-9f Working skeletal development environments surround the erupting teeth. The clefts are volumes that lack the essential elements to form bone. Existing regulatory signaling is derived from the periodontal ligament systems (+++++).

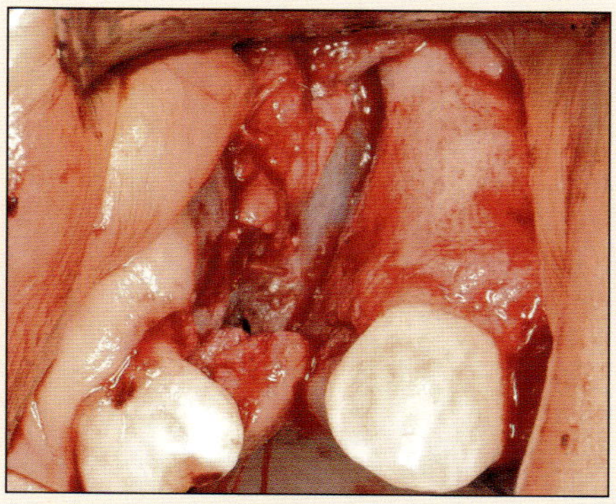

Fig 5-9g Surgical repair of the left cleft exposes the skeletal boundaries of the cleft. The nasal mucosa has been elevated and sutured to create a bone-forming chamber that is isolated from nasal secretions and bacteria. Bone that overlies the primary canine and primary central incisor roots is supported by the periodontal ligament systems of these teeth.

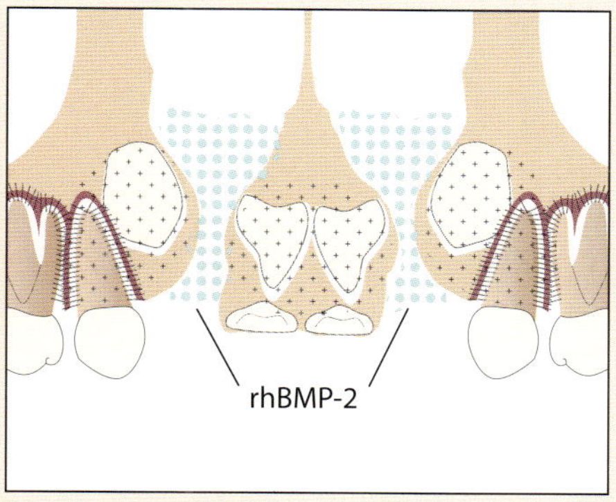

Fig 5-9h The surgical strategy is to use rhBMP-2 to deliver cells to the bone-forming chamber.

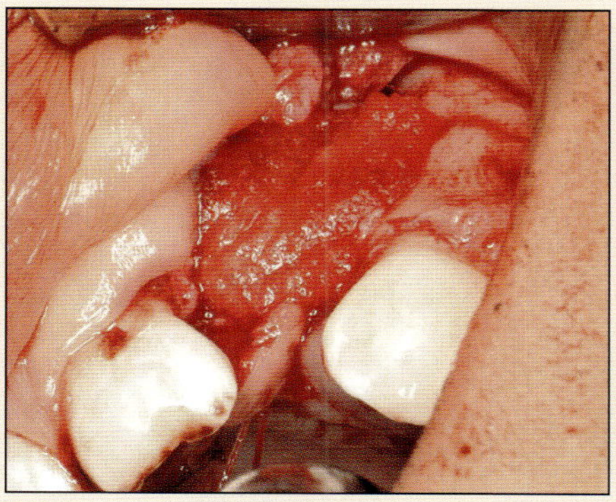

Fig 5-9i A collagen sponge carrying rhBMP-2 fills the gap between the cleft margins.

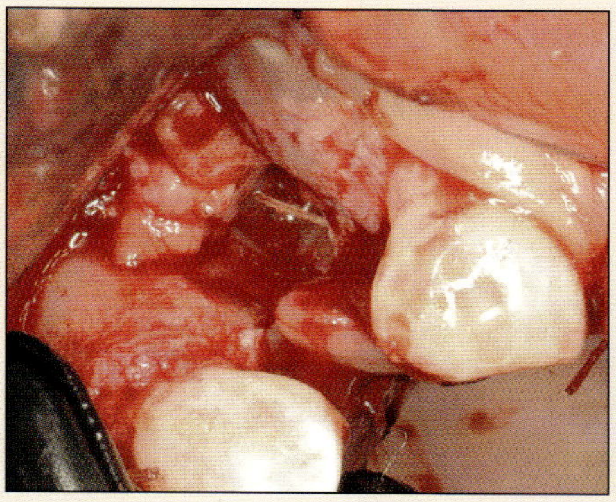

Fig 5-9j The right cleft is managed in the same manner. The bone overlying the roots of the teeth adjacent to the cleft is being regulated by the periodontal ligaments. These ligaments deliver neuromuscular signals to the bone to promote growth.

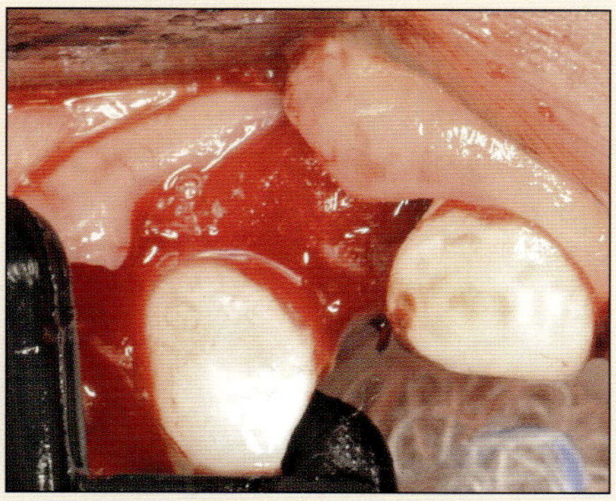

Fig 5-9k A collagen sponge carrying rhBMP-2 is used to fill the chamber created by advancement of the mucosal flaps.

→

ed 3-0 polyglactin 910 sutures that were visible. The rhBMP-2/ACS device was positioned to fill the skeletal discontinuity (see Fig 5-9i). The dose of rhBMP-2 was 2 mg for each cleft.

The right cleft was repaired with similar closure. Visible 4-0 polyglactin 910 sutures closed the nasal floor and palatal mucosa (Fig 5-9j). These sutures were covered by the rhBMP-2 graft. A collagen sponge carrying 2 mg of rhBMP-2 was positioned to fill the cleft discontinuity (Fig 5-9k).

The fabricated surgical construct was a hybrid of anabolic and catabolic activity (Fig 5-9l). Elevation of mucoperiosteal flaps exposed bone at the cleft margins. This initiated a resorptive process. Resorption removed the thin cortex at the repair site, exposing the medullary portion of the alveolus. Simultaneously, the rhBMP-2/ACS device recruited immature cells to the regeneration chamber. These cells were directed down a bone-forming lineage by the rhBMP-2, the influence of the exposed erupting teeth, or both. The net effect was to preferentially form bone rather than fibrous tissue.

The suture lines that overlay the rhBMP-2 sponges healed well (Figs 5-9m and 5-9n). During the initial phase of rhBMP-2 healing, the ACS sponge resorbed and the chamber was filled with new vessels and immature tissue (Fig 5-9o). The physical chamber environment was maintained by the bone adjacent to the clefts and the soft tissue closure at the oral mucosa and nasal floor. In this initial period, there was little neuromuscular input from the teeth, and total resorption of the graft was a risk.

As the paper-thin cortex overlying the developing teeth was resorbed, the young tissue established in the regeneration chamber came under the influence of the teeth and their periodontal ligament systems (Fig 5-9p). Responding to an unknown mechanism, the teeth migrated toward the newly formed, immature bone.

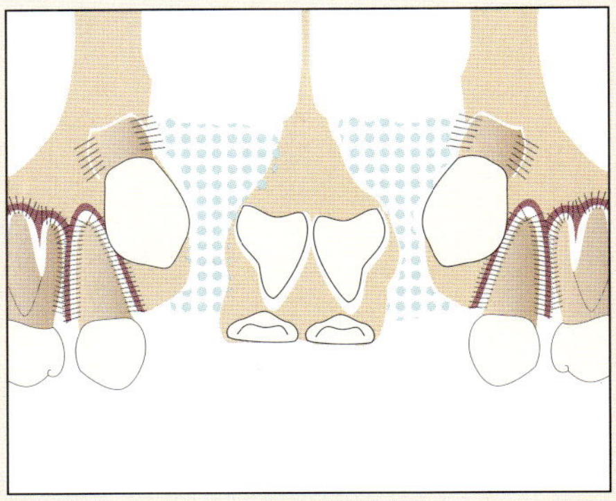

Fig 5-9l The rhBMP-2 draws cells with bone-forming potential into the cleft site. As the bone overlying the roots demineralizes, the Sharpey fibers from the periodontal ligament system come into contact with the amorphous cell mass derived from the rhBMP-2. The Sharpey fibers have the potential to introduce neuromuscular regulation to the environment, which contains cells that require direction to organize into a functional skeletal unit.

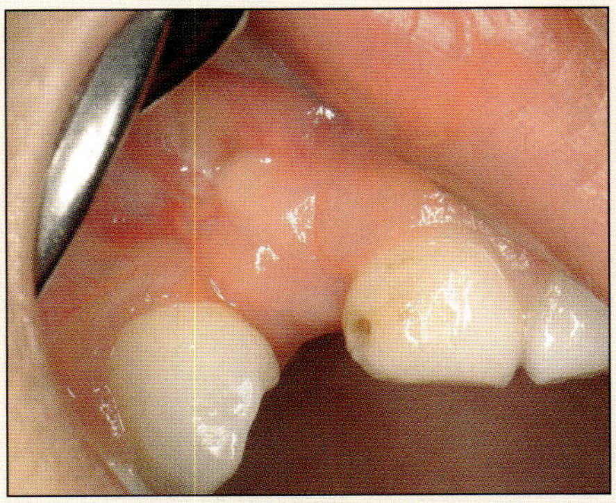

Fig 5-9m After 2 months, the mucosa of the right cleft has healed over the rhBMP-2 graft.

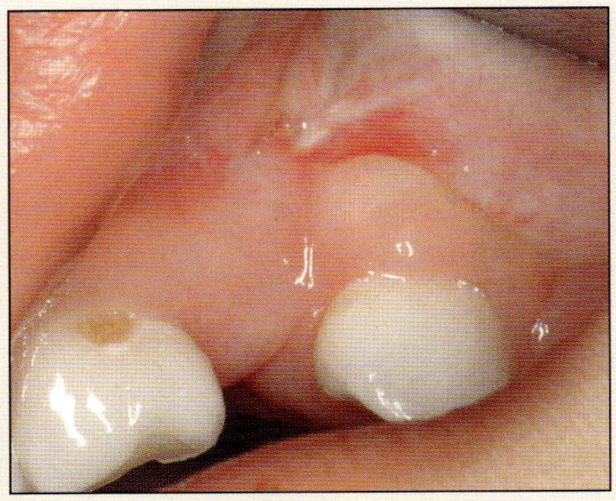

Fig 5-9n The mucosa of the left cleft has also healed, eliminating the oronasal fistula.

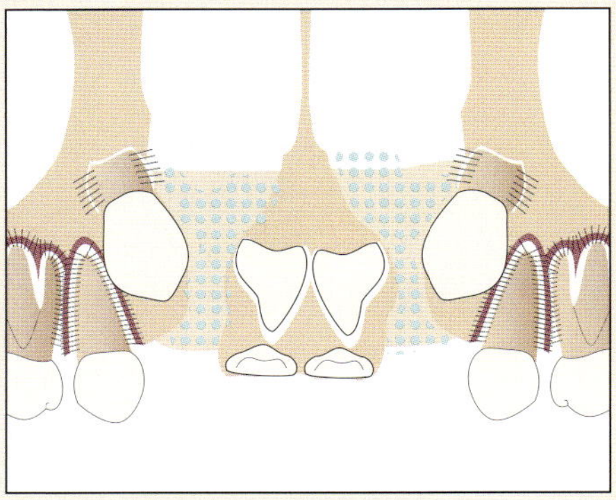

Fig 5-9o The initial response of the rhBMP-2 depends on limited neuromuscular signaling derived from the periodontal ligaments of the adjacent teeth. If the teeth are not healthy or the width of the cleft is large, the intensity of stimulation may be lacking.

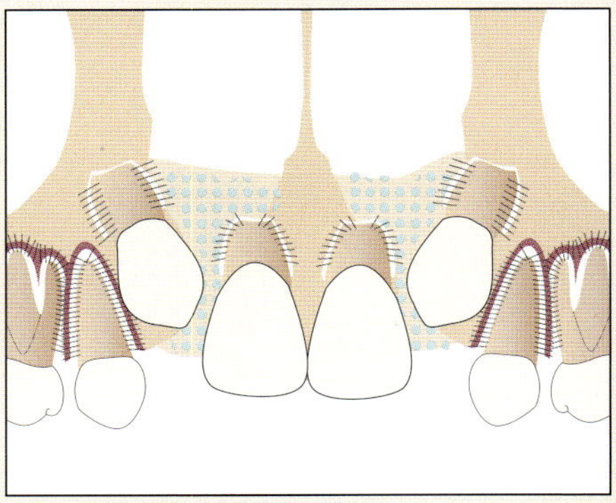

Fig 5-9p The thin cortex overlying the roots demineralizes, and the periodontal ligament system is opened to the regeneration chamber. The mechanism that causes bone to grow in response to dental development is now available to promote growth and organization of the graft.

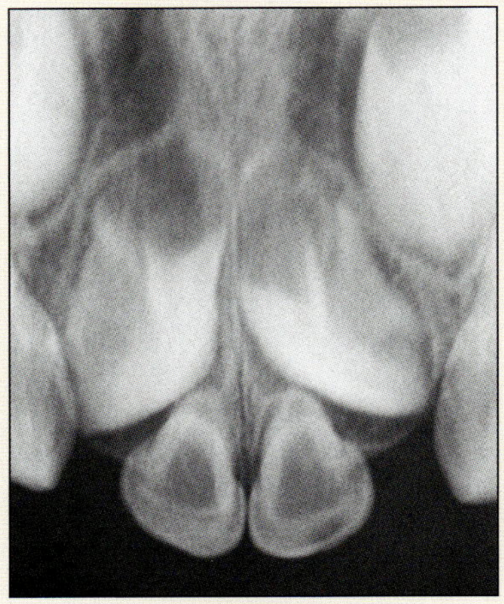

Fig 5-9q Six months after placement of rhBMP-2 in the maxillary clefts, the defects are filled and teeth have migrated into the new bone volume.

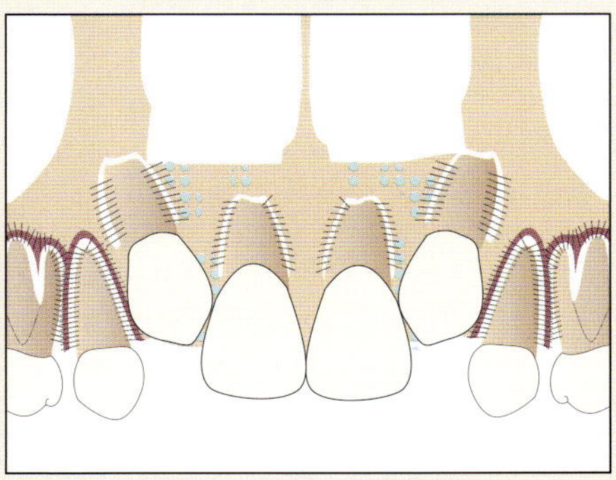

Fig 5-9r The new volume of bone allows normal dental eruption and subsequent normal maxillary development.

→

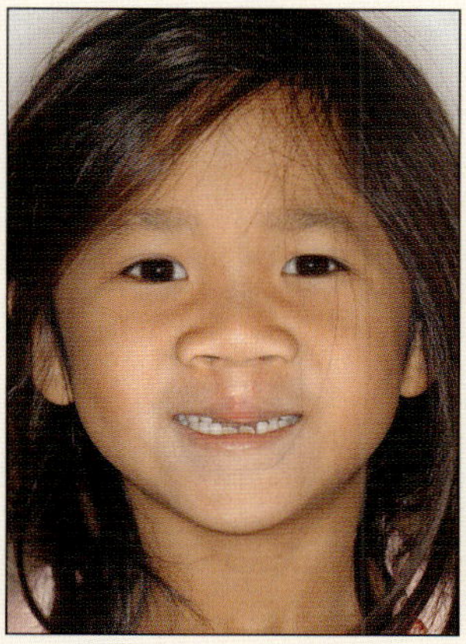

Fig 5-9s The facial appearance of the patient 2 years after surgery is good. The child is now 6 years old.

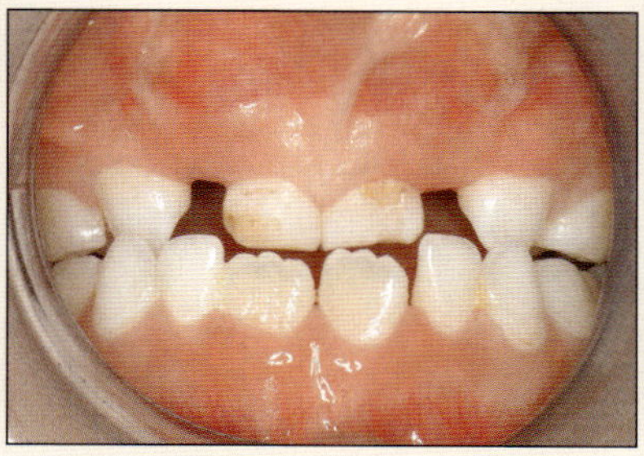

Fig 5-9t The dental arches have continued to develop without orthodontic treatment.

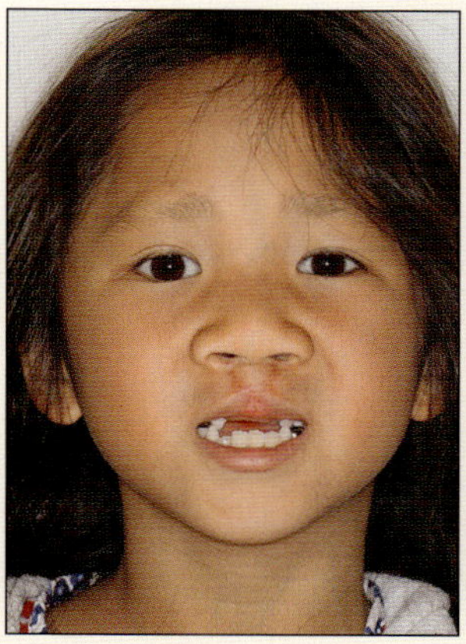

Fig 5-9u The patient's facial appearance continues to be satisfactory 3 years after surgery. The child is now 7 years old.

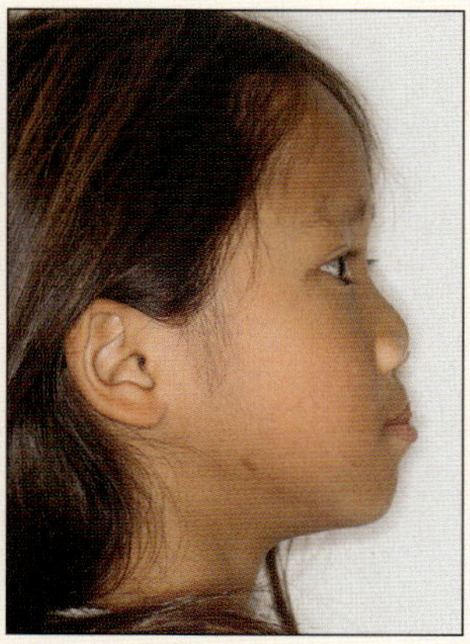

Fig 5-9v The facial profile has been maintained by growth in the absence of orthodontic treatment.

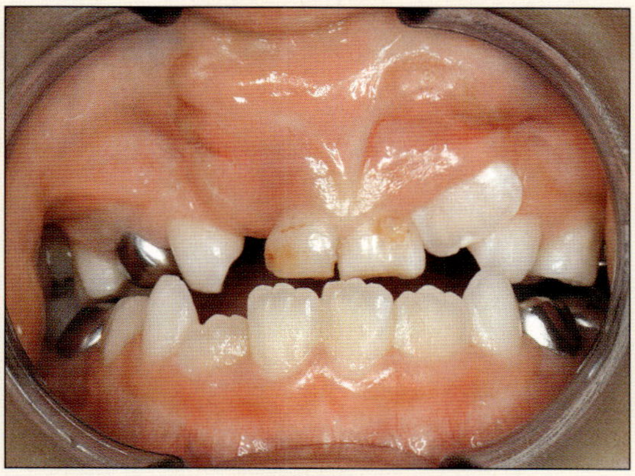

Fig 5-9w Dental arch development has been obstructed by abnormal eruption of the central incisor.

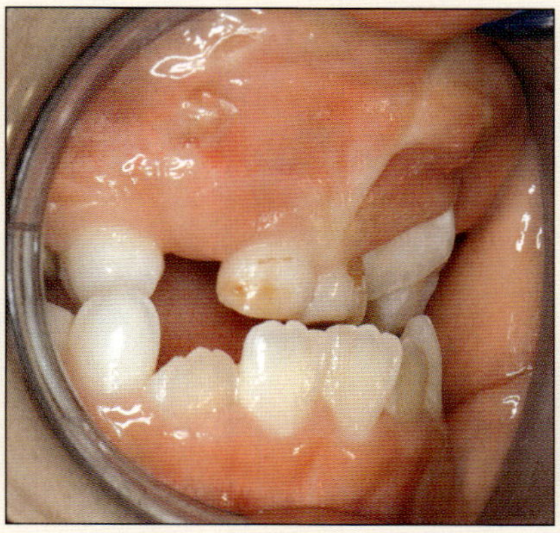

Fig 5-9x The reconstructed alveolar process provides a continuous volume to house the developing permanent teeth.

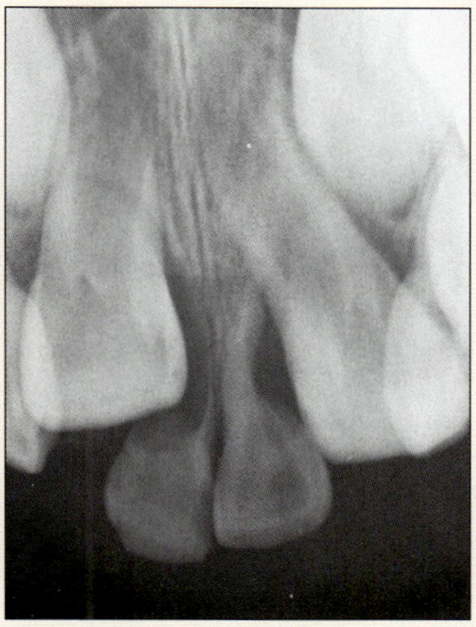

Fig 5-9y A radiograph taken at 7 years of age shows that the permanent central incisors have erupted into the space of the missing lateral incisors. The primary central incisors have been retained.

→

A radiograph taken 6 months after rhBMP-2 grafting revealed that, as the canine teeth repositioned themselves into the bone construct, the new bone tissue responded to the interaction by organization (Fig 5-9q). This initiated a lifelong interaction between the teeth and the bone construct. This interaction was the desired integration of the synthesized skeletal unit into the patient's global physiology. The treatment was not a simple fill of a missing skeletal part. To be successful over the long term, the construct had to be able to participate in the complex regulatory process that maintains morphology in a relative steady state for a lifetime.

The newly established bone volume provided the permanent teeth with a place to erupt and form a complete dental arch (Fig 5-9r). The teeth interacted with the bone to regulate growth, structural organization, and maintenance of morphology.

Two years after surgery, the patient's facial appearance was good and the dental arches had developed without orthodontic intervention (Figs 5-9s and 5-9t). At age 7 years—3 years after surgery—the patient still had a good facial appearance (Figs 5-9u and 5-9v). Ectopic eruption of the permanent left central incisor required intervention (Figs 5-9w and 5-9x). A radiograph taken at 7 years of age showed that the permanent central incisors had erupted into the space of the missing lateral incisors (Fig 5-9y). The primary central incisors had been retained. The primary central incisors were therefore removed to provide a space for the permanent central incisors.

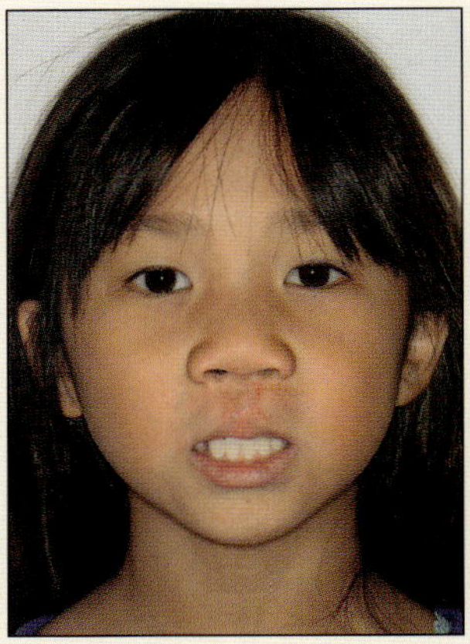

Fig 5-9z The facial appearance of the child at 9 years of age, 5 years after cleft repair with rhBMP-2. No orthodontic treatment has been done.

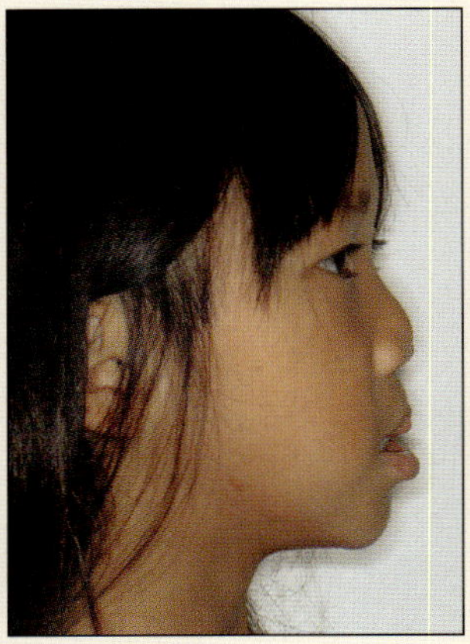

Fig 5-9aa The facial profile shows a tendency toward midfacial retrusion, but the deficiency is limited.

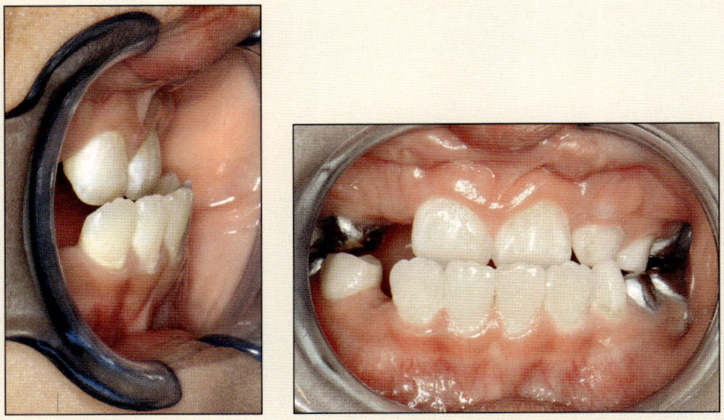

Figs 5-9bb and 5-9cc The occlusion is now Class III. However, the central incisors have erupted and assumed a normal midline position without orthodontic treatment.

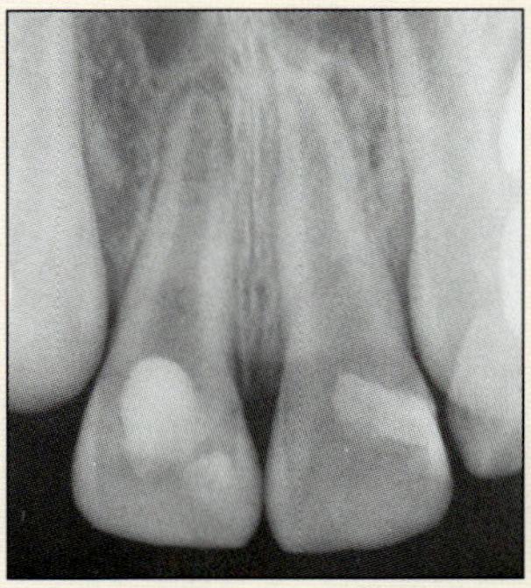

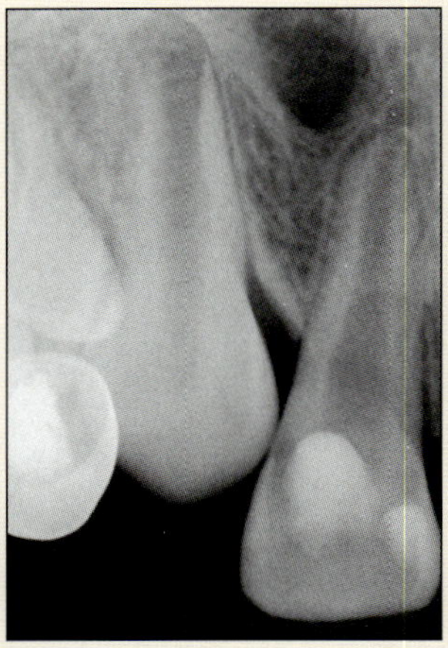

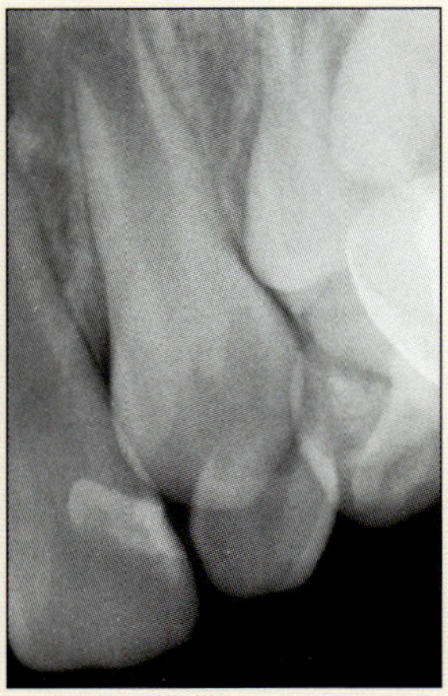

Fig 5-9dd *(far left)* The central incisors have well-developed roots, and the permanent canines have positioned themselves into the lateral incisor sites.

Fig 5-9ee *(left center)* The right alveolar cleft repair site shows normal bone volume and architecture. Both teeth have a well-defined lamina dura, and the trabecular pattern shows that the bone volume is a well-integrated structural ossicle.

Fig 5-9ff *(left)* The repaired left cleft exhibits normal structures and teeth with well-formed roots. The prior presence of the cleft discontinuity is not evident.

The patient was evaluated at age 9 years, 5 years after repair of the bilateral clefts with rhBMP-2 (Figs 5-9z and 5-9aa). The facial profile showed a tendency toward midfacial retrusion. The magnitude of the deficiency was limited, and the etiology was difficult to determine accurately. The state was the net result of the inherent bilateral cleft disorder, repair of the lip and palate, rhBMP-2 repair of the alveolar clefts, congenital absence of maxillary lateral incisors, and lack of any orthodontic treatment.

The occlusion was now Class III. Five years after rhBMP-2 repair, the central incisors had erupted and assumed a normal midline position without orthodontic treatment (Figs 5-9bb and 5-9cc). The central incisors had well-developed roots, and the permanent canines had positioned themselves into the lateral incisor sites (Fig 5-9dd). Radiographs of the alveolar cleft repair sites revealed normal bone volume and architecture (Figs 5-9ee and 5-9ff). Both teeth had a well-defined lamina dura, and the trabecular pattern showed that the bone volume was a well-integrated structural ossicle.

Discussion

These synthesized skeletal constructs are successful because they are engineered to include the essential elements to form and maintain bone. A treatment solution designed and constructed in this manner results in a skeletal unit that is self-assembling in that the environment directs structural organization and maintenance.

Most patients with cleft lip and palate are missing teeth. Typically, the maxillary lateral incisor is missing at the site of the cleft. In some cases, the missing tooth is replaced by a dental prosthesis. The prosthesis may take the form of a removable prosthesis, a tooth-supported fixed prosthesis, or an implant-supported crown. As an alternative, the canine tooth can be directed to erupt into the site of the missing lateral incisor.

Regardless of the treatment course elected, bone must be constructed to eliminate the discontinuity representing the osseous cleft. Grafting procedures with autogenous bone or bone morphogenetic proteins are clinically viable options. With either option of grafting technology, the result will be best if natural eruption of teeth occurs at the cleft site.

Fig 5-10 Bone construction for placement of implants in cleft sites.

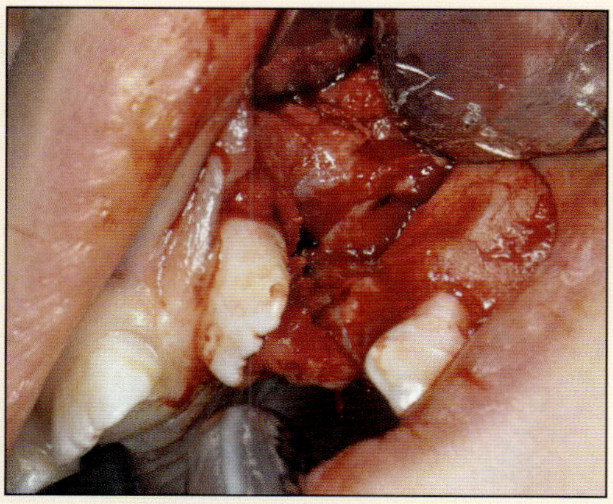

Fig 5-10a A unilateral cleft lip and palate is present in a 7-year-old girl. The surgical plan is to close the oronasal fistula and grow bone across the skeletal discontinuity of the maxillary cleft.

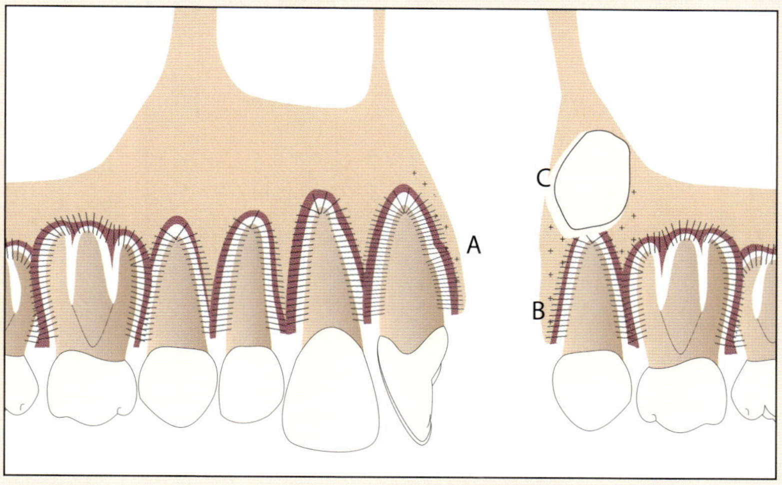

Fig 5-10b Functional analysis of the existing skeleton reveals that the bone at the anterior wall of the defect (A) developed and is maintained under the regulation of the periodontal ligament system of the maxillary left central incisor. Sharpey fibers from the periodontal ligament penetrate the thin layer of bone covering the central incisor root. On the lesser maxillary segment, the bone facing the cleft is under the regulation of the periodontal ligament system of the primary canine (B). At the level of the missing piriform rim, the developing permanent canine (C) is moving to a position that will increasingly influence the bone architecture in its eruption path.

→

Bone Construction for Placement of Implants in Cleft Sites

Natural eruption of teeth results in the formation of bone. The process also promotes optimal organization of the bone that develops. Children with cleft lip and palate are most often missing the lateral incisor at the cleft site. Many orthodontists prefer to form the maxillary dental arch, leaving the missing lateral incisor site open for prosthetic replacement. Dental implants are most often recommended for replacement of the missing lateral incisor tooth.

Two major challenges are associated with this treatment plan. First, the discontinuity defect at the cleft site must be repaired along with closure of the oronasal fistula. Second, a dental implant must be successfully osseointegrated in the synthesized bone segment. Successful osseointegration of the dental implant requires adequate bone volume and normal bone physiology. If this type of treatment plan is to achieve success, preparation of the future implant site must consider both the quantity and quality of the bone segment to be constructed. The following case demonstrates a method to manage these cases in a way that will provide a predictable result.

Case description

A 7-year-old girl with unilateral cleft lip and palate presented for repair of the cleft. The mother's sister had a cleft lip and palate, so the family was knowledgeable about the range of treatment options for repair of the cleft and for replacement of the missing lateral incisor. The teeth adjacent to the cleft were intentionally maintained in an unrotated position (Fig 5-10a). This allowed maintenance of the thin alveolar bone covering the roots facing the cleft discontinuity. The cleft was a funnel-shaped defect in which the width increased at the superior aspect, the nasal base. The nasal mucosa was rotated medially and superiorly and closed primarily with 4-0 polyglactin 910 sutures.

When a procedure to construct bone across a congenital discontinuity is designed, it is important to understand the regulatory mechanisms that have formed and maintain the defect (Fig 5-10b). These same forces will participate in the healing of the graft. In this patient, the osseous cleft walls were formed and maintained by the teeth adjacent to the cleft. The thin layer of bone that covered the root of the maxillary left central incisor was under the regulation of the periodontal apparatus of the tooth. The bone on the distal side of the cleft was regulated by the erupted premolar and unerupted canine. These bone segments had stable cortices and existed in a steady state. The

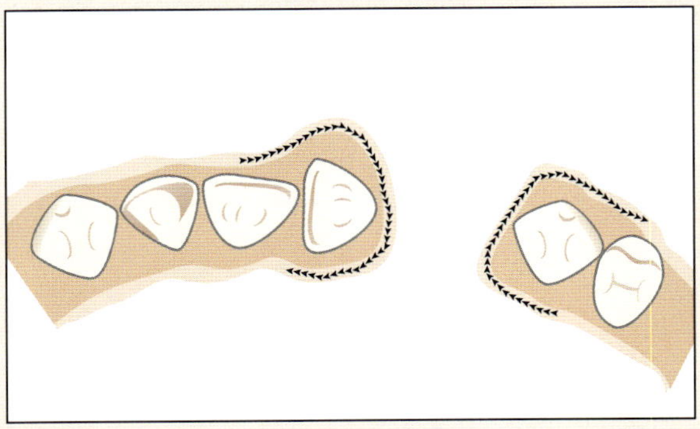

Fig 5-10c From an occlusal viewpoint, the discontinuity is bounded on the mesial and distal walls by well-defined cortical plates. These cortical structures have formed in response to the mechanical forces of the environment and the neuromuscular regulation imposed by the adjacent periodontal ligament systems.

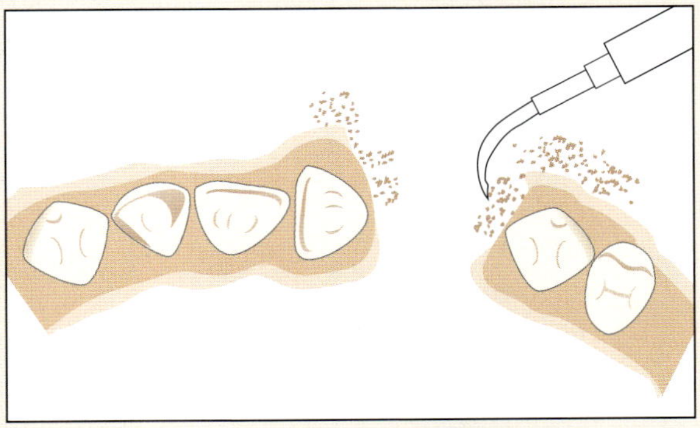

Fig 5-10d Piezosurgery is used to disrupt the integrity of the cortical plates so that the regulatory forces from the periodontal ligament systems can be directed to the graft site.

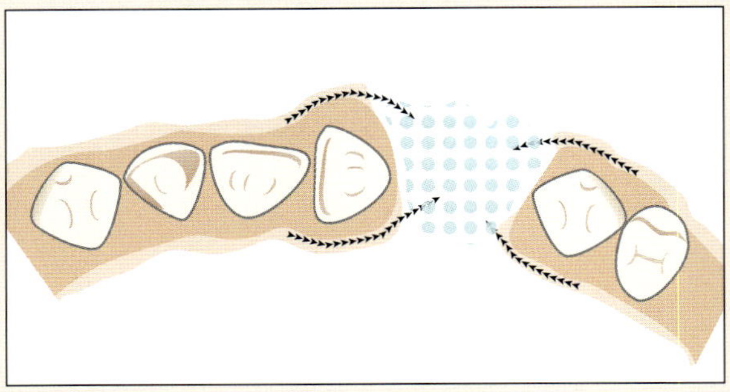

Fig 5-10e Cells introduced to the cleft repair site by rhBMP-2 can be regulated by the exposed Sharpey fibers extending from the periodontal ligaments.

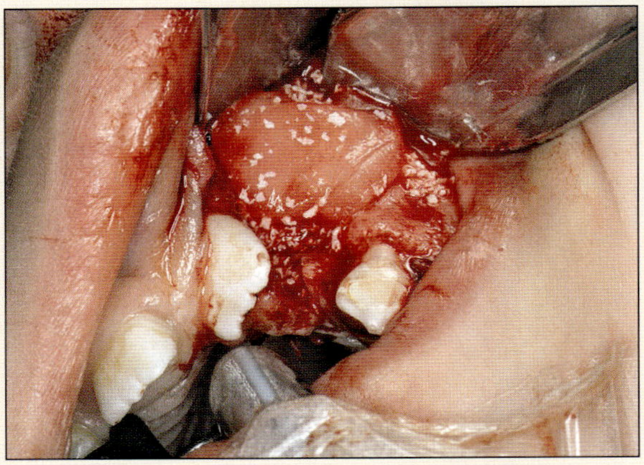

Fig 5-10f The collagen sponge containing rhBMP-2 is intended to introduce cells to the site.

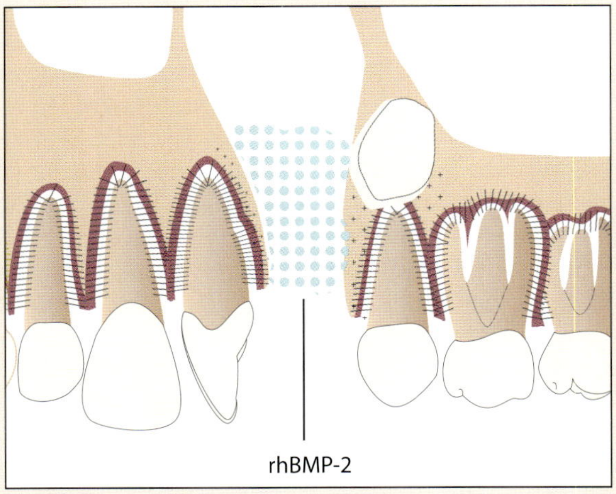

Fig 5-10g After elevation and closure of the mucosal flaps and placement of rhBMP-2, demineralization of the exposed bone allows the regulatory signals to enter the graft site. Existing regulatory signaling is derived from the periodontal ligament systems (+++++).

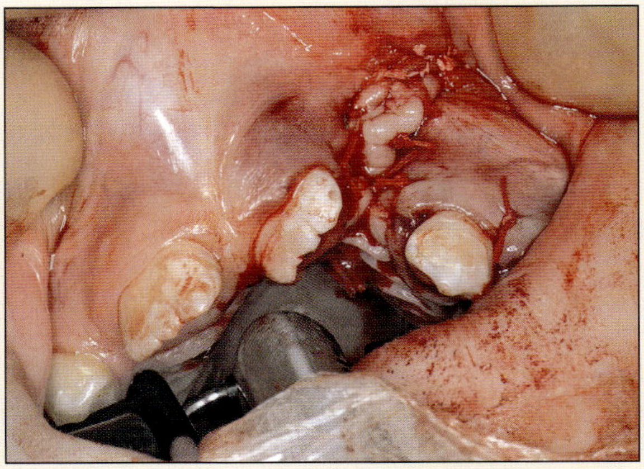

Fig 5-10h Primary closure of the oral and nasal floor mucosa creates a barrier from secretions and bacteria.

→

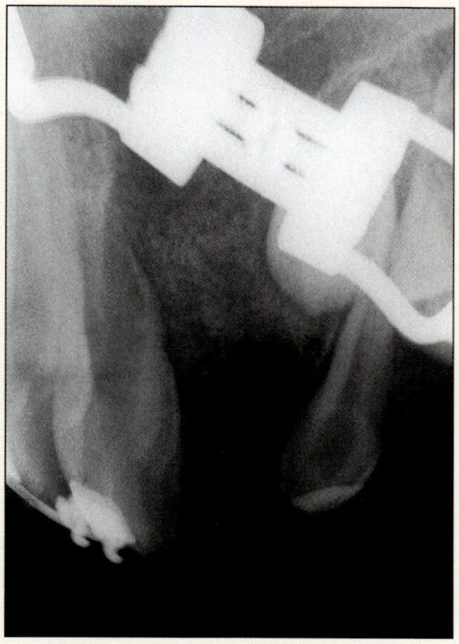

Fig 5-10i A radiograph taken 8 weeks after surgery shows bone filling the cleft site. There is little evidence that the bone is functional or organized.

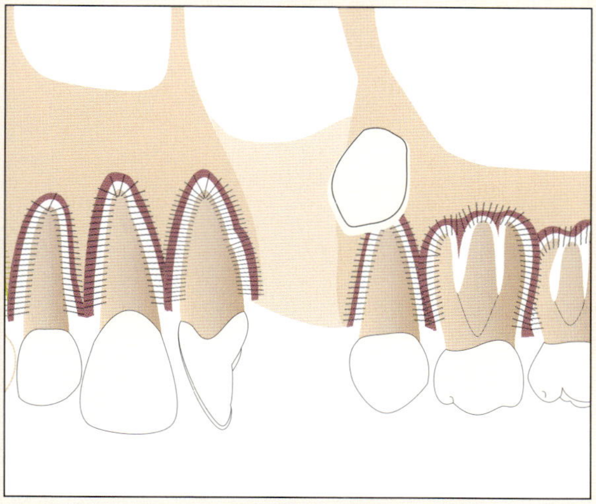

Fig 5-10j Bone fills the alveolar cleft discontinuity.

→

functional forces at the site were distributed within these established structures. The existing cortical plates surrounding the walls of the cleft contained and directed the signaling forces generated by the teeth, muscle attachments, and secondary deformation of the bone under function (Fig 5-10c). The net effect of these functional parameters was a relatively steady state manifested by the presenting skeletal morphology.

If a new morphology was to be developed, the forces that maintained the old form had to be redirected. A piezoelectric surgical instrument was used to remove the cortical bone of the walls of the cleft (Fig 5-10d). The autogenous bone harvested with the piezoelectric surgical instrument was placed as part of the graft.

Removal of the shielding effect of the cortical plates allowed the regulatory signals to be redirected to the graft. These signals were necessary to direct cells introduced by rhBMP-2 to form bone (Fig 5-10e). It was also important to direct the new bone to organize into a skeletal unit that was fully integrated into the skeleton.

The cleft defect was filled with a collagen sponge carrying rhBMP-2 reconstituted at 1 mg/mL (Fig 5-10f). The total dose of rhBMP-2 at this cleft site was 2 mg. Bone harvested from the cleft site and left lateral portion of the maxilla was used as an autogenous graft.

The rhBMP-2 graft was contained within a mechanically stable chamber. The teeth and their periodontal ligament systems housed within the walls of the cleft were a source of neuromuscular signaling to the graft chamber (Fig 5-10g). Exposure of the medullary space by decortication of the cleft walls enhanced the ability of rhBMP-2 to draw bone precursor cells to the bone construction site. The mucosal flaps over the rhBMP-2–containing collagen sponges were closed (Fig 5-10h).

A radiograph obtained 8 weeks after surgery showed development of immature bone (Fig 5-10i). The chamber constructed at the cleft site had the essential components to develop bone (Fig 5-10j). The chamber was mechanically stable and shielded from major disrupting forces. The rhBMP-2 drew cells to the chamber and promoted differentiation toward a bone-forming phenotype. The adjacent and erupting teeth provided neuromuscular-like stimulation to the immature cell mass. The signaling from the adjacent teeth promoted organization of the new bone into a functional skeletal unit.

The canine tooth erupted through the newly formed bone (Fig 5-10k). As the tooth passed into and through the constructed bone, the effect was to modify and organize its architecture. The result was that the volume of the constructed bone increased and the trabecular architecture was refined. A continuous, structural labial cortex developed under the regulation of a newly formed, continuous periosteum (Fig 5-10l).

A radiograph taken at the 3-month follow-up revealed the left canine erupting through the graft into the site of the lateral incisor (Fig 5-10m). As it descended, the periodontal apparatus moved through the graft. The effect on the graft site was to promote volume expansion and maturation of the medullary architecture (Fig 5-10n). Although the orthodontic plan was to open a space at the site of the missing lateral incisor for placement

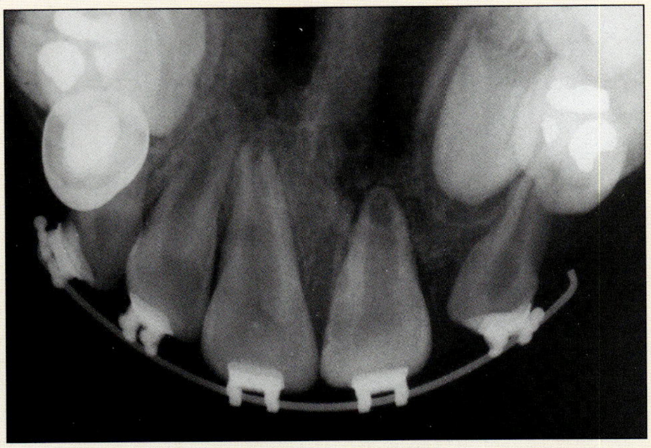

Fig 5-10k A follow-up radiograph taken 10 weeks after surgery shows the permanent canine erupting into the lateral incisor site.

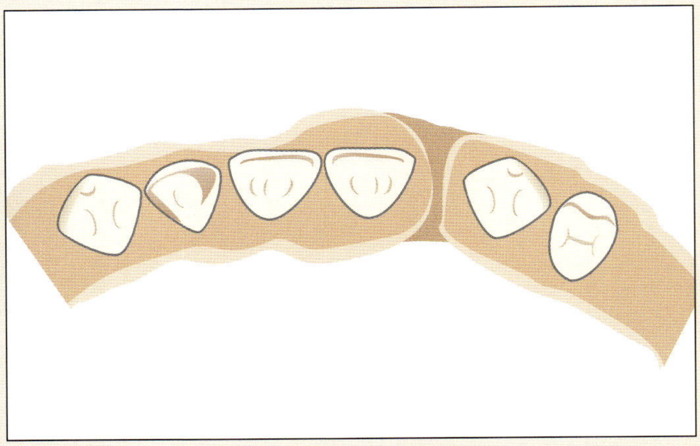

Fig 5-10l Full organization of the constructed alveolar bone segment remains incomplete because it has not been organized by the effects of tooth eruption.

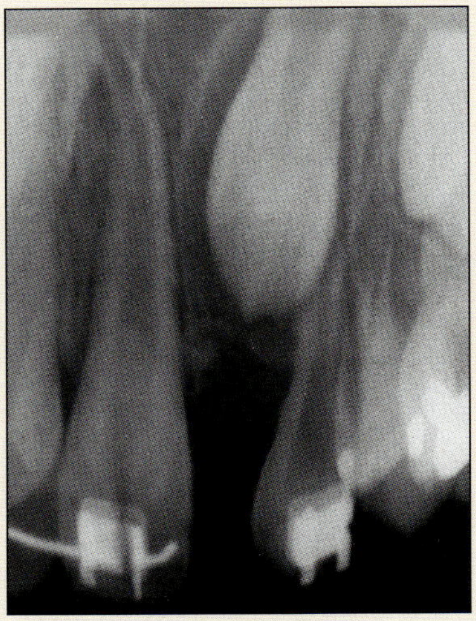

Fig 5-10m The maxillary canine is allowed to erupt normally into the lateral incisor position. The process completes the organization of the bone and allows it to mature into a fully functional skeletal unit.

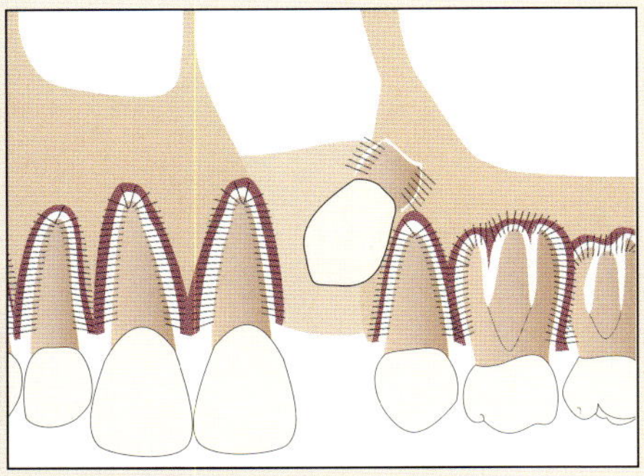

Fig 5-10n The long-term plan is to open a space for a lateral incisor implant, but the canine is allowed to erupt into the lateral incisor site.

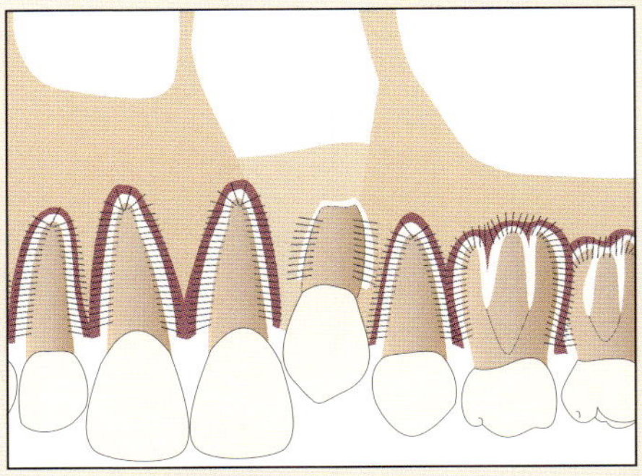

Fig 5-10o With the canine in the lateral incisor position, the structural architecture of the site is completed. This includes the trabecular architecture of the medullary space and the periodontal ligament–Sharpey fiber network surrounding the tooth.

→

of a dental implant, the canine tooth was first directed to erupt into the site of the lateral incisor. This allowed the alveolar bone to mature completely (Fig 5-10o).

Ten years after repair of the alveolar cleft and eruption of the canine into the lateral incisor position, the patient returned for placement of a dental implant (Figs 5-10p and 5-10q). She had undergone another course of orthodontic treatment (Fig 5-10r).

Orthodontic treatment had opened a space at the site of the lateral incisor for placement of a dental implant (Fig 5-10s). This treatment involved moving the canine tooth distally. The lateral incisor site was suitable for placement of the implant (Fig 5-10t). The process of allowing the canine to erupt into the lateral incisor site and then distalizing the canine to its anatomical location allowed full maturation of the bone graft and soft tissue (Fig 5-10u).

Unlike most alveolar bone grafts that have been left for 10 years before implant placement, this site had an adequate quantity and quality of bone and soft tissue for successful osseointegration treatment (Fig 5-10v). The alveolar bone was of good height and width (Fig 5-10w). Distal movement of the canine left behind a volume of bone that had the opportunity to mature and organize.

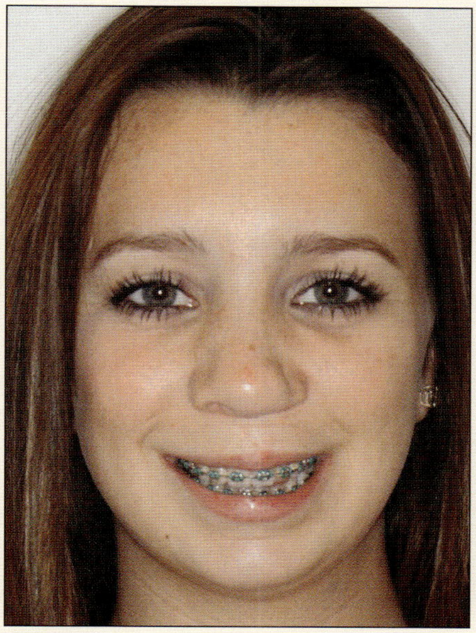

Fig 5-10p Ten years after alveolar cleft repair with rhBMP-2, the patient is 17 years of age.

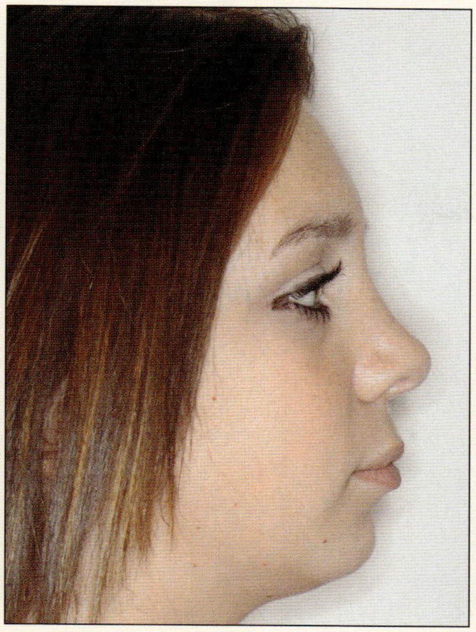

Fig 5-10q Her facial profile shows good maxillary growth.

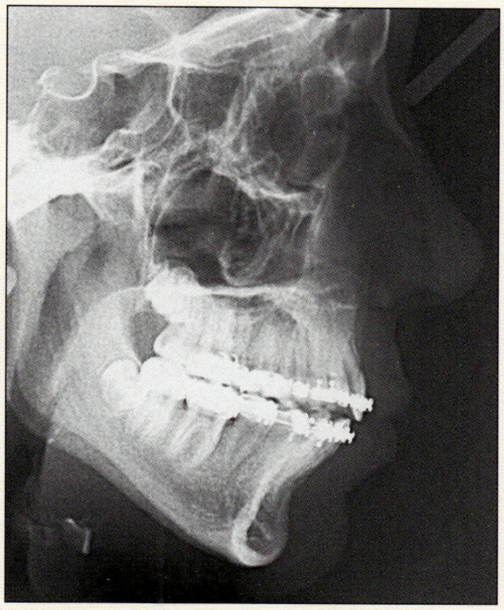

Fig 5-10r The lateral cephalometric radiograph reveals good maxillary projection.

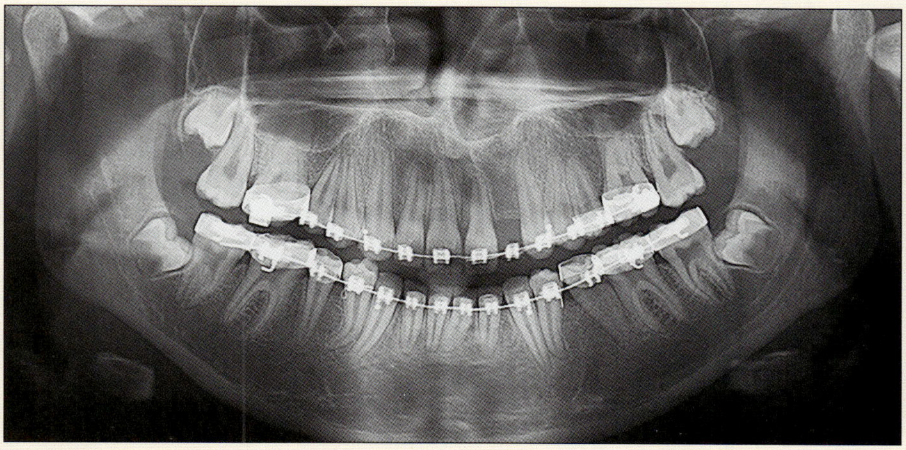

Fig 5-10s The maxillary left lateral incisor site has been opened by orthodontic means.

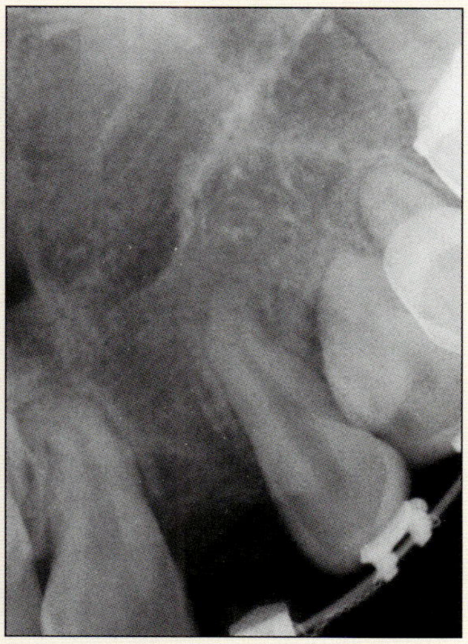

Fig 5-10t The cleft site has been replaced by a skeletal unit with normal functional architecture.

A dental implant was placed to support a single crown (Fig 5-10x). The maturation process created an implant site that required no special surgical or restorative management.

Discussion

When placement of dental implants is planned at alveolar cleft sites, a good implant site requires deliberate sequencing of surgery and orthodontics. If alveolar bone grafting is performed when the patient is 8 years old and the space is left edentulous for 10 years, the site is unlikely to be in an ideal state for implant placement. Augmentation of alveolar cleft repair sites with onlay grafts often provides disappointing results because of multiple challenges specific to the cleft palate disorder. For example, the cleft is the center of a developmental field deficiency, so that even the adjacent existing alveolar bone is affected.[15,16] Simple autogenous grafts placed to repair alveolar clefts are not fully organized unless the volume has experienced dental eruption.

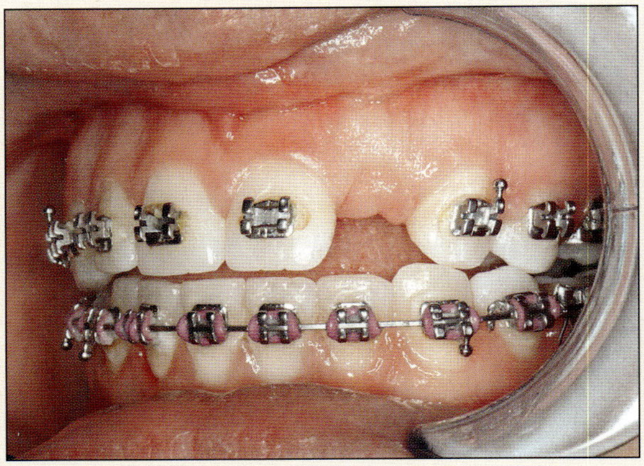

Fig 5-10u Under the influence of the canine eruption into the lateral incisor site, the alveolar housing has developed a normal structure.

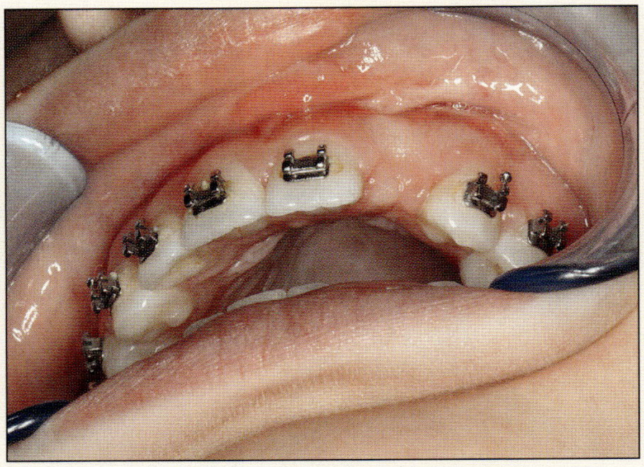

Fig 5-10v The site is suitable for placement of a dental implant.

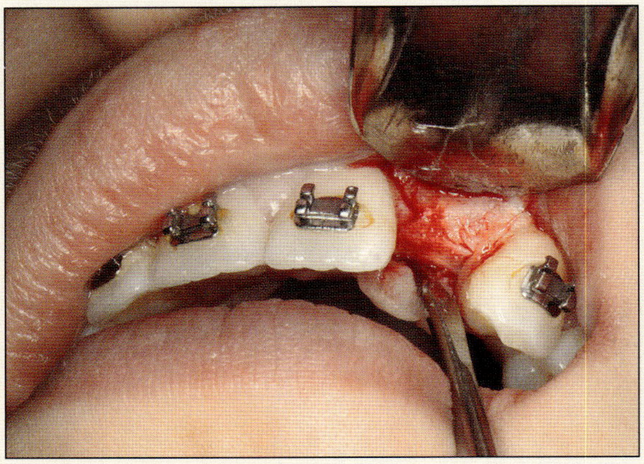

Fig 5-10w The site shows good bone height and normal attachment levels on the adjacent teeth.

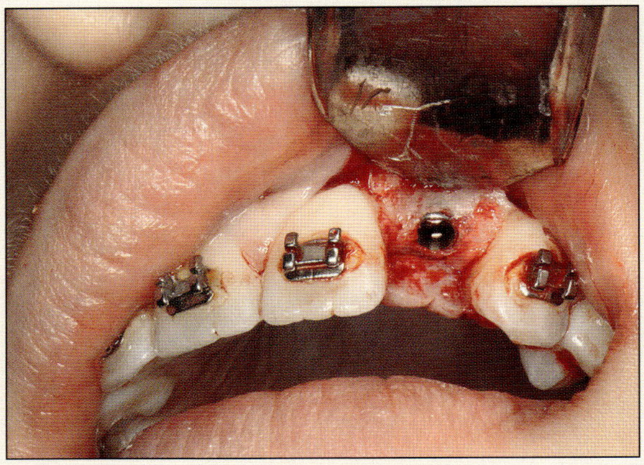

Fig 5-10x A dental implant is placed. The plan is to restore the implant with a single-tooth restoration.

In addition, orthodontic treatment for the Class III tendency often present in patients with clefts places teeth adjacent to the cleft in an expanded and protracted position. In some cases, the presence of teeth positioned labially in the alveolus might benefit healing of an onlay graft. More commonly, there is a degree of periodontal damage to the teeth adjacent to the cleft that will compromise the healing environment.

A major challenge to successful onlay grafting of alveolar cleft repair sites is a deficient quantity and quality of overlying soft tissue. Even if an implant can be placed, there is often a substantial esthetic compromise. Thoughtful sequencing of these cases can avoid many of these obstacles to successful treatment.

Conclusion

Development of the teeth and their functional attachment via ligaments to the surrounding bone has a stimulating and regulating effect on the alveolar bone. Although Sharpey fibers have long been recognized as the interface between bone and skeletal muscle, in recent years the role of Sharpey fibers in the development, growth, maintenance, and repair of bone has become clearer. It is evident that this system is also important in the repair of skeletal injuries and participates in the process of healing after surgical procedures. Thoughtful incorporation of these processes in surgical designs can substantially improve healing and extend the limits of the treatments that surgeons can offer to their patients. An approach that combines dental development, rhBMP-2, and surgical design modifications can be used in children to manage alveolar defects related to cleft lip and palate.

References

1. Holmstrup P. Anatomy of the periodontium. In: Wilson TG Jr, Kornman KS (eds). Fundamentals of Periodontics, ed 2. Chicago: Quintessence, 2003:21–38.
2. Sicher H. The principal fibers of the periodontal membrane. The Bur 1954;55:2–4.
3. Aaron JE. Periosteal Sharpey's fibers: A novel bone matrix regulatory system? Front Endocrinol (Lausanne) 2012;3:98.
4. Aaron JE, Skerry TM. Intramembranous trabecular generation in normal bone. Bone Miner 1994;25:211-230.
5. Urist MR. Bone: Formation by autoinduction. Science 1965;150:893–899.
6. Harvold EP. The theoretical basis for the treatment of hemifacial microsomia. In: Harvold EP, Vargervik K, Chierici G (eds). Treatment of Hemifacial Microsomia. New York: Alan R. Liss, 1983:1–37.
7. Chen CS, Ingber DE. Tensegrity and mechanoregulation: From skeleton to cytoskeleton. Osteoarthritis Cartilage 1999;7:81–94.
8. Ingber DE. Tensegrity: The architectural basis of cellular mechanotransduction. Ann Rev Physiol 1997;59:575–599.
9. Ingber DE. The architecture of life. Sci Am 1998;278:48–57.
10. Ingber DE. Opposing views on tensegrity as a structural framework for understanding cell mechanics. J Appl Physiol 2000;89:1663–1670.
11. Ingber DE. Tensegrity. II. How structural networks influence cellular information processing networks. J Cell Sci 2003;116:1397–1408.
12. Ingber DE. Tensegrity. I. Cell structure and hierarchical systems biology. J Cell Sci 2003;116:1157–1173.
13. Ingber DE. Tensegrity and mechanotransduction. J Bodyw Mov Ther 2008;12:198–200.
14. Ingber DE. Tensegrity-based mechanosensing from macro to micro. Prog Biophys Mol Biol 2008;97:163–179.
15. Carstens MH. Neural tube programming and craniofacial cleft formation. I. The neuromeric organization of the head and neck. Eur J Paediatr Neurol 2004;8:181–210.
16. Carstens MH. Neural tube programming and the pathogenesis of craniofacial clefts. I. The neuromeric organization of the head and neck. Handb Clin Neurol 2008;87:247–276.

6 Using Osteotomies to Generate Bone in Defects of Local Origin

Osteotomy is an important technique in the design and fabrication of bone-forming constructs. When employed properly, osteotomy and repositioning of fragments can create an environment that will support new bone growth and its long-term maintenance. The effects of these procedures alter more than the physical shape of the skeletal unit. When applied properly, the process can change the structural and physiologic dynamics of the region to the advantage of the treatment goal. Disruption of the existing bone architecture offers the opportunity to redirect force distribution within the skeleton to maintain morphology of a new steady state. The result is a new skeletal unit that is integrated into the patient's functional anatomy.

Repositioning of functional elements such as muscle attachments and teeth changes the physiology of the entire region. These potential changes must be engineered into the planned objective of the new bone construct.

Although osteotomy is only a part of a comprehensive bone reconstruction strategy, it is useful to examine the process as a separate topic. There is a wide range of applications of osteotomy in which bone reconstruction is the objective. There are also specific technical challenges that have to be managed. Precision repositioning is required to meet both functional and esthetic objectives. A practical method to achieve safe and predictable repositioning of osteotomy segments is an essential part of surgical design.

This chapter addresses the use of osteotomy as part of a bone-forming construct to manage bone loss with local etiology. Use of osteotomy to manage bone loss complicated by the presence of systemic disorders will be addressed in chapter 7.

Box 6-1 Objectives of osteotomy for the design of bone-forming constructs

- Expand the boundaries and potential volume of the bone-forming environment
- Redirect the existing balance between structural bone and neuromuscular regulation
- Expose the existing cancellous bone to the regeneration chamber, allowing access to cells, growth factors, and mechanical signaling
- Reposition muscle attachments so their effects can be recruited into the new bone construct
- Reposition teeth and their periodontal apparatus so they can be recruited into the neuromuscular signaling process of the new bone construct
- Position bone volume so that it can be properly loaded by osseointegrated implants
- Alter the occlusion to allow creation of self-protective occlusal patterns
- Provide an opportunity to improve esthetic balance of facial morphology

Objectives of Osteotomy for the Design of Bone-Forming Constructs

Within the practice of maxillofacial surgery, osteotomies have become synonymous with orthognathic surgery. Surgeons are therefore familiar with the surgical techniques. Osteotomies performed for most orthognathic procedures have improvement of occlusion or esthetics as the primary goal. Planning and performing osteotomies for the purpose of meeting the design objectives of bone-forming constructs requires additional thought.

From a mechanical standpoint, orthognathic surgery involves creating a discontinuity of the existing skeleton and then moving the mobilized segment to a different position. In general, vascular supply to the bone fragment is maintained by way of a local pedicle. The mobilized fragment may be as small as a segment of the alveolus or as large as the entire midface and orbits. The method of repositioning and fixation may involve intraoperative movement and immobilization with internal hardware. When the movement distance exceeds the confines of the soft tissue pedicle, gradual transport of the segment via distraction osteogenesis may be required.

To optimize the potential of osteotomies as part of the bone reconstruction strategy, it is necessary to look beyond the traditional purpose of osteotomy as it is used in orthognathic surgery. The term *orthognathic* means "to straighten the jaws." The name is derived from its precursor in facial bone surgery as a solution to trauma-related fractures. Experience gained in trauma surgery was eventually extended to management of developmental anomalies. Combined surgical and orthodontic collaboration became orthognathic surgery. The traditional role of osteotomies and orthognathic surgery evolved into a treatment process to alter the physical shape of the facial skeleton to one judged to be more desirable. Included in the list of treatment objectives were occlusion, esthetics, mastication, speech, and jaw mechanics.

The effect of muscle function on the reconfigured skeleton was most often regarded as an obstacle to successful treatment.[1] Relapse was blamed on the action of muscles on the healing skeleton. The recruitment of muscles to support bone formation was not considered as part of conventional surgical design.

The inclusion of osteotomies as part of the bone reconstruction process requires rethinking how these procedures change the physiology of the skeletal system (Box 6-1). Osteotomies allow repositioning of skeletal segments. This process is clear and easy to understand. Traditional orthognathic surgery uses osteotomies to move jaws or jaw segments into positions to meet objectives of function, occlusion, and esthetics. However, movement of skeletal segments has multiple effects that extend beyond the apparent. Rather than to simply alter the shape of the skeletal system, osteotomies for bone reconstruction must create an environment that contributes to bone formation. In addition, the environment must support long-term stability. The resultant bone construct must be able to maintain a steady state over many years. To meet this goal, it is necessary to create a bone construct that is fully integrated into the regulatory support system. Creation of a supportive environment is equally as important as repositioning bones and teeth in a desired shape.

Distraction is a special type of orthognathic surgery. Distraction technology was developed to extend the distance osteotomy fragments could be moved safely. The basic objectives of distraction are the same as orthognathic surgery. The additional benefits important to engineering bone constructs are also the same as with conventional orthognathic surgery. When distraction is incorporated in a bone-forming strategy, the benefit of distance and volume must be balanced against the challenge of precision movement and the complexity of the devices.

Relationship Between Osteotomy and Bone-Forming Constructs

Creation of mechanically stable environments

Bone forms best in an environment of relative mechanical stability. Conventional onlay grafting to raise the vertical height of the alveolar ridge is challenging for multiple reasons. Grafting material placed under elevated mucosa is vulnerable to mechanical forces from the oral cavity. Movement of block or particulate grafts is associated with resorption and failure.[2]

An alternative strategy is to create an osteotomy and elevate the fragment via distraction or immediate repositioning. This process has multiple effects on the bone-forming environment. First, the elevated and fixed bone creates a sheltered chamber at the distraction site. Cells filling the chamber are protected from harmful mechanical forces that are associated with formation of fibrous connective tissue instead of bone.

A second important consequence of osteotomy for ridge elevation is destabilization of the existing architecture. Prior to osteotomy, the skeleton at the deformity site exists in a stable state. Although deficient for the purposes of dental implant placement, the structure itself is self-maintaining. The morphology is being maintained by balanced resorption and deposition under some type of physiologic regulation.

Although the regulatory mechanism is still incompletely understood, the fact that the morphology is able to maintain itself within the dynamics of natural remodeling is evidence that a regulatory strategy exists. The manner in which the physiologic and mechanical processes operate is reflected by the anatomy itself. In the posterior region of the mandible, there is always an external cortex and an internal medullary space. Mechanical integrity of the mandibular body depends on the ability of the intact, circumferential cortex to resist the forces that are distributed.

If mechanical signaling is important in both formation and maintenance of bone, then forces should be directed through the bone-forming construct. Osteotomy disrupts the existing force distribution and allows it to be redirected to the advantage of the bone construct. Disruption of the existing force-distribution pattern is critical to engineering a strategy to exploit the mechanical signaling forces to the benefit of the bone-forming chamber.

A third consequence of osteotomy is the ability to position appropriate bone and soft tissue at the site at which they will be needed during subsequent reconstruction. For example, when cortical plates are elevated for the purpose of posterior mandibular augmentation, mature, viable cortical bone with attached gingiva ends up in the position of the desired new alveolar ridge. Because the bone is already cortical, there is no need for remodeling and healing to convert a cancellous structure into a cortical one.

Establishment of desired alveolar ridge morphology is also part of the engineering design. Normal atrophy of the posterior mandibular ridge is uneven. In general, the lingual aspect of the remaining ridge is taller than the labial side. Dental implants are geometric devices that work best when the insertion site is level. Rotation of the osteotomy segment prior to transport via fixation or distraction allows engineering of a level surface for future implant placement.

Recruitment of neuromuscular input

Designing neuromuscular elements into bone-forming environments is challenging and unfamiliar territory for most oral surgeons. Understanding the role of neuromuscular signaling mechanisms in bone formation is one challenge for the modern surgeon. Incorporating these processes in the surgical design is another obstacle. Osteotomies are critical to the fabrication of bone-forming environments that have appropriate neuromuscular elements.

Scientific understanding of how neuromuscular signaling regulates bone growth and maintenance is incomplete but evolving. Muscle action and the periodontal apparatus of teeth are the most useful sources for introducing neuromuscular regulation to maxillofacial reconstructions at this time.

Muscle delivers regulatory signaling to the skeleton at the point of attachment and to the immediately adjacent area. To be useful in the bone-forming construct, a muscle attachment must exist at the site of reconstruction or be repositioned there. A segment of bone that includes a contained muscle attachment is mobilized through osteotomy and then repositioned. Detachment of muscle insertions from bone and attempted surgical reattachment to a distant site does not produce predictable results.

The objective of repositioning the bone segment and attached muscle is to direct the stimulating signal to the bone-forming chamber. Cells that fill the chamber experience direction by muscle action to form bone tissue and to organize into a functional skeletal structure. Small-level movement introduced by muscle action can result in metabolic changes in bone-forming cells within the chamber.[3] An orchestra of intracellular and extracellular processes result in the formation of bone tissue and its organization into a functional anatomical structure. The same pathway that maintains the steady state regulates morphologic stability long term.

A second vector for transmission of neuromuscular signaling involves teeth and their periodontal apparatus. Bone will form adjacent to erupting teeth. Healthy periodontal ligaments bridging living bone and teeth seem to stimulate bone formation and organization. It is likely that the action of the periodontal ligaments inserting into the alveolar lamina dura is similar to the mechanism of muscle insertions into bone. Both of these systems use Sharpey fibers to establish and maintain anatomical continuity with bone.[4]

Osteotomies can be used to move teeth and their periodontal ligament system into the regeneration chamber. The stimulation introduced by the periodontal structures results in development of bone tissue and organization into mechanical support systems. Another strategy is to use osteotomies or orthodontics to direct developing teeth to erupt through the regeneration chamber. This strategy is time intensive but effective. The erupting tooth improves the quality and quantity of bone through which

Fig 6-1 Use of osteotomy and distraction to create a bone-forming chamber for management of alveolar ridge deficiency.

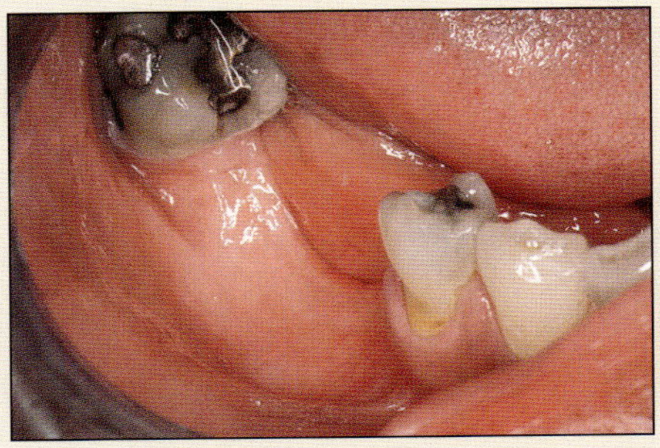

Fig 6-1a Typical mandibular posterior deficiency has developed secondary to tooth loss and atrophy.

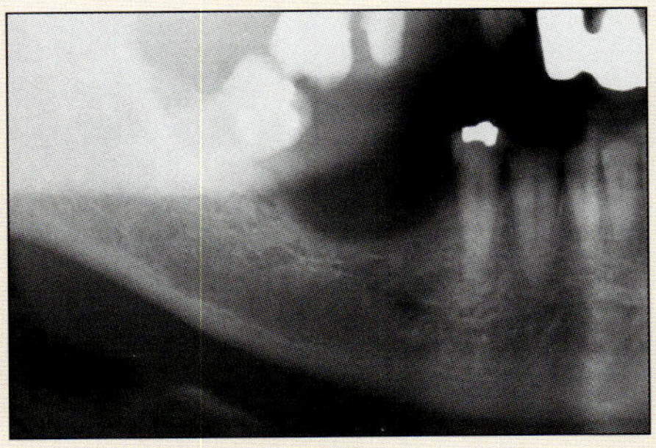

Fig 6-1b Minimal bone overlies the mandibular nerve.

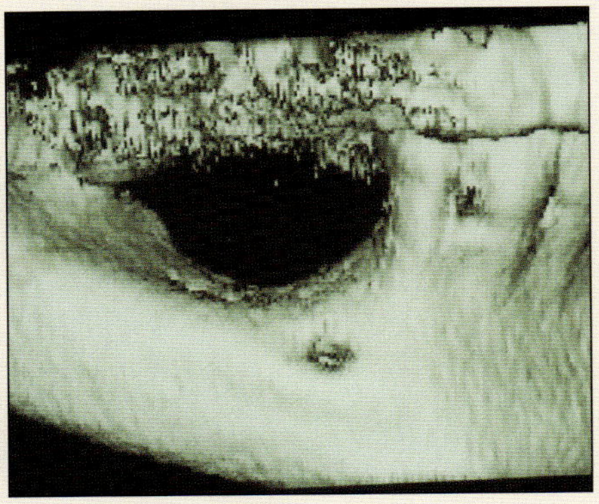

Fig 6-1c Cone beam computed tomography reveals the canted surface of the alveolar ridge.

→

it passes. Even if the tooth is subsequently lost or moved by orthodontics to a site outside the regeneration chamber, the volume and mature organization of the site remain.

There are neuromuscular elements that are beyond current understanding. There is probably a stimulation process working during sinus elevation surgery. Healthy sinus mucosa with normal cilia seems to allow better sinus graft healing than a sinus membrane that is atrophic and without cilia. Whether there is underlying neuromuscular control of sinus cilia is unknown. Does the coordinated motion of sinus cilia involve a mechanism within the individual cells? Is there central nervous system coordination of these cells? These aspects await further research.

Clinical Applications

The case reports in this chapter demonstrate the wide range of applications of osteotomy in bone reconstruction procedures.

Osteotomy to Create a Bone-Forming Chamber

The most basic application of osteotomies in the fabrication of bone-forming constructs is creation of a chamber in which bone can grow. The osteotomy establishes bone discontinuity. Two important goals are met when the continuity of the existing skeleton is disrupted. First, the mobilized segment offers the opportunity to open the potential space across the osteotomy and establish an intramedullary chamber. The space created is the potential regeneration chamber in which bone may fill. Changing the position of a bone fragment creates a space that is sheltered from excessive external forces.

Second, the osteotomy disrupts and redirects the distribution of mechanical forces within the structural bone. To be effective, the osteotomy must disrupt the existing structural configuration of the site to allow local neuromuscular signaling forces to enter the regeneration chamber. The inclusion of neuromuscular regulatory forces in the design of bone-forming environments is a factor that is easily overlooked. Some surgeons believe that graft material has inherent bone growth propensity and will mature without any external stimulus or regulation. To improve the efficacy and predictability of procedures to create skeletal units, it is important that all the factors that contribute to bone formation be optimized as part of the design and fabrication of the bone-forming construct.

The following case demonstrates the use of osteotomy and a distraction device to create a sheltered bone-forming chamber that was designed to increase the height of the alveolar ridge.

Case description

A patient desired dental implants to replace lost premolar and molar teeth. Years of atrophy had resulted in loss of the alveolar process and overlying soft tissue (Fig 6-1a). A radiograph confirmed that there was not enough bone superior to the inferior alveolar nerve to position dental implants (Fig 6-1b). Three-dimensional imaging showed that the crest of the alveolar ridge was canted (Fig 6-1c). The buccal aspect of the ridge was more vertically deficient than the lingual aspect.

A well-defined bone cortex surrounded the medullary space (Fig 6-1d). The buccal cortex showed less vertical atrophy than the labial side. The result was a cant of the superior cortex. A dental implant could not be placed in this bone site without additional bone volume, as a result of both the total vertical volume deficiency and the cant of the superior cortex (Fig 6-1e).

Before this anatomical unit could be modified, it was important to understand the forces that were working to maintain its existing morphology (Fig 6-1f). The atrophic mandible site existed in a steady state. Its morphology of atrophy was maintained as a balance between anabolic and catabolic processes. Regulation of these metabolic processes was partly controlled

Fig 6-1d *(right)* The cortical plate of the alveolar crest overlies a medullary volume. *Blue area* denotes the inferior alveolar nerve. B, buccal; L, labial.

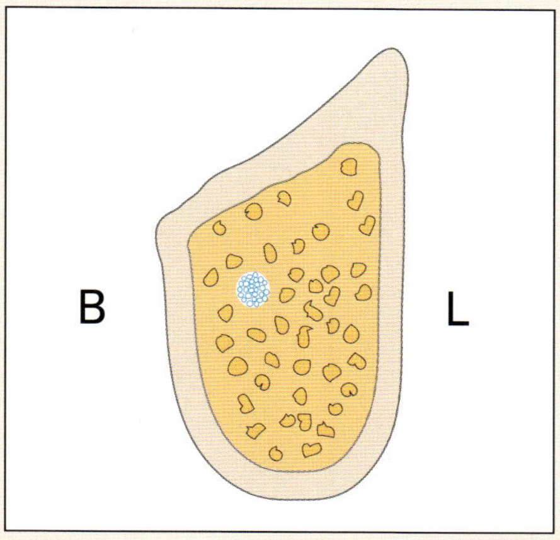

Fig 6-1e *(far right)* The cant of the ridge crest results in a greater need for vertical augmentation on the labial aspect. If placed into this deficient site, an implant would have insufficient bone coverage on its labial surface.

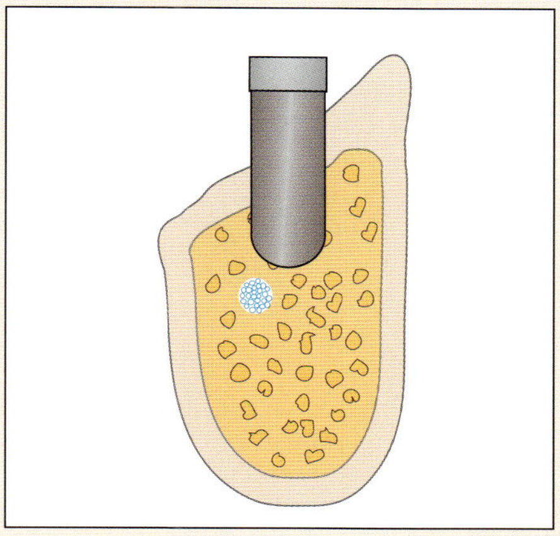

Fig 6-1f *(right)* Analysis of the functional anatomy of the site shows that mechanical forces are absorbed within the cortex that surrounds the mandible. Neuromuscular forces *(arrows)* are introduced to the site from all the muscles that insert on the mandible adjacent to this location. The existing state of atrophy is the net result of functional forces acting at the site. *Red line* denotes the periosteum.

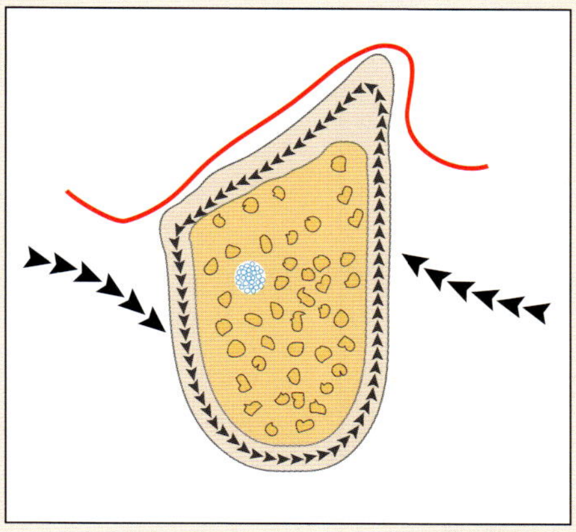

Fig 6-1g *(far right)* If a bone graft *(area under red line)* is placed at the ridge crest for augmentation, the mechanical forces *(arrows)* that determine the site morphology remain unchanged. The signals do not enter the new graft to promote incorporation into the functional anatomy.

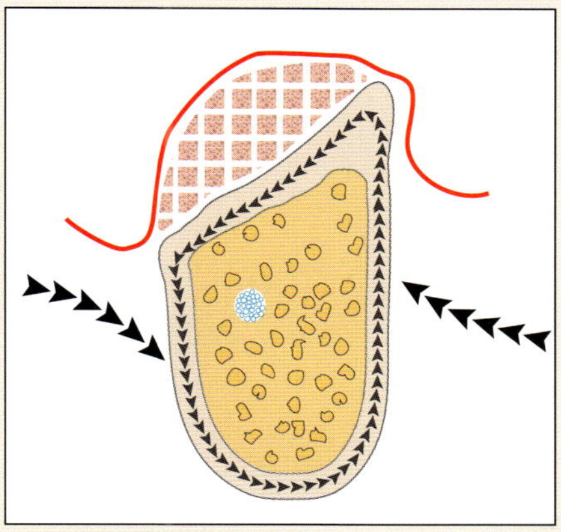

by mechanical signaling from muscles that exerted forces on the mandible. The mylohyoid muscle inserted directly into the lingual cortex adjacent to the potential implant site. Muscles controlled the motion of the mandible during mastication, swallowing, and speech.

The mandible is a semirigid structure that responds to forces of function with distortion. The magnitude of movement ranges from microns to millimeters. Movement causes changes at the tissue level and the cellular level. At the tissue level, the energy of distortion is absorbed by the structural trabeculae and dense cortex. Frost[5] described the relationship between mechanical load and structural bone adaptation. Ingber et al[3] described how physical distortion of individual cells alters their metabolism and may direct protein synthesis.

The cortex experiences these forces most directly. As forces result in slight deflection of the mandibular shape, energy is absorbed preferentially by the cortex. This is due to the peripheral geometry of the cortex as well as its mechanical qualities. If the bone deflects a given amount, the cortex distorts more than the central medullary bone. Sheer force may place the superior cortex in tension and the inferior cortex in compression. This can leave the center of the medullary bone at near-zero stress even though the mandible itself is under high stress. The modus of elasticity of the dense cortex is higher than that of the medullary bone. If the mandible is subjected to force, the energy rises rapidly in the cortex because its modus of elasticity will not allow it to yield to force by distorting easily.

The morphology of the jaw is a functional adaptation. Its process of regulation tends to favor preservation. In the case of maintenance, a steady state is a positive attribute. If the surgeon's objective is to change the existing morphology to one that is more desirable, it is necessary to disrupt the status quo and attempt to reset the steady state in a new configuration. Successful reconstruction, therefore, involves both disruptive and constructive activities.

Grafts are most often placed as onlays (Fig 6-1g). In this strategy, the mucosa is lifted, opening the potential space. Some type of graft material is then inserted under the soft tissue. The hope is that the graft will turn into living bone and then become incorporated into the functional physiology of the site. If the existing regulatory system involving the intact cortex remains, there is no opportunity for the neuromuscular signals to enter the graft site. The graft therefore does not have the advantage of the neuromuscular signaling system that forms and regulates normal skeletal physiology. The tendency is for the graft to resorb and the reconstruction to fail.[6]

Surgeons recognize that drilling small holes into the cortex of the graft bed seems to enhance healing.[7] The rationale for drilling holes is to provide a route for cells in the medullary space to migrate into the healing graft. Other surgeons speculate that

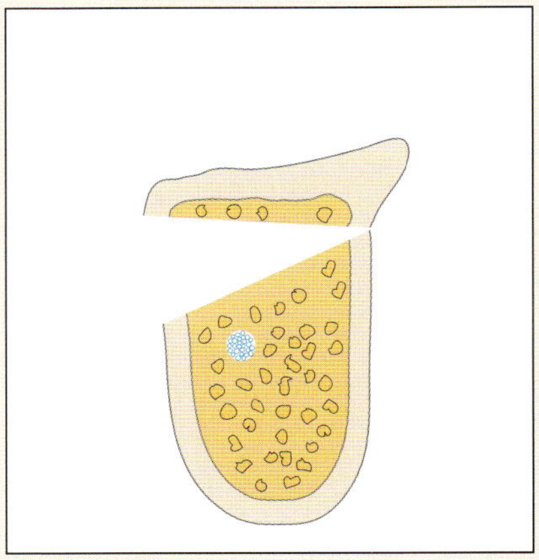

Fig 6-1h An osteotomy that disrupts the cortical continuity changes how forces are distributed within the altered mechanical structure.

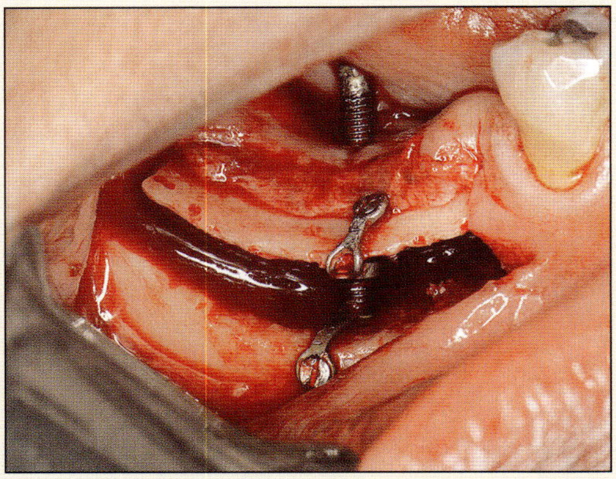

Fig 6-1i A horizontal osteotomy mobilizes the alveolar ridge crest while maintaining its attachment to the overlying soft tissue. A distraction device provides fixation and the ability to alter the position of the fragment postoperatively.

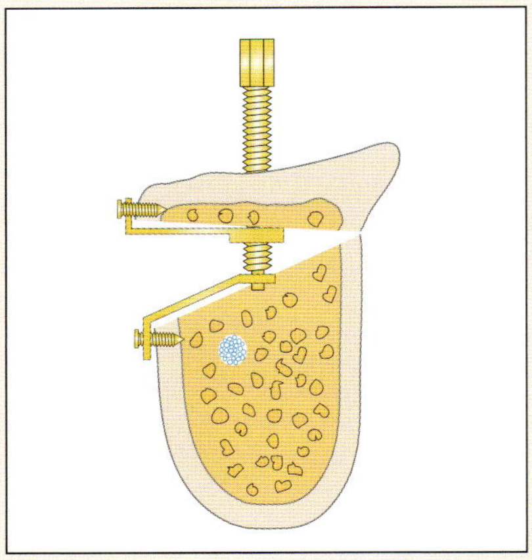

Fig 6-1j The transport fragment is rotated, opening a wedge-shaped chamber within the divided medullary space.

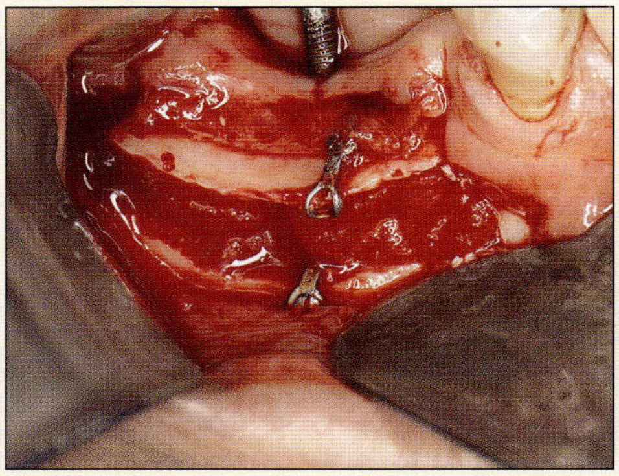

Fig 6-1k The distraction chamber is filled with a collagen sponge carrying rhBMP-2.

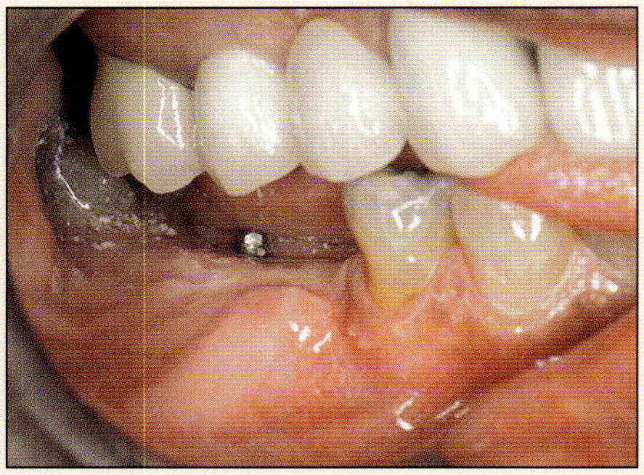

Fig 6-1l The distraction screw allows the transport segment to be elevated after the mucosa has healed.

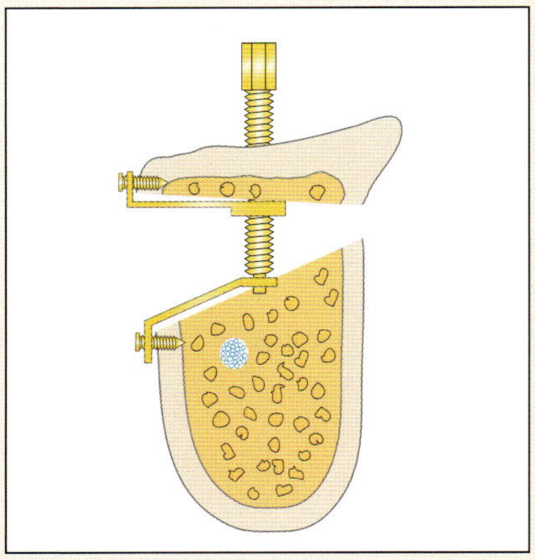

Fig 6-1m The result of the transport process is that the ridge crest is elevated and leveled. The distraction device provides stability so that the volume within the distraction chamber can meet the essential requirements as a bone-forming environment.

→

opening the medullary space to the healing graft site provides a source of blood vessels. It is also possible that drilling holes compromises the existing structure of the cortex to allow signaling through mechanical distortion to direct healing. This may help the graft to heal by partially disrupting the existing force pathways.

Osteotomy establishes a discontinuity of the bone and disrupts the pathway along which forces originally travelled (Fig 6-1h). The viability of the mobilized bone segment is maintained by preserving its connection with the overlying soft tissue. The continuity of the cortex is disrupted, and the cellular medullary space is now open to the regeneration chamber. Displacement of the mobilized segment results in expansion of the regeneration chamber volume. Differential displacement of the bone segment allows establishment of a level platform to place dental implants.

The repositioned segment must be mechanically stabilized. In this patient, a distraction device (LEAD, Stryker Leibinger) was placed to affix the segment (Fig 6-1i). The threaded screw allowed transport of the segment to increase the volume of the regeneration chamber and vertical height of the native cortex. The regeneration chamber created was part of the bone-forming construct. Viability of the bone segment was maintained by the lingually based mucosal flap. Rotational displacement of the segment minimized challenges to the circulation of the pedicle (Fig 6-1j).

The regeneration chamber was filled with recombinant human bone morphogenetic protein 2 (rhBMP-2) carried on absorbable collagen sponges (Fig 6-1k). The collagen sponge would resorb within 2 weeks, leaving the rhBMP-2 in the regeneration chamber. No particulate grafting material was placed as it might have posed a risk to the exposed inferior alveolar nerve. Surrounding the nerve with particulate allogeneic bone graft or hydroxyapatite has been associated with nerve fibrosis.

After the mucosa was allowed to heal for 1 week, the distraction device was activated to raise the cortex ridge and increase

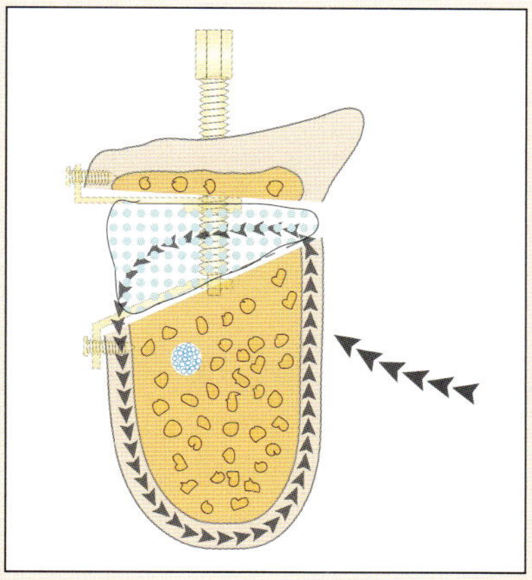

Fig 6-1n Cells introduced as a result of the rhBMP-2/collagen sponge graft require neuromuscular input to promote growth and organization. Disruption of the circumferential cortical continuity allows mechanical forces *(arrows)* to enter the distraction chamber, which contains large numbers of immature cells.

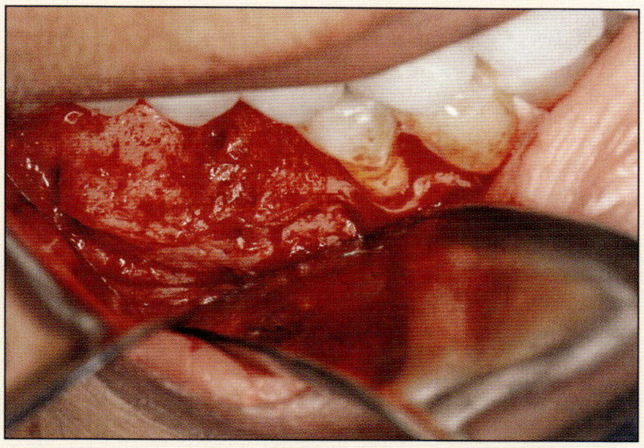

Fig 6-1o Three months after the distraction procedure, the site is opened for placement of dental implants. The transport segment is fused to the existing bone, and the distraction chamber is filled with bone.

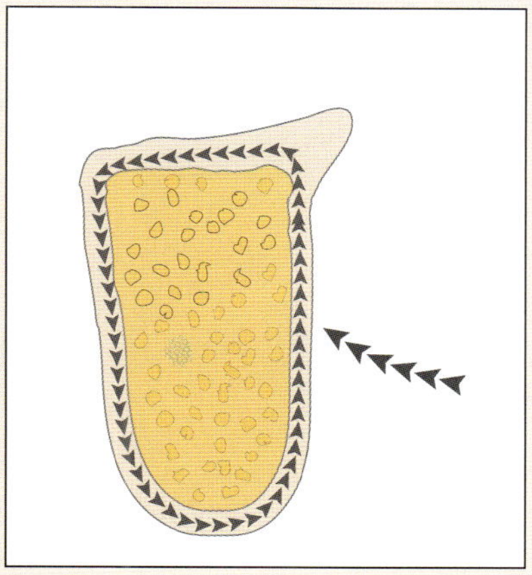

Fig 6-1p The medullary space is markedly increased. A new cortex has formed at the periphery.

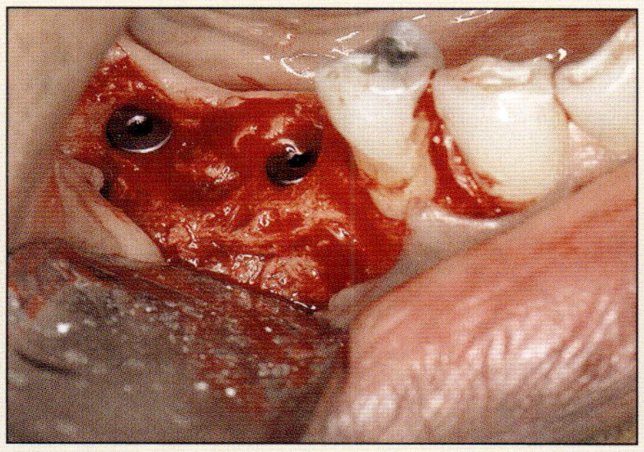

Fig 6-1q Implants are placed through the transported cortex and into the expanded medullary space.

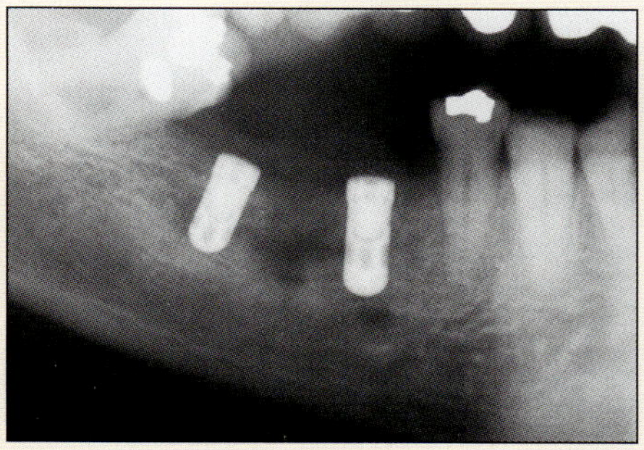

Fig 6-1r Implants have been positioned above the mandibular nerve.

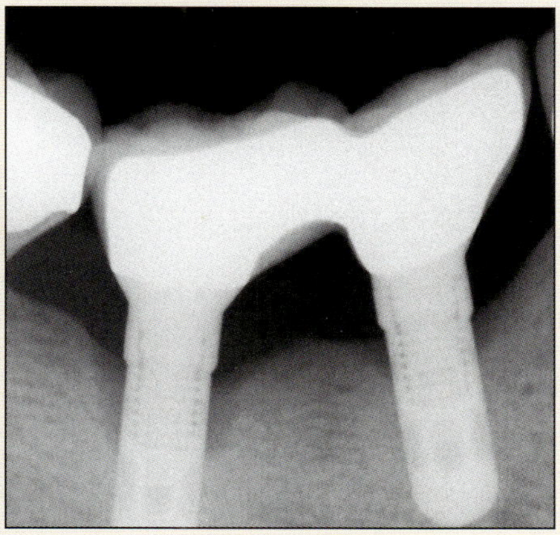

Fig 6-1s A radiograph taken at the 11-year follow-up reveals that the ridge height has been maintained, although the distal implant exhibits some bone loss.

the volume of the regeneration chamber (Fig 6-1l). Once the bone segment reached its final position, the distraction device was used for fixation (Fig 6-1m).

Osteotomy allows creation of a sheltered chamber for bone formation. It also results in disruption of the existing skeletal configuration that confines the neuromuscular signaling stimulus. The disruption of continuity of the cortex changes the mechanical integrity of the mandible and allows forces to enter the graft in the regeneration chamber (Fig 6-1n). These signals direct immature cells to differentiate into bone-forming cells and then to organize into a skeletal organ.

Complete decortication of the superior cortex could have allowed redirection of the neuromuscular signaling to the bone-forming chamber. However, in this patient, osteotomy allowed establishment of a ceiling for the regeneration chamber that was a composite flap. The resulting reconstruction was vascularized, autogenous bone with keratinized mucosa at the future implant site. The transport cortex became the new alveolar crest. The regeneration chamber filled and matured into a medullary structure (Fig 6-1o).

The new mandibular construct formed a circumferential cortex and continuous medullary space (Fig 6-1p). Osteotomy and repositioning of the original alveolar crest cortex were essential steps in the reconstruction process. As long as the original cortex morphology remained, the mechanical forces that regulated bone activity would have followed that path.

The natural history of any successful conventional onlay bone graft follows the same regenerative process. The timeline, however, is prolonged. For a conventional onlay graft to heal and be useful, the cortex at the graft bed must still be resorbed and a new cortex formed at the periphery. Because the graft is unprotected while a new cortex is forming, the graft is vulnerable to resorption.

Implants were placed in the new bone (Figs 6-1q and 6-1r). After 11 years in function, the prosthesis remained stable. The ridge height was maintained, although there had been some bone loss on the distal implant (Fig 6-1s). The new steady state included a newly formed cortex. The implants served to stabilize the regenerated bone environment but were not a replacement for the periodontal ligament system.

Fig 6-2 Incorporation of segmental maxillary osteotomy in a surgical design to manage failed treatment of an impacted canine.

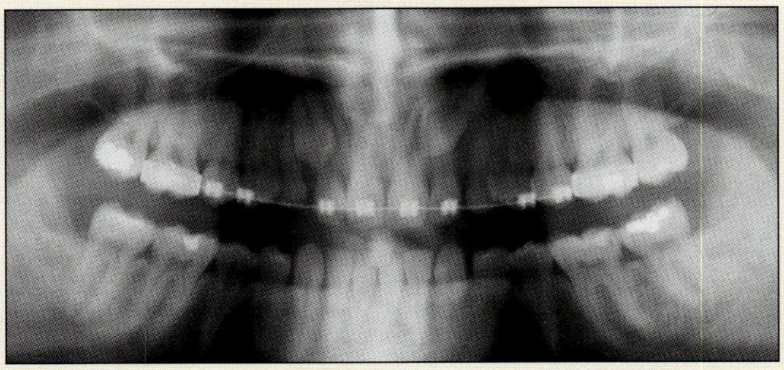

Fig 6-2a The maxillary canines are impacted bilaterally.

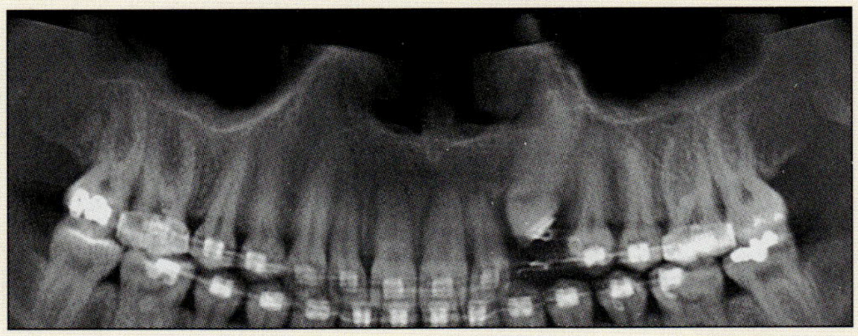

Fig 6-2b Cone beam computed tomography after 3 years of orthodontic treatment reveals that the maxillary left canine has not moved. The left lateral incisor and left premolars have intruded.

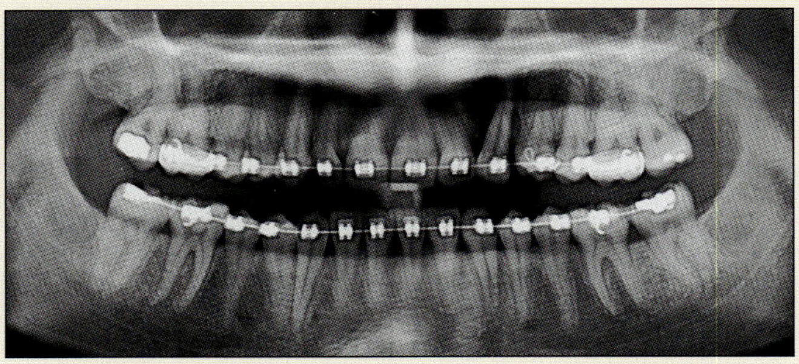

Fig 6-2c The repositioned maxillary left canine is stabilized on the orthodontic archwire.

→

Discussion

Maintenance of morphology is the role of the neuromuscular regulatory system. If a different balance state is not set, the tendency is for the system to return or relapse to the original phenotype. Establishment of a new balance point requires removal of the old one. When the new system has been constructed, it may still have the potential for relapse. In this patient, osteotomy and distraction disrupted the existing patterns and allowed redirection of regulatory forces to create a new steady state.

Segmental Osteotomy to Treat a Defect Resulting from Failed Treatment of an Impacted Canine

Treatment of impacted canine teeth is generally uncomplicated. However, a minority of cases fail to respond to orthodontic traction with bonded chains. Ankylosis is one obstacle to successful orthodontic eruption of an impacted tooth. Collision with teeth already occupying the dental arch can also prevent eruption and result in damage to other teeth. Damage to the site or adjacent teeth may occur during the exposure and bonding procedure. Intentional reimplantation may also result in local damage secondary to surgery or subsequent infection.

When treatment results in a defect involving the alveolar bone, overlying soft tissue, and periodontal structures of the adjacent teeth, the surgical designer should take care to provide a surgical plan that will optimize the chance for successful healing in a compromised environment. The following case presents the treatment of a patient who had undergone multiple unsuccessful surgeries for management of a missing maxillary left canine.

Case description

A 30-year-old woman presented for evaluation and treatment recommendations for her missing maxillary left canine. Other practitioners had performed multiple surgeries on the patient in failed attempts to manage the problem. After each surgical attempt, healing did not occur and the defect became larger. The teeth adjacent to the site developed recession, bone loss, and mobility. She sought a third surgical opinion prior to undergoing a fourth attempt to repair the defect.

Six years prior to her consultation visit, the patient had presented to her orthodontist for evaluation and treatment. Bilaterally impacted maxillary canines were noted on her initial orthodontic records (Fig 6-2a). Following standard practice, the teeth were surgically exposed, and chains were bonded for orthodontic traction. The chains were activated while a complete-arch maxillary orthodontic appliance was used for anchorage.

After 2 years of orthodontic treatment, it was discovered that the maxillary left canine was not moving. The tooth was exposed, a bracket was bonded to it, and a gold chain was attached for orthodontic traction. After 5 months of traction did not yield any movement, the tooth was exposed again and surrounding bone excised. Two additional years of orthodontic traction produced no movement of the impacted canine. The surgeon then exposed the tooth again to remove more tissue. A

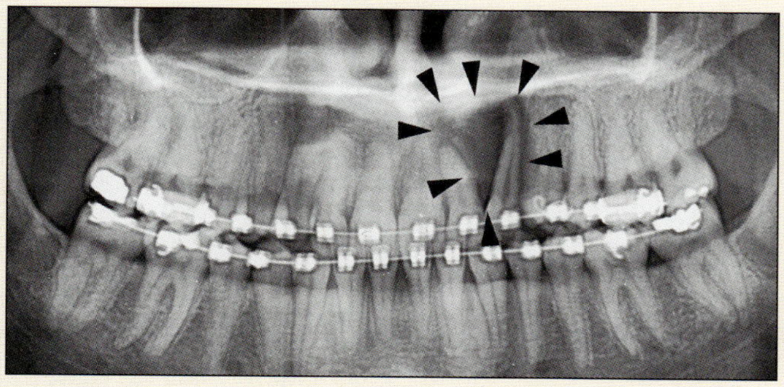

Fig 6-2d Three weeks after intentional reimplantation of the canine tooth, a radiolucency *(arrowheads)* secondary to infection is visible on the radiograph.

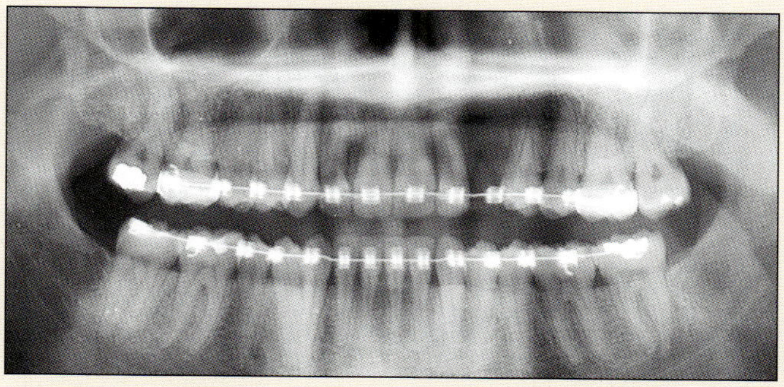

Fig 6-2e Five months after intentional reimplantation, the canine tooth has been extracted and the defect grafted with banked human bone. The radiograph shows that bone loss has extended to involve the lateral incisor and premolar roots.

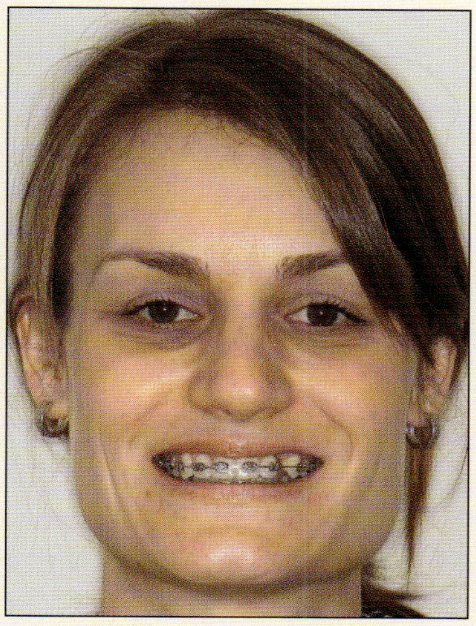

Fig 6-2f Patient as she presented for evaluation following 4 years of orthodontic treatment.

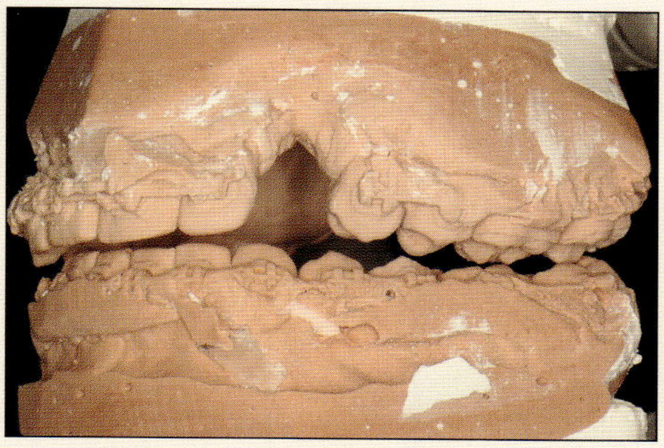

Fig 6-2g Dental casts mounted in centric relation reveal an open bite.

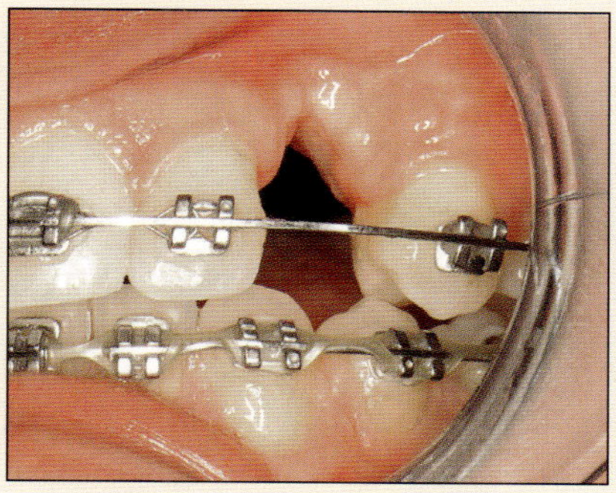

Fig 6-2h Large defect in the alveolar ridge. In centric occlusion, the patient can accommodate into a functional occlusion.

→

follow-up radiograph taken 2 months after the last surgical procedure revealed that orthodontic traction had placed the crown of the canine into close proximity to the lateral incisor root (Fig 6-2b). Bone loss was evident on the lateral incisor root extending to the root apex.

After 4 years of unsuccessful orthodontic traction, the patient presented to a second oral surgeon. The second oral surgeon extracted the tooth, repositioned it in the dental arch, stabilized it to the orthodontic archwire, and placed a banked bone graft (Fig 6-2c). The procedure was a form of intentional reimplantation.

During the 3 weeks following canine repositioning, the site developed infection and drainage (Fig 6-2d). Antibiotic treatment was continued, and the site was observed over the following 4 months. The tooth remained mobile and the site infected, despite multiple courses of antibiotics.

Five months following the reimplantation of the tooth, it remained mobile and infected. The patient returned to the first oral surgeon, who extracted the tooth and grafted the site with banked human bone (Fig 6-2e). Infection at the site persisted after placement of the bone graft. The graft was removed, and the site was allowed to heal. A second attempt at bone grafting was then recommended to the patient. Use of an autogenous graft from the iliac crest was offered as the surgical option. At this point, the patient requested an opinion as to possible alternative treatments.

When the patient presented for evaluation (Fig 6-2f), she wished to know if there were alternatives to bone grafting of the alveolar defect in preparation for dental implant placement. She was concerned about the healing of a bone graft after her past experience with multiple failed oral surgeries. In addition, the maxillary left lateral incisor exhibited gingival recession and mobility. The patient recognized that the lateral incisor appeared worse after each failed procedure. The patient was concerned about losing the lateral incisor as the result of another procedure.

In centric relation, primary occlusion was on the right and left second molars, resulting in an open bite malocclusion (Fig 6-2g). This condition resulted from intrusion of the dental arch when it was used for anchorage to erupt the impacted canine. Dental casts demonstrated that the defect involved both the labial and palatal bone plates.

Clinical examination showed a large defect in the alveolar ridge involving bone and soft tissue (Fig 6-2h). There was gingival recession on the lateral incisor, which exhibited Class I mo-

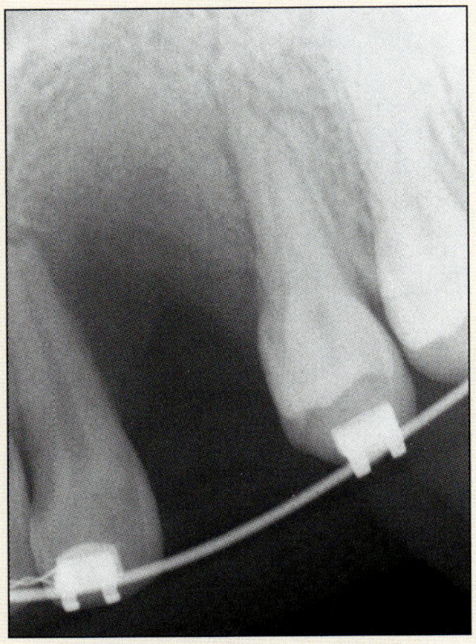

Fig 6-2i A radiograph taken at the third-opinion consultation reveals extensive bone loss on the lateral incisor.

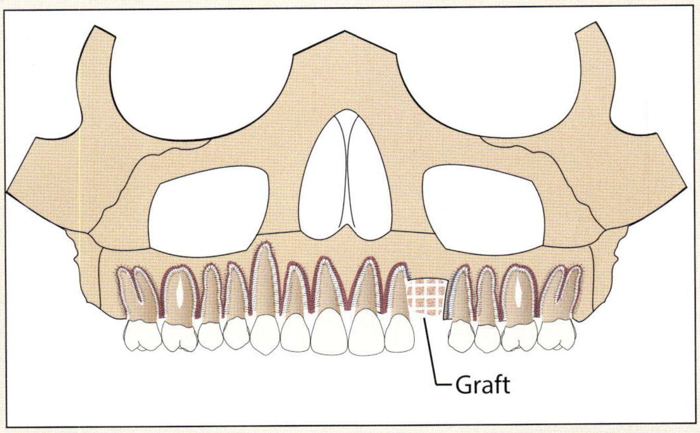

Fig 6-2j A functional analysis of the existing defect defines the limitations of bone grafting in a compromised environment.

→

bility. In centric occlusion, the patient was able to accommodate into a functional occlusion.

A radiograph demonstrated bone loss on the lateral incisor that extended nearly to the root apex (Fig 6-2i). There was some bone loss on the mesial aspect of the premolar as well. The alveolar defect extended apically to the level of the apices of the teeth.

For a conventional bone graft to heal in this site and be maintained in a stable state over the long term, it would have to meet all of the essential requirements for a bone-forming construct (see chapter 1). Healing is always challenged when bone grafts are placed against the exposed lateral incisor root.[8] In the condition in which the patient presented, a bone graft would not heal (Fig 6-2j).

The local environment would not support bone growth because the neuromuscular regulation of the site derived from the periodontal ligament systems of the adjacent teeth, and the distance and vectors of these signaling sources were not configured properly to control growth of a bone graft. The surviving, working periodontal ligament system for the lateral incisor was located too far apically to reach the coronal aspect of the graft. The mesiodistal width of the bone defect was too large for the periodontal signaling to reach the center of a bone graft. This challenge was increased given the damage to the periodontal systems of the adjacent teeth.

The alveolar defect extended through the full labiopalatal dimension and included the labial gingiva and palatal mucosa (Fig 6-2k). Surgical exposure showed that the canine site was narrow and vertically deficient (Fig 6-2l). The lateral incisor root was exposed on its distal surface nearly to the apex. Some labial bone remained, and that was important to the surgical design. There was marked loss of bone on the labial aspect of the first premolar, but the mesial root surface was mostly covered. The palatal soft tissue had collapsed into the alveolar defect. It was scarred and not suitable for creation of advancement flaps.

The width deficiency of the alveolar housing extended beyond the surgical defect to include the entire maxillary arch. This feature was a characteristic of the patient's essential morphology. An onlay graft placed in an attempt to increase the width of this deficient site for a future implant would likely fail or resorb slowly over time, because a constructed skeletal unit cannot exist long term within an environment that cannot support it.

As an alternative to onlay grafting, a strategy combining segmental osteotomy and rhBMP-2 was designed (Fig 6-2m). The objectives were *(1)* replacement of the missing canine, *(2)* management of periodontal damage on the lateral incisor and premolar, *(3)* management of the orthodontic intrusion of the maxillary left posterior teeth, and *(4)* cosmetic and functional correction of the lost gingiva.

A segmental osteotomy was to be used to construct a physical environment that would support regeneration at the defect site. The damaged and deficient alveolar bone at the canine site was to be resected. A horizontal osteotomy leading to the pterygoid plate would prepare the segment for mobilization.

The segment was to be mobilized by luxation from its connection with the lateral and medial pterygoid plates (Fig 6-2n). Fracturing the pterygoid plates with curved osteotomes must be avoided because it exposes the patient to potential surgical complications (see chapter 8). In this patient, the pterygoid plates were to serve as the origin of the muscles that would provide neuromuscular regulation to the healing osteotomy.

Horizontal repositioning of the transport segment would create a physical environment with improved healing potential (Fig 6-2o). The problem of the missing canine was to be resolved by repositioning the teeth and creating a continuous dental arch that would not require a dental implant. The segment was

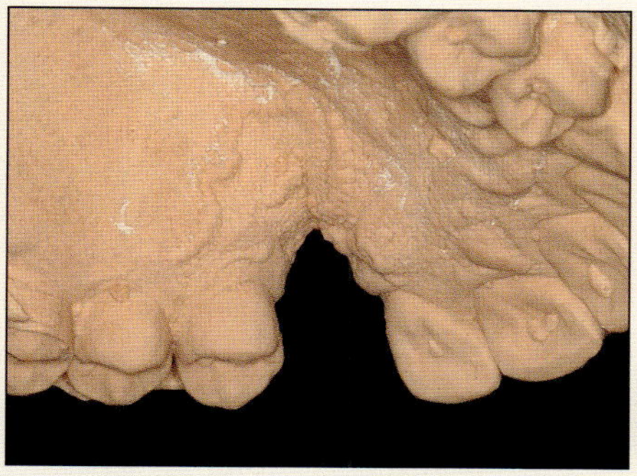

Fig 6-2k The cast demonstrates the cleftlike deformity.

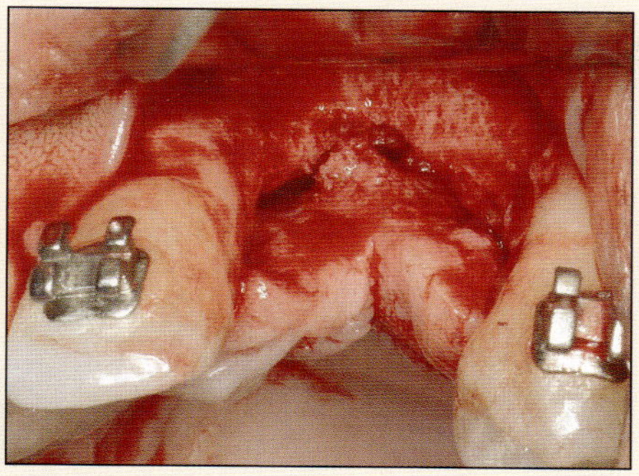

Fig 6-2l Surgical exposure of the adjacent teeth and alveolar ridge reveals the extent of bone loss.

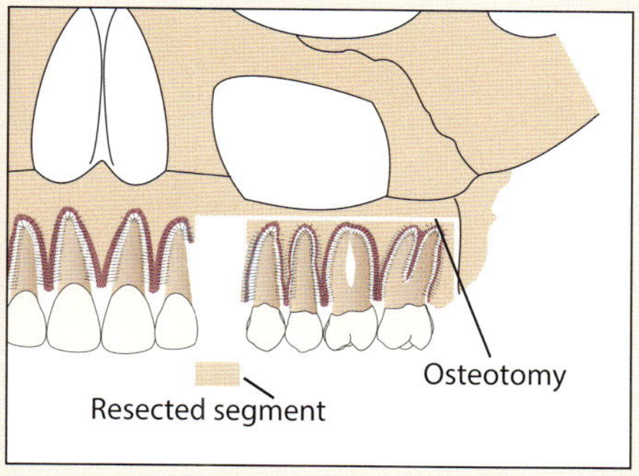

Fig 6-2m The surgical design includes a segmental osteotomy and resection of the damaged ridge.

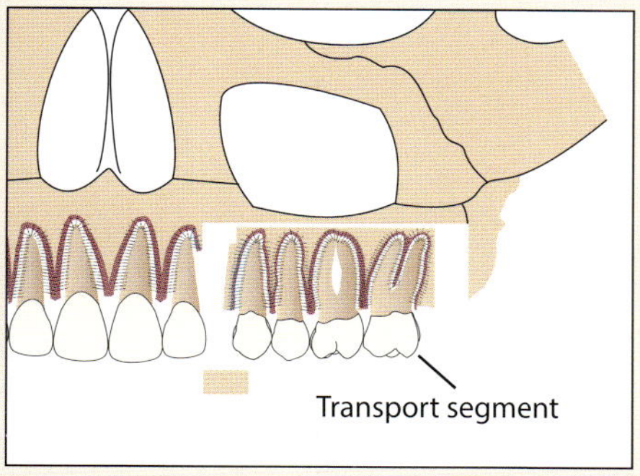

Fig 6-2n The segment will be mobilized, sparing the pterygoid plates.

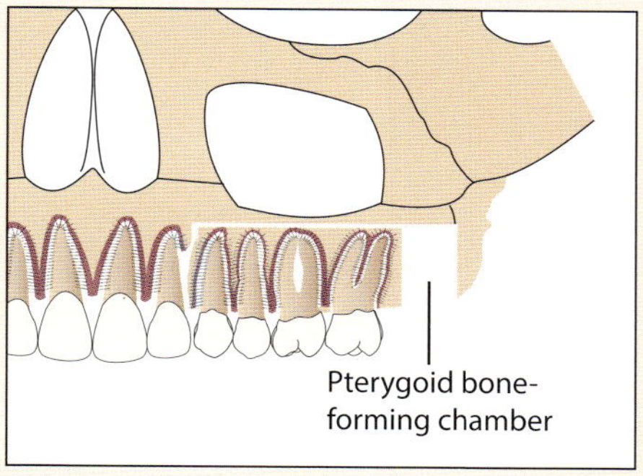

Fig 6-2o The transport segment will be repositioned.

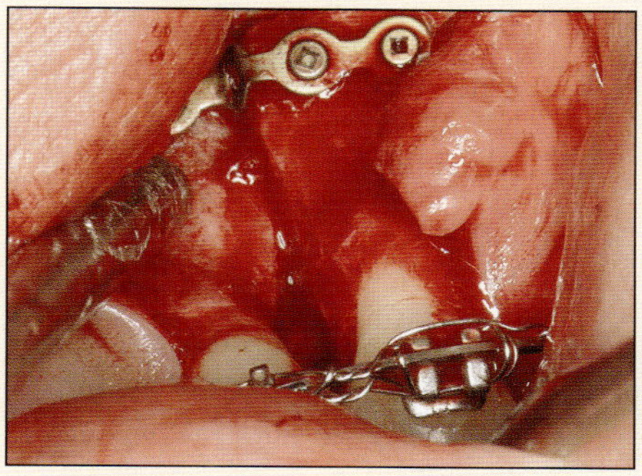

Fig 6-2p A second regeneration site is created at the docking site of the segmental osteotomy.

→

to be repositioned slightly inferiorly to correct the problem of orthodontic intrusion. Protracting the posterior maxilla from the preserved pterygoid plates would open a space with powerful bone-forming capability.

Protraction of maxillary segmental osteotomy created a second regeneration chamber at the docking site (Fig 6-2p). The thin, vertically deficient alveolar bone was resected. This allowed transport of healthy tissue into the site. The segment was displaced laterally and fixed in that position with a bone plate. Lateral displacement of the maxillary segment established a structural and functional unit lateral in the arch to the damaged lateral incisor periodontal apparatus.

The site of most critical regeneration, the labial and distal lateral incisor root, was placed in a relative concavity. The roots of the lateral incisor and premolar were now in a position to deliver neuromuscular signaling to the regeneration chamber. Cells were introduced by an rhBMP-2 device. The bone plate and orthodontic appliance provided relative stability.

Moving the premolar into the missing canine site solved the problem of canine replacement. Long-term success also required reversal of bone loss on the lateral incisor and premolar, union of the osteotomy and regeneration of interproximal bone, and regeneration of gingiva.

A collagen sponge containing rhBMP-2 filled the regeneration chamber at the docking site (Fig 6-2q). The objective was to form bone to cover the exposed labial and distal surfaces of the lateral incisor root. Bone will only grow in the confines of the sheltered and stimulated environment. In this patient, bone would not grow on the labial aspect of the premolar because it was outside the sheltered environment. To be useful long term, the bone had to form a functional periodontal apparatus and lamina dura. Simply filling the site with radiopaque material would not have met the objective of reconstruction. New bone was needed to bridge the osteotomy gap and reverse the bone loss on the mesial root surface of the premolar.

Advancement of the maxillary segment carried labial and palatal soft tissue into the defect, correcting the soft tissue deficiency. A tension-free closure was possible because movement of the segment carried 8 mm of additional vascularized soft tissue into the defect. Two weeks after surgery, the mucosa had healed uneventfully (Fig 6-2r).

The procedure created three unique regions of bone regeneration: the docking site of the segmental osteotomy, the site of the maxillary osteotomy, and the pterygoid site (Fig 6-2s). Each region healed under different physical and regulatory conditions. The segmental osteotomy docking site had the greatest challenge

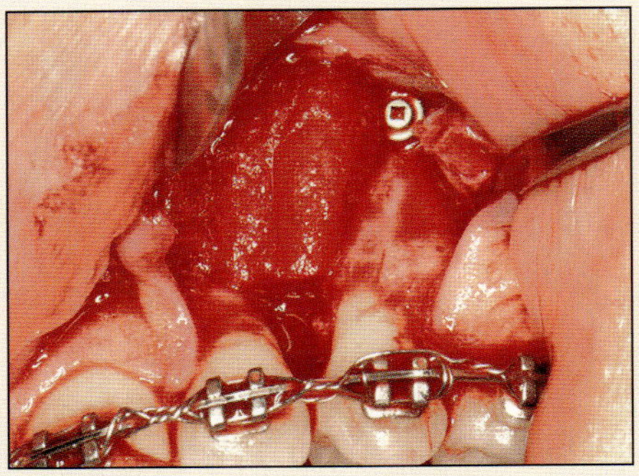

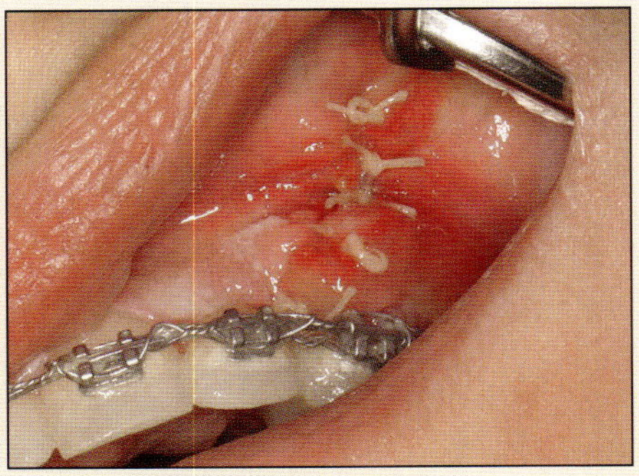

Fig 6-2q *(far left)* A collagen sponge containing rhBMP-2 is placed.

Fig 6-2r *(left)* The limited incision has healed 2 weeks after surgery.

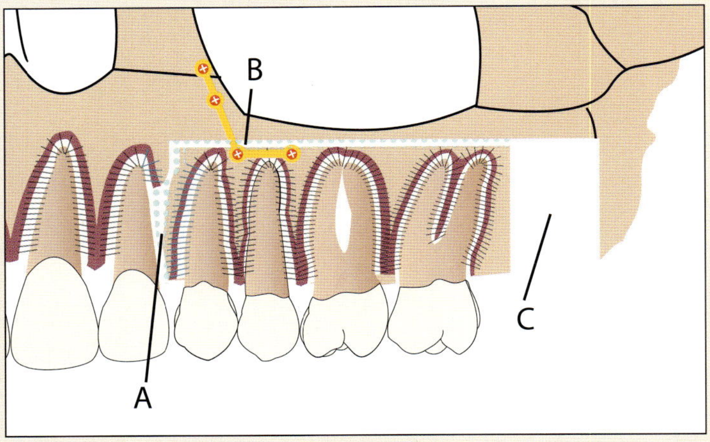

Fig 6-2s The procedure has created docking site, osteotomy, and pterygoid regeneration chambers. The segmental osteotomy docking site (A) has the greatest challenge to successful healing because of periodontal damage from prior failed treatment. The maxillary osteotomy site (B) is expected to show successful healing. Placement of rhBMP-2 has been performed because of the bone gap created by inferior repositioning of the segment. The pterygoid regeneration chamber (C) should heal without grafting or rhBMP-2 because of the proximity of the lateral and medial pterygoid muscle attachments.

→

to successful healing because reversal of the periodontal damage from prior failed treatment would require mechanisms that are incompletely understood. Experience gained through years of orthognathic surgery assured successful healing at the site of the maxillary osteotomy. Healing was enhanced by placement of rhBMP-2 because of the bone gap created by inferior repositioning of the segment. If the skeletal anatomy was preserved, the pterygoid regeneration chamber site was expected to heal without grafting or rhBMP-2 enhancement because of the proximity of the lateral and medial pterygoid muscle attachments.

The radiographic appearance of the defect prior to surgery (see Fig 6-2i) can be contrasted with that 4 months after surgery (Fig 6-2t). At 4 months, radiopacity partially filled the interproximal space. There was no clear sign of a lamina dura, and the opacity was still lower at the ridge crest.

Eight months after segmental osteotomy, the radiopacity extended coronally (Fig 6-2u). The general increase in radiopacity reflected mineralization and consolidation. There was still no clear lamina dura, implying that the interradicular space that was the osteotomy docking site was filling with bone. The radiograph did not confirm how well the periodontal ligament system was responding.

Fourteen months after segmental osteotomy, there was early formation of trabeculae within the endosteal space, reflecting functional remodeling (Fig 6-2v). The cortical bone overlying the mesial aspect of the premolar was resorbing, and the rhBMP-2 graft was now continuous with the periodontal apparatus of the tooth. There were early signs of lamina dura formation at the distal aspect of the lateral incisor.

Although development of stable interradicular bone may be considered successful reconstruction, only regeneration of the periodontal system can produce long-term stability. The appearance of normal bone architecture with a cortex and structural trabeculae provided compelling evidence of functional regeneration. Forty months after segmental osteotomy, there was a clear lamina dura around the root of the lateral incisor, evidence that a functional periodontal apparatus had been created (Fig 6-2w). The trabecular pattern of the newly generated bone appeared the same as the native bone. The surgical process created a volume of bone and soft tissue that produced a functional, physiologic, and esthetic repair of the defect.

Reconstruction consists of more than filling a defect with material. To be successful long term, the newly formed construct must assume the role of a normal structure on the macroscopic, microscopic, and physiologic levels. With the use of alloplastic grafts such as hydroxyapatite, the void can be filled but cannot remodel into normal bone. In this reconstruction, however, the new ossicle consisted of living normal bone created by the influence of rhBMP-2. The resultant, primitive tissue mass consolidated, calcified, and organized its trabecular architecture into a stress-bearing unit. By this process, the amorphous mass of young bone tissue became incorporated into the functional skeletal system of the maxilla.

To be complete, however, the construct had to establish a relationship with adjacent organ systems. In this case, the new ossicle needed to form an anatomical and physiologic relationship with the adjacent teeth. Bone interacts with teeth through the periodontal ligaments and gingival attachment. To be suc-

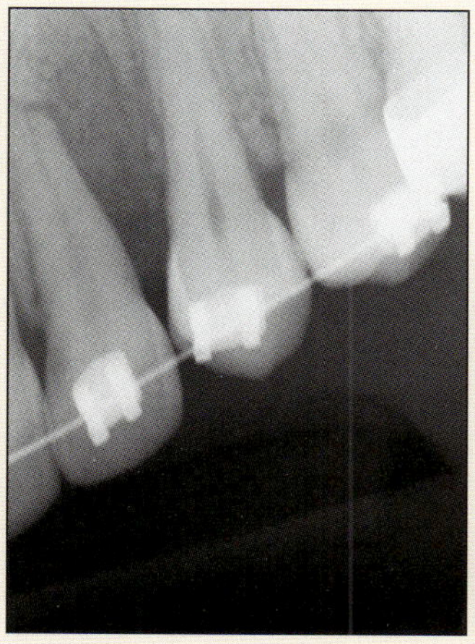

Fig 6-2t Four months after segmental osteotomy, radiopacity partially fills the interproximal space. There is no clear sign of a lamina dura, and the ridge crest is still less radiopaque.

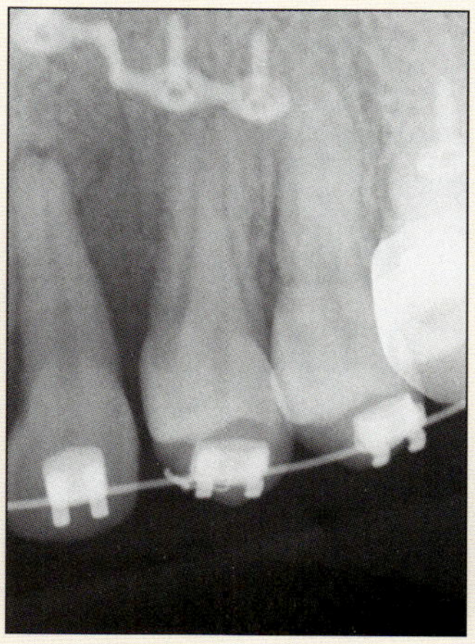

Fig 6-2u Eight months after surgery, the radiopacity extends coronally.

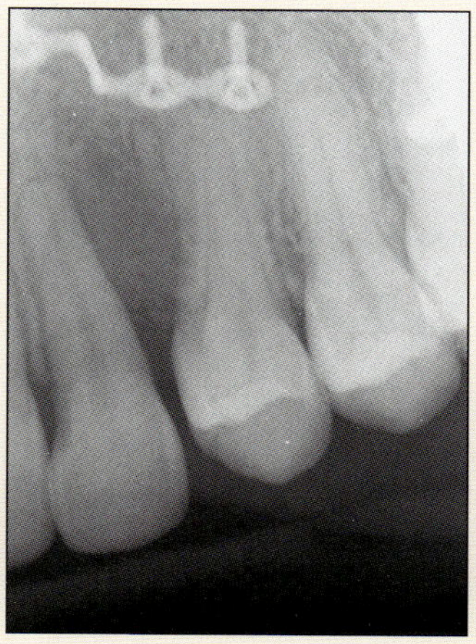

Fig 6-2v Fourteen months after surgery, early formation of trabeculae within the endosteal space reflects functional remodeling. The rhBMP-2 graft is now continuous with the periodontal apparatus of the tooth.

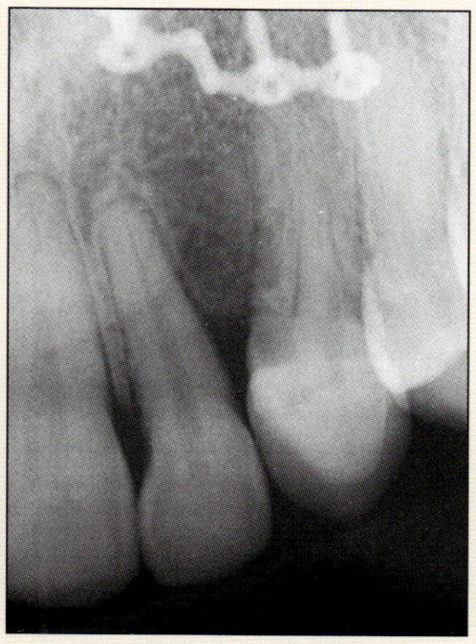

Fig 6-2w Forty months after surgery, there is a clear lamina dura around the root of the lateral incisor, evidence that a functional periodontal apparatus has been created.

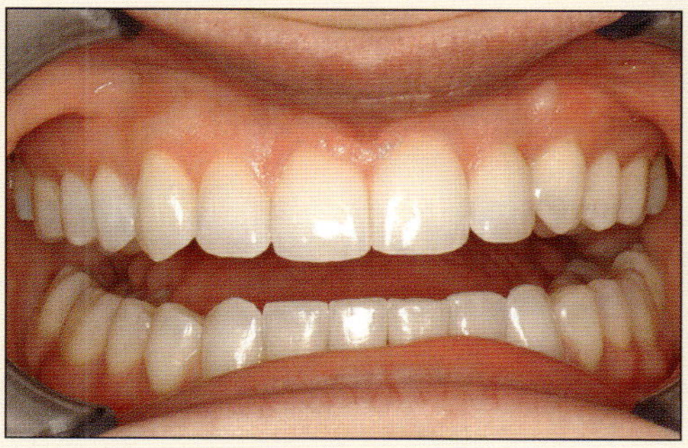

Fig 6-2x The gingiva has a healthy appearance 40 months after osteotomy and rhBMP-2 grafting. The gingiva has healed solely as a result of the osteotomy repositioning.

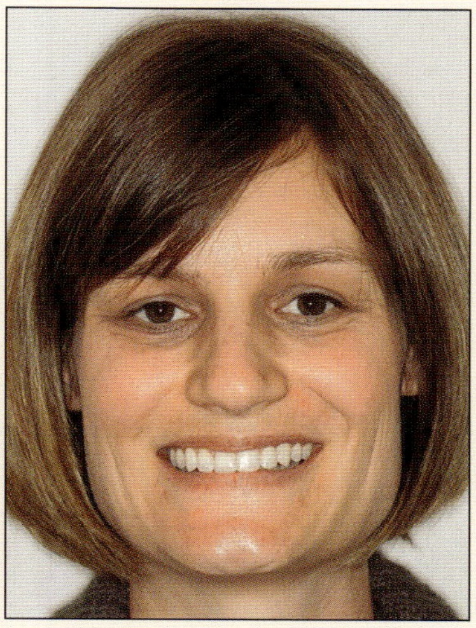

Fig 6-2y The functional and esthetic results of the reconstruction are good 40 months after osteotomy and rhBMP-2 grafting.

cessful long term, the construct had to create and maintain a healthy periodontal apparatus, including periodontal ligament attachments, lamina dura, and stable gingival attachment to the adjacent teeth. As the follow-up radiographs illustrated, maturation of the construct required many months.

The healing response to the surgical approach described was clearly different from the results of the prior procedures. After three grafting failures, it was clear that the basic approach of onlay grafting into this defect was not a predictable process. The basic patient physiology was not changed when the segmental osteotomy and rhBMP-2 procedure was done. The prior procedures likely compromised the ability of the local tissue to heal to some degree. The strategy in this repair was to engineer and build an environment that would support self-assembly of a fully integrated skeletal construct.

As a result of this reconstruction, the patient exhibited a continuous dental arch of natural teeth 40 months after osteotomy and rhBMP-2 grafting (Fig 6-2x). The periodontal damage to the teeth was corrected. The functional and esthetic results were good (Fig 6-2y). The treatment was completed in a single procedure. No additional periodontal surgery was done. The gingiva healed solely as a result of the osteotomy repositioning. The primary source of bone regeneration was the pterygoid bone-forming chamber, which healed without grafting. The docking site requiring periodontal repair healed with the application of rhBMP-2 (2 mg) alone.

Discussion

The conditions of the alveolar defect and the surrounding anatomy in this patient did not provide an environment in which a bone graft was likely to be successful. Even if a volume of viable bone were grafted, it would lack the long-term stability to secure a dental implant for years of function. Placing an autogenous bone graft into the presenting defect would not have addressed the problem of periodontal damage to the lateral incisor. The volume of bone necessary to fill the defect could not be covered with the limited amount of scarred soft tissue at the site. However, despite the challenges of prior surgery, periodontal damage, and underlying skeletal hypoplasia, a procedure can be designed to take advantage of the underlying ability of the body to repair itself.

Improving the long-term prognosis for the lateral incisor tooth was a primary objective of the surgical design. Full regeneration of the osseous socket, periodontal ligament attachments, and gingiva would be the ideal result. If optimal regeneration was to be achieved, it required conditions that met the essential needs of bone-forming constructs. These conditions were designed into the surgical plan as a primary requirement.

Stabilized environment

In this case, a stabilized environment was constructed by moving the tooth-containing alveolar segments into close proximity. The posterior segment was displaced laterally and held in that position by the bone plate. The lateral incisor root was placed in a relative concavity by establishing a stable structure laterally in the dental arch. This provided the labial root surface with a degree of shelter from detrimental forces.

Source of cells

The available population of bone-forming cells was enhanced by placement of rhBMP-2. No particulate graft material was placed because there was no structural need. The objective was to introduce maximum cellular substrate to be available to the limited-intensity neuromuscular input remaining from the damaged periodontal system. Introduction of particulate graft material would be indicated to promote prolonged remodeling or to participate in the mechanical maintenance of volume. The amount of bone needed in this reconstruction was small, however, because the defect was mostly eliminated by repositioning of the osteotomy segment.

Neuromuscular input

Within the alveolar process, the primary source of neuromuscular regulation is the periodontal system. Sharpey fibers that connect the root to the bone penetrate the periosteum to enter the lamina dura. The effect of these fibers may be directly at their superficial attachment to the cortical socket. Mechanical signaling to the cortex may be transmitted through the lamina dura into the medullary space from the endosteal side of the lamina dura. It is possible that the fibers penetrate the lamina dura to reach the endosteal space directly. In any case, neuromuscular signaling involves the periodontal ligament system. Designing a surgical procedure that provides the cells participating in the regeneration with access to periodontal signaling is critical. The challenge in this case was to reverse or manage periodontal damage. The functioning periodontal ligament system of the first premolar tooth was repositioned to place it into the site needing regeneration. As the bone overlying the mesial root of the first premolar demineralizes, the Sharpey fibers contained within become exposed. These fibers are then available to deliver regulatory signaling to immature bone-forming cells attracted to the site by rhBMP-2.

Absence of pathology

Infection at the regeneration site must be avoided. Isolation of the healing site from repeated oral contamination is one method to avoid infection. In this patient, transportation of viable soft tissue into the bone-forming site allowed a tension-free soft tissue closure. Placement of nonvital bone particles in a wound is always a risk. Use of rhBMP-2 carried on a collagen sponge in this patient limited the potential for infection inherent to particulate grafts.

Summary

In summary, a segmental maxillary osteotomy can be incorporated in a surgical design to address the defects of *(1)* a missing tooth, *(2)* missing alveolar bone, *(3)* deficient gingiva, *(4)* periodontal damage, and *(5)* intrusion of teeth in a single procedure. The surgical plan must be analyzed prior to surgery to verify that it can meet all of the essential requirements for bone formation. In addition to promoting initial successful healing of the bone construct, the design provides elements that will allow the site to function in a steady state for years. A reconstruction in which the dental arch consists of all natural teeth surrounded by native bone has inherent stability.

Osteotomy in a Bone-Forming Construct to Manage Congenital Deficiencies

The design and fabrication of bone-forming constructs for developmental deficiencies require special attention. Osteotomies may be necessary to establish an environment that will support bone formation and long-term maintenance. Bone deficiencies that are congenital have no precursor structure. This means that the neuromuscular matrix that directs formation of the missing structures in utero is itself compromised. The intensity and scope of the deficiency vary with each patient.

The visible manifestation of the underlying deficiency is the cleft of the lip, maxillary discontinuity, and cleft palate. It is critical to recognize that compromise of the adjacent physiology extends outward from the bone discontinuity. Cleft palate is best thought of as a field disorder rather than an anatomical variation.[4] Approaching the problem as a discrete mechanical repair underestimates the challenge to successful healing. The neuromuscular elements that can be recruited in the patient

Fig 6-3 Use of an osteotomy to manage congenital deficiencies.

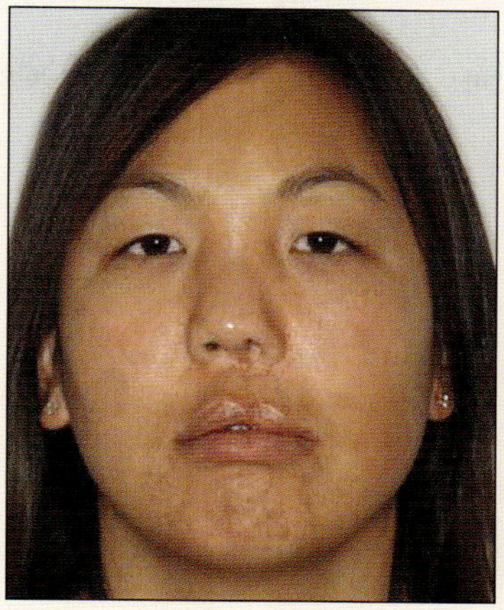

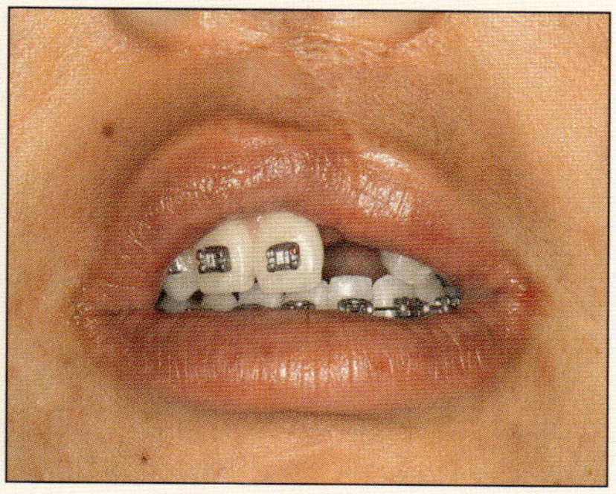

Fig 6-3a *(right)* A 27-year-old woman presents with a patent alveolar cleft, a missing lateral incisor, and an oronasal fistula.

Fig 6-3b *(far right)* The patient's smile shows substantial remaining asymmetry.

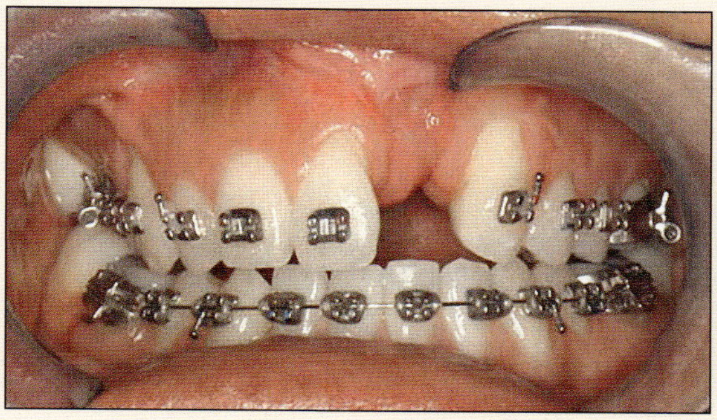

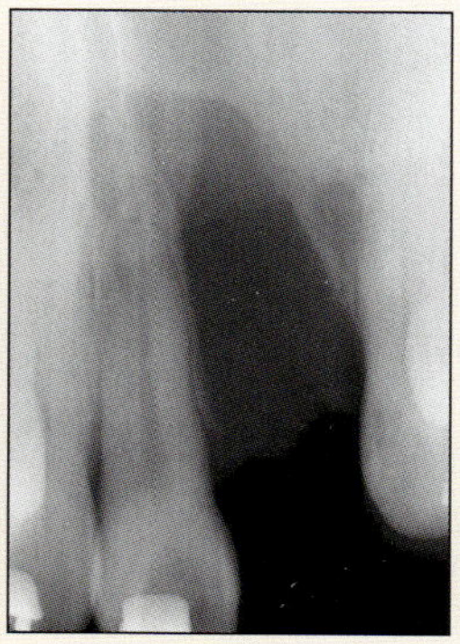

Fig 6-3c *(right)* Despite years of treatment, the patient presents with substantial malocclusion, a missing tooth, and compromised esthetics prior to surgery.

Fig 6-3d *(far right)* A radiograph shows the compromised condition of the teeth.

→

with alveolar atrophy or traumatic bone loss do not operate at the same intensity in developmental anomalies. Engineering of successful bone-forming systems in these patients requires establishment of conditions that are within the capability of the compromised environment to successfully heal.

The cleft itself is a manifestation of a primary deficiency in the neuromuscular system. This discontinuity of the maxilla that is visible on a radiograph is the focus of a wider deficiency that extends to the adjacent soft tissue and bone. Tooth proximity across a congenital cleft may not supply the neuromuscular signaling to promote healing and maintenance of a bone graft. Osteotomy and segment transport is one method to establish neuromuscular support processes in the skeletal discontinuity site. This approach was used successfully in a patient who had undergone multiple failed attempts at grafting.

Case description

A 27-year-old woman who presented for initial evaluation and treatment recommendations wished to know if a dental implant could be placed for management of a congenitally missing maxillary lateral incisor. Her past medical history included cleft lip and palate (Fig 6-3a). The lip and palate were repaired when she was a young child. Repair of the alveolar cleft was complicated by multiple failed procedures. This left a discontinuity defect in the maxilla that extended to the nasal cavity. A removable prosthesis was used to provide a prosthetic lateral incisor and to obturate the oronasal fistula. Her dentist thought that, given the history of failed bone graft repairs of the alveolar cleft, the use of rhBMP-2 might offer the potential for successful bone reconstruction.

She underwent conventional staged treatment that included orthodontics. The maxillary left central incisor was positioned at the normal site of the right incisor (Fig 6-3b). The first bone graft involved harvesting a cranial graft from the outer cortex of the calvarium. The graft failed to heal and was lost. In a second surgery, cancellous bone from the patient's iliac crest was used as the graft. The second bone graft failed to heal and was lost. In a third reconstructive attempt, a tongue flap was placed to transfer additional soft tissue to the site in preparation for the third autogenous bone grafting attempt. The tongue flap procedure failed, and the oronasal fistula remained patent. The patient then presented for an evaluation for possible alternative treatment. The patient presented with a large discontinuity defect through the left maxilla (Figs 6-3c and 6-3d).

The patient's past treatment course was complicated by failure of alveolar cleft bone grafting on multiple occasions. Autogenous bone was used in each of the grafting attempts. The procedures were performed in a standard fashion by experienced surgeons. Persistent discontinuity of the maxilla prevented the completion of orthodontic treatment and formation of the maxillary dental arch.

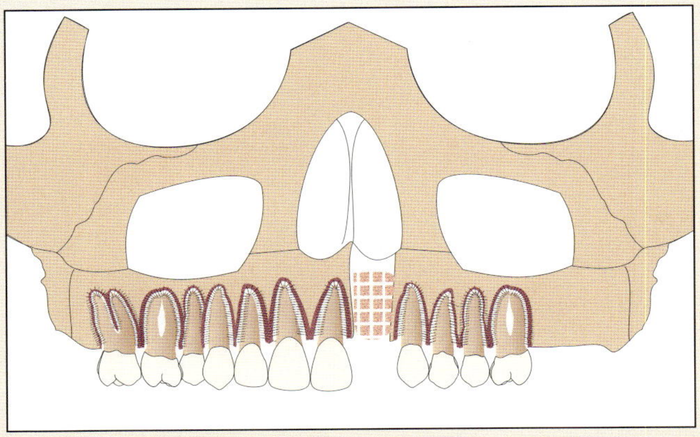

Fig 6-3e The large distance between the roots of the teeth adjacent to the cleft is an obstacle to successful graft healing. Neuromuscular signaling from the periodontal systems of these teeth will not reach the center of the defect.

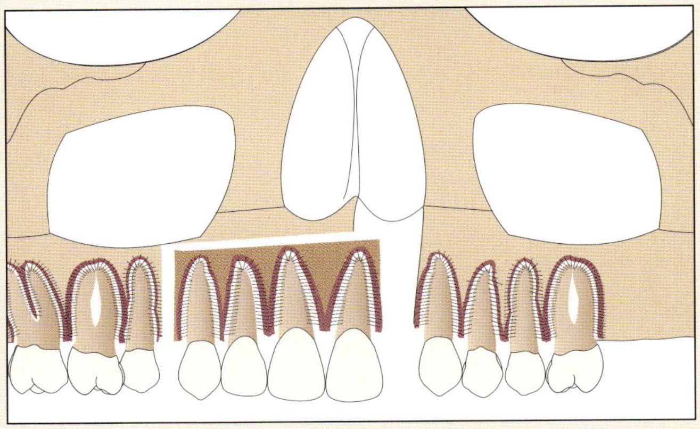

Fig 6-3f The proposed reconstruction uses a segmental osteotomy to carry an intact skeletal system to the defect.

→

After many years of surgical and orthodontic treatment, the patient remained with a substantial malocclusion, a missing tooth, and compromised esthetics (see Fig 6-3c). The two maxillary central incisors were 8 mm to the right of the facial midline. The maxillary left central incisor occupied the position of a normal maxillary right central incisor. The lip contour was also distorted.

The skeletal deficiency represented a typical cleft maxilla. There was compromise of the periodontal systems of the teeth adjacent to the cleft. Bone graft failures, particularly in adult dentition, often result in further periodontal damage. Lack of alveolar bone prevented orthodontic correction of the midline. There was moderate crowding of the maxillary right posterior teeth.

Functional analysis of the defect included analysis of how the existing morphology was maintained (Fig 6-3e). The regulatory forces that maintained the open cleft in a steady state would also affect the healing after surgery. These factors were operating during the prior surgeries, so their effect on a conventional bone grafting procedure was known. Before a viable surgical plan could be designed, the cause of the prior failures had to be understood.

To be successful, the surgical design had to include all of the essential elements for a bone-forming construct. In two of the prior reconstructive attempts, autogenous bone was used as a graft. In general, these grafts would provide a source of cells and a mechanically stable environment for bone to grow. However, the roots adjacent to the cleft were probably too far apart to recruit neuromuscular signaling from the periodontal systems into the healing graft site. It was also possible that poor healing of the soft tissue closure exposed the graft to oral bacteria. Failure of the tongue flap to heal suggested that simple closure of the repair site with advanced mucosa flaps was likely to fail as well.

At the time the patient presented, the primary interest was the possible use of rhBMP-2 to grow bone across the cleft. If rhBMP-2 were to be used in this case, it would only have the capacity to deliver cells with bone-forming potential to the site. A source of neuromuscular signaling was still needed if a complete bone-forming construct was to be assembled. The distance between the periodontal systems of the central incisor and the canine was too great to allow the stimulating effect to reach the central aspect of the regeneration chamber. Failure would be the expected outcome if rhBMP-2 were used in the existing site.

The skeleton adjacent to the cleft maintained a stable morphology because of its relationship with intact teeth. These teeth and their periodontal structures provided the neuromuscular direction to maintain their surrounding alveolar housing in a steady state. The strategy in this case was to use osteotomy to mobilize an intact skeletal system and to transport it into the cleft defect (Fig 6-3f). To be effective, the osteotomy segment must contain all of the elements that are lacking at the cleft site. In this case, the osteotomy segment would carry an intact skeletal unit including teeth, periodontal apparatus, and the osseous alveolar process.

A thin layer of bone covered the root of the left central incisor. Any surgical treatment would predispose this compromised periodontal state to further damage. When a procedure to manage this type of situation is designed, the bone-forming construct must provide a protective environment to limit the risk of damaging the periodontal attachment structures. In addition, healing of the donor site must be part of the surgical design. In this patient, the skeletal unit was to be displaced at the expense of the posterior maxilla.

Piezoelectric surgery created a maxillary segmental osteotomy (Fig 6-3g). This required minimal access and resulted in a mobilized maxillary segment with limited trauma to the bone and adjacent soft tissue. Vertical interdental osteotomy through the posterior maxilla was used to establish discontinuity (Fig 6-3h). This vertical bone cut became the site of the posterior regeneration chamber.

Transport of the segment was to be accomplished with the aid of a Liou distraction device (KLS-Martin). After the device was mounted across the docking site (Fig 6-3i), it was gradually closed. This pulled the fragment from right to left, closing the osseous alveolar cleft. The movement opened an alveolar defect in the posterior region.

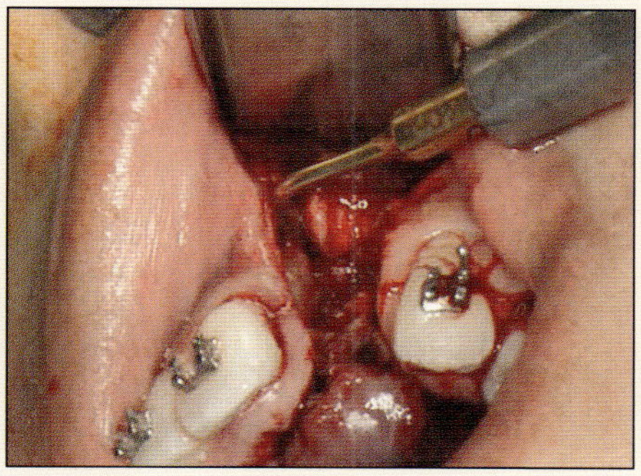

Fig 6-3g Piezoelectric surgery creates a maxillary segmental osteotomy.

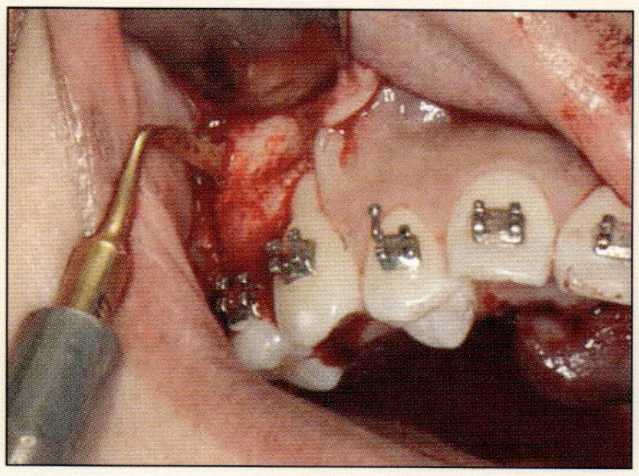

Fig 6-3h There is limited access for the vertical interdental osteotomy.

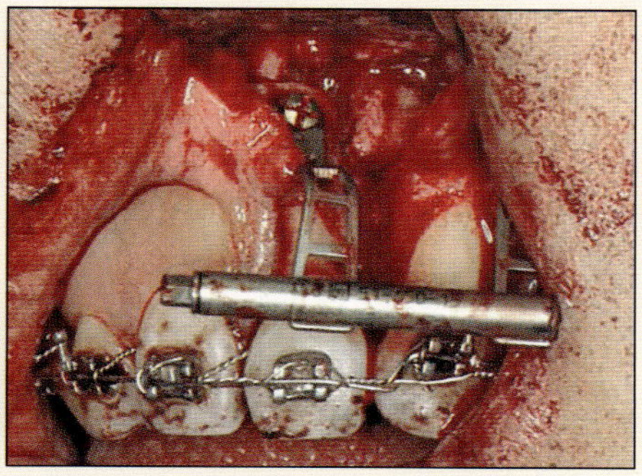

Fig 6-3i A Liou distraction device is mounted across the cleft.

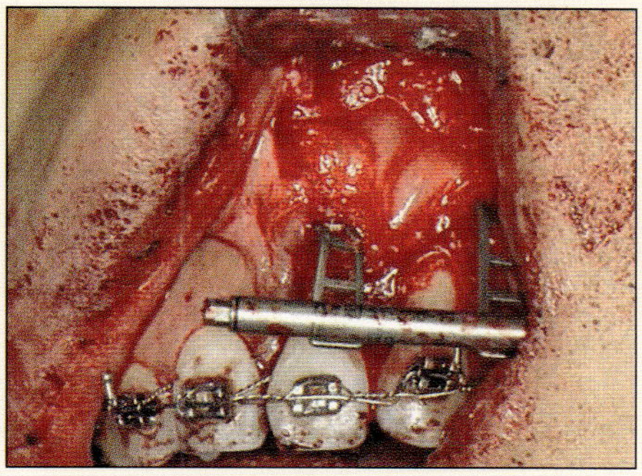

Fig 6-3j The docking site is filled with rhBMP-2.

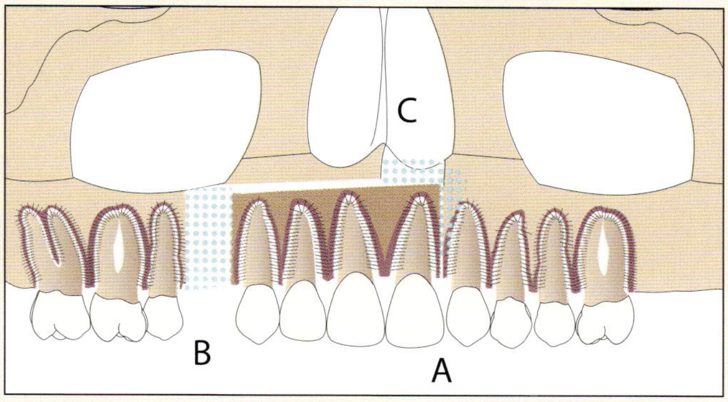

Fig 6-3k Collagen sponges containing rhBMP-2 are placed at the cleft site (A), the distraction chamber (B), and the nasal aperture (C). Site A is the primary focus of the bone construction challenge. The rhBMP-2 graft increases the number of available bone-forming cells. Site B is the donor site. Although the distance between the roots has been increased, the signaling intensity is less compromised and can reach the center of the regeneration chamber. Site C is now supported by the presence of an intact structural bone system.

In the case of patients with developmental disorders, the donor site osteotomy must be positioned at a distance from the site needing regeneration. For optimal healing, the regeneration chamber should not be positioned within the compromised developmental field that created the anatomical defect being treated.[9] After each incremental activation of the distraction device, the integrity of the pedicle is reevaluated. If there is sign of vascular or mechanical compromise of the pedicle, the distraction device is turned in reverse. Use of distraction devices for this application allows the surgeon the option of completing the transport process intraoperatively. It also offers the alternative of observing a latency period and activating the distraction device postoperatively.

In this patient, the device was activated over about 30 minutes, closing the cleft. The cleft gap was nearly eliminated by the repositioning maneuver. The roots of the teeth were now in close proximity. The volume requirement for successful osseous union was greatly reduced. This placed a limited demand on the host healing ability and required a minimal dose of rhBMP-2. A collagen sponge containing rhBMP-2 was placed over the docking site that was the previous open cleft (Fig 6-3j).

Collagen sponges containing rhBMP-2 were placed to enhance the healing response at the cleft site, the distraction chamber, and the nasal aperture (Fig 6-3k). The primary healing challenge was at the cleft site, where rhBMP-2 sponges were placed at the docking site and as an onlay over the labial cortex. The donor site represented a distraction chamber, where rhBMP-2 would be helpful in promoting bone formation. The third site of grafting was the nasal floor and piriform rim.

At the cleft site, the transport of the osteotomy segment brought the edges of the original cleft into physical contact. The rhBMP-2 increased the number of available bone-forming cells. The periodontal apparatus of the approximated teeth was now in a position to provide neuromuscular direction to the cells creating the union. Although the signaling capacity was less than normal, drawing the sources of stimulation into close proximity enabled the site to exploit the bone-forming potential. At the donor site, although the distance between the roots was increased, the signaling intensity was less compromised and could reach the center of the regeneration chamber. The site of the nasal floor and piriform rim was now supported by the presence of an intact structural bone system. Adding a volume

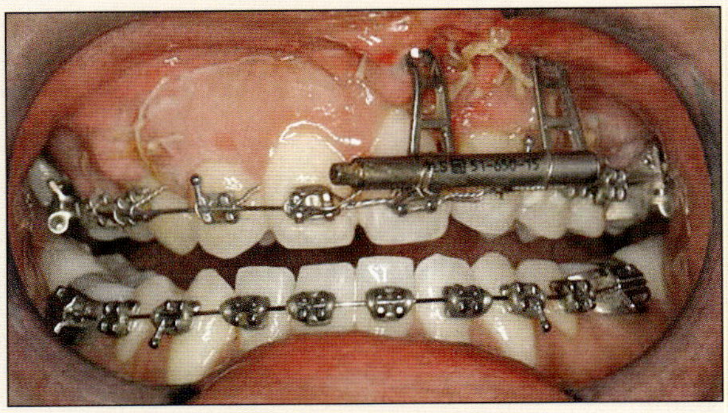

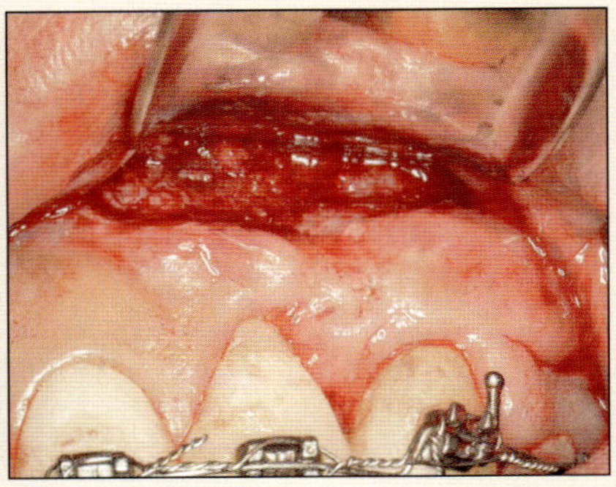

Fig 6-3l *(far left)* Four weeks after segmental osteotomy with rhBMP-2 grafting, soft tissue healing is uncomplicated.

Fig 6-3m *(left)* The cleft site demonstrates osseous union after 6 weeks.

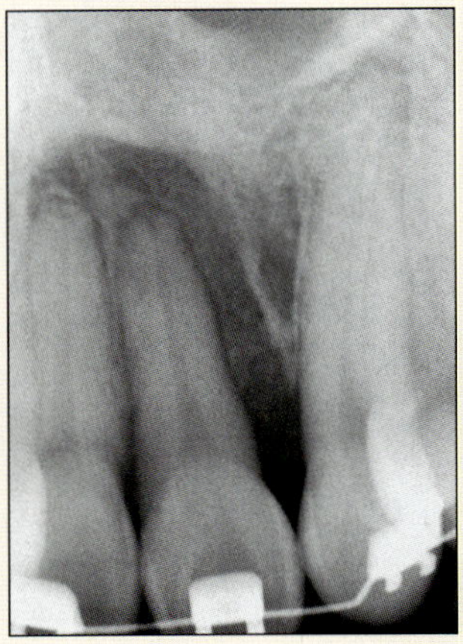

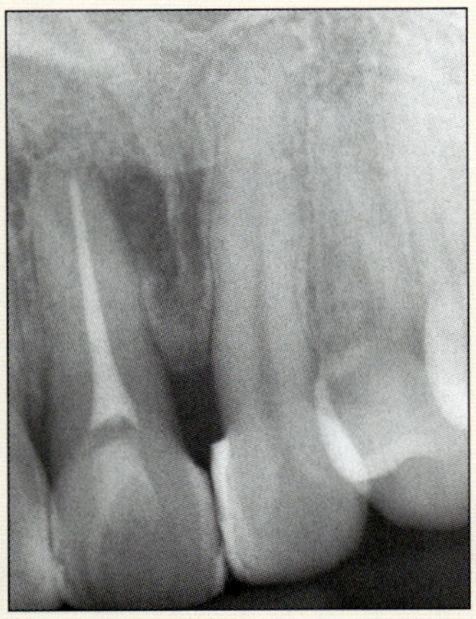

Fig 6-3n *(far left)* A radiograph taken 9 months after surgery shows fill of the bone across the cleft.

Fig 6-3o *(left)* A radiograph taken 7 years after surgery reveals consolidation and organization of the cleft repair site.

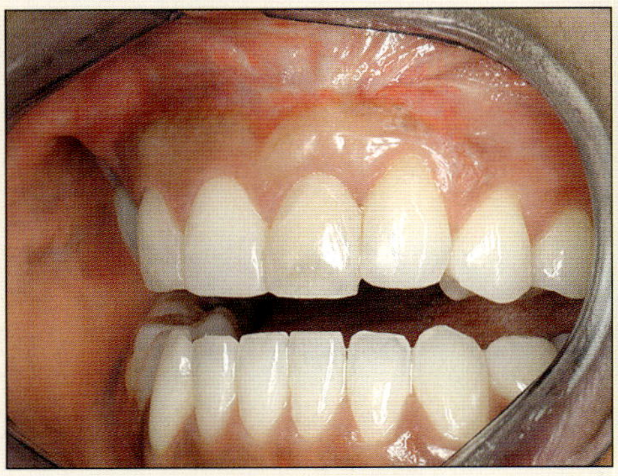

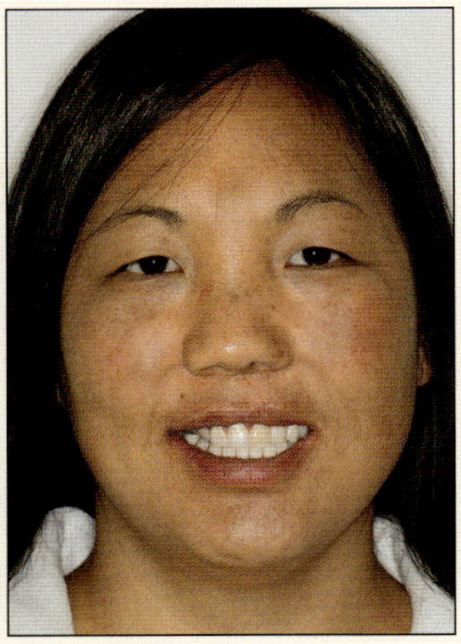

Fig 6-3p *(far left)* The result of the treatment plan is a complete dental arch of natural teeth. Note the periodontal health.

Fig 6-3q *(left)* Facial appearance 7 years after surgery. The facial and dental asymmetry have been corrected as part of the cleft site repair.

of bone at this site would be helpful in establishing a better base for nasal reconstruction.

Four weeks after surgery, the soft tissue healing was uncomplicated (Fig 6-3l). This was a contrast to the findings after prior surgeries. The maxillary central incisors had been transported to the midline. At that time, the distraction device was removed and the cleft site examined. Full and complete bone healing across the cleft was found (Fig 6-3m). There was no clinical sign of the original cleft.

A postoperative radiograph taken at 9 months showed fill of the bone across the cleft and the maintenance of lamina dura on the adjacent teeth (Fig 6-3n). Seven years after surgery, the bone that bridged the original cleft was consolidated and organized (Fig 6-3o). There was a mature cortex at the ridge crest that could support an interdental papilla. The periodontal health of the site remained stable (Fig 6-3p).

Osteotomy was used to rehabilitate this challenging problem of maxillary cleft discontinuity after three failed reconstructive procedures. In response to this new treatment approach, consolidation and osseous union required 6 weeks. There was no need to harvest bone grafts or to use banked bone. The teeth were transported into a position that could be managed by conventional orthodontic treatment. The dental arch was complete and consisted of all natural teeth (Fig 6-3q).

Discussion

Although bone grafting of alveolar clefts is a viable treatment option for many patients, success is challenged by the complex nature of congenital deficiencies. In this patient, use of a segmental maxillary osteotomy to fabricate a bone-forming construct provided a better treatment outcome than conventional methods. When designing and engineering these procedures, the surgeon is required to rethink how these disorders came to be and thereby to refine the diagnosis. Osteotomies, when combined with healing-enhancing agents such as rhBMP-2, can offer improved results with greatly reduced morbidity.

Osteotomy to Correct a Defect Resulting from Failed Orthodontic Extrusion

Management of any clinical problem should follow a deliberate and logical sequence of steps. Too often the surgeon starts by conceptualizing a treatment course based on the physical deformity that presents. Failed treatment is most often the result of an inadequate understanding of the disorder being confronted.

Accurate and comprehensive diagnosis is the first step in determining the range of treatment options. Diagnosis is more than a physical description of the presenting disorder. Diagnosis includes etiology and how the patient has accommodated to the deformity. Instead of focusing on the absence of a segment of bone or missing teeth, the clinician must understand the physiology of the structures that border the defect. In the case of a skeletal defect, the surgeon must understand how the bone bordering the defect is being maintained. The same physiology that establishes a steady state of bone morphology on the bone bordering the defect will directly impact how a graft heals. Much attention has been directed at the type of graft material placed in the defect. Not enough study has been invested in understanding how the environment in which the graft is placed impacts the healing.

The following case involves a history of treatment failure and the presentation of one strategy to manage a missing skeletal segment. It is important to analyze and understand why the prior treatments failed. The same environment and general physiology that produced the prior failure will be acting on the new treatment plan. Thoughtful retrospective analysis of past treatments is valuable in establishing a full diagnosis.

Case description

A 33-year-old patient presented with missing maxillary right first premolar, canine, and lateral incisor teeth. The first premolar had been removed in anticipation of erupting the impacted canine under traction by a bonded gold chain. However, the canine did not form a functional periodontal apparatus during eruption, and the erupting canine and the root of the lateral incisor collided. As a result, both the canine and lateral incisor were lost (Fig 6-4a).

In addition to the three missing teeth, there was substantial damage to the soft tissue. Beneath the soft tissue deficiency was a large defect in the alveolar process extending to the nasal floor. A second oral surgeon placed an autogenous graft from the mandibular ramus. The graft did not heal and was lost.

Radiographic examination showed a major defect (Figs 6-4b and 6-4c). The bone loss extended to the nasal floor, so vertical distraction was not an option. The condition of the roots of the adjacent teeth was compromised. Prior grafting with autogenous bone failed. Further autogenous bone grafting was likely to further compromise the periodontium of the remaining teeth. The site was difficult to graft because the gap was large, the central portion of the defect lacked neuromuscular stimulation potential, the roots had preexisting damage, and the site was in a cosmetic zone.

Before a bone reconstruction plan could be engineered, the forces that maintained the existing defect had to be identified and understood (Fig 6-4d). Following the loss of the canine and lateral incisor, the maxillary segment established a form maintained in a steady state. This defect was maintained through a dynamic process of bone resorption and deposition. Each site along the defect was controlled by its own regulatory process.

The bone of the alveolar process is chiefly regulated by teeth with healthy periodontal structures. In this case, point A was a thin layer of bone covering the mesial aspect of the second premolar. The bone was maintained under the influence of the periodontal apparatus of the tooth. Without the tooth and its periodontal structures, the bone at point A would resorb and disappear. The bone at point B was maintained in a similar way. The bone at point C was controlled by the maxillary sinus and possibly the lining of the maxillary sinus. The bone at points D and E was under the control of the nasal structures including the nasal mucosa and nasal septum.

All of the regulating processes surrounding the defect maintained the deformity in a steady state. When cells with bone-forming potential were introduced into the defect, the influence of the stimulating forces at play in the surrounding bone were insufficient to direct the cells to form bone. When an autogenous bone graft was placed in this defect, the graft failed chiefly because the stimulating forces at the periphery could not reach the immature cells and direct them to form bone.

Loss of both the canine and lateral incisor posed a challenge because of the combined functional and cosmetic requirements of these teeth. One strategy to increase the stimulatory forces in the center of the bone graft site would have been to reposition the sources of stimulation toward the center. In this case, a segmental maxillary osteotomy could have been considered to transport the maxillary posterior segment anteriorly (Fig 6-4e). This type of change would have multiple effects on the environment of the defect. The stimulating potential of the periodontal systems of the teeth adjacent to the defect would have been stronger because the distance to the center of the graft site would have been shorter. The anterior transport of the maxillary segment also would have moved gingival tissue into the defect. The addition of keratinized soft tissue to surround the graft would have supported healing. If segmental protraction of the maxillary segment had been done prior to the first attempt at bone grafting, the potential for success would have been higher.

Although it would have been surgically possible to protract the segment extending from the third molar to the second premolar anteriorly, the second premolar did not meet the cos-

Fig 6-4 Management of a large defect caused by a failed attempt at orthodontic extrusion and subsequent failed bone grafting.

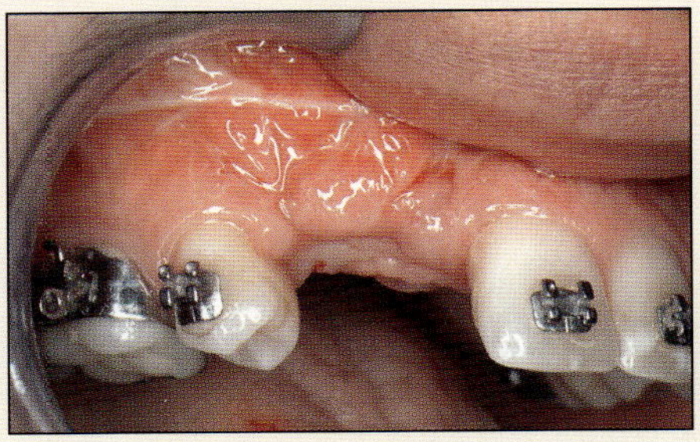

Fig 6-4a As a result of unsuccessful management of an impacted canine, the first premolar, canine, and lateral incisor have been lost. The bone defect extends vertically to the nasal floor. The labial and palatal plates have been lost. There is periodontal damage on the teeth adjacent to the defect.

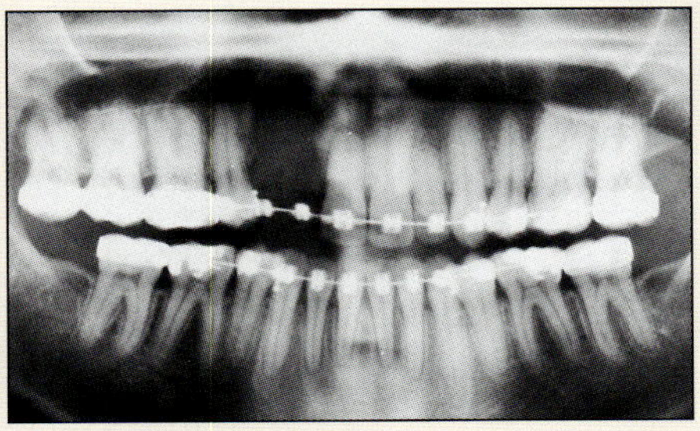

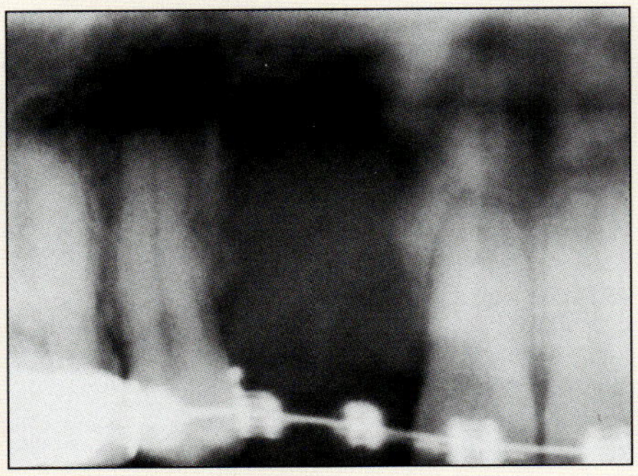

Figs 6-4b and 6-4c Radiographs reveal the extent of the defect.

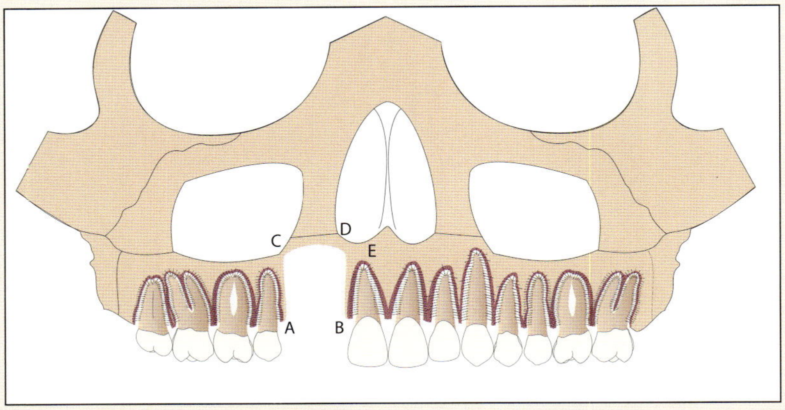

Fig 6-4d Functional analysis of the existing defect indicates the sources of neuromuscular regulation that are stabilizing the existing morphology. Point A is a thin layer of bone covering the mesial aspect of the second premolar. The bone is maintained under the influence of the periodontal apparatus of the tooth. The bone at point B is maintained in a similar way. The bone at point C is controlled by the maxillary sinus and possibly the lining of the maxillary sinus. The bone at points D and E is under the control of the nasal structures, including the nasal mucosa and nasal septum.

→

metic requirements of a lateral incisor. In addition, a segmental osteotomy involving the hemimaxilla usually requires general anesthesia, which the patient wished to avoid.

The selected treatment option was an osteotomy and horizontal repositioning of a single-tooth segment (Fig 6-4f). A single tooth and its periodontal apparatus would be mobilized with osteotomy and transported with distraction to the center of the defect.

Under local anesthesia, a single-tooth osteotomy mobilized the maxillary right second premolar in a segment of alveolar bone (Fig 6-4g). A Liou cleft palate distractor was mounted to transport the segment. The distraction site between the sites of the first molar and second premolar was filled with rhBMP-2. The docking site between the second premolar and central incisor was filled with a collagen sponge carrying rhBMP-2. The vascular supply was maintained by the soft tissue.

The result of the osteotomy and transport process was that the large defect was divided into two smaller ones (Fig 6-4h). Cells were introduced into the site using rhBMP-2. Because the rhBMP-2 was placed at the time of osteotomy, more protein could be placed in the docking site than in the distraction chamber. As the transport segment moved anteriorly, the concentration of rhBMP-2 decreased in the distraction chamber and increased in the docking chamber. The periodontal structures of the three teeth bordering the two regeneration chambers acted on the cells provided by the rhBMP-2 devices. The distances confronted by the single-tooth sites seemed to be narrow enough to effect the direction of stimulating forces from the teeth. The cells contained within the anterior bone growth chamber received regulatory signaling from the periodontal systems of the second premolar and the central incisor. The posterior chamber received input from the first molar and the second premolar (Fig 6-4i).

At the time of surgery, the soft tissue was closed and the distractor was left without activation for 7 days (Fig 6-4j). Following this 7-day latency period, the distractor was activated by 1 mm every other day. The transport vector was controlled by guidance of the orthodontic archwire. This process was continued for 1 week, after which the second premolar tooth had been transported to the center of the original defect (Fig 6-4k).

Both of the regeneration chambers consolidated with bone, and the periodontal structures remained intact. The density of

Fig 6-4e *(right)* One strategy to decrease the defect volume and move the periodontal ligament systems of the second premolar and central incisor into closer proximity is a segmental maxillary osteotomy.

Fig 6-4f *(far right)* A single-tooth distraction transport segment is another option. The molar teeth can be left relatively undisturbed.

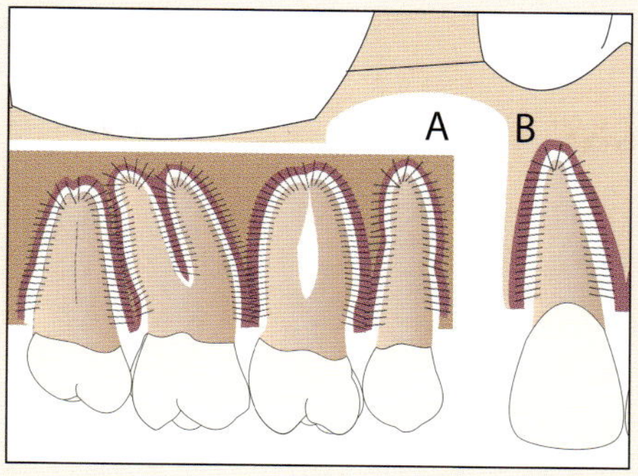

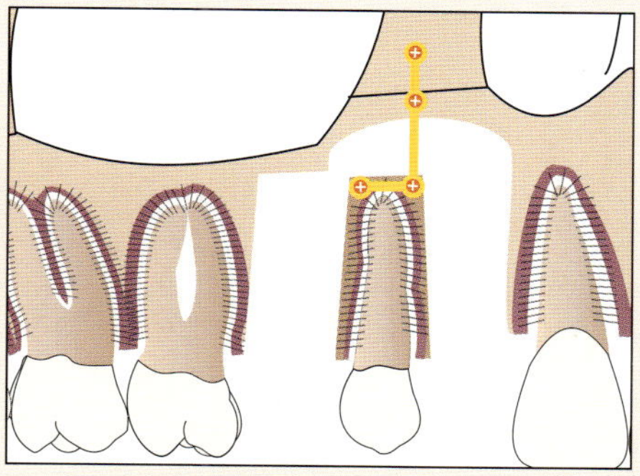

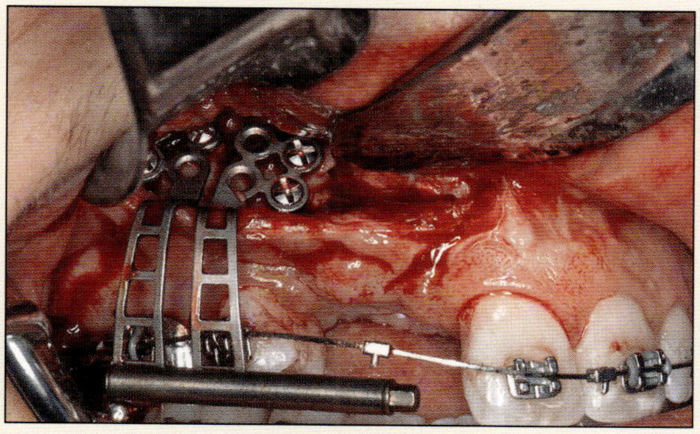

Fig 6-4g The single-tooth transport segment is mobilized and prepared for distraction.

Fig 6-4h *(right)* The strategy is to open a distraction chamber between the molar and premolar. The volume between the premolar and incisor will be decreased. Both sites will be filled with rhBMP-2.

Fig 6-4i *(far right)* The periodontal ligament and Sharpey fiber systems of the four teeth adjacent to the two bone-forming chambers will provide the neuromuscular input to cells recruited by rhBMP-2. The cells contained within the anterior bone growth chamber receive regulatory signaling from the periodontal systems of the second premolar (A) and the central incisor (B). The posterior chamber receives input from the first molar (C) and the second premolar (D).

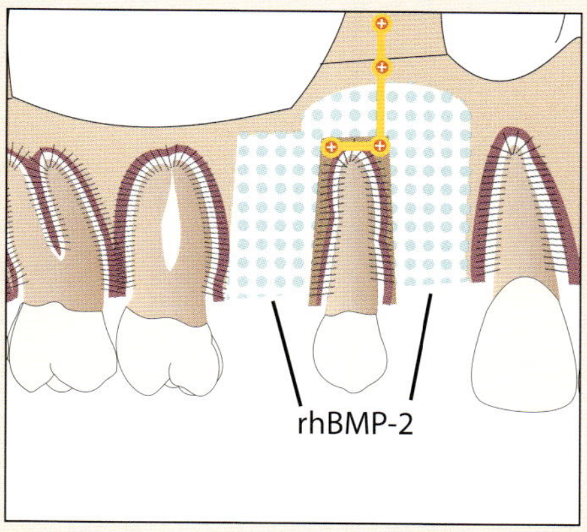

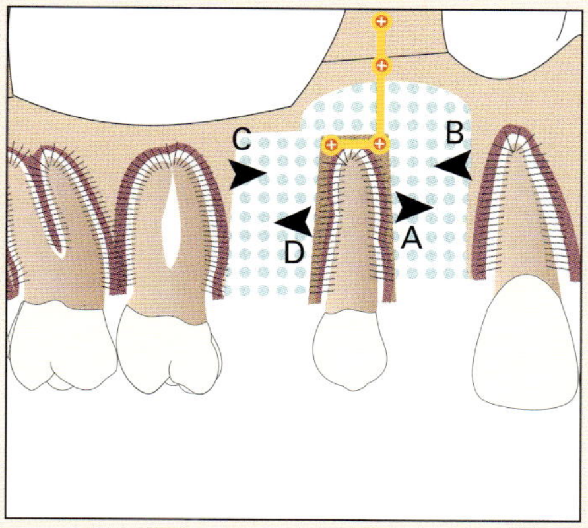

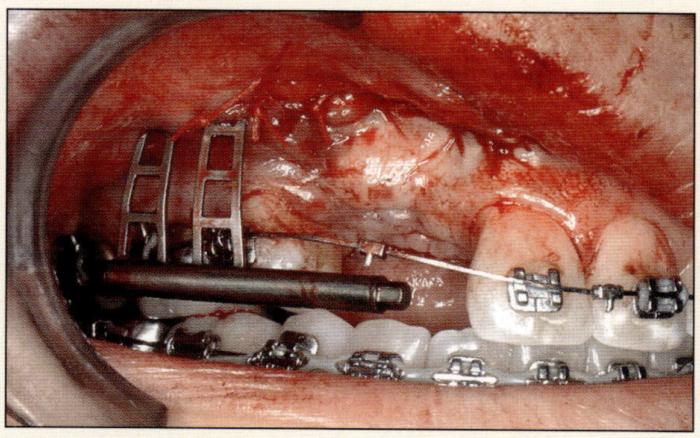

Fig 6-4j The wound is closed, beginning a 7-day latency period.

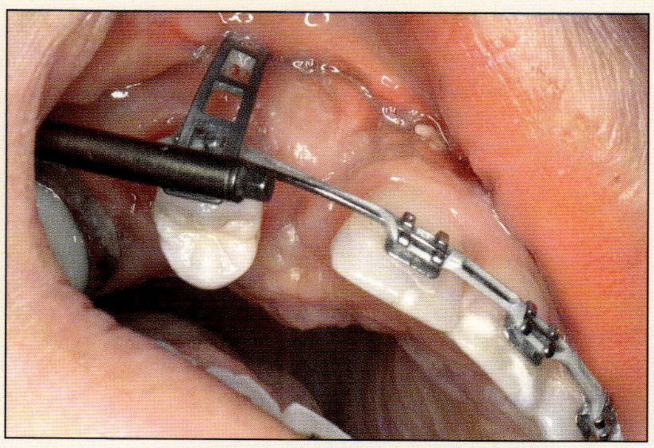

Fig 6-4k The second premolar is transported, under the control of the distraction device, to the center of the defect.

→

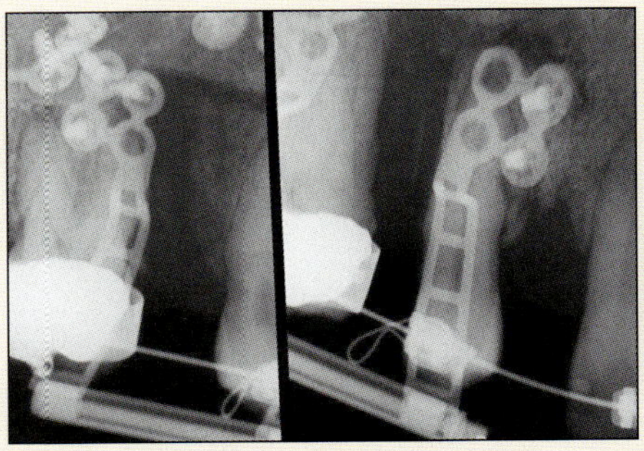

Fig 6-4l Radiolucent gaps are visible adjacent to the transported second premolar.

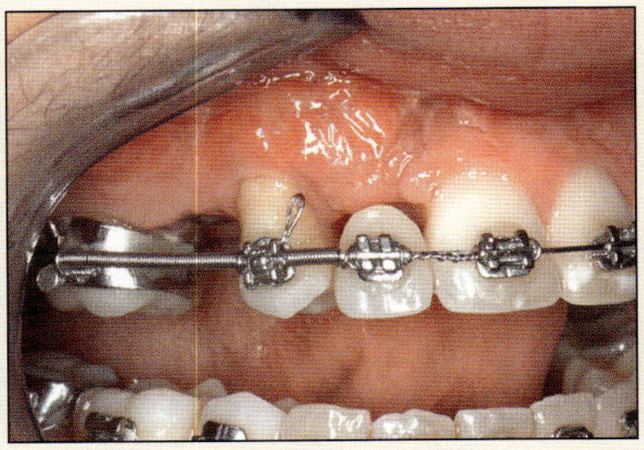

Fig 6-4m The archwire is used to supplement fixation after the distraction device is removed.

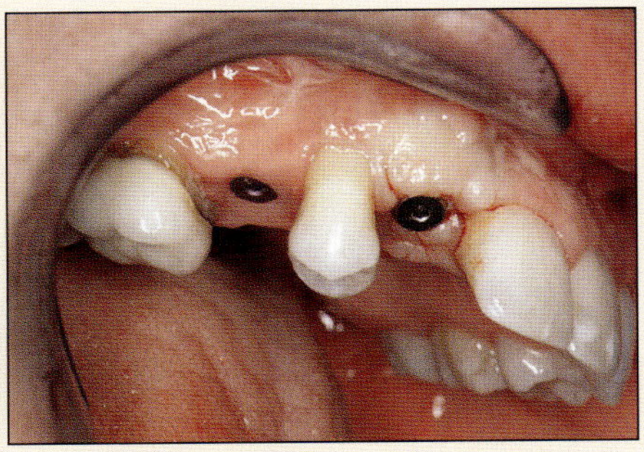

Fig 6-4n Both sites have consolidated with bone, and implants are placed.

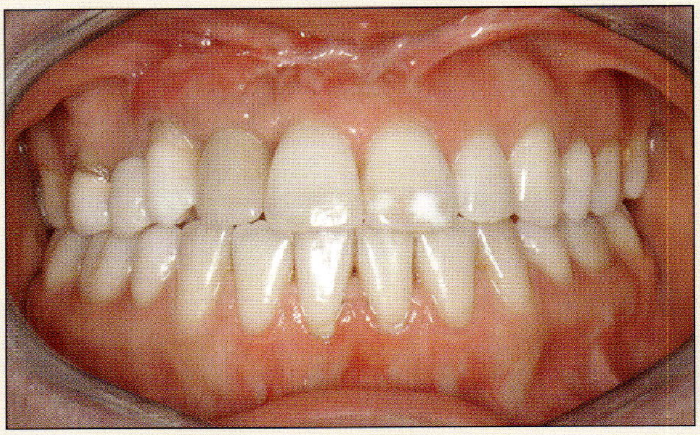

Fig 6-4o The dental arch has been restored.

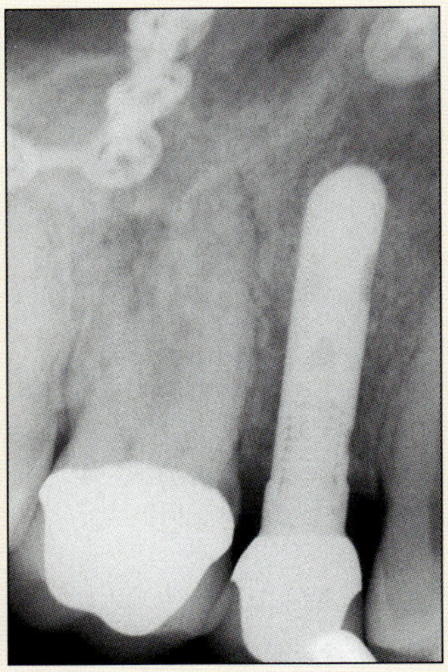

Fig 6-4p Six months after placement, the second premolar implant appears stable and osseointegrated in the constructed bone volume.

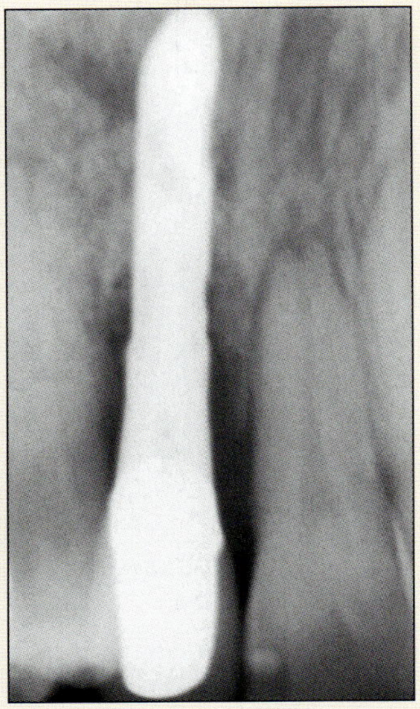

Fig 6-4q Six months after placement, the lateral incisor implant appears stable at the docking site.

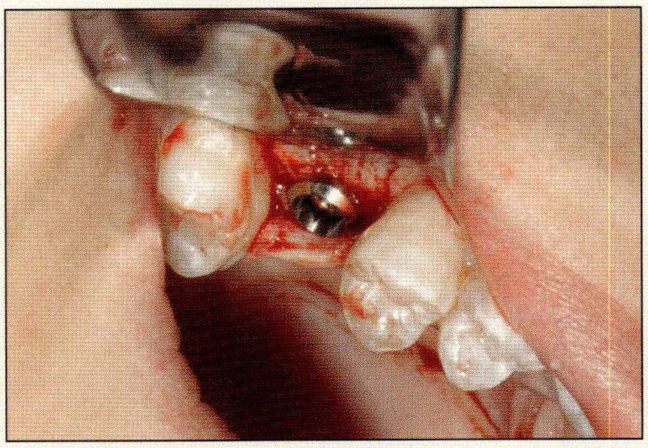

Fig 6-4r The second premolar implant has developed mobility after 2 years in function and is replaced with a new implant.

the newly formed bone was higher in the healed defect than at the donor site. This may have been due to the relative concentrations of rhBMP-2 in the two chambers. As the second premolar was transported anteriorly by distraction, the concentration of rhBMP-2 at the donor site decreased as the volume increased. The opposite situation took place in the defect site. As the transport segment moved anteriorly, the defect chamber volume decreased and the rhBMP-2 concentration increased. However, the actual reason for the difference in bone density is unknown and may have been related to the different anatomical locations within the functional skeleton.

Radiographs taken 3 weeks after surgery revealed that the single-tooth transport segment docked anteriorly (Fig 6-4l). The distraction chamber did not show signs of calcification at that time. The collagen sponge with rhBMP-2 partially filled the gap.

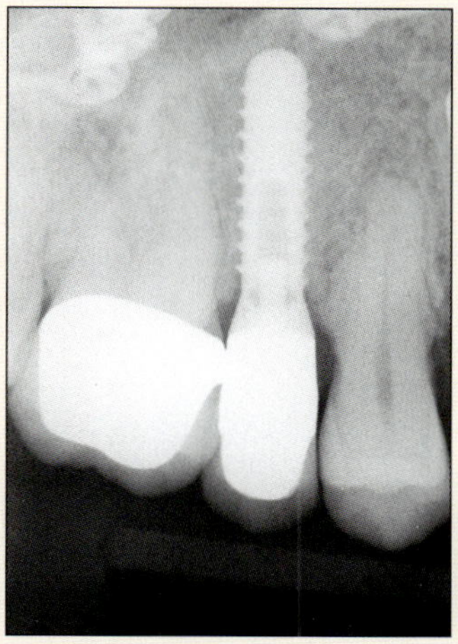

Fig 6-4s Replacement second premolar implant after 6 years in function.

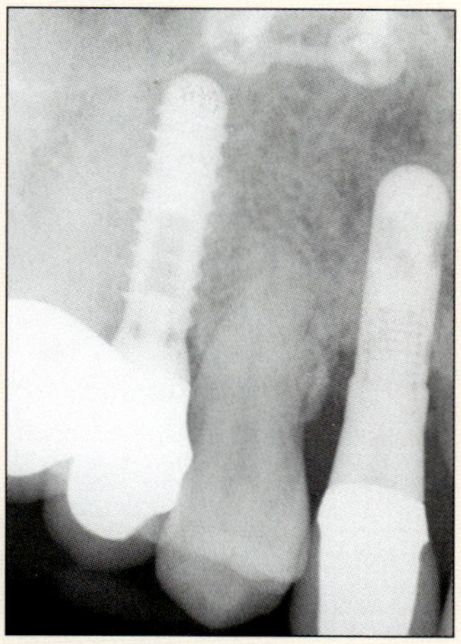

Fig 6-4t Lateral incisor implant after 8 years in function. The bone level remains at the level of the implant's polished collar.

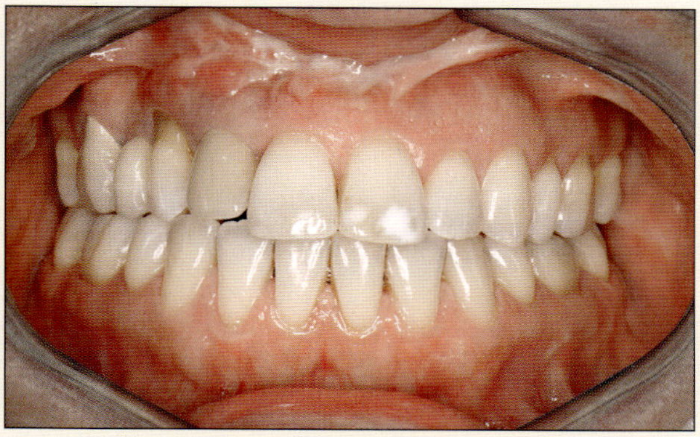

Fig 6-4u The dental arch reconstruction remains satisfactory at the 8-year follow-up.

Following successful transport, the distraction device was removed and the archwire was modified to serve as a fixation device (Fig 6-4m). Following 11 months of consolidation time, two dental implants were placed (Fig 6-4n). After 6 months to allow for osseointegration, the dental implants were restored (Fig 6-4o). The second premolar distraction site was consolidating, and the implant had healed (Fig 6-4p). The docking site at the right lateral incisor had consolidated, and the implant appeared to be healed (Fig 6-4q).

Two years after the second premolar implant was restored, the implant developed mobility. Examination on removal of the failed implant showed the bone to be intact. A new implant was placed (Fig 6-4r). The revised reconstruction did not require bone augmentation. The replacement implant integrated and was restored.

Six years after placement of the second implant at the site of the second premolar, the restoration and anchoring bone were intact (Fig 6-4s). The transported premolar was in good condition, and the bone level appeared stable. After 8 years, the implant at the docking site was functional and stable. Bone was near the level of the polished collar of the implant (Fig 6-4t). The appearance of the dental arch remained satisfactory 8 years after surgery (Fig 6-4u).

Discussion

Typical treatment of impacted canines involves surgical exposure of the crown and bonding of a gold chain for orthodontic traction. Most canines respond well to this management, but occasionally there are complications. Delay in recognizing that the impacted tooth is not responding to treatment increases the magnitude of the resultant defect.

The realization that the submerged tooth is not moving properly is a challenge because, unlike with erupted teeth, the orthodontist cannot visualize the crown and its changing position. The response to traction can only be followed with standardized plain dental radiographs or cone beam computed tomography. Frequent radiographic assessment of progress is not within the normal practice of everyday orthodontics. Detection of eruption failure may take months or years.

The only visible hardware in this approach is the end of the gold chain and the anchoring orthodontic archwire. The movement of the gold chain links can be deceptive. Over time, elastic traction moves the gold chain links closer to the archwire. The assumption is often made that the movement is due to the coronal eruption of the canine crown. The orthodontist or dental assistants may not realize that the movement is relative and that what they see is actually impaction of the anchoring dental arch.

This situation is further complicated by the simultaneous changes in the growing patient. These patients most often remain in occlusion because slow changes in the occlusion allow the neuromuscular matrix and temporomandibular joints to accommodate by developing a centric relation–centric occlusion shift.

Ankylosis is most often cited as the reason an impacted canine does not erupt under orthodontic traction. In many cases, however, surgical findings at the time of exposure and bonding verify that the tooth is mobile. Even when eruption failure is discovered and the tooth is extracted, many impacted canines show gross mobility at the time of surgery. In other cases, the tooth moves under traction but no periodontal structures are formed. In this way, the tooth is slowly extracted by the orthodontic appliance. A major defect in the alveolar process may be the result.

In the most severe cases, eruption of the canine takes a path that collides with the root of the lateral incisor, resulting in the loss of both teeth. Even if the damage to the lateral incisor root and periodontal structures is not complete, the resulting defect may limit the potential to graft the lost canine site for implant placement. In the case presented, the defect involved the adjacent lateral incisor, damaging its periodontal structures and root. As a result, both the canine and lateral incisor were lost.

The defect that this patient presented with could not be predictably reconstructed with conventional bone grafting to a state in which stable implants could be placed. The prior bone graft failed because the environment into which it was placed did not have the necessary elements to support initial healing or to integrate a new bone construct into the physiology of the region. Even if a graft could have been placed with the aid of a titanium mesh cage, the construct would have tended to resorb after the cage was removed. As the construct relapsed, implants placed in the unstable portion of housing would develop labial dehiscence and periodontal failure.

The alveolar process of the maxilla is vulnerable to resorption because it lacks powerful muscle attachments that provide neuromuscular stimulation to the bone. Without underlying muscle-directed regulation of bone metabolism, the volume of alveolar bone in the maxilla is disproportionately dependent on the periodontal attachment of healthy teeth to maintain the morphology of the alveolar bone. This is true during the lifelong process of maintaining existing natural bone as well as when healing of an alveolar bone construct is desired. A source of continued neuromuscular stimulation to the bone is essential to the long-term stability of the skeletal unit.

In this patient, the wide edentulous span between the second premolar and central incisor teeth caused a deficiency of stimulation potential in the center of the gap. Loss of both labial and palatal cortices created a defect that lacked confining walls. Establishment and maintenance of mechanical stability of a defect this large were difficult but essential. The basic strategy was to engineer an environment that would support bone growth and maintenance. This was accomplished by transporting the second premolar, along with its periodontal apparatus and alveolar housing.

Osteotomy for Reconstruction of a Traumatic Deformity

Trauma is a common cause of many of the defects that present to oral and maxillofacial surgeons. Simple fractures are amenable to repair by repositioning of the skeletal units and stabilization until healing can occur. In other cases, the injury results in the loss of a segment of the facial skeleton. In this situation, fracture reduction is not possible because anatomical parts are missing or damaged beyond the ability to heal.

Many traumatic deformities involve both bone and soft tissue deficiency. These composite defects are difficult to manage by grafting one tissue type at a time because a stable skeletal unit is an organized system in which each tissue type supports the other. The orchestration of the interaction requires some type of neuromuscular input. Jaws derive this regulation from muscular signaling to bone insertions, periodontal attachments, or both. Engineering analysis of possible rehabilitation strategies must include how the reconstruction materials will interact with the physiologic environment in which they are intended to function.

The specific design of the bone-forming construct should optimize the capabilities of the substrate and the environment. The substrate may include bone grafts, transported bone segments, adjacent cells, or cells induced by morphogenetic agents. The environment consists of existing anatomical boundaries, existing dental and neuromuscular elements, a surgically constructed physical environment, or a surgically constructed source of neuromuscular signaling. The following case demonstrates successful treatment of a traumatic defect despite the magnitude of volume deficiency and the difficulty in meeting the requirement of neuromuscular regulation for the new bone construct.

Case description

A 25-year-old woman presented after a recent bicycle accident had caused trauma to her face and teeth. The maxillary left lateral incisor was avulsed and lost at the scene of the accident. She was taken to the emergency department for medical evaluation, repair of facial lacerations, and stabilization of luxated maxillary incisors. The oral surgeon who evaluated the patient at her initial presentation at the emergency department attempted to reposition the luxated teeth and stabilize them by bonding a surgical wire.

Her general dentist later referred the patient for management of failing reimplanted incisors and placement of dental implants. As the patient recovered from the pain and swelling of the initial injury, it became clear that reconstruction would pose challenges for the patient, surgeon, and restorative dentist (Figs 6-5a to 6-5e). The posterior occlusion was Class III on both sides. The alveolar process fracture combined with the loss of the left lateral incisor increased the Class III interarch relationship. The condition of the central incisors and their supportive periodontium was poor. The patient had an anterior open bite tendency, and the central incisors were in reverse articulation. Root exposure on the left central incisor reflected the loss of alveolar bone across the anterior maxilla.

Six weeks after the injury, abscesses formed around the failed central incisor roots (Fig 6-5f). The two teeth were removed, and the extraction sites were treated with rhBMP-2. During removal of the teeth, examination revealed that the alveolar bone was comminuted. The labial and palatal plates were resorbed, resulting in a defect without containment walls.

The challenge in rehabilitating this type of defect is often underestimated. Although the initial presentation suggested management with conventional ridge preservation technology and dental implants, the deficiencies in the underlying environment complicated healing and long-term stability. In this case, the damaged alveolar housing would resorb despite ridge preservation procedures. The obstacles to successful treatment were the magnitude of volume deficiency and the difficulty in meeting the requirement of neuromuscular regulation for any new bone construct.

Following loss of both maxillary central incisors and the left lateral incisor, the alveolar process would be expected to remodel into a predictable configuration (Fig 6-5g). Resorption would remove the portion of the alveolus that had been damaged and lacked regulation from a stimulating source. The bone would resorb until it encountered new stimulatory forces, the right lateral incisor (tooth 12) and left canine (tooth 23). A line between these two teeth would become the post-trauma stable boundary. The maxilla would not continue to resorb beyond this line unless the right lateral incisor and left canine were compromised or lost.

Fig 6-5 Use of osteotomy to manage a traumatic defect.

Fig 6-5a *(right)* Facial appearance 3 weeks after a bicycle accident.

Fig 6-5b *(far right)* Oral condition 3 weeks after the injury. The luxated teeth had been repositioned and stabilized at the time of the accident.

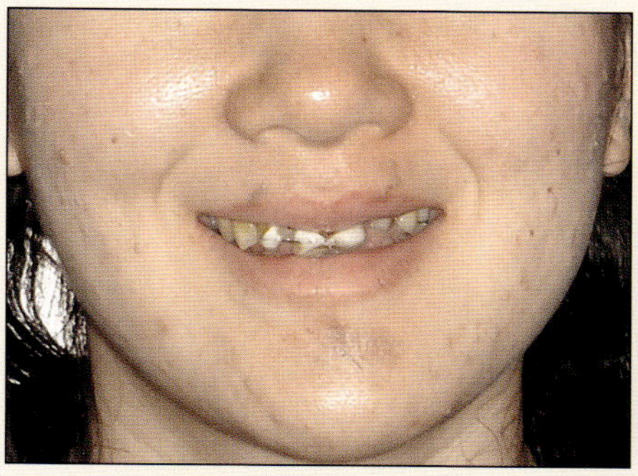

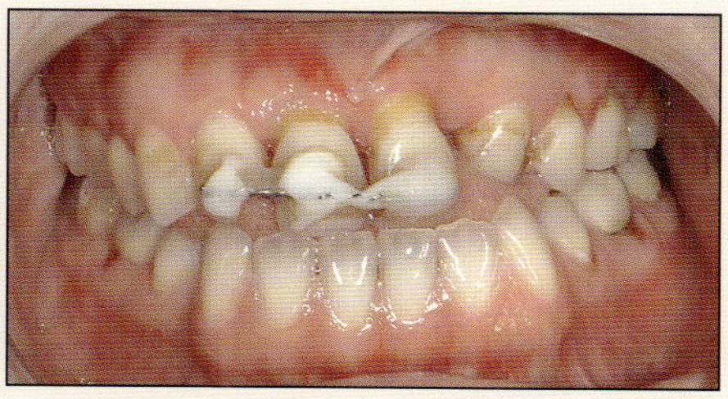

Fig 6-5c *(right)* Lateral view of the right side of the dental arch shows a Class III occlusion and retrusion of the anterior maxillary alveolus.

Fig 6-5d *(far right)* Left-side occlusion.

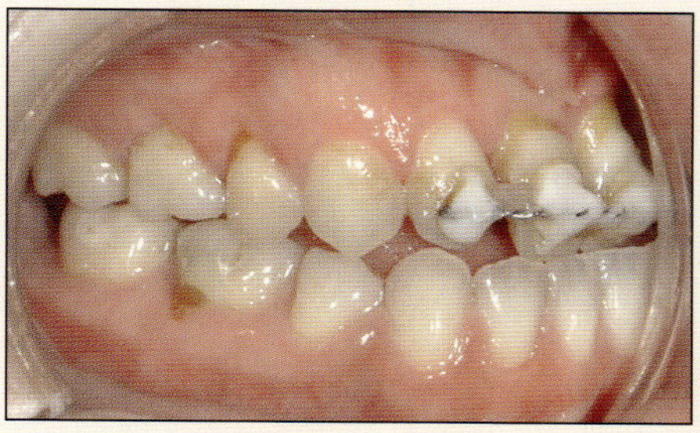

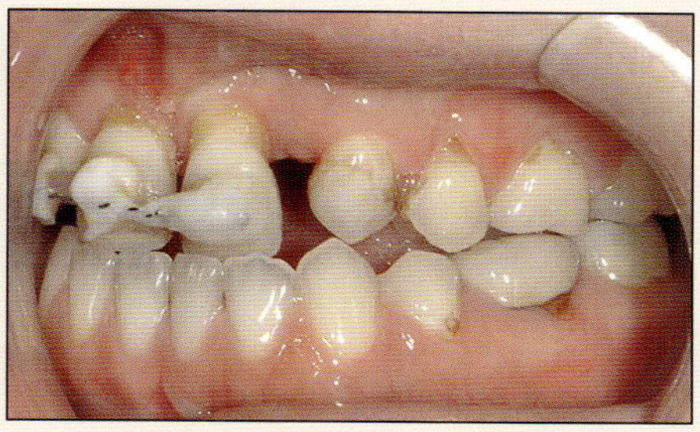

Fig 6-5e *(right)* Occlusal perspective of the maxillary arch form.

Fig 6-5f *(far right)* Six weeks after the injury, infection surrounds the central incisors.

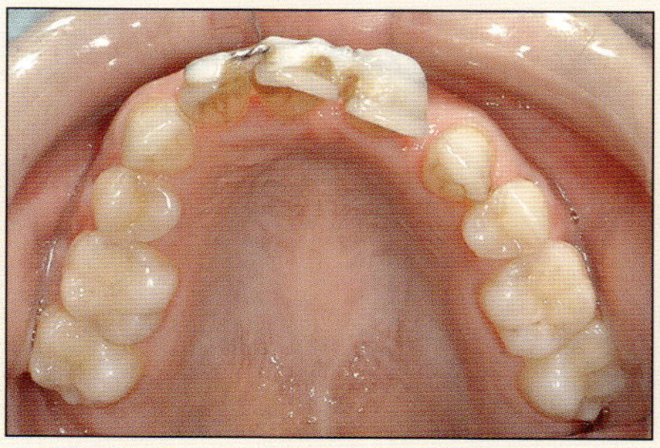

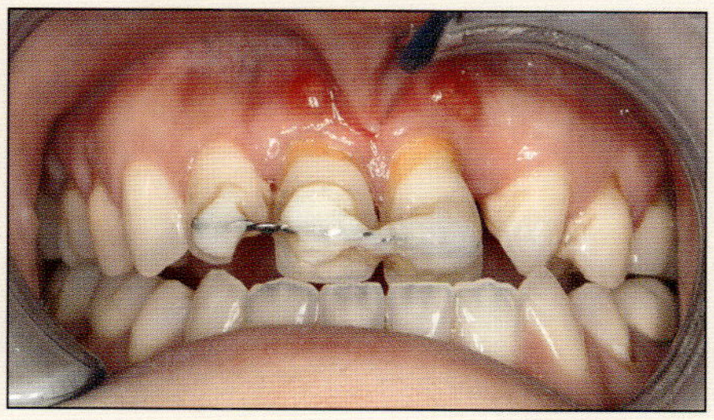

→

A portion of the ridge deficiency could be attributed to maxillary retrusion. The skeletal and dental Class III deformity had to be corrected if the goal of Class I incisor relationships was to be attained (Fig 6-5h).

If the goal were set at placing dental implants or fixed partial pontics to replace the central incisors, a substantial volume of bone would be required (Fig 6-5i). A mass of bone equivalent to a new alveolar process would have to be added to repair anterior and coronal deficiency. Soft tissue was also needed as part of the reconstruction. Creation of a bone construct that would resist resorption over years of service was the greatest challenge. The volume of the construct to be designed was defined by a comparison of the starting position of the ridge and the objective (Fig 6-5j).

When the design of this bone-forming construct was engineered, a method had to be included to alter the regulation of bone volume and position. As the patient presented, the right lateral incisor and left lateral canine established this boundary. To be successful, a new stable boundary had to be established to support the anterior bone volume augmentation (Fig 6-5k).

If a self-regulating bone construct was to be built, new neuromuscular elements had to be placed at or anterior to the line of the required stable boundary (Fig 6-5l). This would create a new stable boundary in the anterior position. Bone and implants housed within this boundary would be supported in their healing and maintenance.

Use of osteotomies would be one method to transport a regulating unit to the desired position. In this case, a four-piece Le Fort I maxillary osteotomy would be used to mobilize and reposition maxillary segments and the contained teeth (Fig 6-5m). The right lateral incisor, housed in the maxillary right segmental osteotomy, would be protracted to position A (see Fig 6-5l). The left canine, housed in the maxillary left osteotomy, would be protracted to position B. This would create a bone-forming chamber containing all of the essential elements to grow and maintain an integrated skeletal unit.

This design had limitations. If the stimulating units, the right lateral incisor and left canine, were successfully positioned, the stable boundary would only extend between them (Fig 6-5n). The regulatory influence of these teeth did not extend further anteriorly. The alveolar convexity needed to anatomically house the implants replacing the central incisors would still be somewhat deficient. One option would be to compensate for the deficiency with the prosthesis design. In this case, the dental implants would have to be positioned palatal to the anatomical location.

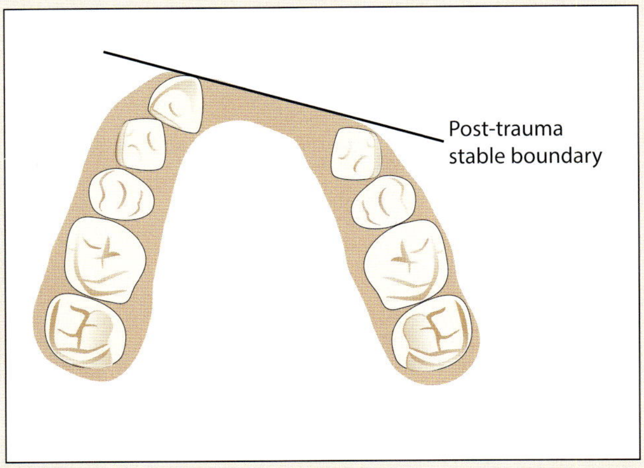

Fig 6-5g Functional analysis of the anatomical elements that maintain the existing morphology. A line between the remaining stimulatory forces, the right lateral incisor and left canine, becomes the post-trauma stable boundary.

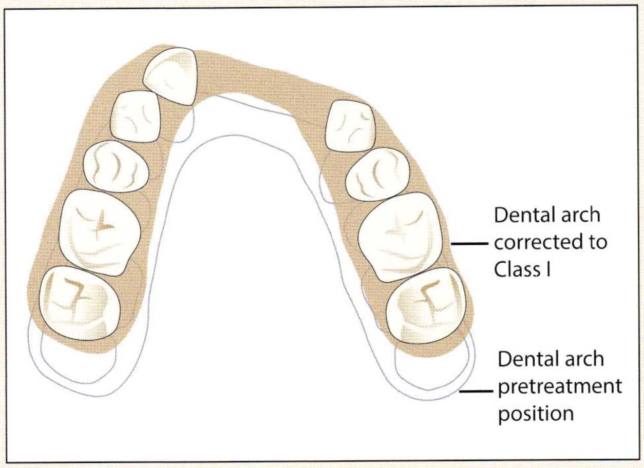

Fig 6-5h Correction of Class III maxillary retrusion would partially fill the anterior alveolar deficiency.

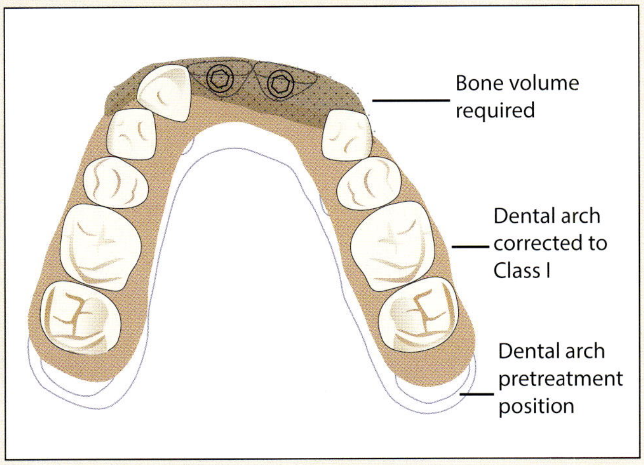

Fig 6-5i Projection of the bone volume required to position implants to replace the maxillary central incisors beyond maxillary bone protraction by Le Fort I osteotomy.

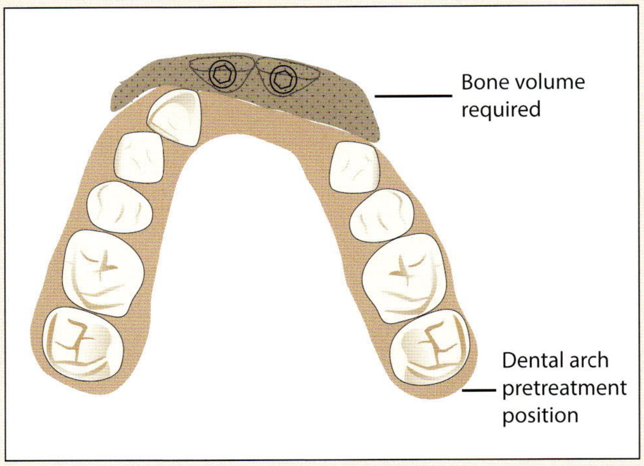

Fig 6-5j Total bone augmentation required to meet the restorative dental objective.

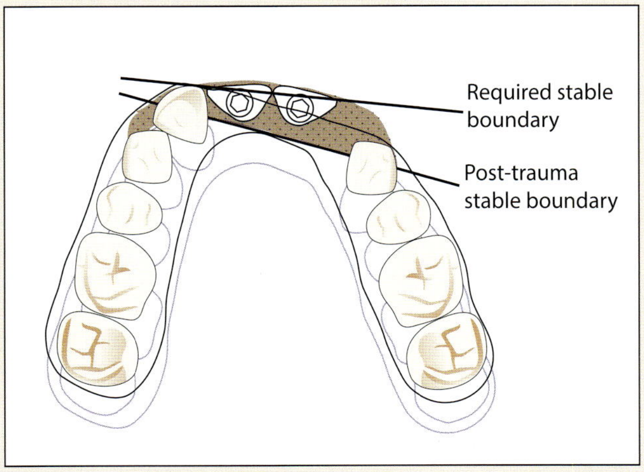

Fig 6-5k Engineering objective that will provide a stable site for central incisor implants.

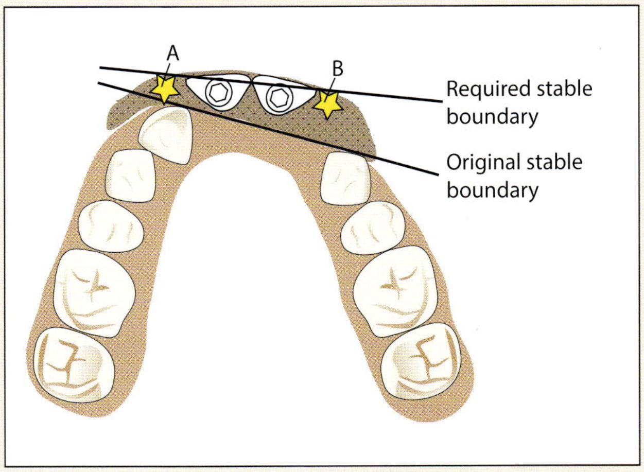

Fig 6-5l If a functional bone volume is to be constructed, a source of neuromuscular input must be positioned to maintain stability. The position of the regulatory source (points A and B) must be at or anterior to the line of the required stable boundary.

→

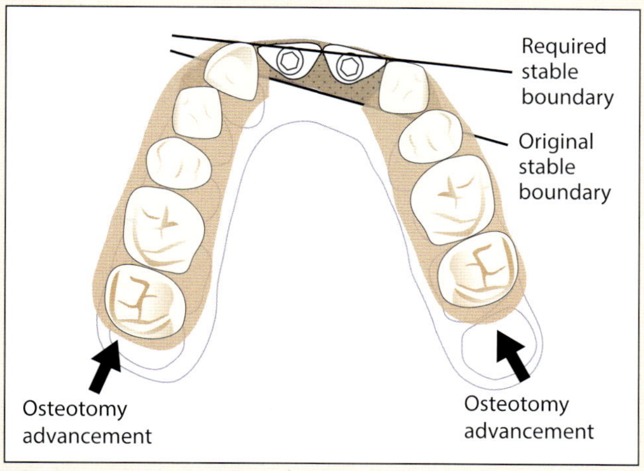

Fig 6-5m Because teeth are the only practical source of neuromuscular signaling within the alveolar process, the plan must allow positioning of healthy periodontal ligament and Sharpey fiber systems at the required stable boundary.

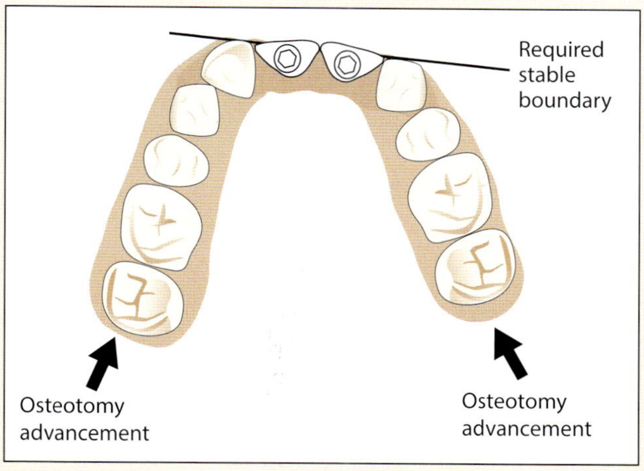

Fig 6-5n Projection of the surgical design.

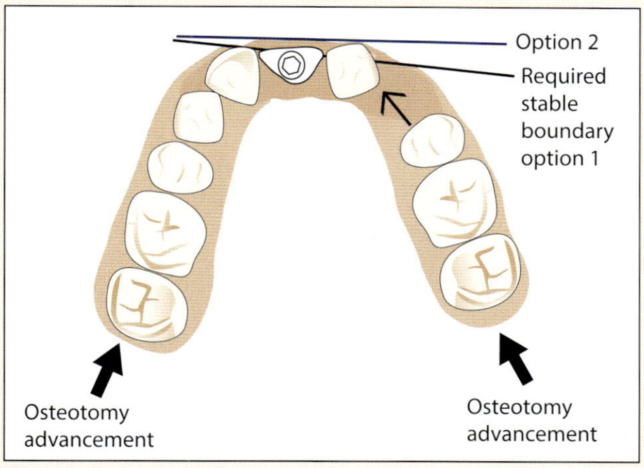

Fig 6-5o An alternative design (option 2) would transport the maxillary left canine to the central incisor position.

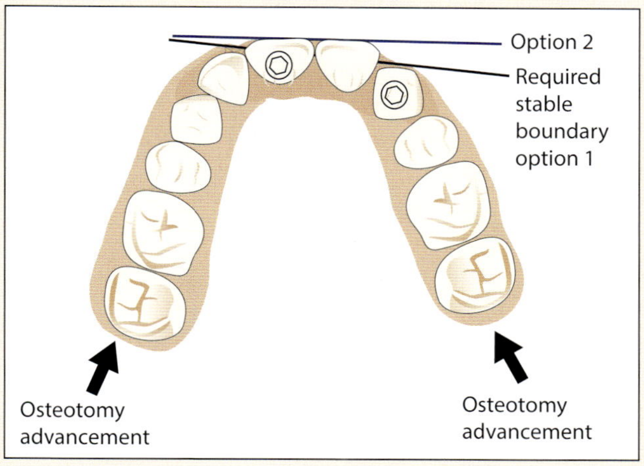

Fig 6-5p Moving the canine to the central incisor position would have benefits but would require substantially longer orthodontic treatment.

If the position of the stable boundary was to be moved further anterior, then a regulating unit must be located to support it. One strategy would be to move the left canine into the left central incisor position orthodontically (Fig 6-5o). If successful, it would result in the further protraction of the stable boundary.

Orthodontic movement of the left canine to the left central incisor position would have theoretical benefits (Fig 6-5p). However, there would also be potential hazards. Moving the previously damaged tooth orthodontically would pose a risk of root resorption. The process would involve months of orthodontic treatment. If the tooth were to develop ankylosis before full repositioning was achieved, extraction might be necessary. In addition, if the canine were repositioned as the central incisor, it would require substantial restorative modification.

The selected treatment option involved Le Fort I maxillary osteotomy (Fig 6-5q). Because the primary bone-forming chamber was at the pterygomaxillary junction, damage to the pterygoid plates had to be avoided. To mechanically luxate the maxilla from the pterygoid plates, a maxillary mobilizing instrument was used (Fig 6-5r).

Purchase on the maxilla was from the dental arch below and the nasal floor above (Fig 6-5s). Use of pterygoid chisels would have risked damaging the pterygoid plates and adjacent structures because the vector of the instrument's impact was not aligned with the pterygomaxillary suture. Preservation of the muscle attachments to intact pterygoid plates was important in the bone-forming process.

After the maxilla was downfractured, the surgeon had a direct view of the nasal floor and maxillary sinus floors. Piezoelectric surgery was used to divide the maxilla into four segments (Fig 6-5t). Each of these segments was planned for three-dimensional repositioning to meet the engineering and design objectives. Each segment had to maintain a profusing pedicle to remain viable. Piezoelectric surgery allowed creation of osteotomies while sparing the underlying mucosa (Fig 6-5u).

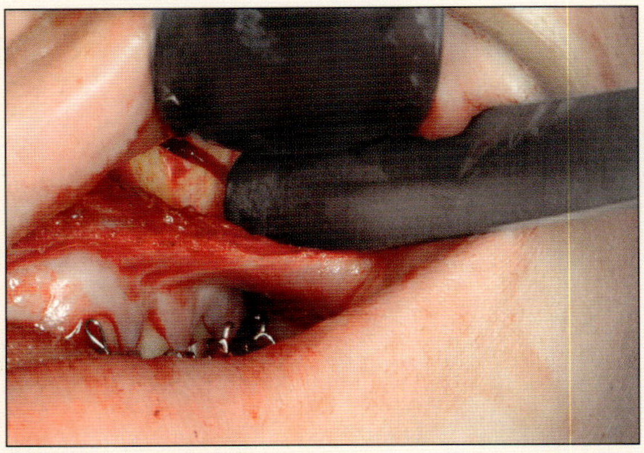

Fig 6-5q Le Fort I osteotomy prepares the maxilla for mobilization.

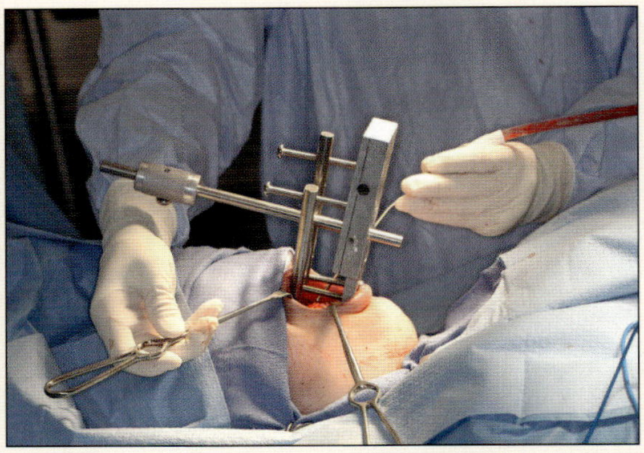

Fig 6-5r A mobilizing instrument allows separation of the posterior maxilla from its fusion with the pterygoid plates without direct osteotomy.

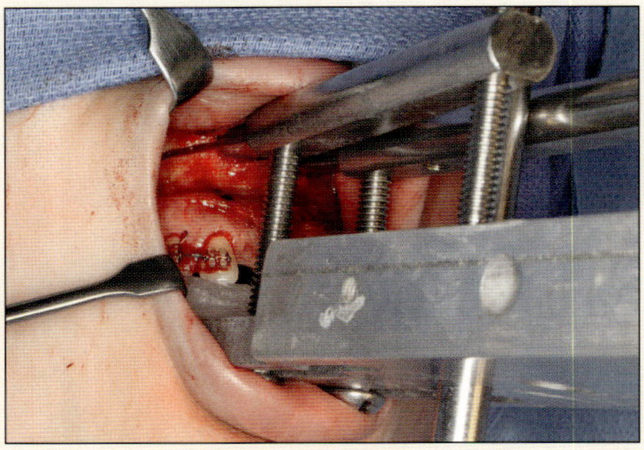

Fig 6-5s Protracting force is applied to the maxilla.

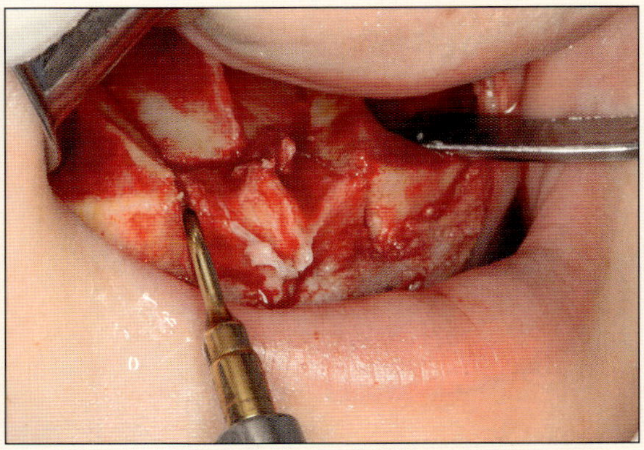

Fig 6-5t Piezoelectric surgery is used to divide the downfractured maxilla into four segments.

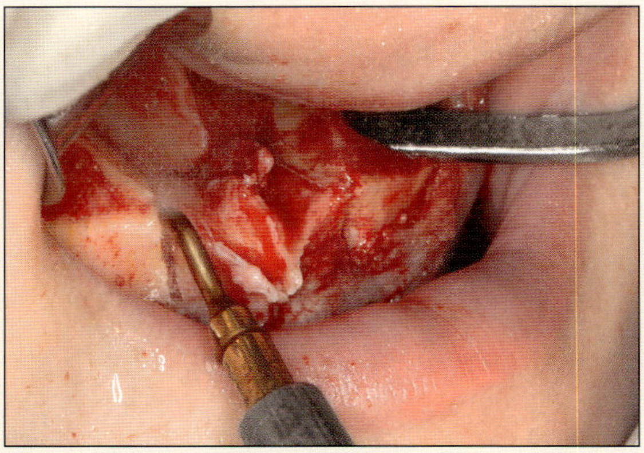

Fig 6-5u The piezoelectric surgical instrument makes precise bone cuts without damaging the adjacent soft tissue.

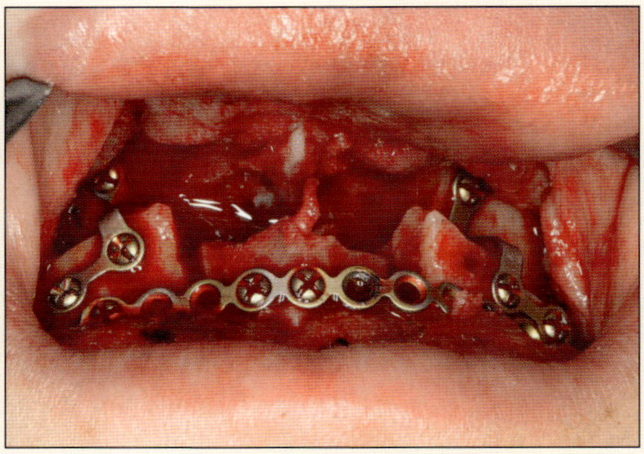

Fig 6-5v The four maxillary segments are positioned using acrylic splints made on articulator-mounted casts and then fixated using titanium plates and screws.

→

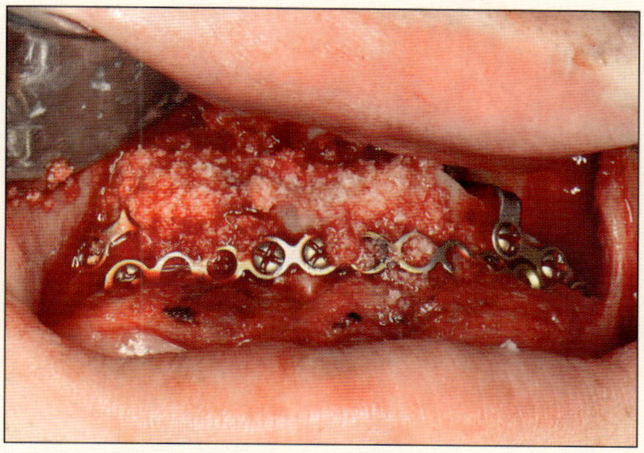

Fig 6-5w Cancellous chips carrying rhBMP-2 fill the voids resulting from the osteotomy segments.

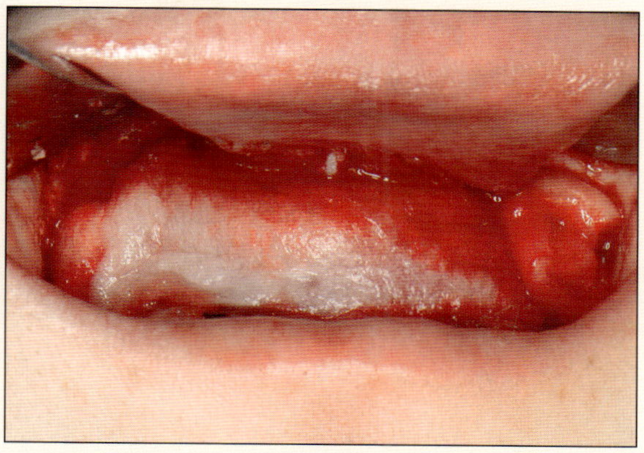

Fig 6-5x Collagen sponges with rhBMP-2 are used to fill the steps created by the maxillary advancement and to cover the cancellous graft.

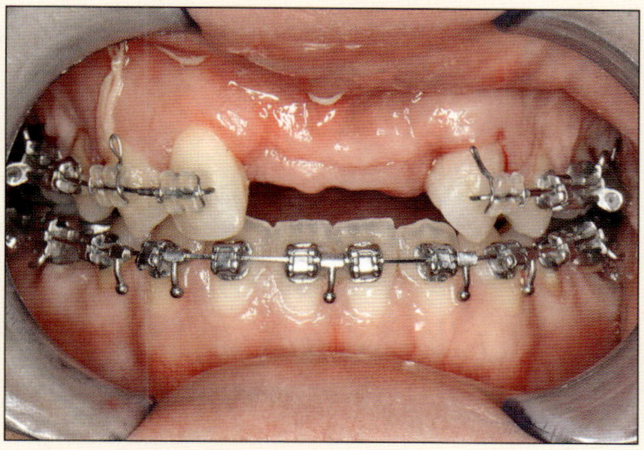

Fig 6-5y Appearance 3 weeks after Le Fort I maxillary osteotomy.

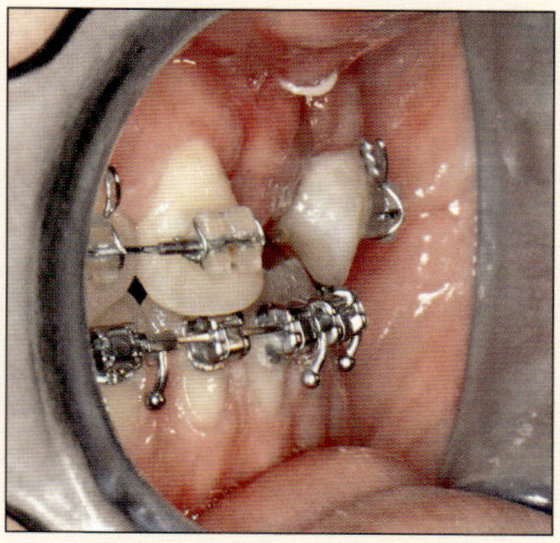

Fig 6-5z Protraction with Le Fort I osteotomy has improved the occlusion and ridge relationships.

→

Splints and cranial headframe–based navigation were used to reposition and stabilize the maxillary segments with bone plates (Fig 6-5v). The amount of protraction of the maxillary segments was reflected in the large steps in the bone. The anterior segment was repositioned inferiorly to compensate for vertical alveolar resorption. The amount of inferior repositioning of the anterior segment was limited by the impact on the damaged teeth adjacent to the transported segment. The space above the anterior segment represented the donor site. It became the regeneration chamber to regrow the bone.

Cancellous chips from the bone bank with rhBMP-2 were used to fill the regeneration chamber and gaps (Fig 6-5w). Collagen sponges soaked with rhBMP-2 were used to fill the steps created by the maxillary advancement and to cover the cancellous graft (Fig 6-5x).

The patient was reexamined 3 weeks after Le Fort I maxillary osteotomy (Fig 6-5y). Protraction with Le Fort I osteotomy had improved the occlusion and ridge relationships (Fig 6-5z).

After 4 months of healing of the osteotomy and graft, dental implants were placed (Fig 6-5aa). After 4 months to establish osseointegration, the implants were restored (Figs 6-5bb to 6-5ee). The posterior occlusion was corrected, and the maxillary ridge reconstruction allowed placement of crowns with good interdental papilla form. An esthetic smile was restored (Figs 6-5ff to 6-5hh).

Discussion

Treatment planning for dental implants in patients with anterior maxillary deficiencies requires special attention. These defects may have resulted from trauma, deficient development, or bone loss related to periodontal failure. The common feature of these cases is relative retrusion of the anterior maxillary edentulous ridge into a Class III relationship. This configuration challenges the surgeon's ability to position implants that will allow placement of a prosthesis that will meet mechanical and esthetic requirements.

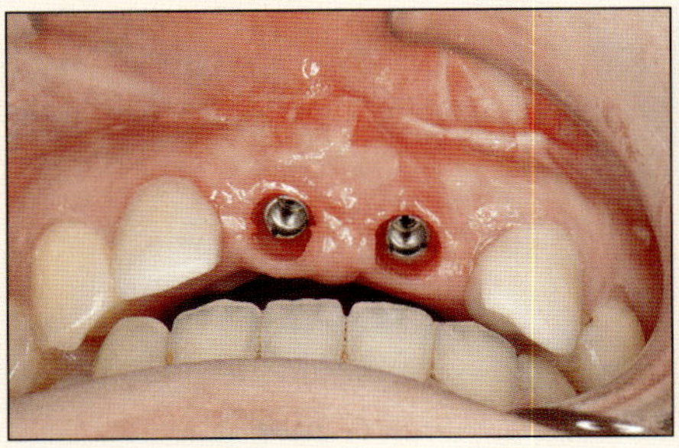

Fig 6-5aa Implants in place.

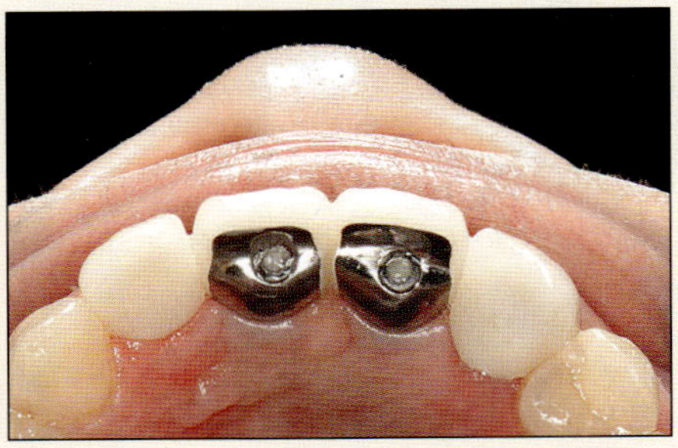

Fig 6-5bb Screw-retained implant crowns in the reconstructed alveolus.

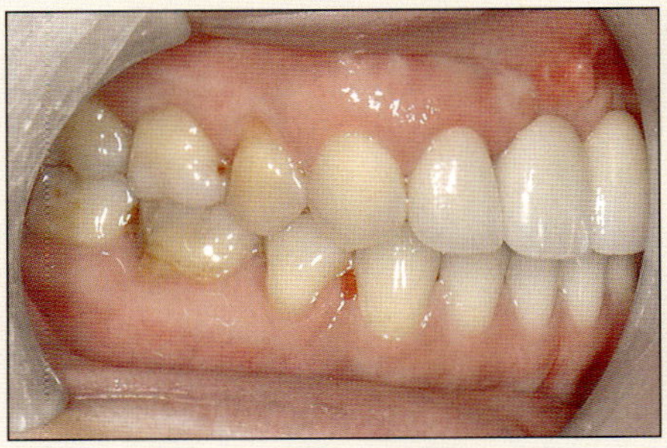

Fig 6-5cc Right occlusion. Osteotomies have corrected the retruded ridge position, the vertical loss of ridge height, and the gingival deficiency, allowing a straightforward implant restoration.

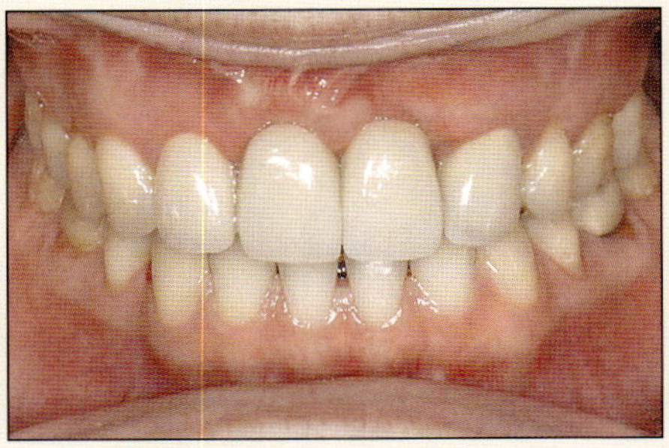

Fig 6-5dd Anterior crowns and reconstructed maxilla.

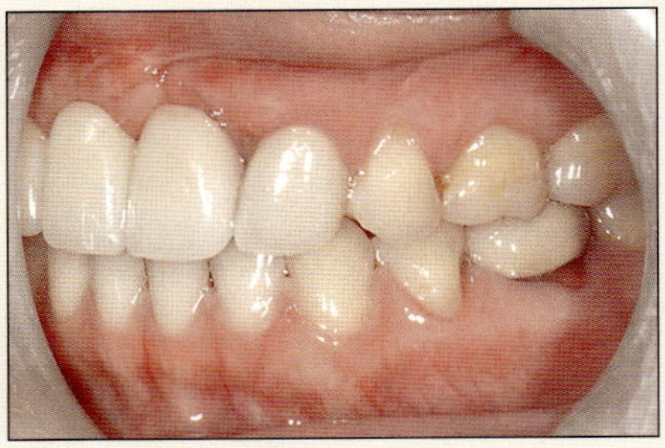

Fig 6-5ee Left occlusion.

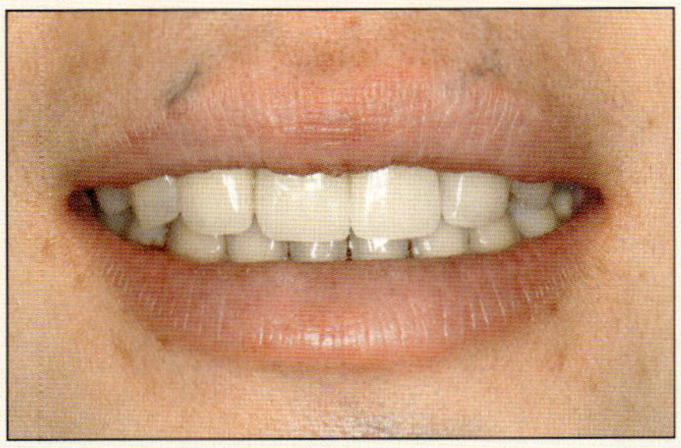

Fig 6-5ff Restoration of the patient's smile.

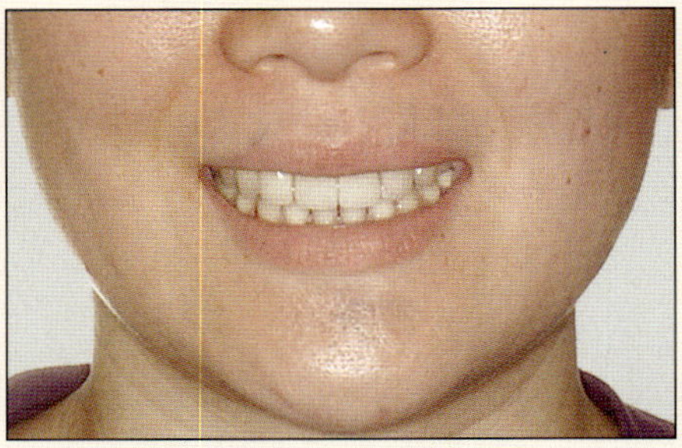

Fig 6-5gg Facial appearance after healing from surgery and placement of definitive implant crowns.

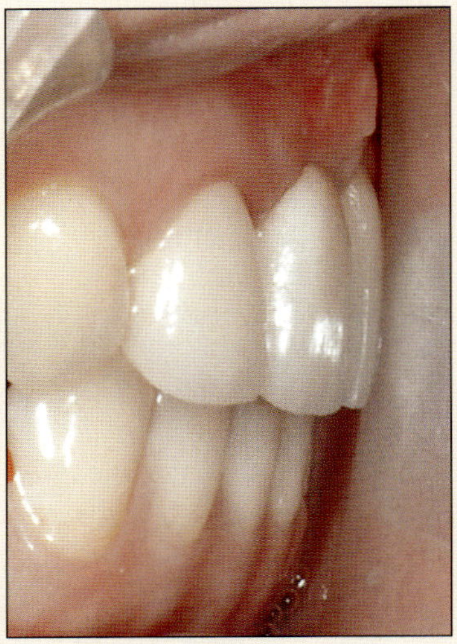

Fig 6-5hh Lateral view shows that the labial projection and alveolar height have been restored.

After recognizing that incisor implants cannot be placed unless more bone is available, many surgeons will choose the course of onlay grafting. This is a familiar process that directly addresses the geometric problem of inadequate bone volume. The f aw in this approach is that it ignores the regulatory mechanisms that are necessary to maintain bone in a steady state over the long term. The maxillary alveolar process assumes its familiar curvilinear form in response to dental eruption. It is maintained for years by the regulatory effect of the teeth and their periodontal ligament systems. The ability of the maxillary arch to maintain its anterior projection is dependent on the presence and health of the anterior teeth. Without the teeth, the ridge tends to resorb, resulting in retrusion of the edentulous segment.

The presence of dental implants may help to maintain bone volume, but only in a specific, limited manner. Bone that extends beyond the stimulating influence of the natural teeth is at risk of resorption. If implants are placed in this zone, the cylinders may become exposed as remodeling results in resorption along their labial surfaces. Radiographs may not detect the slow thinning to bone covering the labial aspect of the implants until the implant is compromised.

In this patient, severe bone and soft tissue deficiency challenged successful reconstruction of the anterior maxilla. The alveolar ridge was both retruded and vertically deficient. The soft tissue was deficient and damaged. The defect in the anterior maxilla had to be reconstructed so the existing regulating mechanisms could promote maintenance of the bone and soft tissue volume for many years.

If the projected bone volume lacks a source of neuromuscular regulation, the surgical plan must correct the deficiency by repositioning a mechanism into the bone construct. The possible sources of neuromuscular input are dictated by the surgical engineering phase and are the product of basic science. The mechanism employed and the manner in which it is applied are determined by the surgical designer and become part of the surgical plan.

In this patient, a surgical plan involving a Le Fort I maxillary osteotomy in four segments was elected because it had the potential to reposition bone volume and periodontal systems into a relationship that would meet the requirements of the bone-forming construct. The vulnerable region of the reconstruction was the maxilla at the potential location of the central incisors. This area projected anteriorly beyond the dental arch, so all of its neuromuscular signaling was delivered from the palatal aspect. To optimize the stability of this region, the surgical plan repositioned natural teeth in the lateral incisor sites.

The vertical deficiency at the central incisor sites would have compromised the esthetic result if not corrected. Bone and soft tissue were delivered to that site by repositioning of the anterior segmental osteotomy in an inferior direction. This corrected the anatomical defect at the expense of the bone at the piriform rim. This defect was grafted with rhBMP-2.

Although the Le Fort I osteotomy procedure requires general anesthesia, it produces a comprehensive reconstruction in a single surgery. Placement of implants is all that is necessary to complete the treatment. The placement of natural teeth into the bone-forming construct offers the potential for self-regulation of the reconstruction and long-term stability.

Conclusion

Osteotomy is an important part of the design and fabrication of bone-forming constructs. The utilization of osteotomy and repositioning of functional elements such as muscle attachments and teeth can create an environment that will support and maintain new bone growth. The objective of repositioning the bone segment and attached muscle is twofold: The elevated and fixed bone creates a sheltered chamber at the distraction site so that cells filling the chamber are protected from harmful mechanical forces, and the stimulation introduced by the periodontal structures results in development of bone tissue and organization into mechanical support systems.

References

1. Epker BN. Modified sagittal ramus osteotomy. In: Epker BN (ed). Dentofacial Deformities: Surgical-Orthodontic Correction. St Louis: Mosby, 1980:84–85.
2. Meyer U, Wiesmann HP, Meyer T, et al. Microstructural investigations of strain-related collagen mineralization. Br J Oral Maxillofac Surg 2001;39:381–389.
3. Ingber DE, Dike L, Hansen L, et al. Cellular tensegrity: Exploring how mechanical changes in the cytoskeleton regulate cell growth, migration, and tissue pattern during morphogenesis. Int Rev Cytol 1994;150:173–224.
4. Aaron JE. Periosteal Sharpey's fibers: A novel bone matrix regulatory system? Front Endocrinol (Lausanne) 2012;3:98.
5. Frost HM. Dynamics of bone remodelling. In: Frost HM (ed). Bone Biodynamics. Boston: Little, Brown, 1964:315–347.
6. Harvold EP. The theoretical basis for the treatment of hemifacial microsomia. In: Harvold EP, Vargervik K, Chierici G (eds). Treatment of Hemifacial Microsomia. New York: Alan R. Liss, 1983.
7. Wang HL, Boyapati L. "PASS" principles for predictable bone regeneration. Implant Dent 2006;15:8–17.
8. Schallhorn RG. Postoperative problems associated with iliac transplants. J Periodontol 1972;43:3–9.
9. Carstens MH. Neural tube programming and the pathogenesis of craniofacial clefts. I. The neuromeric organization of the head and neck. Handb Clin Neurol 2008;87:247–276.

7 Using Osteotomies to Generate Bone in Patients with Systemic Disorders

Some of the most challenging skeletal deformities are cases that combine an anatomical defect with an underlying systemic deficiency. The bone deficiency might appear ordinary and amenable to straightforward surgical treatment. Many of these patients present with a history of multiple failed attempts to repair the problem with conventional surgery.

This group of patients includes a wide range of special conditions. Advanced age itself can be considered a special obstacle to successful healing. Patients with multiple systemic congenital anomalies may exhibit deficiencies in the healing of their soft tissue. Patients with clefts of the facial midline respond poorly to conventional bone grafting. Some patients present with healing that is compromised as a result of radiation therapy to manage malignancies.

Special attention to the specific healing challenge in each of these cases is needed to create a successful surgical design. Osteotomies are often needed as part of the design of the bone-forming construct.

Clinical Applications

The cases in this chapter demonstrate the important role osteotomy can play in bone-forming constructs for patients with systemic challenges.

Osteotomy for Bone Construction in a Patient of Advanced Age

Advanced age is generally considered a risk factor when the potential for a successful surgical outcome is assessed. A defect that may respond favorably to surgical repair at age 6 years may not heal at age 16 or 66 years. Repair of developmental maxillary clefts is an example of a procedure that is most successful in children but often fails in young adults. Surgeons recommend repair of alveolar clefts before the eruption of the permanent canine teeth to take advantage of the enhanced healing capability of the child. Alveolar bone grafting success rates are at least 93% when performed before age 6 years.

Some patients do not have the opportunity to have these defects repaired as children; as they age, their surgical options are limited. Removable prosthetic appliances are used to replace missing teeth and to obturate the oronasal fistula. This situation poses multiple functional challenges that tend to increase over time. The teeth adjacent to the cleft often deteriorate because of their compromised alveolar housing. Prosthetic appliances may exert unfavorable forces on the anchoring teeth. Most of these patients will experience failure of their prosthesis during their lifetime, and many will present as adults to reevaluate their treatment options.

Experience has shown that conventional free bone grafting of an alveolar cleft in a 65-year-old patient is unlikely to be successful. For these mature adults, successful surgical design and construction depend on an understanding of the mechanisms that maintain the deficient skeleton in a relatively steady state. Only the functioning mechanisms can be recruited into the engineering and design of the surgical plan.

A young child in the early developmental stage is in the process of tooth eruption. This process develops the alveolar process and can be recruited to enhance the growth and organization of bone grafts. The adult does not have the tooth development process to enhance bone growth. The adult does have functioning neuromuscular systems operating in two key sites. The periodontal systems of the teeth adjacent to the cleft are the most important source of neuromuscular regulation within the alveolar process. The neuromuscular complex operating at the pterygomaxillary junction is the other critical system that can be used in the design of the surgical plan.

Bone-forming constructs designed to have enhanced healing potential can extend the opportunity for successful surgical repair to older patients. The following case is an example of designing a surgical plan that optimizes the potential for successful healing by recognizing that healing potential for facial bones is preserved in specific locations and is minimally compromised by advanced age.

Case description

A 65-year-old woman with an unrepaired cleft of the maxilla was referred for bone grafting of the alveolar cleft, closure of the oronasal fistula, and placement of a dental implant (Fig 7-1a). For most of her life, the patient accommodated to the missing lateral incisor tooth and oronasal communication by using a removable prosthesis. The partial denture replaced the missing lateral incisor and obturated the fistula. The instability of the teeth adjacent to the cleft became a concern to the patient, and she wished to know if bone could be constructed to improve the prognosis of the teeth and to support a dental implant.

Current standard management of the osseous discontinuity of the maxilla associated with cleft lip and palate is to repair the site when the patient is aged 4 to 8 years. After patients reach the age of 15 years, the risk of bone graft failure increases markedly. In a patient aged 65 years, the prognosis for a successful and functional bone graft repair is very poor. Age alone is not a contraindication to conventional bone graft construction; however, if a surgical procedure was to be designed to construct a site for placement of an osseointegrated implant, multiple obstacles needed to be addressed and the associated risk of failure accepted.

The other challenging factors were the large osseous defect at the nasal floor, the nasal fistula, and the compromised periodontal condition of the teeth adjacent to the cleft. In addition, the cleft was the manifestation of a developmental field defect. The physiologic anomaly extended farther than the bone discontinuity. This would challenge the healing process. Even if a bone graft could be successfully healed in the site, the new skeletal unit would always lack the full functional integration with the physiology of the adjacent skeleton. This would compromise the long-term stability of osseointegration.

Because there were clear, substantial challenges to bone graft repair and dental implant placement, alternative strategies had to be considered. The panoramic radiograph revealed typical features of cleft lip and palate (Fig 7-1b). The teeth adjacent to the cleft had minimal bone covering their roots. The volume of the bone deficiency increased superiorly. Within the alveolar process, the periodontal systems were the chief source of neuromuscular input. The surgical design chosen would use the bone-growing potential of the pterygomaxillary junction (Fig 7-1c). This strategy is not age dependent, so it is useful in many situations.

The root of the central incisor had incomplete bone coverage of the surface facing the cleft (Fig 7-1d). Cleft-related maxillary hypoplasia challenged the ability to position the teeth in a Class I occlusion (Fig 7-1e). The oronasal fistula extended through the labial and palatal aspects of the cleft site (Fig 7-1f).

The strategy chosen to overcome these challenges was to perform a segmental maxillary osteotomy to advance the lesser segment (Fig 7-1g). As a result of the repositioning of the segmental osteotomy, the alveolar cleft would be closed. The roots of the central incisor and canine would be placed in close proximity. The anterior movement of the maxillary segment would

Fig 7-1 Use of osteotomy to create a successful bone-forming construct in a patient with multiple challenges, including advanced age, a developmental defect, and periodontal compromise.

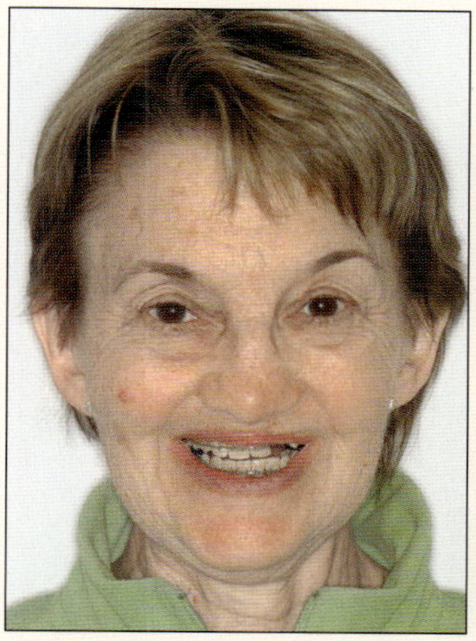

Fig 7-1a A 65-year-old woman with unrepaired cleft of the maxilla was referred for bone graft repair of the cleft and placement of a dental implant for the congenitally missing lateral incisor.

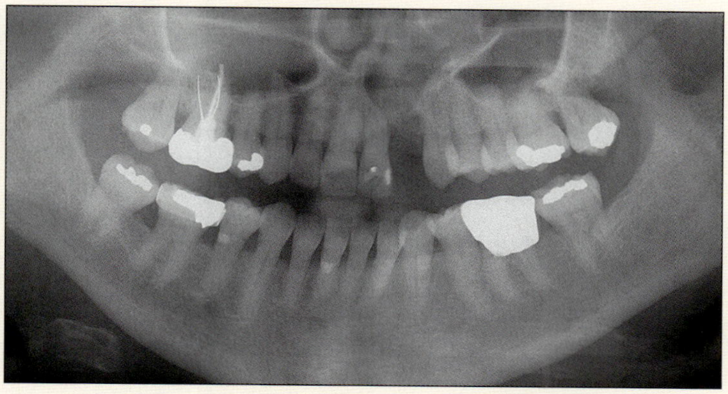

Fig 7-1b The radiograph shows a typical bone defect associated with cleft lip and palate.

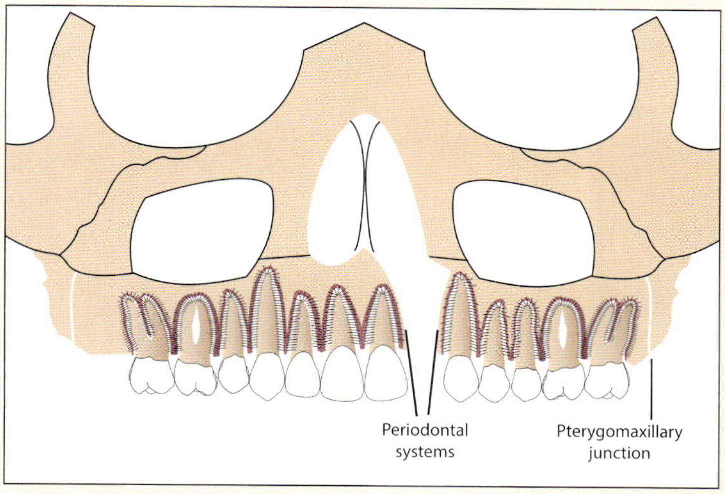

Fig 7-1c Functional analysis of the existing defect defines the elements that maintain the discontinuity in a steady state. The periodontal ligament systems of the teeth adjacent to the cleft established and maintain the local bone volume. These sources of neuromuscular regulation will also control the performance of the constructed bone-forming chambers.

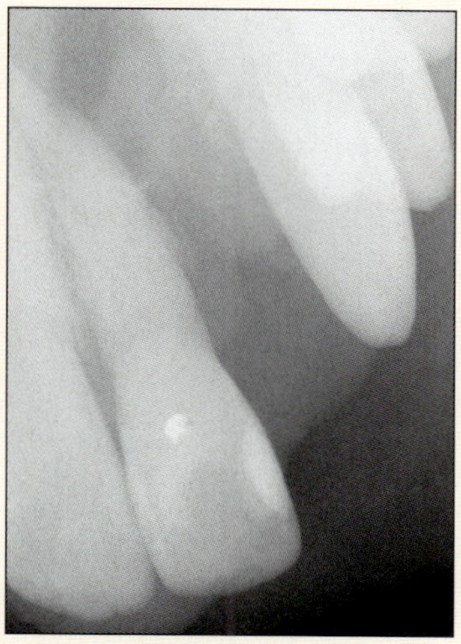

Fig 7-1d The radiograph shows typical periodontal compromise of the teeth adjacent to the cleft.

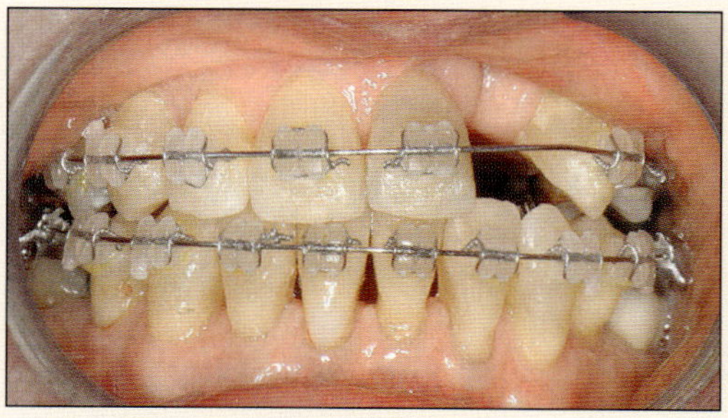

Fig 7-1e Cleft-related maxillary hypoplasia challenges the ability to position the teeth in a Class I occlusion.

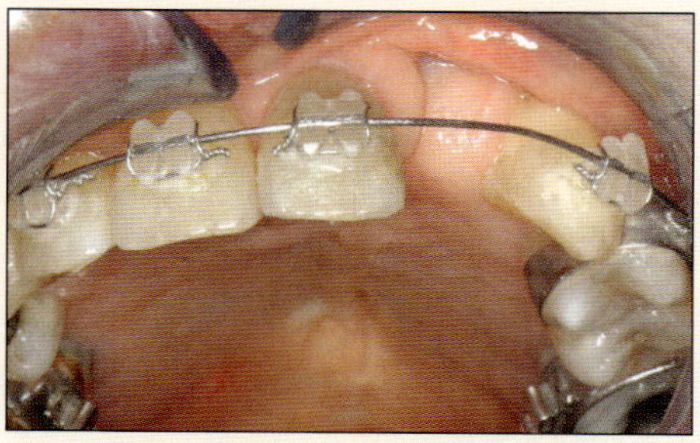

Fig 7-1f The oronasal fistula extends through the labial and palatal aspects of the cleft site.

→

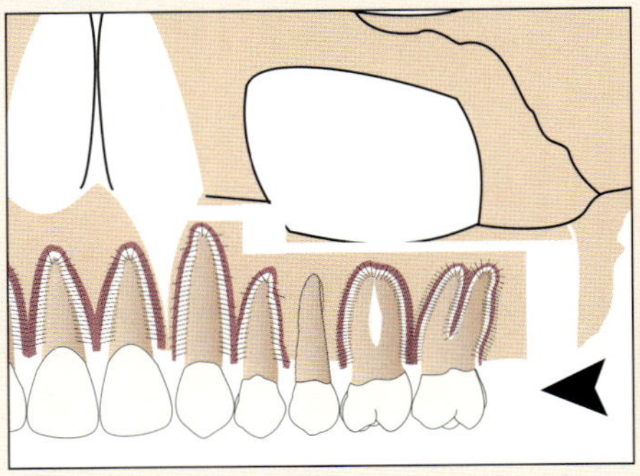

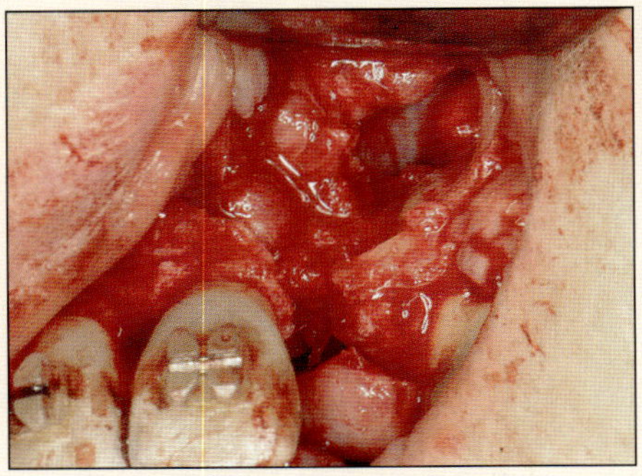

Fig 7-1g *(far left)* The treatment strategy involves segmental maxillary osteotomy.

Fig 7-1h *(left)* Surgical findings after mobilization of the segmental osteotomy. The bone defect increases in width in the apical region.

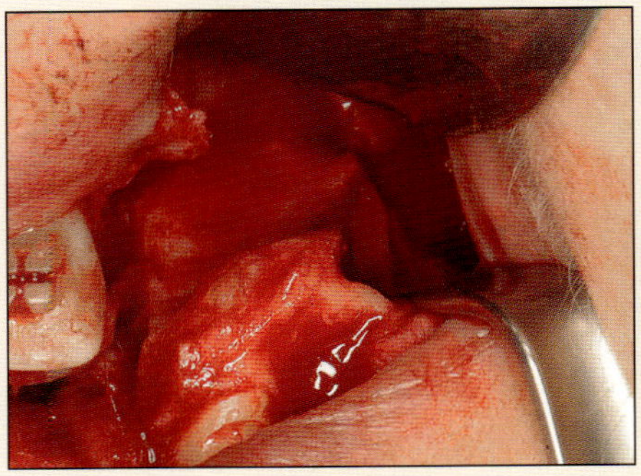

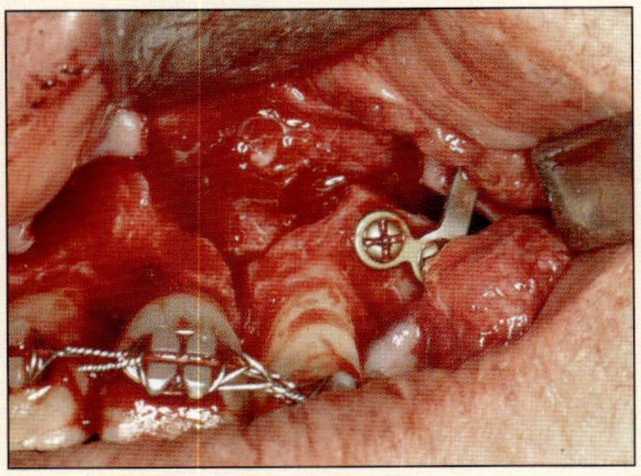

Fig 7-1i *(far left)* The maxillary segment is luxated to separate the pterygomaxillary junction without damaging the pterygoid plates.

Fig 7-1j *(left)* The segment is protracted and docked with the anterior maxilla. A titanium bone plate and the orthodontic appliance provide fixation.

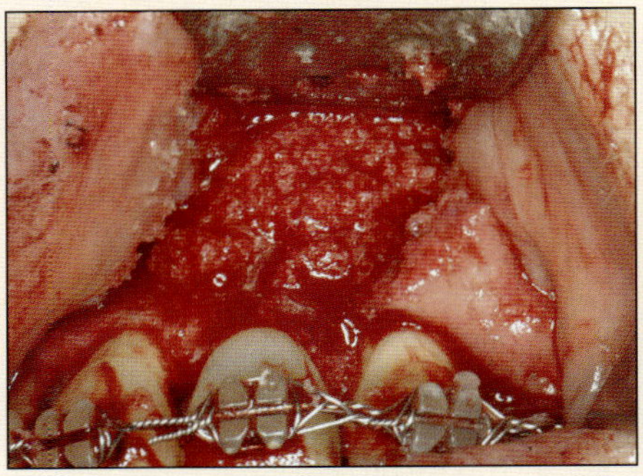

Fig 7-1k Cancellous bone particles reconstituted in rhBMP-2 are positioned to construct the nasal rim and the apical aspect of the alveolar process.

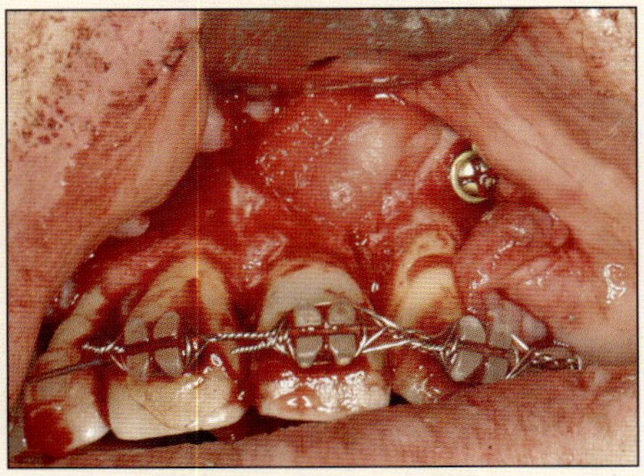

Fig 7-1l The bone graft is covered with a collagen sponge carrying rhBMP-2.

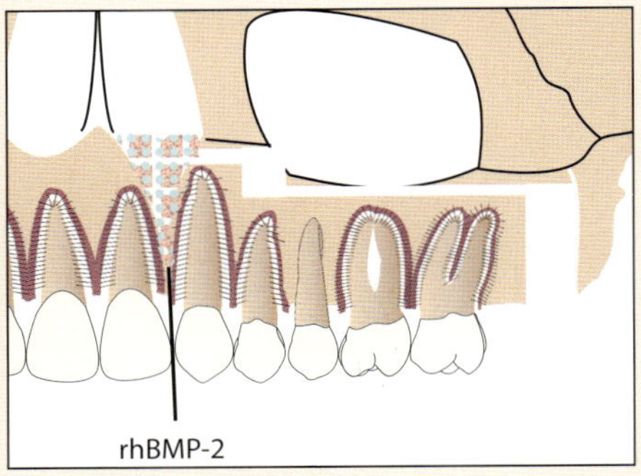

Fig 7-1m The cleft docking site and the piriform rims are grafted with a combination of rhBMP-2, solvent-dehydrated cancellous bone particles, and collagen sponges. No grafting material is necessary at the pterygomaxillary chamber. →

open a pterygomaxillary regeneration chamber. The pterygoid bone-forming chamber site would heal rapidly without grafting. The neuromuscular input would be supplied by the muscle originating from the pterygoid plates.

During surgery, mucosal flaps were raised and the maxillary left segment was mobilized. The osteotomy through the left lateral portion of the maxilla penetrated the maxillary sinus. Instrumentation to mobilize the segment gained access through the cut sinus membrane. The lumen of the maxillary sinus could be seen through this access route (Fig 7-1h).

Protraction of the mobilized segment met resistance from the scar tissue of the prior palate repair. Adequate mobilization of the segment had to be achieved without damaging the attached mucosal pedicle. The pterygomaxillary junction had to be disarticulated without damaging the pterygoid plate (Fig 7-1i). Maintenance of the muscle attachments to an intact pterygoid plate complex was important because the muscles were to provide the primary neuromuscular input in the regeneration chamber created between the posterior maxilla and the pterygoid plates.

The maxillary osteotomy segment was protracted and stabilized (Fig 7-1j). The cleft gap was obliterated by the anterior movement of the segment. The funnel-shaped bone defect that remained was in the apical region. A single titanium bone plate stabilized the bone segment.

The roots of the maxillary left central incisor and canine were now in close proximity. This configuration would provide the necessary neuromuscular input in the collapsed cleft and promote bone formation. The region of the missing nasal aperture was now a region of relative mechanical stability. Bone formation in this region was supported by the apices of the central incisor and canine roots. A bone graft with recombinant human bone morphogenetic protein 2 (rhBMP-2) enhancement would

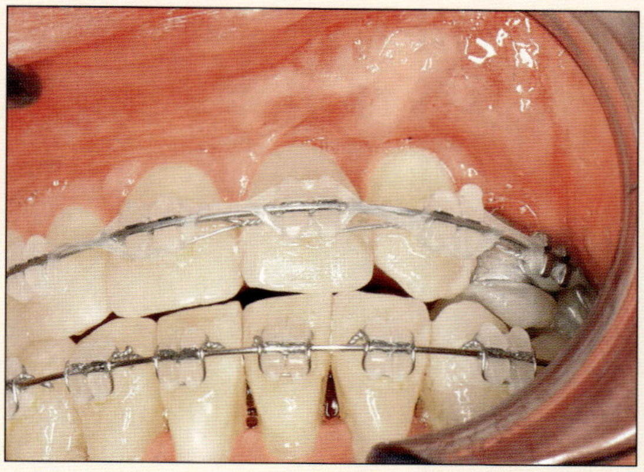

Fig 7-1n *(right)* Healing of the segmental osteotomy after 1 month.

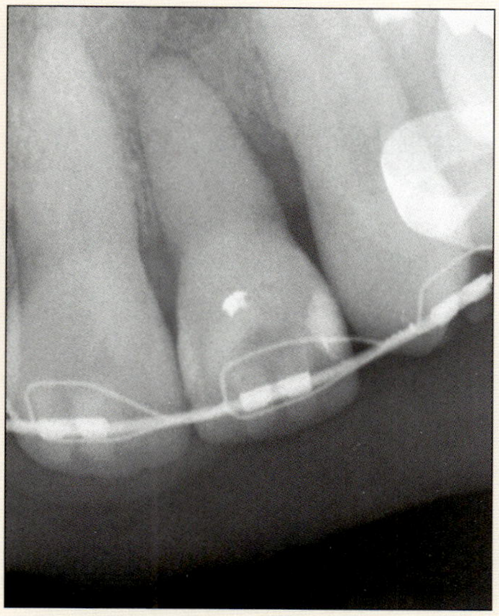

Fig 7-1o *(far right)* A radiograph of the repair site 3 months after surgery shows evidence of bone growth, but it lacks a lamina dura and an organized trabecular pattern.

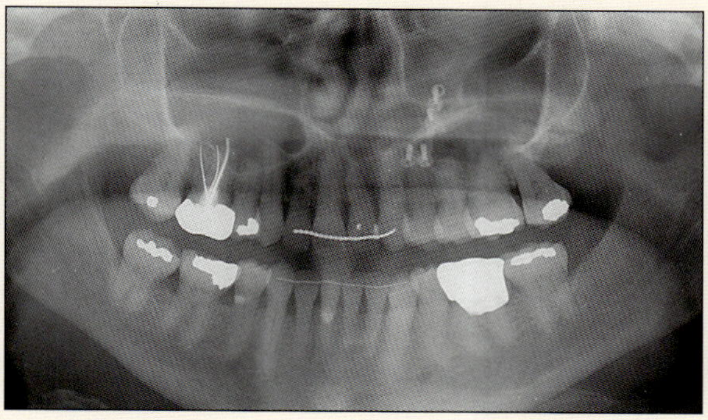

Fig 7-1p *(right)* A radiograph taken 13 months after surgery shows a continuous dental arch and no sign of the alveolar cleft.

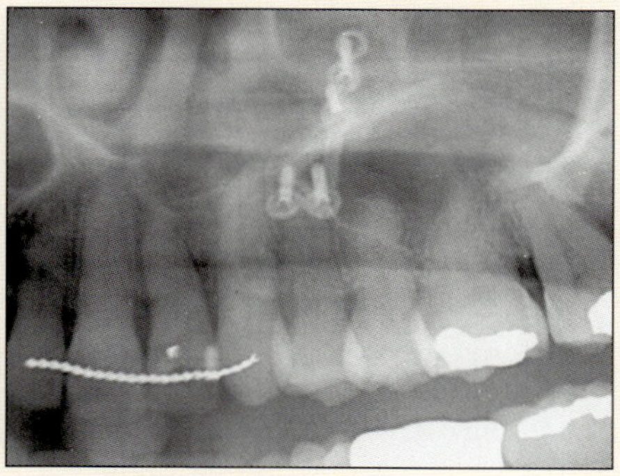

Fig 7-1q *(far right)* A magnified view of the cleft site shows normal bone architecture and good bone levels on the teeth adjacent to the repair.

→

provide additional cells for bone formation in that region. The most important bone-forming site in the chamber was opened between the maxillary tuberosity and the pterygoid plates. Placement of rhBMP-2 carried on absorbable collagen sponges (ACSs) enhanced bone formation in the pterygoid junction and the lateral maxilla.

Solvent-dehydrated cancellous bone particles (Puros, Zimmer Dental) reconstituted in rhBMP-2 were positioned to construct the nasal rim and the apical aspect of the alveolar process (Fig 7-1k). The graft consisted of 1 mL of cancellous particles and 2 mg of rhBMP-2 in 1 mL of sterile water.

The bone graft was covered with a collagen sponge (Integra Life Sciences) containing 2 mg of rhBMP-2 in 2 mL of sterile water (Fig 7-1l). The rhBMP-2/ACS preparation was placed against the lateral maxilla and in the pterygomaxillary junction. Neuromuscular signaling was weak in the lateral maxilla above the premolar teeth. The rhBMP-2/ACS device was placed to cover this osteotomy gap to assure that bone would bridge the discontinuity at this location (Fig 7-1m).

Healing of the mucosal repair of the oronasal fistula was complete at the 1-month follow-up (Fig 7-1n). Two months after surgery, the osteotomy segment was stable (Fig 7-1o).

Radiographs taken 13 months after surgery showed the cleft site to be filled with bone (Figs 7-1p and 7-1q).

Four years after surgery, the dental arch and periodontium remained stable (Fig 7-1r). As a result of the segmental osteotomy and rhBMP-2 grafting, the patient had full repair of the cleft, oronasal fistula, and missing lateral incisor. No dental implants were needed because the result was a continuous arch of natural teeth. The palatal fistula that had been present for 65 years remained closed (Fig 7-1s).

At the 4-year follow-up, the bone constructed across the cleft showed structural and physiologic organization (Fig 7-1t). A clear lamina dura had formed, indicating that the periodontal ligaments of the left central incisor and canine were interacting with the newly formed bone. Trabecular morphology within the interradicular bone indicated that the bone was responding to functional loading. The constructed bone was now fully integrated into the physiology of the native skeleton.

Discussion

Standard treatment for a patient with a cleft palate and missing lateral incisor is to place a bone graft at the defect and then

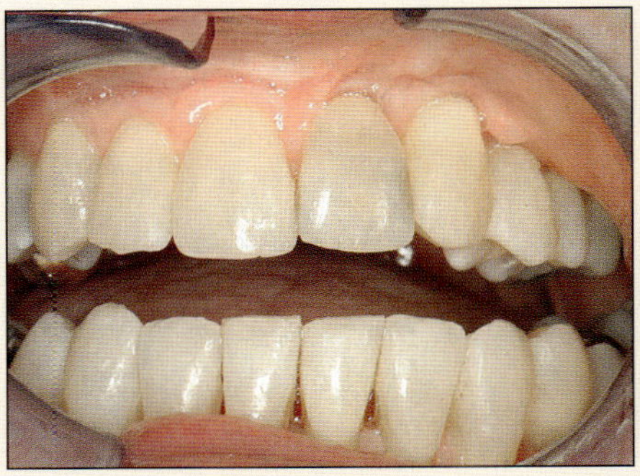

Fig 7-1r Oral appearance 4 years after surgery. The treatment has resulted in a continuous dental arch so that a dental implant is not necessary.

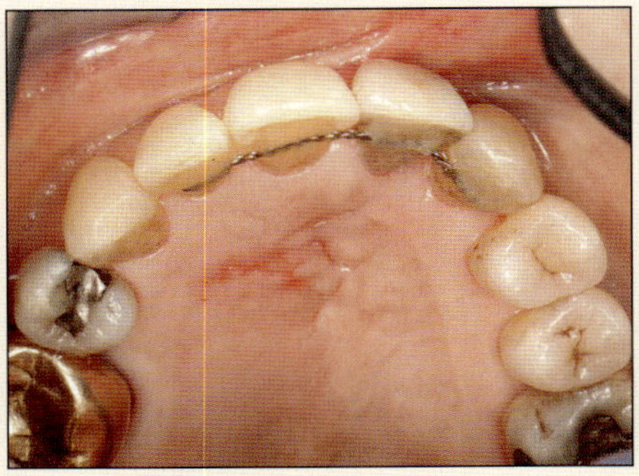

Fig 7-1s Palatal examination at the 4-year follow-up shows stable closure of the oronasal fistula.

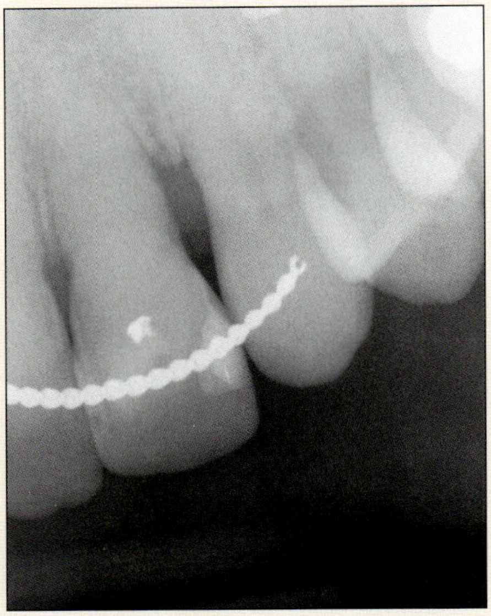

Fig 7-1t A radiograph of the repair site at 4 years shows that the graft has organized and exhibits normal structural architecture.

place a dental implant. In some cases, that protocol cannot be followed. When designing bone-forming procedures for an older patient, the surgeon must compensate for the limited efficiency of the patient's mechanisms to control bone growth. Use of the pterygomaxillary junction to supply bone, accomplished through an indirect, segmental osteotomy strategy, can provide predictable healing in patients challenged by aging.

Designing Surgery for a Compromised Healing Environment

Managing dentoalveolar defects in patients with complex developmental anomalies poses a special challenge. These patients present with an oral deficiency that may appear to be an ordinary cleft because that is what the physical examination shows. The surgical designer must understand that the etiology of cleft disorders is not uniform.[1] The underlying embryology varies and is incompletely understood.

Patients with multisystem developmental anomalies often demonstrate increased difficulty healing after oral surgery. When surgical procedures for these patients are designed, modification of the conventional procedures may be indicated to limit the risk of failure. These children present with a history of multiple surgical failures. The challenge becomes to carefully design an alternative treatment approach, convince the patient and family as to the logic of the alternative treatment, and manage repair of tissues that are damaged from the prior surgical attempts.

In the following case, a conventional bone grafting procedure was attempted first. The procedure was performed by an excellent surgeon using the iliac crest as the donor site. The surgical designer for the second surgery had the advantage of being able to study how the patient responded to the standard procedure. The soft tissue closure did not heal, and then the autogenous bone graft experienced resorption. Analysis of the pattern of healing deficiency allowed development of a new surgical plan that addressed the most likely causes of failure.

Most surgeons performing these craniofacial procedures follow well-established, standard procedures. When surgery is performed in an intact environment, successful healing is the usual outcome. Variation in surgical outcomes is largely dependent on deficiencies in individual patients' healing responses. The technical ability to execute a procedure is an important factor but cannot compensate for inherent challenges of underlying healing deficiencies.

Recognition of the patients likely to present exceptional resistance to healing of a surgical incursion can be difficult. Healing deficiencies may be obvious or occult. The size of the defect is one of the first issues the designer of surgery considers because it presents on the clinical examination and radiographs. The age of the patient is a factor in projecting the expected healing response. How the patient responded to prior surgery in the area provides an important in situ assessment of healing ability. If success is to be realized, the surgical design must adhere to the same requirements as any bone-forming system. The challenge for the surgical designer is to achieve success by deliberate and thoughtful planning.

Fig 7-2 Design of a bone-forming construct in a patient with a complex developmental anomaly and a compromised healing environment.

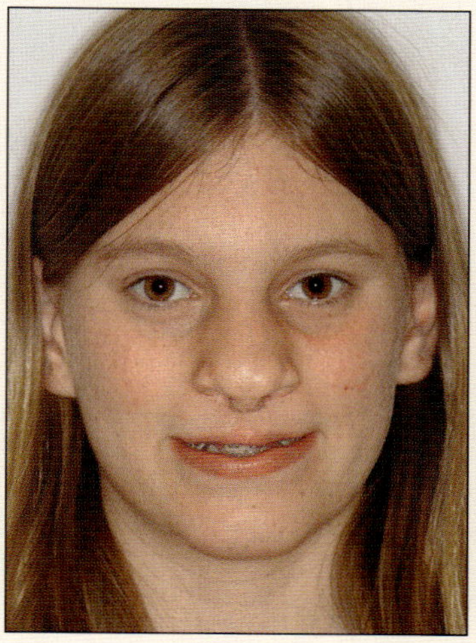

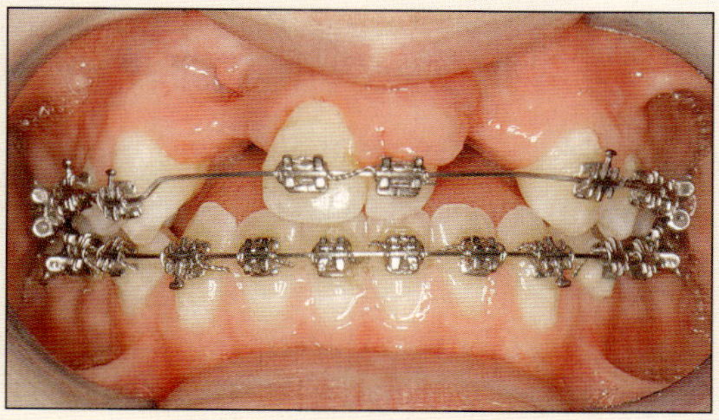

Fig 7-2a *(right)* A 14-year-old girl presented with bilateral cleft lip and palate and missing teeth.

Fig 7-2b *(far right)* Oral examination reveals missing teeth, a hypoplastic incisor, and bilateral alveolar clefts.

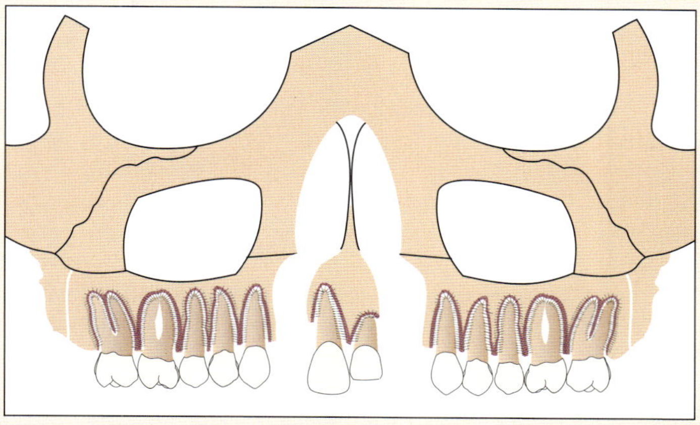

Fig 7-2c The bilateral maxillary clefts divide the maxilla into three alveolar segments.

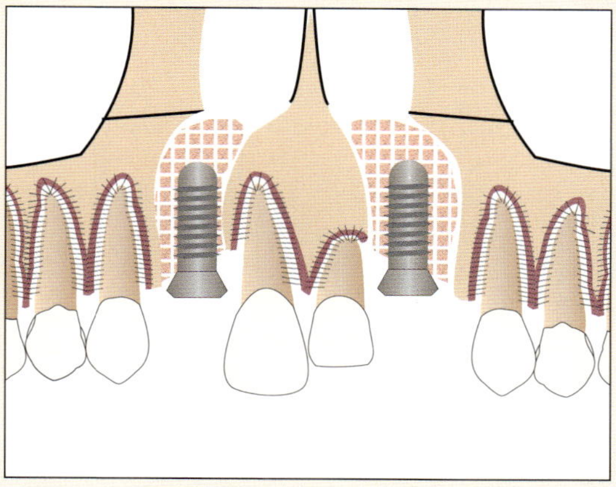

Fig 7-2d Typical management of alveolar clefts involves placement of bone grafts and dental implants.

→

Case description

A 14-year-old girl presented for evaluation and treatment recommendations for the management of bilateral cleft lip and palate (Fig 7-2a). She desired repair of her maxillary clefts so dental implants could be placed for congenitally missing teeth. The patient also had complex congenital heart disease for which she had undergone corrective surgery. The nature of her heart condition demanded special care for anesthesia management.

Oral examination showed missing teeth, a hypoplastic incisor, bilateral alveolar clefts, and deficient soft tissue (Fig 7-2b). The clefts divided the maxilla into three alveolar segments (Fig 7-2c). The discontinuity extended apically to the nasal cavity. There was an associated deficiency in soft tissue, and fistulas connected the oral cavity to the nasal cavity.

The original plan to replace the missing lateral incisors followed standard management protocols, including placement of bone grafts and dental implants (Fig 7-2d). The standard protocol requires successful completion of three treatment stages. The first stage involves placement and healing of bone grafts to establish osseous continuity. Mucosa flaps are advanced to cover the grafts. During the second stage of treatment, dental implants are placed in the healed bone graft. They must heal with an osseointegrated interface to be of long-term service. The third stage is placement of a prosthesis that meets functional and esthetic objectives.

In this case, standard surgical management was initiated by the prior surgeon. That treatment involved harvesting a cancellous bone graft from the patient's iliac crest. The graft site was prepared to receive the bone graft by elevation and advancement of mucoperiosteal flaps in a manner that would allow a tension-free closure. In this case, the mucosa did not heal, resulting in exposure of the bone graft and its eventual loss. The soft tissue was managed by an exceptional plastic surgeon with extensive experience in these cases. There were no unusual technical problems with the surgery. However, healing of the mucosa did not occur in a normal fashion.

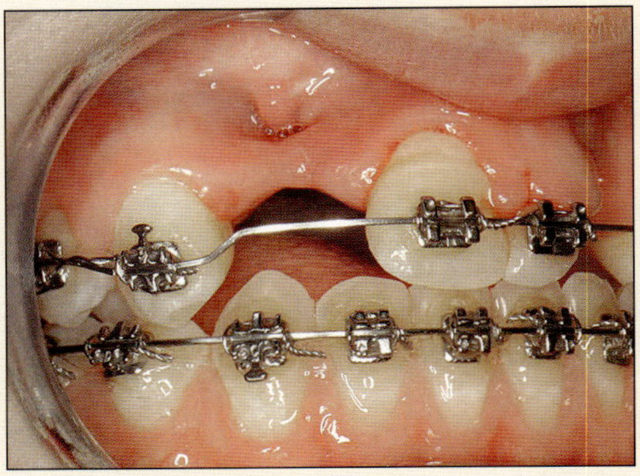

Fig 7-2e The right alveolar cleft has thin, friable mucosa.

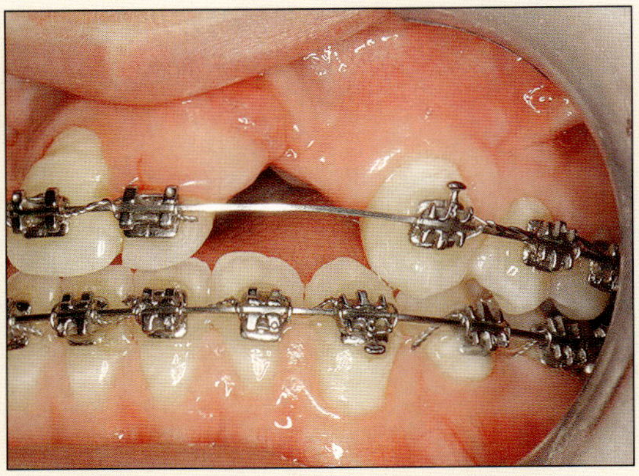

Fig 7-2f The soft tissues overlying the left alveolar cleft are also compromised. The mucosa adjacent to the oronasal fistula is inflamed. The left central incisor is hypoplastic.

→

Healing deficiency is not unusual for patients who have concomitant systemic developmental anomalies. The coincidence of facial and heart developmental disorders has been recognized for years.[2] The underlying physiologic commonality is poorly understood and probably complex. The surgeon was correct in assuming that the mucosa would respond the same way if the surgery were repeated. Because the patient experienced healing complications that prevented a successful outcome, the first surgeon referred the patient for possible alternative management strategies.

The initial examination revealed the compromised quality and quantity of the soft tissue overlying both the right and left clefts (Figs 7-2e and 7-2f). The friable quality of the mucosa in these patients reflects a systemic abnormality of the tissue itself. It is more than a local effect from the cleft. The etiology of this condition is unknown. It is possible that the abnormality was related to a problem of embryogenesis or development. It is also possible that neonatal development was compromised by the challenges of cardiac deficiency and prolonged hospitalization. For treatment to be successful, the compromised nature of the soft tissue had to be taken into account when the surgical design was created.

A radiograph of the right cleft showed that the roots of the teeth adjacent to the cleft were covered by a thin layer of alveolar bone (Fig 7-2g). If successful repair of the cleft was to be attained, the periodontal ligament systems of these teeth had to be recruited to provide neuromuscular signaling into graft material used to bridge the discontinuity. A source of neuromuscular regulation in the construction site was essential for successful bone formation, and the periodontal system was the only option in this section of the alveolar process. In the current configuration, the distance between the roots was too large to allow regulatory signaling effects to reach the center of the defect. To be effective, the surgical design had to move the periodontal systems into closer proximity.

The radiograph of the left alveolar cleft revealed a combined problem of bone deficiency and periodontal compromise (Fig 7-2h). The left central incisor was hypoplastic and had bone loss extending to the root apex. Given the lack of bone surrounding the left central incisor, its prognosis was poor. The first premolar had a well-developed root and periodontal system. The intact periodontal system of the first premolar could potentially deliver neuromuscular signaling to a bone-forming construct, but the potential contribution from the left central incisor was limited. Many surgeons believe that an exposed root in the cleft is a liability to grafting and that such teeth should be extracted.[3] In this case, the decision was made to incorporate all of the remaining periodontal ligament fibers and their Sharpey fiber extensions in the existing bone to deliver essential neuromuscular signaling to the bone-forming construct.

As an alternative to conventional bone grafting, segmental osteotomies were included in the surgical plan (Fig 7-2i). This strategy involved creating two transport segments. The segments would be protracted horizontally to fill the alveolar cleft defects at points A and B. Regeneration chambers would be opened posteriorly at points C and D. The transport process would deliver 8 mm of mucosa to each alveolar cleft site. This was expected to allow closure of the mucosa without tension. Because the mucosa was being transported with the alveolar segment, forces resisting advancement would be absorbed by the transport segment.

A sequence of overlapping events was expected to occur at the right-side cleft repair site (see Fig 7-2i, site A). The rhBMP-2 would draw cells to the site. Sharpey fibers inserted in the root cementum would traverse the periodontal ligament space to reach the thin layer of bone that covered the root facing the cleft. The fibers would penetrate the thin cortical plate and be involved in the maintenance of the bone. These fibers had the potential to introduce mechanical signals to the graft site and direct the behavior of the bone-forming cells. Drawing the two roots into close proximity would increase the potential signaling intensity and decrease the mass of bone needed to establish an osseous union.

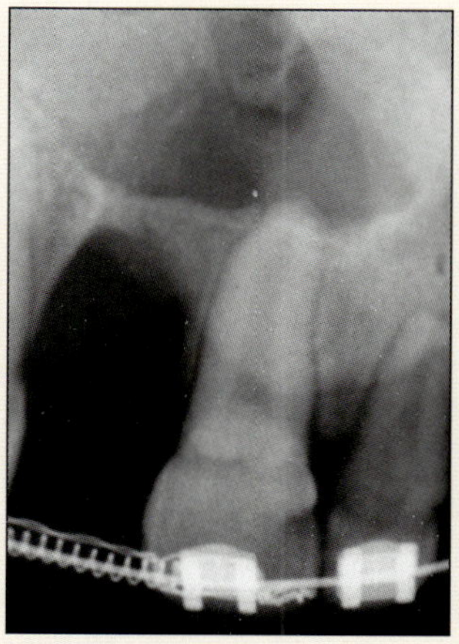

Fig 7-2g Radiographic appearance of the right alveolar cleft.

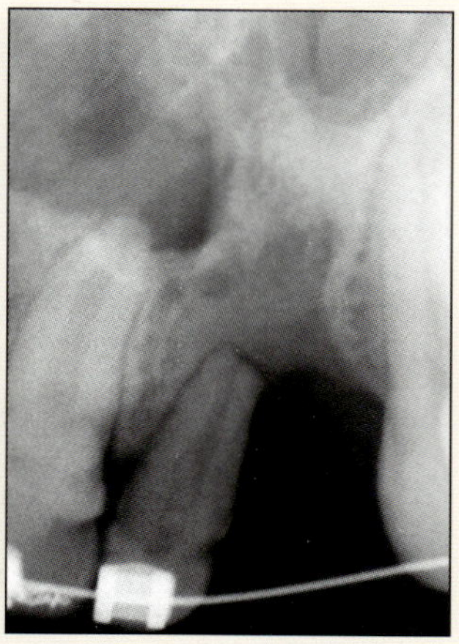

Fig 7-2h Radiographic appearance of the left alveolar cleft and hypoplastic tooth.

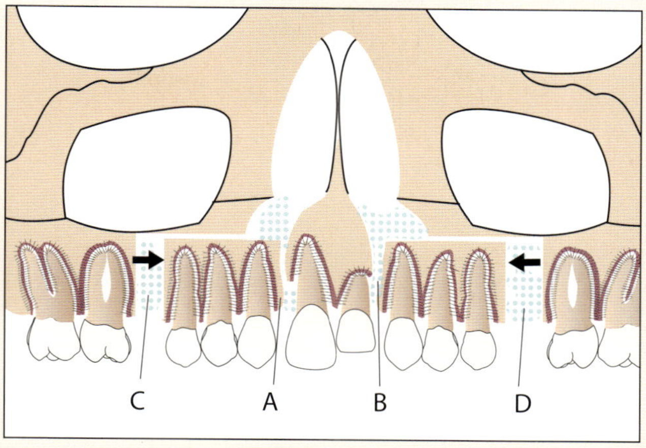

Fig 7-2i The proposed surgical design involves creating two transport segments. The segments will be protracted horizontally to fill the alveolar cleft defects at points A and B. Regeneration chambers will be opened posteriorly at points C and D.

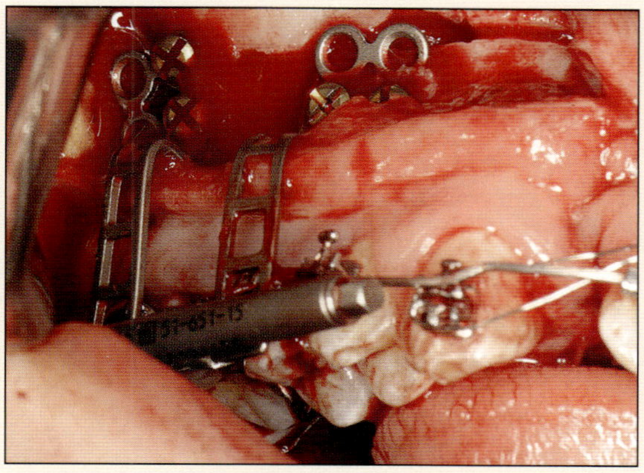

Fig 7-2j The right segmental osteotomy is completed, and the distraction device is placed.

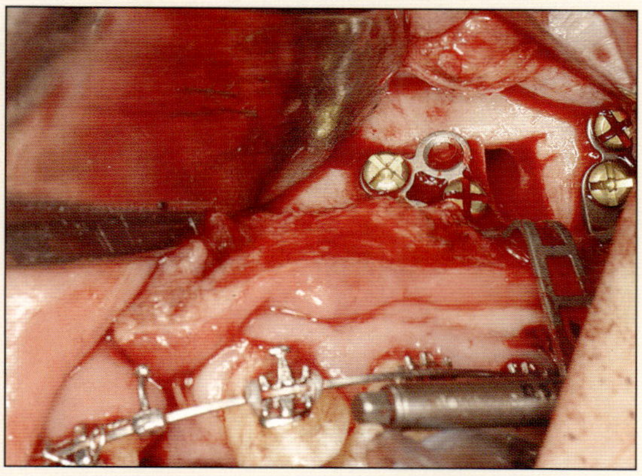

Fig 7-2k After osteotomies create the left transport segment, the distraction device is placed.

Closure of the right cleft required distraction because of the resistance of the past surgery scar tissue and the delicate nature of the mucosa. An incision in the vestibule provided access to create the transport segment on the right side. The horizontal incision spared the mucosa labial to the incisive bone segment to preserve its vascular supply. A Liou distraction device (KLS Martin) was affixed to the zygomatic buttress in the posterior region and to the transport segment in the anterior region (Fig 7-2j).

A minimal-access osteotomy was performed with piezoelectric surgery on the left side. A horizontal osteotomy at the Le Fort I level joined the vertical interdental osteotomy to the lateral nasal aperture. A Liou distraction device was mounted to transport the segment (Fig 7-2k).

There were two sites on the left side that required placement of rhBMP-2 to supply bone-forming cells (Fig 7-2l). In the space between the left incisor and the left canine was the site of the prior failed bone graft. Protraction of the left transport segment moved the roots and periodontal systems of these two teeth into closer proximity. The osseous walls of the cleft were exposed by elevation of the mucoperiosteum. Collagen sponges containing rhBMP-2 were placed between the walls of the cleft. As the distraction device was activated, the segment was transported anteriorly, closing the space between the cleft walls. The collagen sponge was compressed between the converging walls, concentrating the dose of rhBMP-2 into a small volume. Experience has shown that this process will result in bone formation across the docking site.[4]

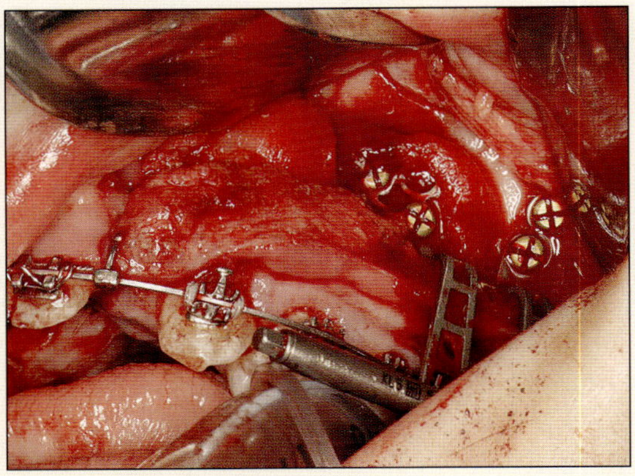

Fig 7-2l To supply bone-forming cells, rhBMP-2–containing collagen sponges are placed in two sites on the left side.

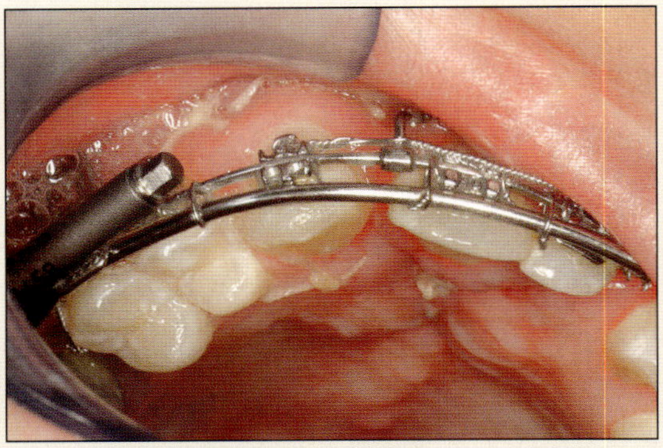

Fig 7-2m The right segment is fully protracted to close the cleft, and the palatal fistula is repaired.

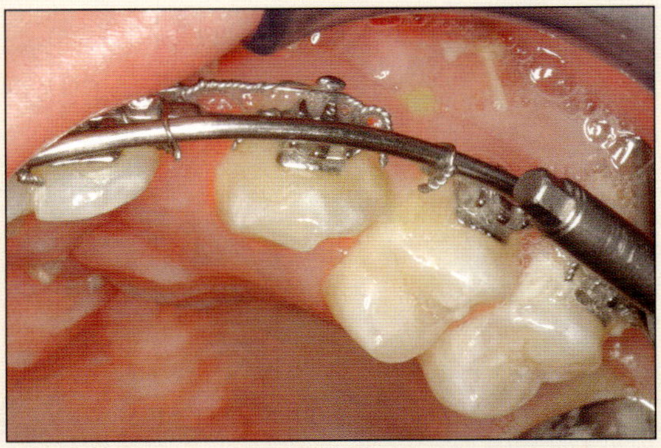

Fig 7-2n After segmental osteotomy repositioning on the left side, a space corresponding to the width of a normal central incisor remains.

→

As the transport segment moved anteriorly, the vertical osteotomy in the posterior region opened. This site was planned for placement of a dental implant. To meet this goal, a substantial bone volume had to be grown at the site to provide a stable environment for the natural teeth and a future dental implant. Unlike the cleft site in the anterior, the posterior distraction chamber was not at the center of the developmental field deficiency. If cells were delivered to the site, the periodontal systems of the adjacent teeth would supply enough neuromuscular regulation to direct bone to form and organize.

Repositioning of the transport segments was completed at the time of surgery. The distraction devices were used to protract and fixate the transport segments but were not used for delayed, gradual movement. To control the transport vector, a 0.035-inch round orthodontic wire bent to the dental arch form engaged the facebow tubes on the molar brackets. This provided a stable anchorage point to apply lateral traction on the transport segments.

With the segments in the protracted position, additional palatal soft tissue was available to repair the oronasal fistula with a tension-free primary closure. The right canine was nearly in contact with the incisor (Fig 7-2m). The remaining space was maintained for later orthodontic closure because it preserved the thin layer of bone that covered the mesial root of the canine and the distal root of the incisor. Within these thin bone segments were the periodontal fibers between the root cementum and the lamina dura. These were an important source of neuromuscular regulation of bone formation across the cleft.

On the left side, repositioning of the transport segment was stopped at a position corresponding to the width of a normal central incisor (Fig 7-2n).

Eight weeks after segmental osteotomies and rhBMP-2 placement, the patient was returned to the operating room for removal of the distraction devices. Her cardiac condition dictated that the procedure be done in the hospital operating room setting with anesthesia and cardiology support. As a result of the osteotomies and rhBMP-2 treatment, the continuity of the maxilla had been restored. Both the distraction sites and the cleft closure sites had healed with bony unions. Surgical examination showed that the graft fully filled the site of the right cleft (Fig 7-2o). The volume of the graft established a mass of viable bone for periodontal support of the teeth.

The cleft on the left side was filled with viable bone (Fig 7-2p). The condition of the hypoplastic incisor had been improved by the growth of additional bone around its compromised root. There was no evidence that the exposed root interfered with

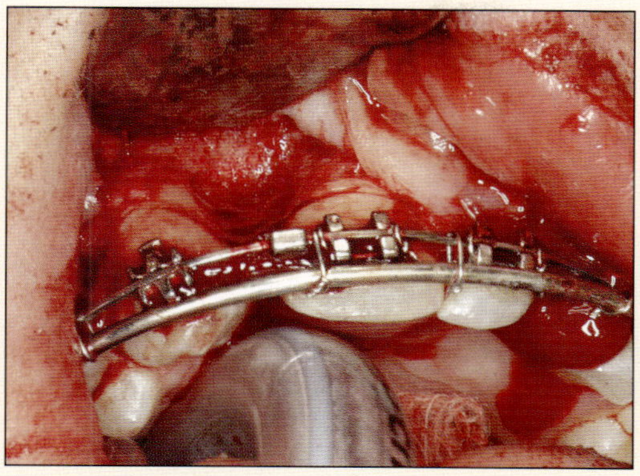

Fig 7-2o Bone has grown across the right cleft after 8 weeks.

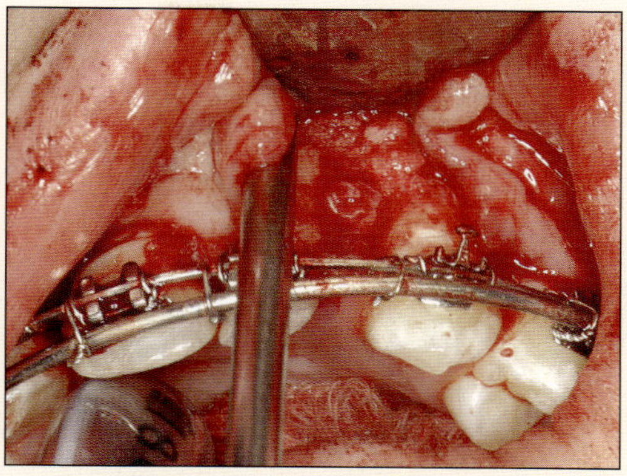

Fig 7-2p The left-side alveolar cleft has filled with viable bone 8 weeks after segmental osteotomies.

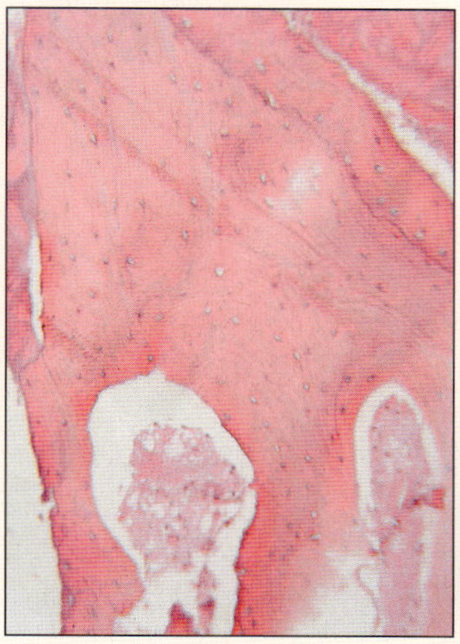

Fig 7-2q Histologic appearance of bone grown at the cleft repair site shows normal organization (hematoxylin and eosin, original magnification ×40).

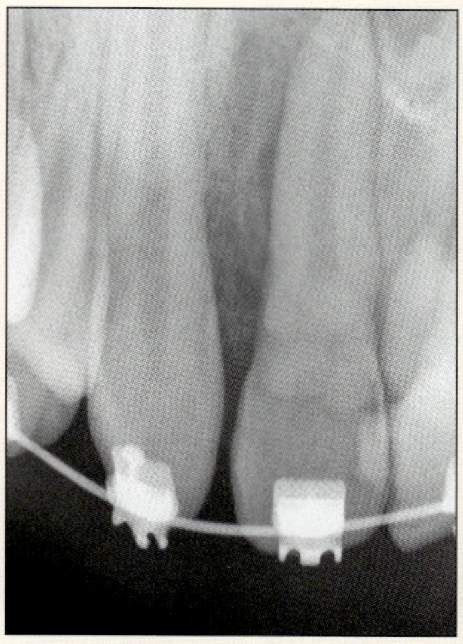

Fig 7-2r A radiograph of the right cleft repair site after 12 weeks reveals that the cleft is no longer visible.

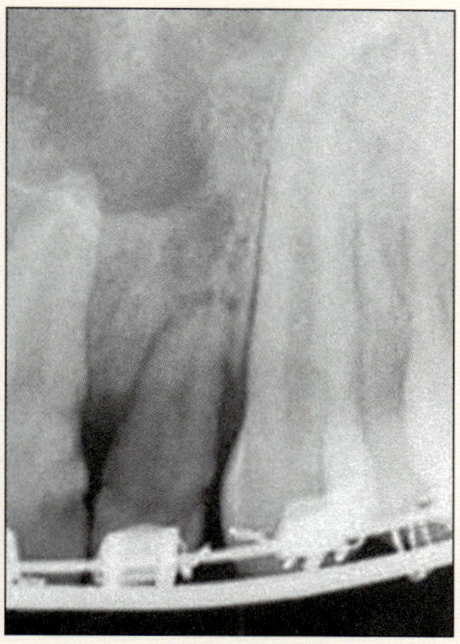

Fig 7-2s On the left side, after 12 weeks, the alveolar cleft has been filled and the bone levels on the mesial surface of the left canine are good.

→

bone formation at the site. Histologic examination of a portion of bone recovered from the cleft repair site confirmed that the process yielded viable bone (Fig 7-2q).

A radiograph of the right cleft repair site 12 weeks after surgery revealed complete fill of the cleft defect (Fig 7-2r). The cleft was no longer visible.

A radiograph of the left cleft repair site 12 weeks after the surgery showed the condition of the bone mass and the effect of the adjacent teeth (Fig 7-2s). The hypoplastic tooth had some bone formation at the apex of the root. The alveolar cleft had been filled, and the bone levels on the mesial surface of the left canine were good.

To complete the dental arch continuity, two dental implants were placed and restored (Fig 7-2t). Three years after the maxillary surgery, the implant on the right side was placed in the osteotomy opened during transport of the segmental osteotomy. The space created by the left segmental osteotomy was closed with orthodontic treatment. At the same time, the left central incisor failed and was replaced with a dental implant and crown. Even though the hypoplastic maxillary left central incisor failed and needed replacement, it served an important role in the surgical design. Healing of the bone graft at the left maxillary cleft utilized the tooth's periodontal ligament system to promote organization into a functional skeletal unit.

Nine years after the surgery and placement of rhBMP-2 grafts, the patient's condition remained resolved (Figs 7-2u to 7-2x). Her periodontal health was stable.

Discussion

This case emphasizes the need to direct special vigilance to the diagnostic phase of the treatment process. The physical findings when the patient initially presented were not particularly alarming. From an anatomical standpoint, it would have seemed

Fig 7-2t *(right)* Follow-up radiograph taken 9 years after segmental osteotomies. The restoration was completed with two dental implants 3 years after osteotomy surgery.

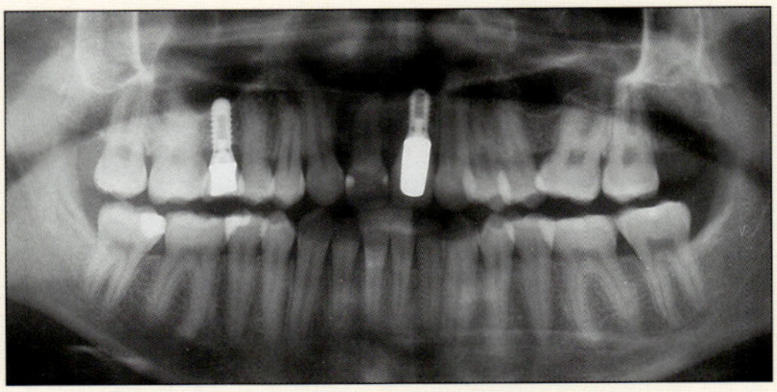

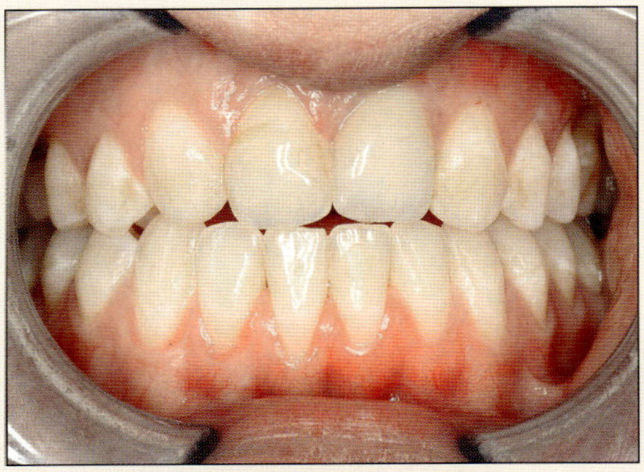

Figs 7-2u to 7-2x The dental arch and periodontal health of the patient remain stable 9 years after cleft repair with segmental osteotomies.

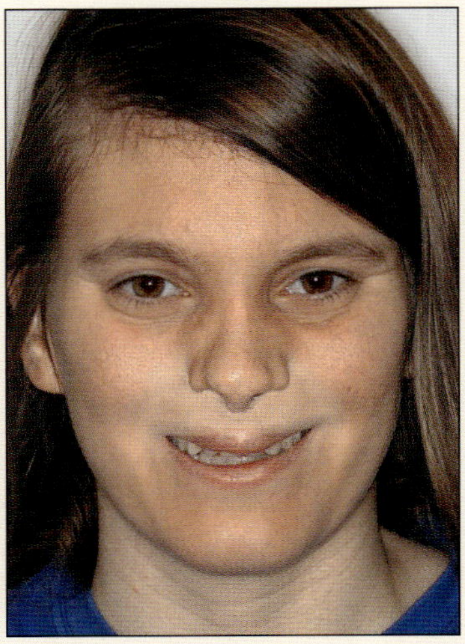

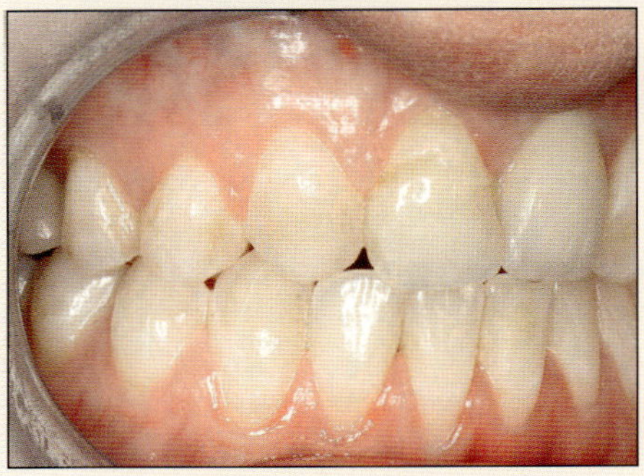

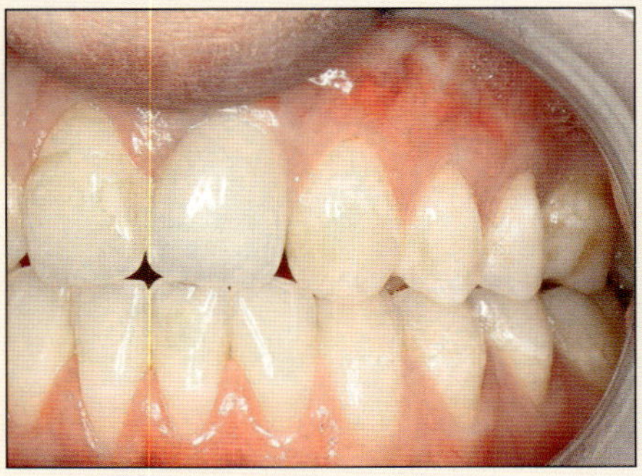

reasonable to perform a standard alveolar cleft repair with an autogenous bone graft in anticipation of replacing the missing teeth with dental implants. However, this patient's mucosal healing response was compromised. This is a common finding in patients with complex, multisystem developmental anomalies. When a constructive design is created, the obstacle of impaired soft tissue healing must be considered.

Successful and stable growth of bone to repair a skeletofacial bone defect can be expected if the surgical plan includes all of the essential elements for bone formation. One of the essential requirements of a bone-forming construct is the absence of pathology. Infection is always a risk when oral surgery is performed because the wound is always contaminated.

To limit the risk of infection, the regeneration site is isolated from the oral cavity by the mucosal closure. If the soft tissue covering a graft or osteotomy fails to heal along the incision line or breaks down, the bone-forming environment is compromised by invasion of bacteria and secretions. Therefore, a critical aspect of the diagnosis is to recognize when mucosal healing will be abnormal. This will direct the surgical designer to formulate a strategy that limits the dependence of this healing deficiency. If successful treatment is to be achieved, the surgical plan must depend minimally on the integrity of the soft tissue closure.

Osteotomies allow repositioning of jaw segments and their associated soft tissue. The result of segment repositioning in this patient was that an additional 8 mm of soft tissue was advanced into the cleft site on both sides. This relative redundancy of soft tissue allowed healing because the tissue was not challenged by a closure under tension.

The remaining essential elements of the bone-forming construct were designed into the system by familiar methods. The environment was stabilized by orthodontic appliances and the distraction devices. Cells were introduced through the application of rhBMP-2 delivered on collagen sponges. Neuromuscular input was supplied by the periodontal ligament systems of the teeth adjacent to the clefts. Because the intensity of periodontally derived neuromuscular signaling diminishes over distance, the roots of the teeth adjacent to the clefts were transported into close proximity by intraoperative osteotomy segment repositioning. Even in the compromised environment, the properly designed and constructed bone-forming chambers delivered stable bone growth and unions within 8 weeks.

Osteotomy to Grow Bone after Multiple Failed Grafting Attempts

The patient who presents with a history of multiple failed attempts at bone grafting represents a special type of risk factor. When a surgical procedure is being designed for a patient who has experienced problems with healing, a sequential analysis of possible causes of failure must be completed before a new treatment plan can be considered. If a specific cause of the prior failures can be identified, the challenge is to find a surgical design that can limit the impact of the deficiency on the successful healing of the construct.

In this patient, the first two surgical repairs involved conventional alveolar bone grafting. Failure to heal demonstrated that the environment in which the bone graft was placed did not support bone growth. For the third attempt at construction, a surgical design was created to alter the environment of the cleft site in order to achieve bone healing. To address the issue of maxillary hypoplasia, a Le Fort I maxillary osteotomy was used to open regeneration chambers at the right and left pterygomaxillary junctions.

Case description

A patient presented for treatment when she was 14 years old (Fig 7-3a). The prior care for her bilateral cleft lip and palate was provided at another craniofacial center. Orthodontic care that expanded the maxillary dental arch had been provided. Orthodontics was followed by two attempts to graft the bilateral maxillary clefts. In one surgery, cancellous bone was harvested from the iliac crest and used to graft the cleft sites. The graft did not heal and resorbed. In a second surgery, autogenous bone from the outer cortex of the calvarium was used to graft the bilateral cleft defects again. This graft also failed to heal.

At the time the patient presented, she complained about bone pieces that continued to extrude through the gingiva. Examination and radiographs showed unconsolidated bone fragments within the soft tissue (Figs 7-3b to 7-3d). Oral examination showed a freely mobile incisive bone segment, anterior maxillary hypoplasia, and expanded maxillary posterior segments. Fragments of the failed bone graft were extruding through the fistulas.

To realize successful healing of a bone graft, the space in which it is placed must be supportive. In their current state, the maxillary fragments would not support bone graft healing (Fig 7-3e). The spatial relationships of the maxillary segments were incorrect. The roots of the teeth adjacent to the clefts were too far apart and were at different vertical heights. Regardless of the quality and quantity of bone grafting material used, healing would be unlikely in this situation.

When grafting introduces cells to the bone discontinuity, regulation of the new tissue is necessary for growth and organization. The periodontal ligament systems of the adjacent teeth were the primary source of supportive signaling in the patient's cleft anomaly. Even in normal anatomy, the muscle attachments that supply neuromuscular regulation to this region are weak. The cleft disorder impaired the regulatory mechanism by disrupting the functional anatomy of both the bone and muscle systems at the site. In this compromised state, optimum recruitment of the periodontal systems would be critical for successful bone healing.

With the intercanine width expanded to this degree, the neuromuscular regulatory effect of the periodontal ligaments would have minimal intensity in the center of the defect. The apical position of the incisive bone segment further decreased the ability of these teeth to support growth of a graft.

Even if a graft achieved continuity across the cleft, the physiology of the segment would always be compromised. Bone that exists in an unsupportive environment is not a good site for placement of dental implants.

The maxillary cast that was made following two failed bone grafting surgeries revealed maxillary deficiency and marked distortion of the dental arch form (Fig 7-3f). The presurgical orthodontic preparation had compromised the potential for successful graft site healing by excessive expansion of the dentoalveolar segments (Fig 7-3g). Because conventional grafts generally resorb and lose volume during the consolidation process, some surgeons try to overbuild the graft to compensate for collapse. The flaw in this strategy is that the host environment must first tolerate the graft before the consolidation process can begin.

In this patient, grafting in the excessively expanded site was tried twice and failed bilaterally on both attempts. The most likely cause of graft failure was the absence of effective neuromuscular signaling into the graft site. This type of orthodontic expansion prior to graft placement displaces the teeth adjacent to the regeneration chamber. As the teeth are moved farther apart, the magnitude of periodontal signaling in the center of the regeneration chamber is diminished. Both autogenous iliac crest and autogenous calvarium have the capability to recruit cells to the regeneration chamber. However, neuromuscular signaling from the periodontal systems of the teeth is necessary to direct the consolidation and organization process.

Expansion of the segments may also challenge the ability to obtain closure of the nasal floor and oral mucosa. Nasal bacteria and secretions must be isolated from the regeneration chamber. Thus, despite the repeated use of good bone grafting material, the construction failed because of the limitations of the surgical design.

The distal root angulation of the maxillary right canine further compromised its capability to supply signaling to the regeneration chamber. The incisive bone segment had been displaced apically so it was not at the same level as the posterior segments. To be most efficient, the periodontal systems of the central incisors should be at the same level as those of the canines. The orthodontic and surgical plans should be coordinated so that design of the regeneration chamber optimally supports bone growth, consolidation, and organization.

Radiographs confirmed that the prior calvarium bone graft had failed and pieces of graft were extruding through the fistulas (see Figs 7-3c and 7-3d). The repeated grafting attempts resulted in scarring of the soft tissue that compromised its viability. The thin layer of bone that covered the root of the left central incisor was compromised when the mucosa was elevated during the bone grafting procedure. Success in these constructions depends heavily on the condition of the periodontal systems of

Fig 7-3 Use of osteotomy to achieve bone growth after multiple failed grafting attempts.

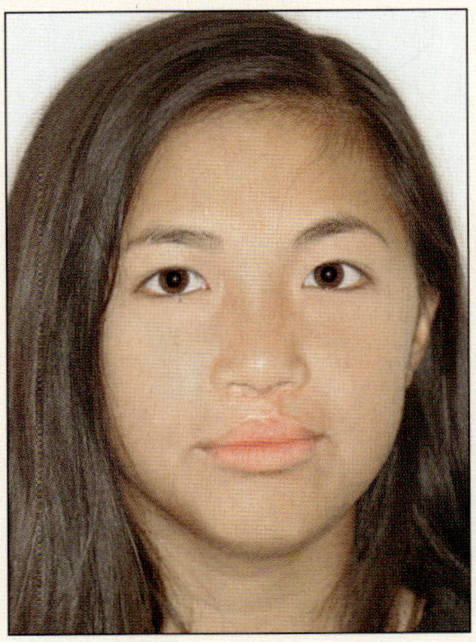

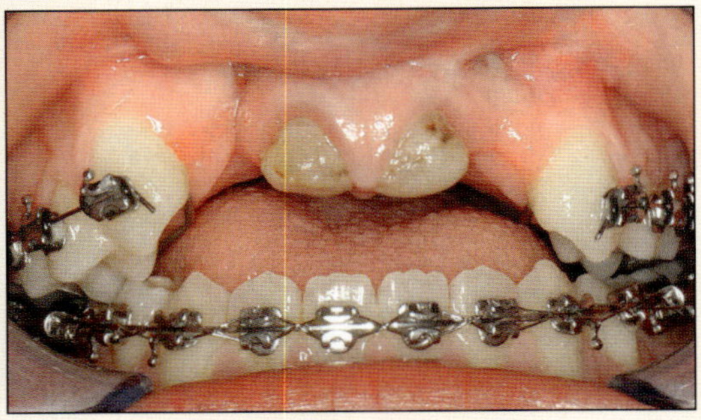

Fig 7-3a *(far left)* A 14-year-old girl presents for management of missing teeth and bone at the anterior maxilla.

Fig 7-3b *(left)* Oral examination shows a freely mobile incisive bone segment, anterior maxillary hypoplasia, and expanded maxillary posterior segments. Fragments of the failed bone graft are extruding through the fistulas.

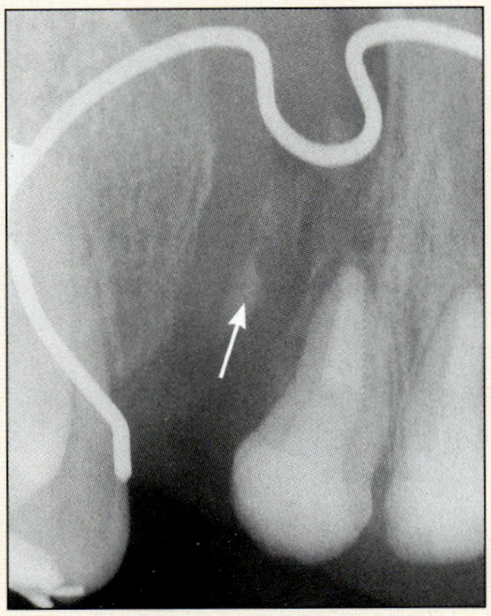

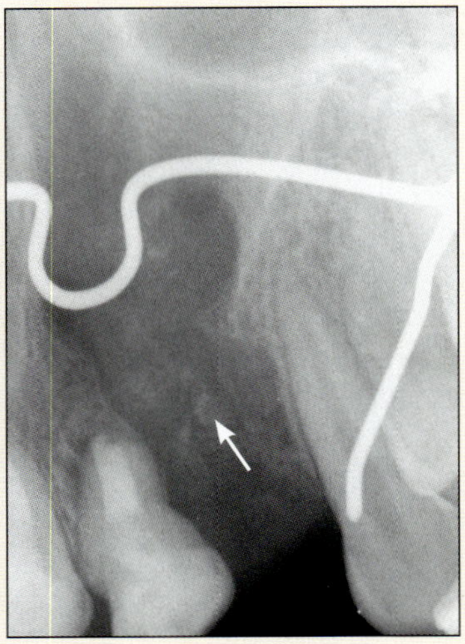

Fig 7-3c *(far left)* A radiograph of the right cleft shows a sequestrum from the failed calvarium bone graft being extruded through the fistula *(arrow)*.

Fig 7-3d *(left)* A radiograph of the left cleft shows graft fragments in the soft tissue *(arrow)*.

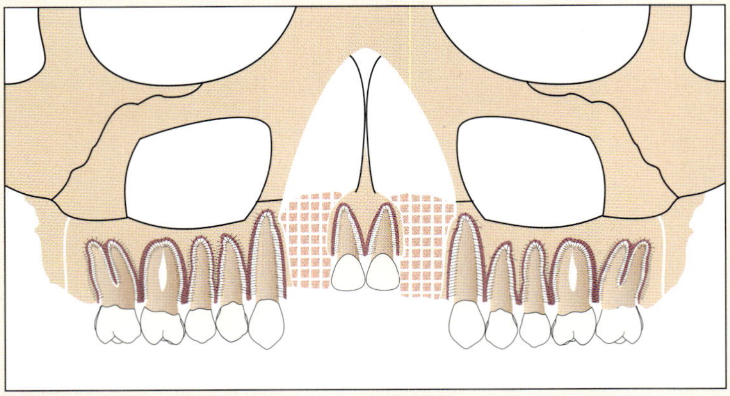

Fig 7-3e In the existing conditions, the challenges to successful repair include the magnitude of the defects and the incorrect alignment of the segments.

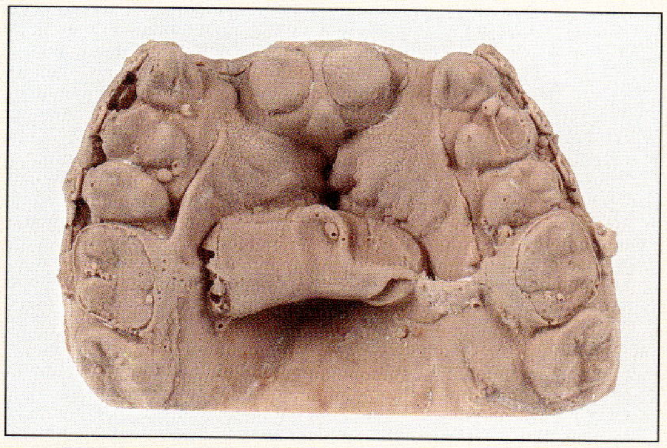

Fig 7-3f A maxillary cast prepared after two failed bone grafting surgeries demonstrates maxillary deficiency and marked distortion of the dental arch form.

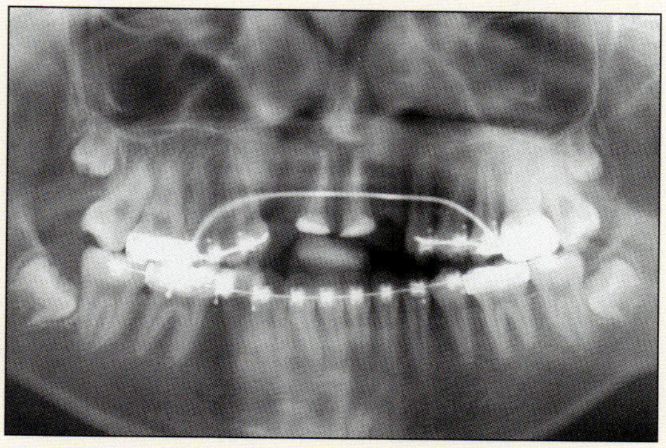

Fig 7-3g A panoramic radiograph shows widening of the clefts by orthodontic expansion.

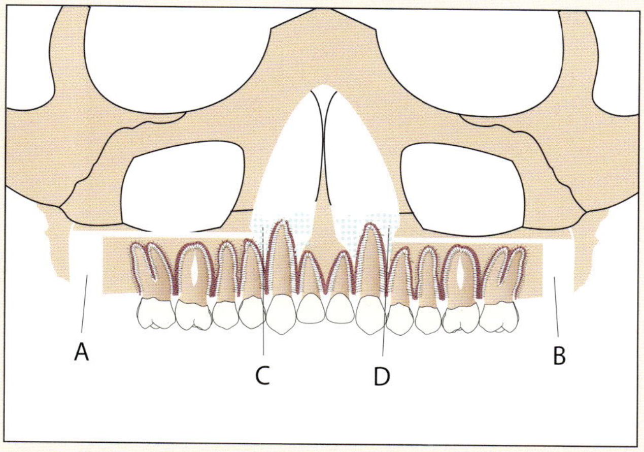

Fig 7-3h The alternative surgical design proposes construction of four bone regeneration sites. After the maxilla is mobilized with a Le Fort I osteotomy, the posterior maxillary segments will be protracted, opening pterygomaxillary chambers at points A and B that are expected to predictably fill with bone without the need for grafting. The maxillary segment will be moved under traction into alignment with the posterior segments, creating regeneration chambers at points C and D. Healing at sites C and D has failed before, and these sites are at the center of the developmental field defect, so rhBMP-2 will be placed to supply cells.

→

the teeth adjacent to the cleft. Maintenance of a healthy, functioning periodontal system at these teeth must be a priority for the pediatric dentist, orthodontist, and surgeon.

The failure of autogenous bone grafting of the alveolar clefts after two surgical attempts demonstrated that the design of that procedure was deficient. The failure occurred because the essential conditions for bone formation were not met by the surgical design. Regardless of the care taken when the surgical plan was executed, the environment would not support bone growth.

To be successful, a surgical design must address the anatomical deficiency in a manner that meets functional and esthetic objectives. The surgical design must also include the essential elements for bone growth. An alternative surgical design developed for this patient had the potential of successful healing (Fig 7-3h). The design proposed construction of four bone regeneration sites. The maxilla was to be mobilized at the Le Fort I level. The posterior maxillary segments would be protracted, opening gaps at points A and B. These pterygomaxillary regeneration chambers were expected to predictably fill with bone without the need for grafting. The mechanism for this process is described in chapter 8.

The maxillary segment was to be moved under traction into alignment with the posterior segments. This would create regeneration chambers at points C and D. Moving the roots of the canines into close proximity to the roots of the central incisors would decrease the volume of the graft and allow stimulating signals from the periodontal systems to regulate the growth and organization of the graft site. However, because they were sites of previous grafting failure and were at the center of the developmental field defect, rhBMP-2 would be placed to supply cells to the regeneration chambers at points C and D.

In accordance with the surgical design, the maxilla was mobilized at the Le Fort I level. Four regeneration chambers were created by repositioning the maxillary segments. Each chamber had to meet the essential criteria for bone formation. The anterior chambers that represented the alveolar cleft had already demonstrated the propensity for graft failure. In both of the prior surgeries, autogenous bone was used as the source of cells. Those surgeries did not fail because of a lack of a source of cells. The revised surgical design included no autogenous grafting material at all. The strategy was to construct an environment with all of the essential elements for bone formation.

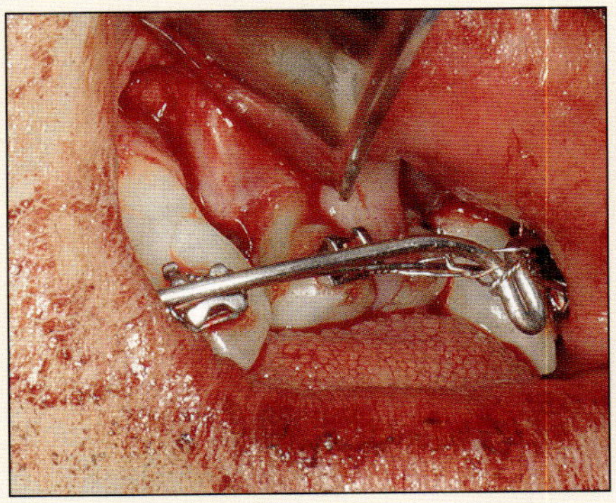

Fig 7-3i Repositioning of maxillary fragments closes the right alveolar cleft.

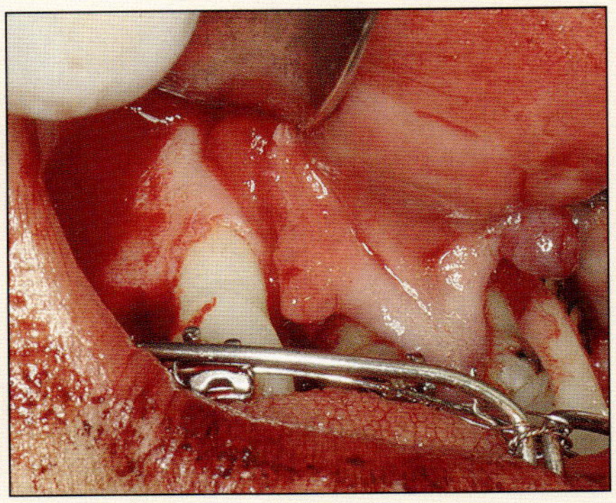

Fig 7-3j A graft of rhBMP-2 on a collagen sponge overlies the closed right alveolar cleft site.

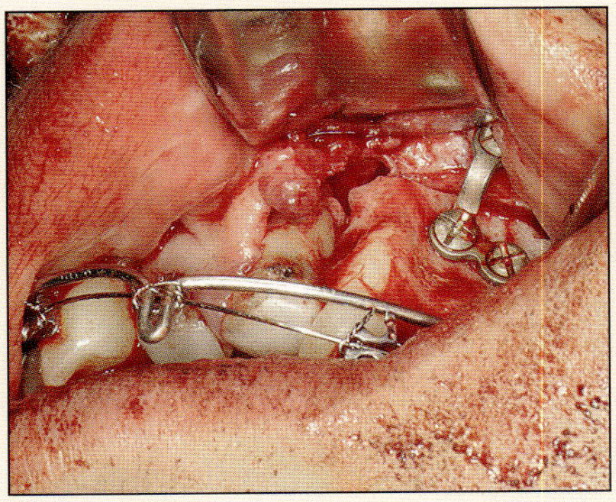

Fig 7-3k The segments have been repositioned at the left alveolar cleft site.

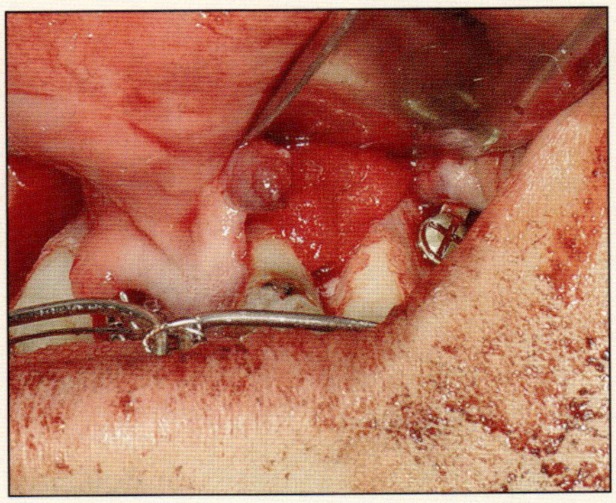

Fig 7-3l The rhBMP-2/ACS material is placed at the left cleft site.

→

The incisive bone segment that contained the two central incisors was protracted and repositioned inferiorly (Fig 7-3i). The objective was to place the periodontal systems of the central incisors and canines into close proximity. Correction of the vertical levels of the periodontal attachments was important. Prior to fixation of the segments in this position, the nasal and palatal aspects of the fistula were repaired with tension-free sutures. There was no space remaining for placement of particulate bone grafting material.

The posterior regeneration chamber was located between the posterior maxilla and the intact pterygoid plates. This region will regenerate predictably without the need for grafting. The entire maxillary complex was protracted and repositioned into a functional occlusion. Correct positioning was verified by indicators on a headframe mounted on the cranium.

The closed right cleft site was covered with rhBMP-2 on an ACS (Fig 7-3j). The sponge was 20 × 20 mm and contained 1 mg of rhBMP-2 in 1 mL of sterile water. This was a contrast to the two prior surgeries, which required harvesting of bone from the patient's iliac crest and calvarium.

The left alveolar cleft was managed in a similar fashion (Fig 7-3k). The segments were repositioned to align the periodontal systems of the central incisor and canine in close proximity. The maxillary complex was repositioned and then fixated with titanium bone plates. A small volume remained for placement of the rhBMP-2/ACS material. The rhBMP-2/ACS material was positioned in the cleft and as an onlay (Fig 7-3l). The suture line overlay the sponge material. On the left side, 2.0 mg of rhBMP-2 in 1.5 mL of sterile water was placed within the 20 × 30–mm collagen sponge.

Two weeks after surgery, the suture lines were intact with dehiscence (Fig 7-3m). Six months after surgery, the gingiva had healed without recurrence of the fistulas (Fig 7-3n).

The former right and left cleft sites were filled with new bone. The regeneration chambers at the pterygomaxillary disjunctions (A and B) filled with bone without the need for grafting (Fig 7-3o).

Repair sites in which rhBMP-2 is placed without particulate graft material follow a typical sequence of healing. Initially, the cortices of the cleft margins are resorbed and the space fills with a radiopaque material that lacks normal structural features. The lamina dura on the adjacent teeth becomes poorly defined. There is no cortical outline at the alveolar crest or the nasal rim. The repair site at the right cleft exemplified this sequence 6 months after surgery (Fig 7-3p).

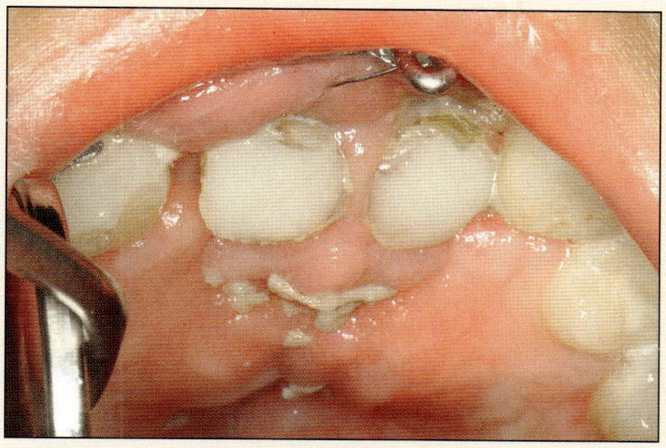

Fig 7-3m Two weeks after surgery, the suture lines are intact with dehiscence.

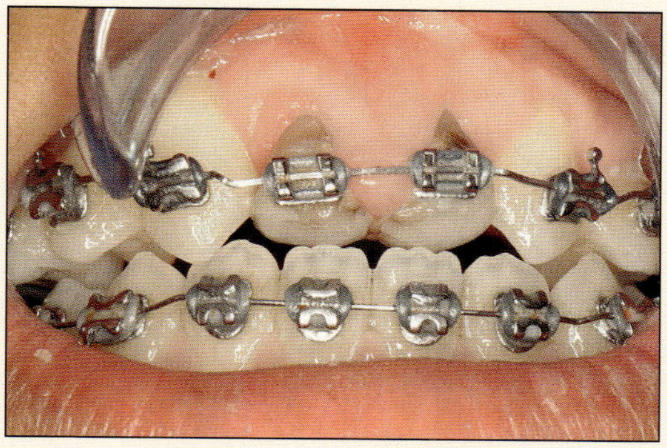

Fig 7-3n Six months after surgery, the gingiva has healed without recurrence of the fistulas.

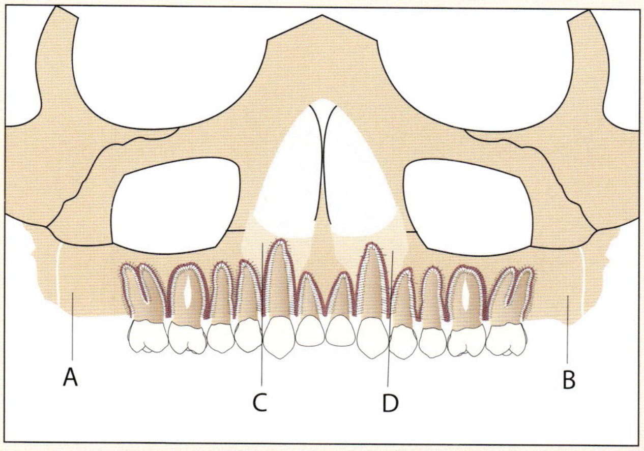

Fig 7-3o The clefts at points C and D are filled with new bone. The regeneration chambers at the pterygomaxillary disjunctions (A and B) have filled with bone without the need for grafting.

The left side showed features similar to those on the right side (Fig 7-3q). There was calcified tissue at the original cleft site, but the architecture lacked signs of structural integration.

After 6 years in function, the newly constructed bone on the right side showed signs of functional integration (Fig 7-3r). There was defined lamina dura around the roots, indicating a functioning periodontal ligament system. The crest of the alveolus had a cortical outline, as did the constructed nasal rim. The trabecular pattern had matured and was similar to that of the native bone.

The left cleft showed full consolidation at the 6-year follow-up (Fig 7-3s). The repair site had matured and demonstrated an active, functional architecture. There was a cortical outline at the alveolar ridge crest that was continuous with the lamina dura of the teeth. A periapical lesion required endodontic treatment.

A panoramic radiograph taken 8 years after surgery revealed that the Le Fort I–level osteotomies had healed (Fig 7-3t). The regeneration chambers between the posterior maxilla and pterygoid plates showed continuous bone formation even though no grafting was done at those sites.

In this strategy for construction, the decision was made to close the cleft defects using a segmental Le Fort I osteotomy. Two prior failed attempts to repair the alveolar clefts with bone grafting demonstrated that the deficiency of the sites involved more than a lack of cells. Even if a bone graft had healed at the site, the lack of neuromuscular support was likely to result in graft resorption and failure of osseointegrated implants. In this patient, the need for dental implants had been avoided (Figs 7-3u and 7-3v). If a tooth failed in the future, the alveolar bone that was constructed was suitable for implant treatment.

Discussion

Patients with cleft lip and palate make up the largest proportion of cases treated by craniofacial centers. Alveolar clefts are therefore a familiar problem that presents regularly to the maxillofacial surgeon. Surgeons often forego the formal treatment-planning process that starts with a comprehensive examination and diagnosis. Instead, the process starts at surgery scheduling. The surgical procedure is dictated by an incomplete assessment of the defect. Because most of these patients respond to placement of an autogenous bone graft, all patients are routed down that path.

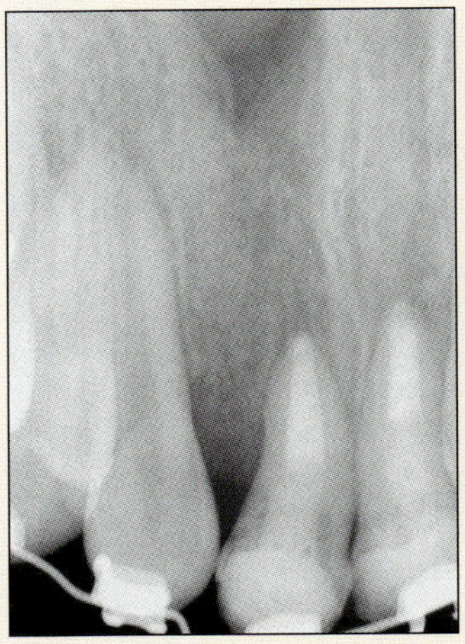

Fig 7-3p Right side 6 months after surgery.

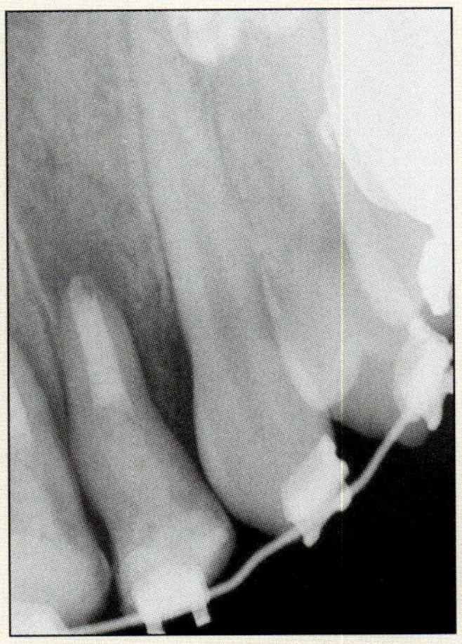

Fig 7-3q Left side 6 months after surgery.

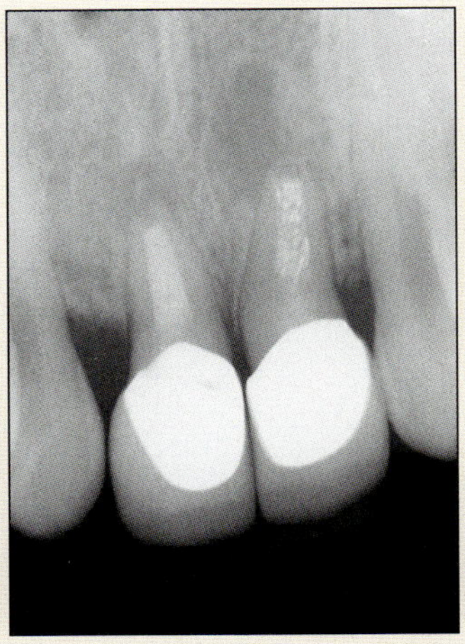

Fig 7-3r Right cleft site after 6 years.

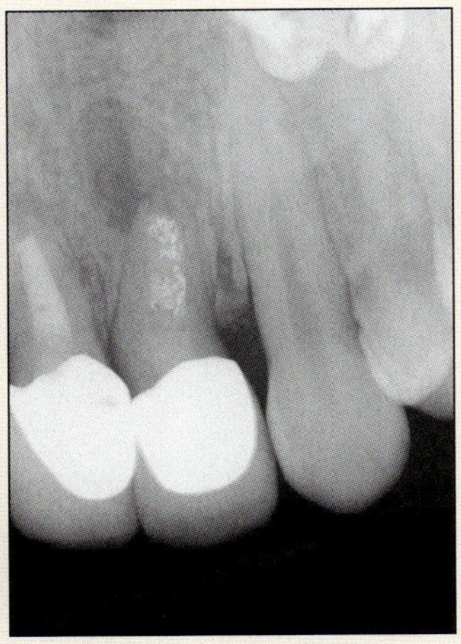

Fig 7-3s Left cleft site after 6 years.

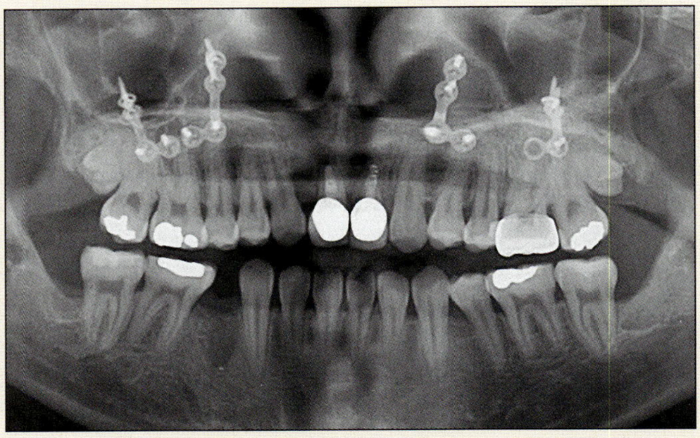

Fig 7-3t Panoramic radiograph 8 years after surgery.

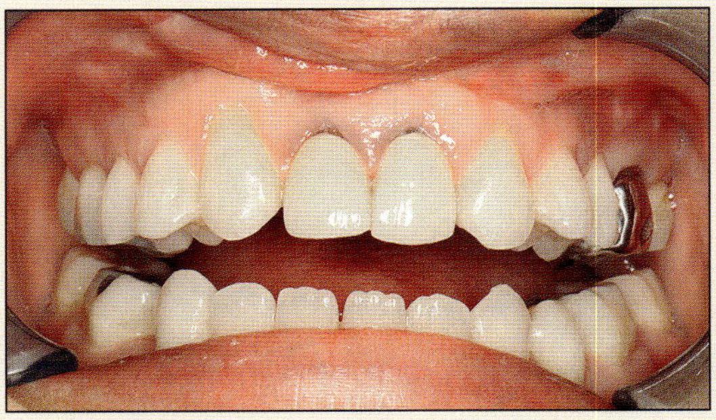

Fig 7-3u Intraoral view 8 years after surgery.

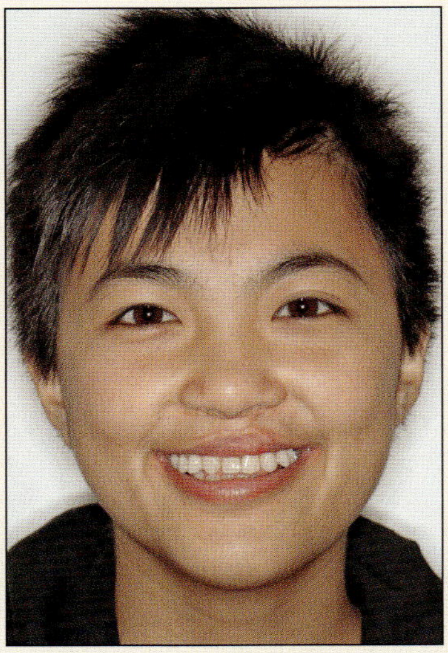

Fig 7-3v Patient's facial appearance at 8-year postsurgery follow-up.

In this case, the physical environment in which the graft was placed could not support bone growth. The essential requirements for a bone-forming construct were not in place. After the first surgery failed on both sides, a second surgery was performed in the same environment. Predictably, the second surgery also failed. This case demonstrates the importance of beginning with a comprehensive diagnosis. The available sources of neuromuscular signaling must be recognized and included in the design of the bone-forming construct. In this case, repositioning of the periodontal systems of the teeth adjacent to the cleft was necessary to make regulatory signaling available to the cells that would be provided to the regeneration chamber by rhBMP-2.

Fig 7-4 Use of Le Fort I osteotomy to manage a large midline facial cleft.

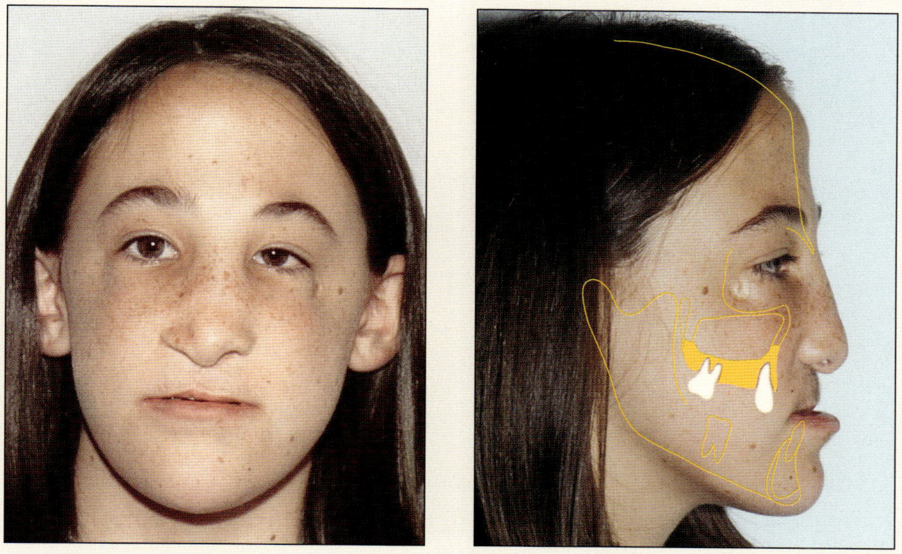

Fig 7-4a A 14-year-old girl with a rare congenital midline facial cleft presents for management of missing teeth and maxillary bone.

Fig 7-4b Superimposition of the lateral cephalometric study and a lateral facial photograph shows the magnitude of maxillary retrusion.

→

Le Fort I Osteotomy to Treat a Major Developmental Field Defect

Large midline facial clefts represent some of the most challenging management problems that confront maxillofacial surgeons. The construct must meet the requirements of viability, durability under function, and esthetics. These patients present as children. The treatment must accommodate growth and many years of service. In addition to the obvious absence of anatomical structures, the etiology and development process of these deficiencies place unique demands on the strategy of management and surgical design.

These congenital skeletal defects are derived from primary agenesis and are resistant to surgical techniques used for conventional reconstruction. The structures did not develop in utero because the anatomical field did not contain the essential elements for bone formation. If a graft is placed in this defective field, it will fail to heal and integrate into the existing skeletal system if the essential elements are still absent.

When these patients first present, the environment in which bone is needed is unsupportive of healing. The oral cavity, nasal cavity, and maxillary sinuses do not offer a source of vascular supply, cells, or neuromuscular input. These cavities introduce a variety of bacteria that do not favor bone growth. Complete construction implies the placement of natural teeth– or dental implant–supported prostheses. The dental construction must meet the demands of mastication, speech, esthetics, and long-term durability.

To meet the objectives of skeletal unit construction, it is critical to design a bone-forming construct with the greatest healing potential. In the following case, osteotomies are used to create a bone-forming construct to fill the anatomical defect.

Case description

A 14-year-old girl presented with a developmental midline facial cleft (Fig 7-4a). The structural deficiency involved a cleft lip, absent incisive bone, missing maxillary anterior teeth, absent midline nasal structures, olfactory nerve dysfunction, and pituitary gland dysfunction. The dental and facial deficiencies were the manifestation of the primary origin of the disorder in the central nervous system. The midline brain-related involvement of the olfactory nerve and the pituitary gland were consistent with the primary central nervous system etiology of this problem.

The midface was hypoplastic and retruded (Fig 7-4b). The soft tissues of the midface and nose were unsupported. Although the anterior maxilla was absent, the right and left posterior maxillary segments had developed. The primary developmental field defect caused midline structural hypoplasia. These anatomical structures did not form because the field lacked the essential elements necessary for development. Both the teeth and the precursors for innervated muscles were absent from this field. Without neuromuscular input from teeth or muscle attachments, the skeletal structure could not form.

The developmental fields lateral to the central defect were less affected. Although hypoplastic, these segments contained all of the essential elements for growing and maintaining a skeletal unit. These two small skeletal units would become the substrate from which the absent portion of the maxilla would be generated.

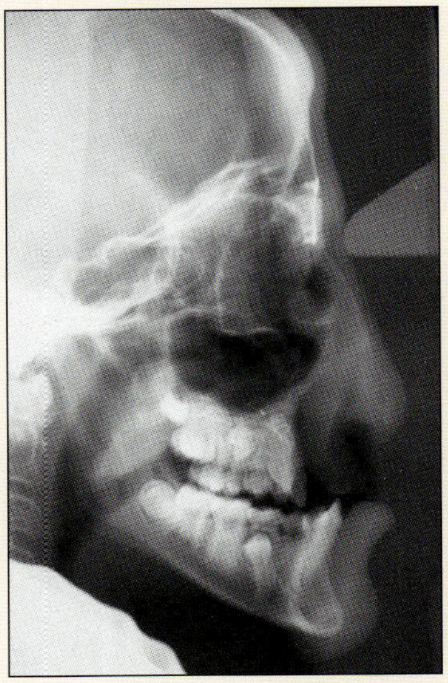

Fig 7-4c The lateral cephalometric radiograph shows the maxillomandibular dental arch discrepancy.

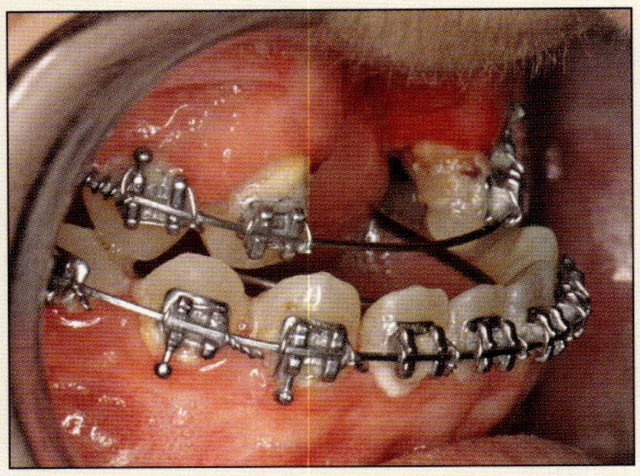

Fig 7-4d Oral examination shows the malocclusion. (Reprinted from Chin et al[4] with permission.)

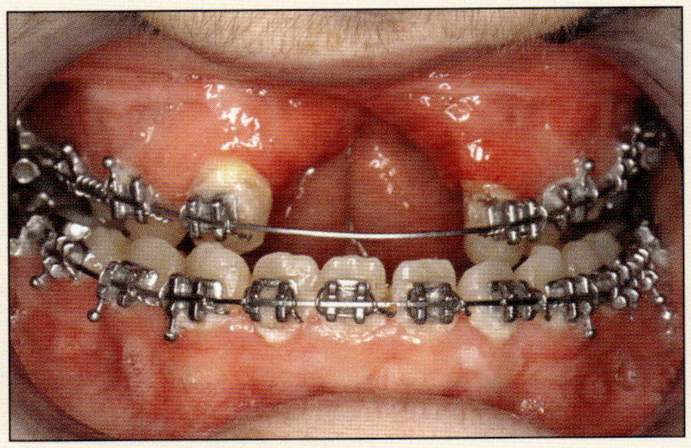

Fig 7-4e Agenesis of the premaxilla.

→

A lateral cephalometric radiograph taken at age 12 years (ie, 2 years earlier) showed severe, pan-midfacial hypoplasia (Fig 7-4c). The Class III maxillomandibular relationship was complicated by agenesis of the premaxillary bone.

Oral examination revealed the magnitude of the defect and the challenge that would be involved in constructing a complete maxilla (Fig 7-4d). The posterior maxillary segments were Class III and in a crossbite malocclusion. The anterior maxilla was completely absent of bone, soft tissue, and teeth (Fig 7-4e). Superior to the midline maxillary discontinuity was the nasal cavity.

In the past, use of a removable dental prosthesis would have been the most common treatment. Use of a partial denture with this Class III maxillomandibular relationship would have placed damaging leverage on the prosthesis and anchoring posterior maxillary teeth. Experience has shown that, over time, the maxillary abutment teeth would fail, leaving the patient in a progressive, worsening dental condition.

This patient presented after an autogenous bone graft had been attempted. Although a portion of the graft remained at the nasal floor, a very large volume of bone and soft tissue was lacking (Fig 7-4f). One strategy would have been to surgically transfer bone and soft tissue to fill the volume deficiency in the form of another graft (Fig 7-4g). This approach, however, would be expected to perform poorly because of the compromised healing potential of the cleft environment. Simple placement of bone tissue or cells in the deficient volume would fail because the field lacked any underlying regulatory mechanism. The conditions that gave rise to the cleft itself would also operate on a surgically inserted graft.

An alternative strategy was to expand the existing, adjacent skeletal structures (Fig 7-4h). This concept borrows from the principles of distraction osteogenesis as described by Ilizarov,[5–8] a Russian orthopedist. Application of the formal protocol for orthopedic distraction osteogenesis was not feasible or necessary in this situation. What was relevant was the essential concept of promoting healing in an unfavorable site by transporting an existing, viable skeletal segment to the defect. Another important lesson from Ilizarov's strategies[5–8] was the basic principle of positioning the donor site osteotomy in a region of high healing potential.

Before a bone-forming construct could be designed for this deficiency, it was necessary to understand how the existing bone segments maintained their own morphology. The fact that these segments formed in the embryo and continued to exist in a steady state implied that an underlying regulatory process was operating. Any surgical intervention had to preserve the mechanisms that were involved in the formation of this section of the skeleton.

The main volume of the segment consisted of the alveolar process. This volume of bone and soft tissue was developed under the influence of the developing and erupting teeth. The stability and the ability to maintain the morphology over the long term depend on the health and location of these teeth. The teeth and periodontal apparatus (A and B) are essential to the physiology of this anatomical unit (see Fig 7-4h). Posterior to the alveolar region is the union of the maxilla to the pterygoid region (C). This region shares regulatory mechanisms with the cranial base. The posterior maxilla and pterygoid region form, grow, and are maintained because of the underlying stability of the skull base. The system of investing muscles and the brain itself contribute to the stability of the anatomical region. At the anterior aspect, the alveolar segment was continuous with the piriform buttress (D). This is a structural skeletal region that gains its stability from adjacent muscles and the functional nasal airway. The mechanism by which respiration regulates the morphology of the nasal cavity is incompletely understood.

Fig 7-4f Three-dimensional computed tomography study reveals the absence of skeletal structures in the facial midline.

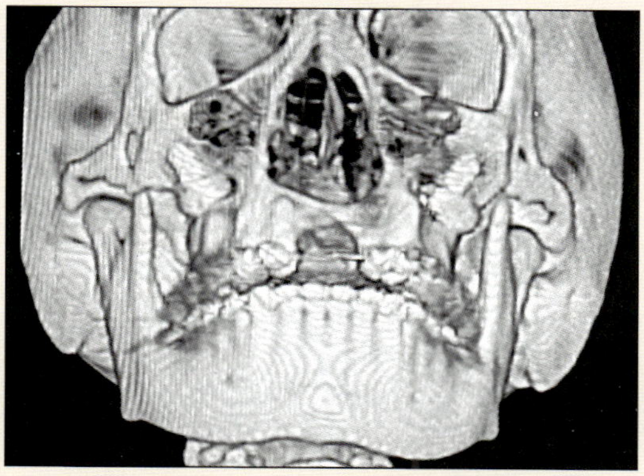

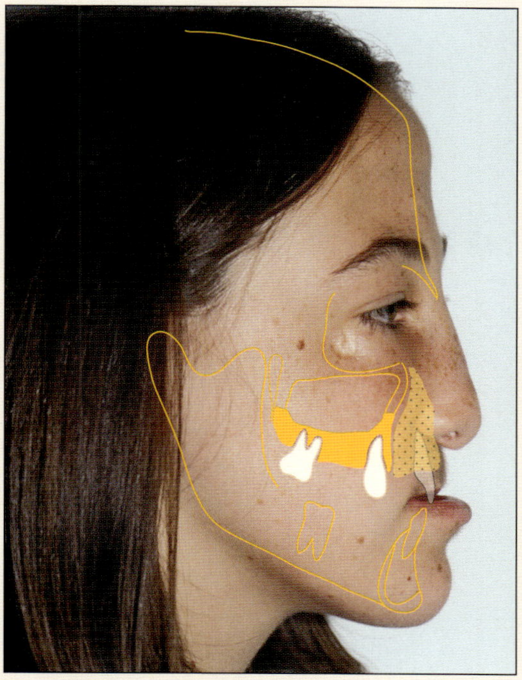

Fig 7-4g Graphic projection of the bone volume and position needed to address the midfacial deficiency. (Modified from Chin et al[4] with permission.)

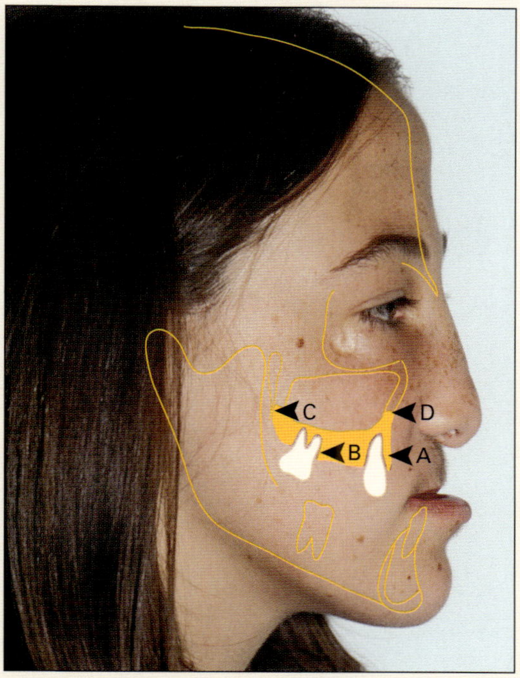

Fig 7-4h Functional analysis defines the elements that are operating to maintain the existing hypoplastic midface. Points A and B are the periodontal ligament systems that maintain the alveolar housings for these teeth. Point C is the intact pterygomaxillary junction, which is under the regulation of the muscle that originates at the pterygoid plates. Point D is the piriform buttress, which is under the regulation of the facial muscles and nasal structures.

→

If the native skeleton that bordered the discontinuity could be enlarged, the resulting volume could be used to fill the cleft defect. Enlargement of each posterior maxillary segment can be accomplished by transporting either a segment or the whole skeletal unit.

One option was to mobilize the maxillary segment at the Le Fort I level and protract it into the anterior volume deficiency (Fig 7-4i). As the maxillary segment is displaced from its original position, the osteotomy kerf is opened into a space-occupying chamber (Fig 7-4j). This newly created compartment then becomes the chamber in which bone would form. Its ability to fill with bone depended on how well the basic requirements for bone formation were met. The chamber at point A was the primary bone-forming site. It was fully bound by viable soft tissue. The anterior and posterior walls of the chamber were the posterior maxilla and pterygoid plates, respectively. The posterior maxilla has neuromuscular input from the molar teeth. The pterygoid plate region receives input from the skull base musculature, the lateral pterygoid muscles, and the skull base itself. The skull base and calvarium are under the regulatory sphere of the brain and dura mater.

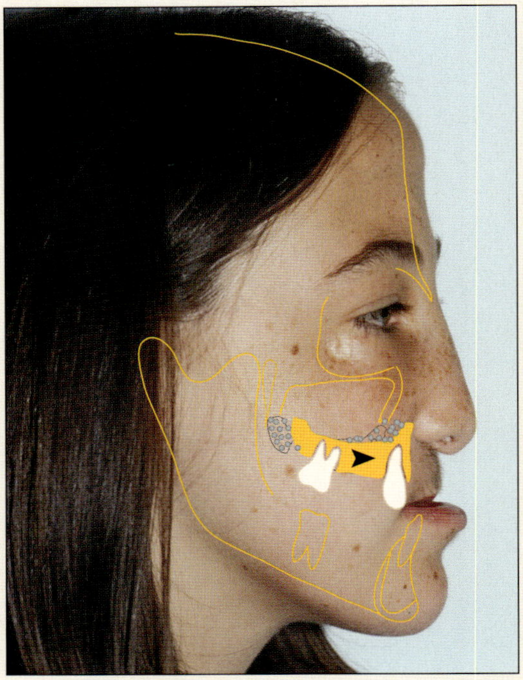

Fig 7-4i One treatment strategy is to fill the deficient volume by protracting the maxilla anteriorly *(arrowhead)*.

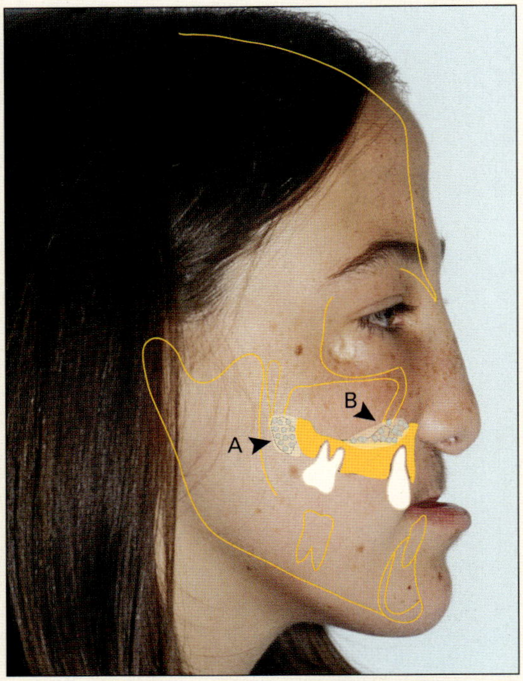

Fig 7-4j Moving the maxilla anteriorly at the Le Fort I level opens a bone-forming chamber at the pterygomaxillary junction (A). The piriform buttress (B) is a secondary bone-forming site.

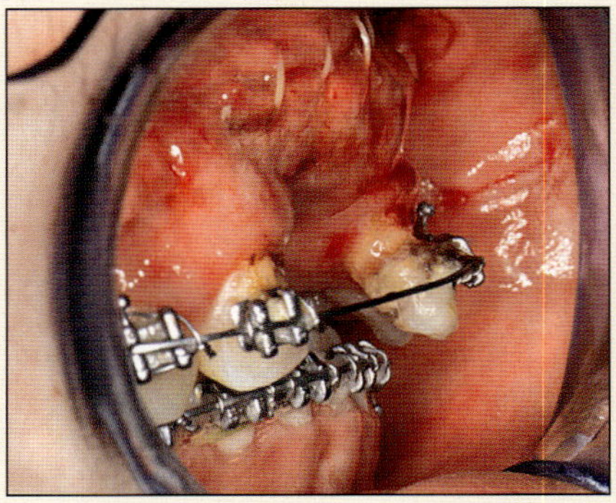

Fig 7-4k The maxilla has been repositioned by Le Fort I advancement.

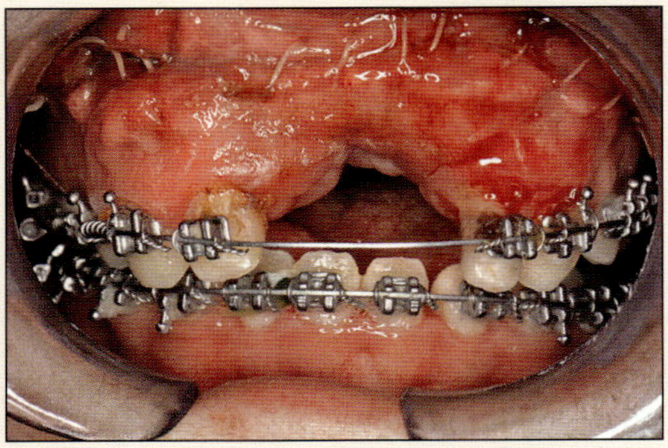

Fig 7-4l The maxillary advancement has moved the teeth and their periodontal ligament systems into a better position. The mucosa shows substantial vascular congestion in response to the tension of protraction. The midline maxillary deficiency remains.

→

The two posterior maxillary segments were mobilized at the Le Fort I level and transported anteriorly with internal distraction devices (Fig 7-4k). Multiple prior oral surgeries resulted in scar tissue and resistance to immediate protraction of the maxilla where internal fixation could be used. Intraoperative findings showed vascular congestion with moderate manual maxillary protraction. Chin internal distraction devices (Lorenz/Biomet) were placed to allow gradual postoperative protraction. The result was that the occlusion more closely represented a Class I relationship.

Although the posterior occlusion was improved, the central alveolar discontinuity remained, and teeth were still missing (Fig 7-4l). Compromised healing of the soft tissue was apparent despite the use of gradual protraction with distraction devices.

To address the problem of discontinuity across the cleft, the healed maxilla underwent a second distraction procedure (Fig 7-4m). Conventional bone grafting was not a good option. In the author's experience, conventional autogenous bone grafting fails even in narrow midline clefts. The origin of the cleft was the developmental absence of critical neuromuscular elements.

Fig 7-4m The unique physiologic deficiency of the midline facial cleft demands a special surgical design. Conventional bone grafting is not an option.

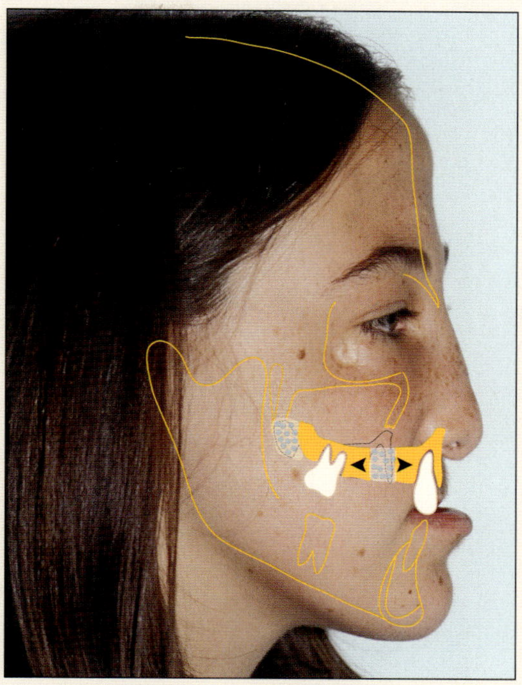

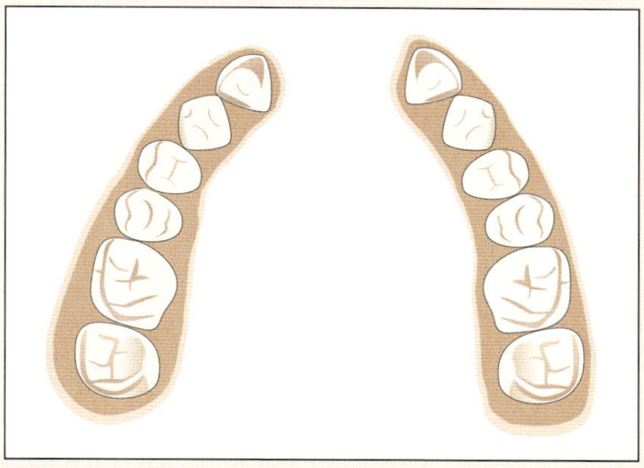

Fig 7-4n Functional analysis of the midline maxillary cleft from the occlusal aspect.

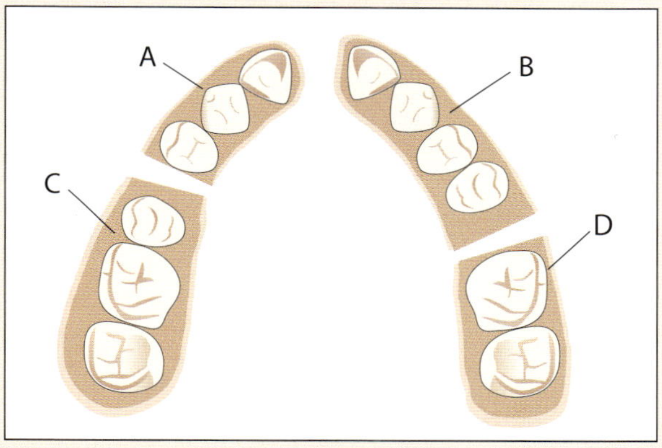

Fig 7-4o The surgical strategy creates four maxillary segments for horizontal repositioning with distraction: Points A and B are the transport segments, while distraction chambers will open at points C and D. The objective is to transport a source of neuromuscular signaling to the deficient skeletal volume.

→

Normally, developing teeth, periodontal structures, and cranial nerve–based innervation would have resulted in the formation of the incisive bone. If successful engineered growth of this missing skeletal unit is to be accomplished, all of the deficient bone-forming elements must be supplied. In this case, the strategy was to transport existing dentoalveolar units to the defect.

The use of transport distraction to close the discontinuity represented a geometric challenge (Fig 7-4n). The discontinuity was at the center of the defective developmental field. The bone at the cleft margin was formed and maintained under the influence of the terminal incisor teeth and their periodontal ligaments.

Osteotomies were to be created through each maxillary segment (Fig 7-4o). The design of the transport segments (points A and B) had to fulfill the requirement to be self-sustaining anatomical units. Each unit had to retain a neuromuscular element that can provide input to the surrounding bone long term. In this case, the teeth and their periodontal apparatus satisfied this requirement. The volume of alveolar bone carried cells as well as an organized trabecular architecture.

The distraction chambers would open at points C and D. These sites were outside the developmental field defect and had osteogenic potential. The osteotomy opened the medullary space

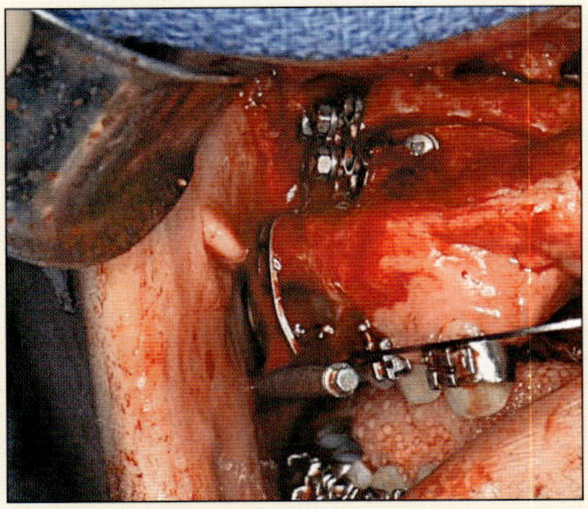

Fig 7-4p The right maxillary transport segment is mobilized, and a Liou cleft distractor is mounted. A similar procedure prepares the left maxillary segment for distraction.

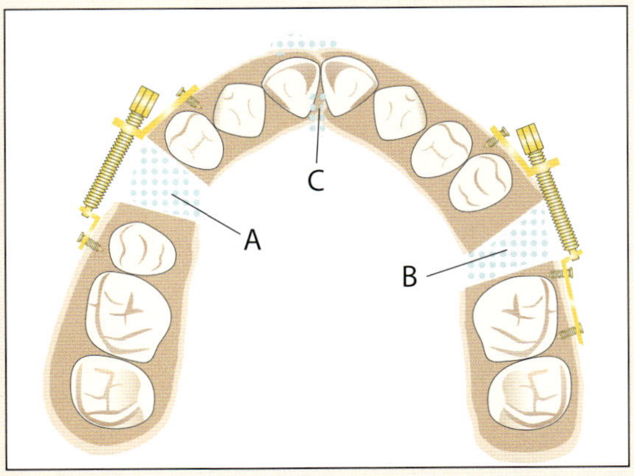

Fig 7-4q The strategy is to open distraction chambers at points A and B. Point C becomes the docking site. All three sites are treated with rhBMP-2 carried on ACSs.

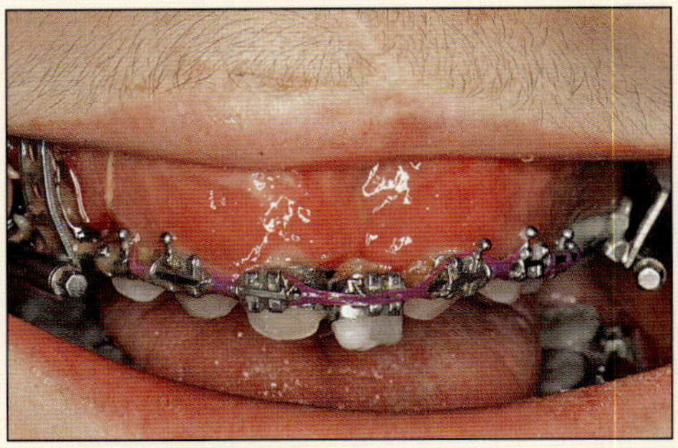

Fig 7-4r Following successful transport, the teeth in the transport segments dock in the midline.

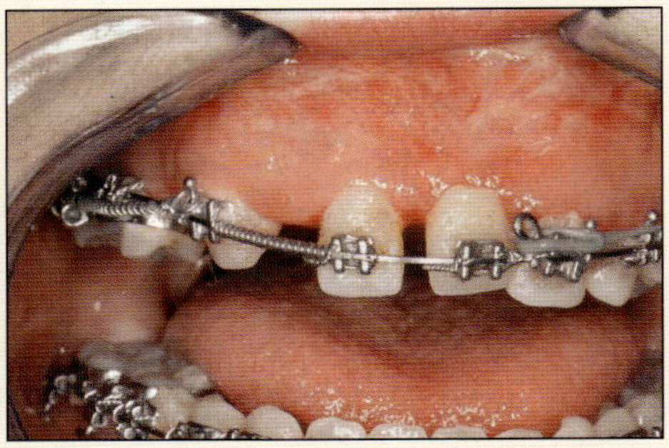

Fig 7-4s Orthodontic treatment refines the occlusion.

→

to the distraction chamber so that cells and vessels had direct access. The teeth adjacent to the chambers would provide neuromuscular input to maintain their own surrounding bone and to stimulate the cells introduced to the chamber to grow bone and consolidate into a functional ossicle.

Transport of the segments required distraction because the soft tissue pedicles were previously operated-on mucosa (Fig 7-4p). To maintain vascular integrity, the transport rate was limited to 2 mm per day. Liou distractors were used for this procedure. The devices were modified with titanium mesh to extend the reach of the anchoring plates.

Bone morphogenetic protein (Infuse, Medtronic) was placed in both distraction chambers and the docking site to supply cells for bone healing (Fig 7-4q). The lateral purchase of the distraction device on the anchoring and transport segments resulted in a curvilinear transport path. This created the shape of the dental arch. The stability of the distraction chambers and the docking site was established with the distraction devices and orthodontic appliance. All of the essential requirements for bone formation were met.

As a result of the segmental distraction process, the midline discontinuity was closed. Teeth within the two transport segments docked in the midline (Fig 7-4r). Orthodontic treatment developed the dental arch and occlusion (Fig 7-4s). Midfacial retrusion was corrected with the combination of Le Fort I maxillary advancement and bilateral segmental distraction osteogenesis (Fig 7-4t). Mandibular surgery was not necessary.

The facial appearance and occlusion remained stable at the 7-year follow-up (Fig 7-4u). The patient's facial appearance 12 years after surgery reflects the stability of the result (Figs 7-4v and 7-4w). The occlusion also remained stable at the 12-year follow-up (Fig 7-4x).

Discussion

In patients with major developmental field defects, surgeons tend to focus on the obvious structural deficiency and underestimate the global impact of the primary developmental etiology. Successful engineering of a bone-forming construct must take into account that the developmental field deficien-

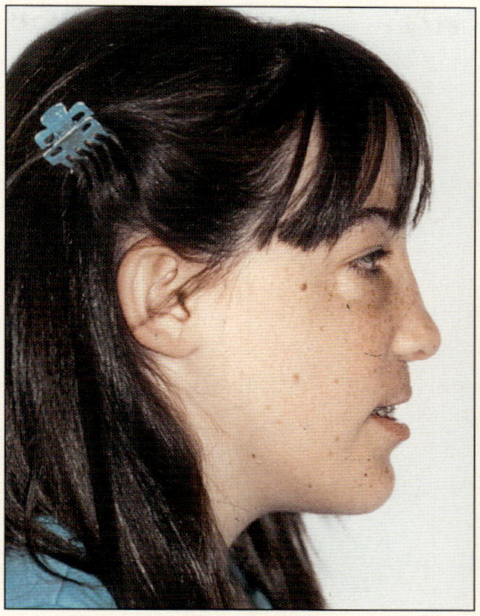

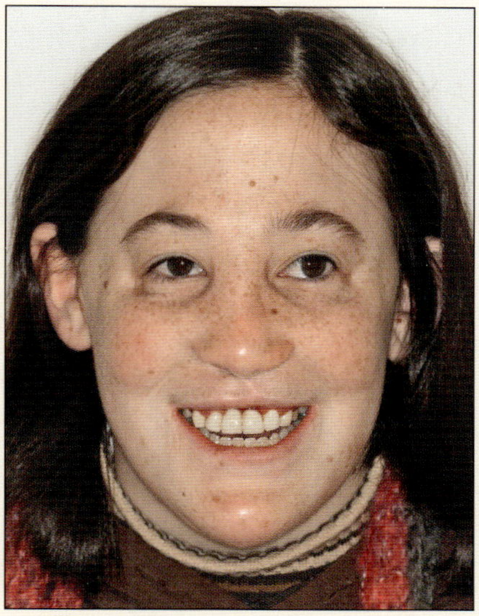

Fig 7-4t *(right)* The facial balance is improved as a result of maxillary construction. The mandible has not received any surgical treatment.

Fig 7-4u *(far right)* The facial appearance and occlusion remain stable at the 7-year follow-up.

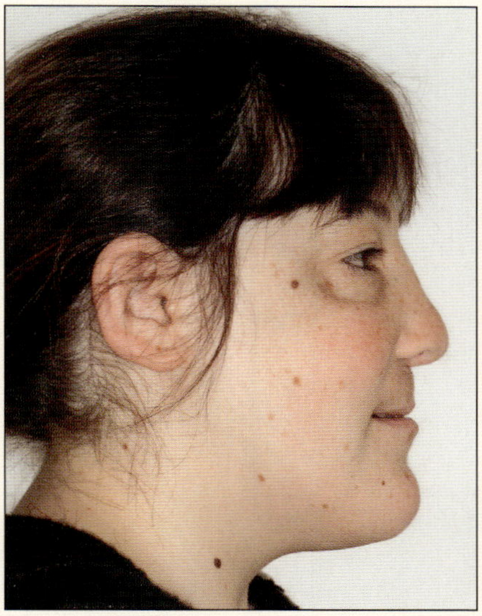

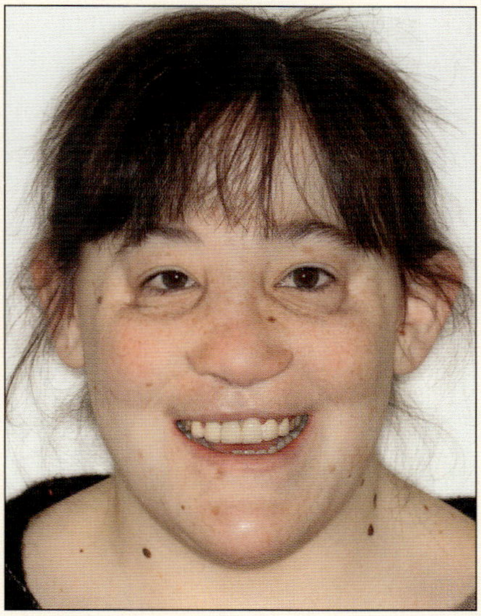

Fig 7-4v *(right)* Facial profile 12 years after surgery.

Fig 7-4w *(far right)* Facial appearance 12 years after surgery.

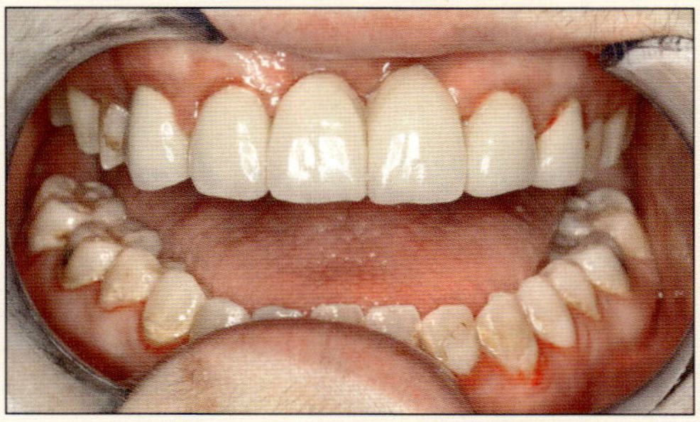

Fig 7-4x *(right)* Dental arches 12 years after surgery.

cy results from a primary central nervous system abnormality. This underlying deficiency in neuromuscular regulation must be addressed; simple replacement of bone volume with grafting will be unsuccessful. Any construct that lacks neuromuscular regulation will either fail to consolidate into a viable skeletal unit or slowly resorb over time. When a bone-forming construct is designed for these very-difficult-to-heal defects, inclusion of Ilizarov's principles of distraction osteogenesis[5–8] in the engineering process can extend the reconstructive possibilities by decreasing the healing demand on the host.

Le Fort III Osteotomy for Bone Formation after Radiation Therapy

Radiation therapy is a primary treatment modality for management of malignancies. Altering the pathologic physiology of the malignant process is the goal of radiation oncology. If treatment is successful, the destructive behavior of the malignant cells is halted or at least slowed. However, the effect of radiation is not limited to the tumor cells. Because delivery of radiation has geometric and physiologic limitations, adjacent tissue is also damaged. This results in a radial zone of diminishing tissue damage with the tumor target as the center.

Reconstructive surgical treatments must compensate for the impaired healing potential of these tissues. The tissue adjacent to the missing structures often does not respond normally to surgical incursion. Surgeons recognize that radiation results in compromised vascular supply in the tissue adjacent to the reconstruction zone. Impairment of neuromuscular regulation of the region is less well understood.

In the past, surgeons developed strategies to promote healing of augmentation procedures within ischemic fields. Hyperbaric oxygen therapy is one approach to prepare a potential graft site for enhanced healing. In a different approach, pectoralis major muscle flaps are used to transfer an intact anatomical segment to the deficient field. The muscle pedicle maintains vascular supply and tissue viability. Free flaps exploit the technology of microvascular anastomosis to allow transfer of composite flaps from distant donor sites. The use of free fibula flaps has become standard practice for reconstruction of facial deficiencies.

Radiation impacts children by slowing or arresting normal growth within the deficient field. Growth impairment results in primary and secondary deficiencies that challenge rehabilitation. Radiation in infants can be lifesaving, but the secondary effects emerge as the child develops. Midfacial growth impairment is manifested as severe Class III jaw and facial patterns. Teeth in the radiation zone may fail to develop. This results in a primary problem of edentulism. The secondary problem is the failure of the alveolar bone to develop in the presence of developing teeth.

Osteotomies are an important tool for managing the multiple challenges that these patients face. The following case demonstrates use of a modified Le Fort III osteotomy approach in a patient whose healing capabilities were compromised by previous radiation therapy.

Case description

This 19-year-old woman presented with severe midfacial hypoplasia (Fig 7-5a). At age 5 years she was diagnosed with a pharyngeal rhabdomyosarcoma. The malignant lesion was treated with 60 Gy of radiation to the midface. As a side effect of radiation treatment, her maxillary teeth failed to develop and she was left with an edentulous maxilla. As another result of radiation, the maxilla and midface failed to grow, resulting in three-dimensional hypoplasia of the bone and soft tissue. The loss of facial vertical dimension increased the restorative challenge by increasing the Class III maxillomandibular relationship. The conditions made it difficult to achieve functional stability for a maxillary denture.

The Class III maxillomandibular relationship posed a mechanical challenge to either removable or implant prosthodontics (Fig 7-5b). Reconstruction with onlay grafting was contraindicated by multiple factors. It was not feasible to onlay bone to the existing maxilla because of the large volume required and the lack of mucosa to house it. In addition, after a patient undergoes radiation therapy, vascular impairment and tissue ischemia must be factored into the engineering design. Elevation of large mucoperiosteal flaps to expose a maxilla that was within the central portal of radiation delivery presented a risk of osteoradionecrosis and poor soft tissue healing. To mitigate this risk, surgical designers must extend their range of options to find potential solutions that present more acceptable risks while optimizing the benefits.

Because the defect included both bone and soft tissue, technology that would transfer bone and soft tissue coverage at the same time was considered. Local composite flap options would have involved mobilizing a portion of the local facial skeleton and transporting it to the defect. Distant composite flaps, such as fibula free flaps, were also an option but would have required a donor site and microvascular anastomosis. It is important for the surgeon to consider each option sequentially to determine the potential for success and the potential risks.

Le Fort I osteotomy for segment protraction is a type of composite flap. It could have potentially satisfied the requirements of delivering bone and soft tissue to the defect and simultaneously creating a regeneration chamber at the donor site. In this patient, however, the maxilla was in the primary portal of radiation delivery. It was difficult to assess the degree of local vascular damage that might compromise the Le Fort I pedicle. In addition, the healing potential of the bone adjacent to the osteotomy might have been impaired. Osteoradionecrosis or impaired healing was a high risk if a Le Fort I osteotomy were used.

As an alternative to the Le Fort I osteotomy, a Le Fort III osteotomy was analyzed for its feasibility, potential success, and risks. The Le Fort III procedure (Fig 7-5c) is also a composite flap with the potential to transport bone and soft tissue coverage to the defect.

A reconstructive procedure involving a Le Fort III osteotomy would avoid some of the hazards specific to this patient's condition. However, the inherent risks and potential complications of the Le Fort III procedure were more concerning than those of the Le Fort I design. The Le Fort III osteotomy mobilizes a major portion of the facial skeleton, and the bone cuts are in close proximity to the eyes and brain. These specific risks had to be analyzed and mitigated if possible.

Figure 7-5c shows one pattern of osteotomy designed to exploit the underlying neuromuscular regulating mechanisms that operate in the midface. Positioning osteotomies distant from the primary radiation ports decreases the risk of osteoradionecrosis. The conventional Le Fort III osteotomy is modified by cutting vertically through the largest mass of the malar bone. Engineering requirements dictate this change in the surgical technique. To preserve vascular supply to the mobilized segment, minimal tissue is reflected. This compromise creates a challenge of access to create and mobilize the segment and to place the distraction device. Engineering requirements dic-

Fig 7-5 Modified Le Fort III osteotomy after radiation therapy.

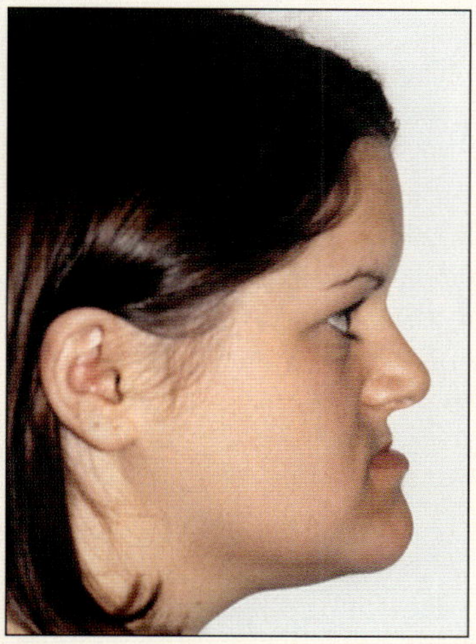

Fig 7-5a A 19-year-old woman presented with missing teeth and midfacial hypoplasia secondary to radiation therapy.

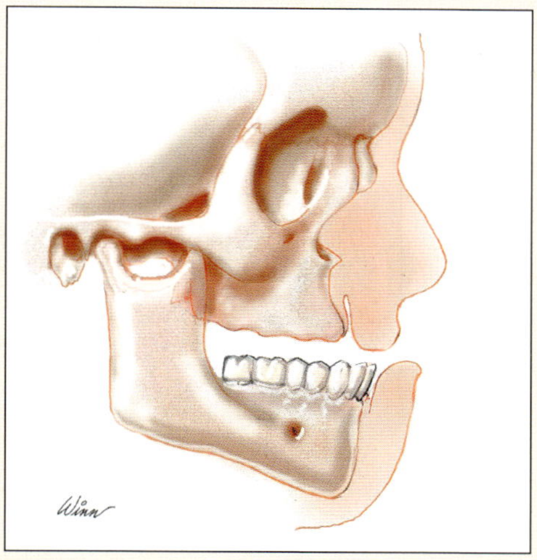

Fig 7-5b Representation of maxillary deficiency and absence of permanent maxillary teeth.

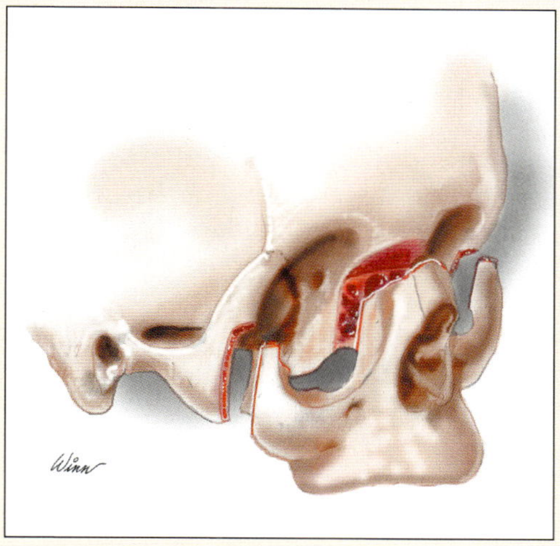

Fig 7-5c Representation of Le Fort III osteotomy to allow protraction of a viable skeletal segment.

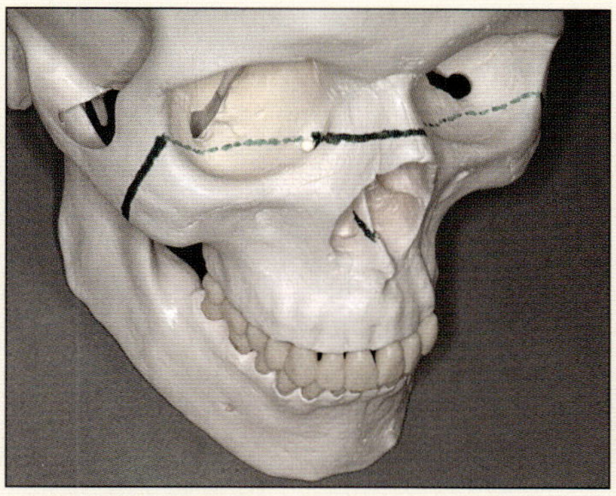

Fig 7-5d The osteotomy plan is outlined on a skull model.

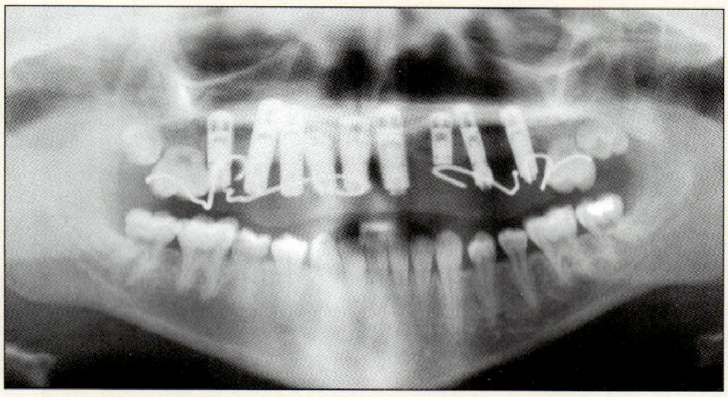

Fig 7-5e Dental implants have been placed in multiple stages.

tate that the anchorage points for the distraction mechanism have adequate mechanical strength to handle the pressure of segment protraction. In this type of procedure, the anchorage points at the malar osteotomy must endure pressures of at least 10 kg without failure. If the malar segment attached to the maxilla fractures during Le Fort III mobilization, the distraction and fixation strategy cannot be completed.

In this patient, the osteotomy through the malar bone was to be moved anteriorly and canted downward versus the Frankfort plane (Fig 7-5d). This would decrease the need for soft tissue reflection and allow transoral placement, operation, and removal of the distraction device. The osteotomy across the nasal aperture was moved inferiorly to avoid the risk of cranial base damage at the cribriform plate.

The edentulous state of the maxilla posed two surgical problems. The midface mobilizing technique requires anchorage to the dental arch and the nasal floor. Implants were needed to safely mobilize the midface. The second engineering problem of the edentulous maxilla involved the possible need for maxillomandibular fixation. In some cases, the expected plan for a distraction osteogenesis procedure must be modified intraoperatively to a conventional osteotomy. Maxillomandibular fixation must be maintained as an option should the need arise. The presence of healed dental implants is necessary to preserve this option.

Nine dental implants were placed in multiple stages (Fig 7-5e). Because of the history of radiation therapy, the healing potential for osseointegrated implants was unknown. Initially, two implants were placed to study the healing response. One of these two implants failed to heal and was removed. One implant successfully osseointegrated. The site of the failed implant was carefully followed and was found to heal. Implants were then added in a staged manner. All of the subsequent implants osseointegrated.

Because the maxilla remained in an extreme Class III position, the implants were not suitable for placement of a fixed prosthesis. The patient was maintained in a provisional denture.

For surgical planning and preparation, the implants were uncovered and abutments were placed. Impressions and jaw relation records were obtained for orthognathic cast surgery and splint fabrication. Custom splints engaged the implants and the midface mobilizing instrument to apply controlled, safe, yet adequate leverage to complete the Le Fort III osteotomy.

A midface mobilizing device was used to complete the Le Fort III osteotomy (Fig 7-5f). The pterygomaxillary junction was not cut directly. Instead, the mobilizing instrument created the separation. The pterygoid plates and muscle attachments were preserved. This preserved the mechanical integrity of the medial wall of the regeneration chamber and the critical neuromuscular input from the medial pterygoid muscle attachment. Use of the nasal floor and dental arch (in this case, dental implants) to apply leverage for mobilization of the Le Fort III segment avoided the risk of separating the malar bone from the maxilla.

The Le Fort III osteotomy established discontinuity between the midface and the cranial base structures (Fig 7-5g). The transport segment included the maxilla, zygomatic buttress, infraorbital rim, anterior orbital floor, lateral piriform aperture, and osseointegrated implants. This special osteotomy divided the malar bones, leaving half attached to the midfacial fragment and half attached to the lateral orbit.

As the mobilized midface was transported, chambers that were intended to fill with bone were opened. Bone morphogenetic proteins and growth factors were not placed in these fields of prior malignancy. The chamber at point A was bounded by the cranial base at the superior, posterior, and medial walls (see Fig 7-5g). The anterior wall was the posterior maxilla. Mucosa enclosed the remaining sides of the chamber. Neuromuscular input was delivered by the musculature inserting into the skull base and the cranium under the regulation of the brain and dura mater. The medial pterygoid muscle takes its origin from the lateral aspect of the pterygoid plate. This was the medial wall of the chamber. The posterior maxilla also benefited from the only four surviving maxillary teeth that were well positioned in the maxillary tuberosity. At point B, a chamber that was bounded by the cut surfaces of the malar bone was opened. The masseter muscle uses this structure as its origin. Cells had access to the chambers through the exposed medullary bone, invading new vessels, and the adjacent muscles. At point C, the cut orbital rim was under the regulation of the periorbital muscles of facial expression.

The distraction device was placed with minimal access (Fig 7-5h). To be effective, the device needed to provide transport and rigid anchorage for many months.

Even without the benefit of growth factors, morphogenetic proteins, or bone grafting, the osteotomy healed and remained stable (Fig 7-5i). The facial appearance was satisfactory 1 year following Le Fort III midfacial advancement (Fig 7-5j). The facial appearance remained stable 5 years after surgery (Fig 7-5k). The patient's implant-borne fixed partial denture was still in function after 5 years (Fig 7-5l). Successful correction of a major skeletal defect had been achieved using an osteotomy and creation of a bone-forming chamber at the donor site. The ridge relationship was Class I (Fig 7-5m).

Fifteen years after surgery, the facial appearance and dental prosthesis remained stable (Figs 7-5n and 7-5o). The long-term maintenance of the prosthesis was greatly facilitated by preparation of the skeletal base. The treatment strategy met all of the essential requirements to promote optimal bone formation and maintenance. This allowed the prosthesis to meet the functional and esthetic goals.

Discussion

The destructive behavior of radiation therapy affects healthy tissue adjacent to the tumor cells. Reconstruction of skeletal defects is challenged by both the anatomical defect and the compromise of the surrounding tissue environment. To increase the potential that reconstructive treatment will be successful, it is important to sequentially analyze the procedure from each aspect. If an anatomical or physiologic deficiency can be identified, modification of the procedure should be considered to minimize the impact each compromise will have on the performance of the bone-forming construct. For example, the Le Fort III procedure has the potential to transport bone with soft tissue coverage to the defect. In this patient, the procedure was modified to help preserve the vascular supply and diminish the risk of osteoradionecrosis in the patient's compromised tissues.

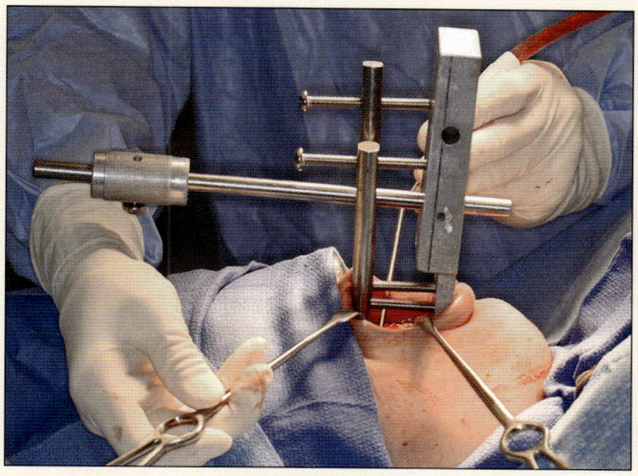

Fig 7-5f A midface mobilizing instrument mobilizes the Le Fort III osteotomy with minimal access and tissue reflection.

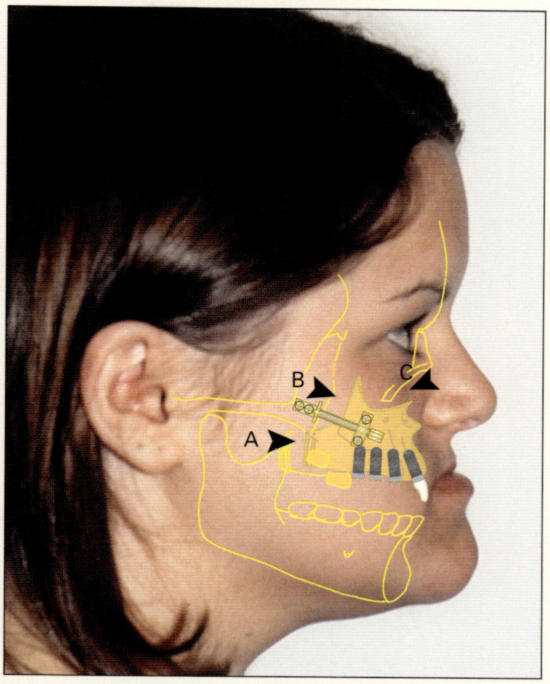

Fig 7-5g The surgery is designed to open three bone-forming chambers. Point A is the pterygomaxillary junction, point B is the divided malar bone, and point C is the nasal aperture and orbital floor.

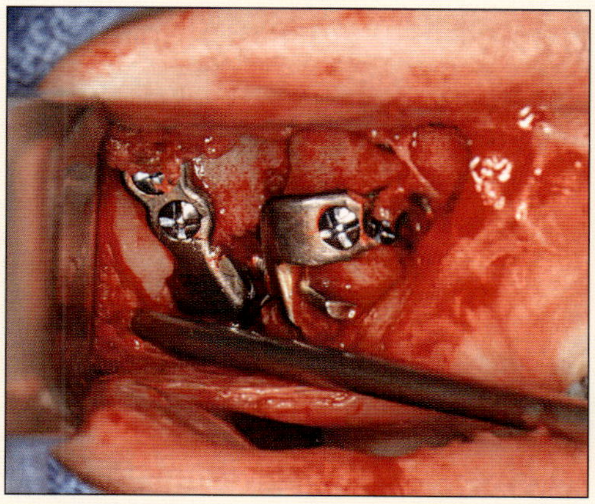

Fig 7-5h The distraction device (Chin Midface) is mounted for midfacial protraction (shown in use in a different patient).

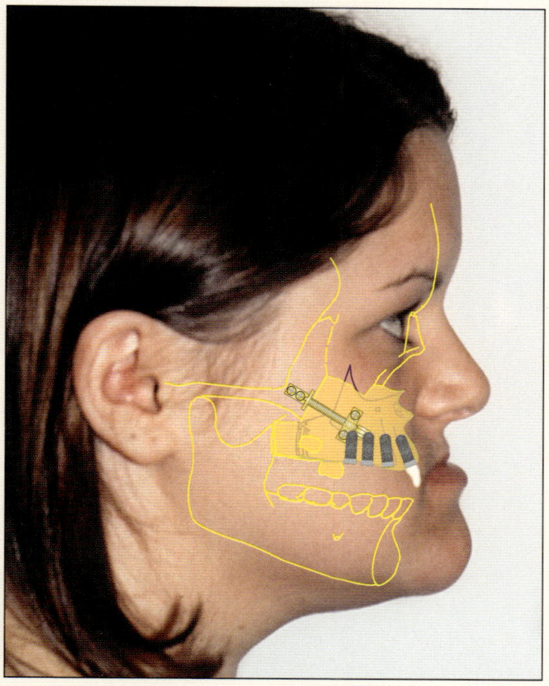

Fig 7-5i The bone-forming chambers fill with structural bone without the benefit of grafting or growth factors.

→

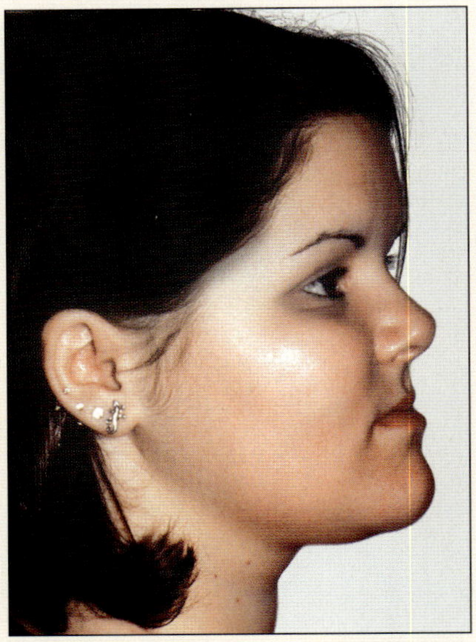

Fig 7-5j Facial appearance 1 year following Le Fort III midfacial advancement.

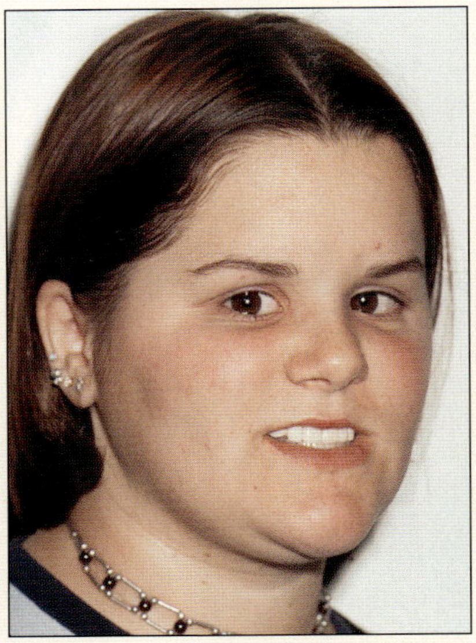

Fig 7-5k Facial appearance at the 5-year follow-up.

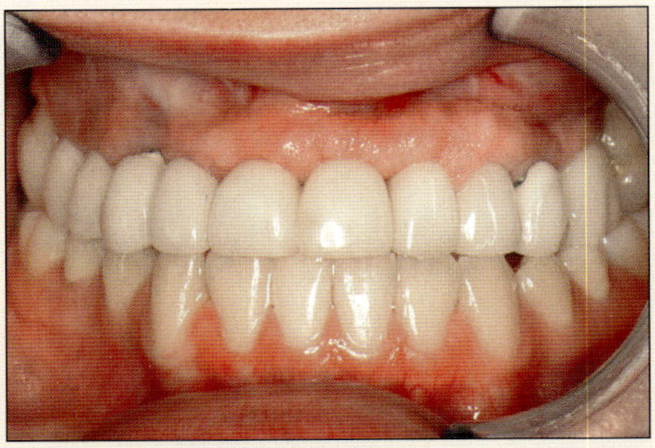

Fig 7-5l The fixed prosthesis is stable and functional at the 5-year follow-up.

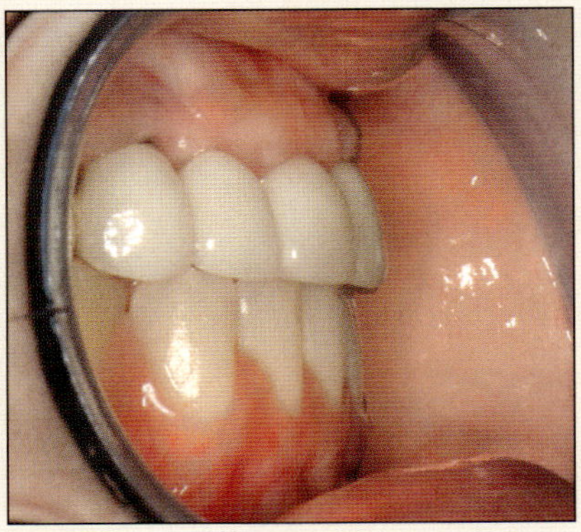

Fig 7-5m The maxillary ridge has been protracted into a Class I relationship with the natural mandibular arch.

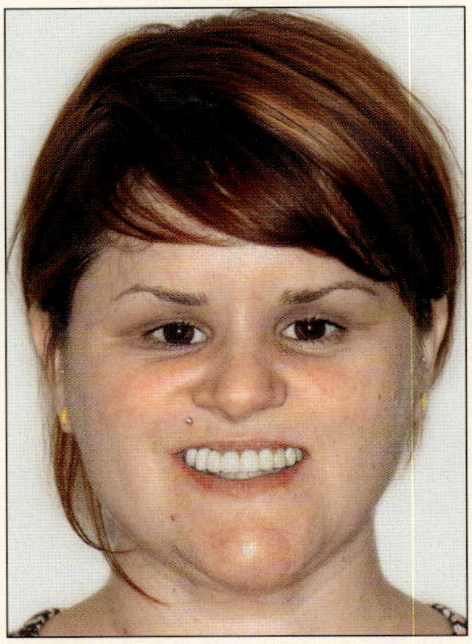

Fig 7-5n The facial appearance remains stable at the 15-year follow-up.

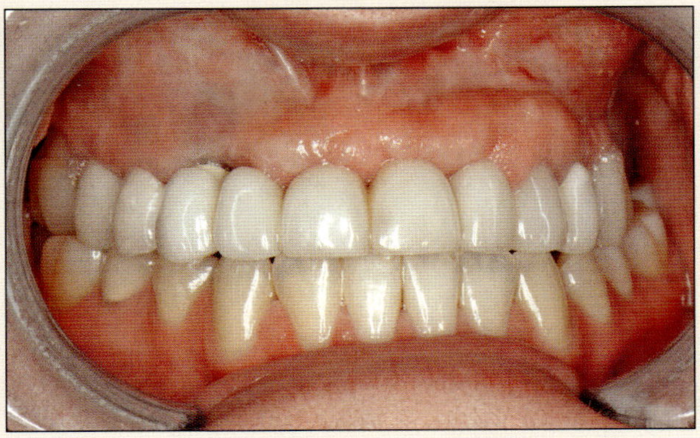

Fig 7-5o After 15 years in function, the implant-supported maxillary prosthesis continues to meet its functional and esthetic objectives.

Conclusion

It is important to recognize that some defects of the jaws that appear simple and familiar at first evaluation exist within deficient physiologic systems. These patients share a common challenge in that their dentoalveolar disorder is impacted by processes that operate at a distance from the anatomical defect in question. Some of the systemic disorders are readily recognized and understood. Other disorders involve anatomical systems that are difficult to visualize or have biologic processes that are at the limit of current science.

Surgery that would be expected to heal in a patient with normal biologic systems has substantial risk of failure in these cases. To avoid complications and disappointment, surgical designs should be followed that deliberately minimize the negative impact of these disorders on the healing process. In each case, the potential healing obstacles were identified and a surgical design established to mitigate the physiologic challenges.

Deliberate and sequential design of surgical treatment plans for these patients allows for the full range of treatment options to be considered. With each design option, the benefits and potential risks can be identified and compared with other plans. If a design reveals a weakness with one of the essential elements of the bone-forming construct, an alternative plan can be considered. Even if there are no better options, the design process can at least identify a level of risk the surgeon and patient must consider before proceeding to surgery.

References

1. Carstens MH. Neural tube programming and the pathogenesis of craniofacial clefts. I. The neuromeric organization of the head and neck. Handb Clin Neurol 2008;87:247–276.
2. Geis N, Seto B, Bartoshesky L, Lewis MB, Pashayan HM. The prevalence of congenital heart disease among the population of a metropolitan cleft lip and palate clinic. Cleft Palate J 1981;18:19–23.
3. Schallhorn RG. Postoperative problems associated with iliac transplants. J Periodontol 1972;43:3–9.
4. Chin M, Ng T, Tom W, Carstens M. Repair of alveolar clefts with recombinant human bone morphogenetic protein (rhBMP-2) in patients with clefts. J Craniofac Surg 2005;16:778–789.
5. Ilizarov GA, Ir'ianov IuM. The characteristics of osteogenesis under conditions of stretch tension [in Russian]. Biull Eksp Biol Med 1991;111:194–196.
6. Ilizarov GA. Clinical application of the tension-stress effect for limb lengthening. Clin Orthop Relat Res 1990;(250):8–26.
7. Ilizarov GA. The tension-stress effect on the genesis and growth of tissues. 2. The influence of the rate and frequency of distraction. Clin Orthop Relat Res 1989;(239):263–285.
8. Ilizarov GA. The tension-stress effect on the genesis and growth of tissues. 1. The influence of stability of fixation and soft-tissue preservation. Clin Orthop Relat Res 1989;(238):249–281.

8 Bone-Forming Constructs for Major Skeletal Reconstruction

Some clinical problems require construction of large volumes of bone. The surgical designer must recognize that these cases are not suitable for bone-forming constructs that operate primarily within the alveolar process. When a large volume of bone is necessary or the local healing capability is compromised, the bone-forming construct may need to use the major facial muscle systems to deliver high-intensity neuromuscular stimulation. Within the mandible, two major muscle systems are available to supply neuromuscular regulation to bone-forming constructs. In the symphysis, the attachment of the genioglossus muscle provides important stimulation to grafts that involve the mandibular midline. When bone is needed for reconstruction of the body of the mandible, the mylohyoid muscle provides important signaling to a constructed bone-forming environment. Without specific and deliberate surgical design that exploits the action of this muscle attachment system, grafts involving the mandibular body are prone to failure.

Within the midface skeleton, the most potent source of neuromuscular regulation is the pterygoid muscle system that originates at the cranial base. When a bone-forming construct incorporates the pterygoid muscles to deliver neuromuscular input, large volumes can be generated.

Although the concept of bone-forming environments is theoretical, practical application must take the form of a specific surgical procedure. The surgical designer's mission is to distill general principles into a technique that a surgeon can execute. In the case of facial reconstruction, some design solutions can be applied broadly to many types of cases. These strategies are very useful because they have been shown to solve difficult problems in a predictable and effective manner. These design elements are the workhorses of this treatment approach. It is worthwhile to examine these strategies in detail.

The essential elements of a bone-forming construct have been proposed in the form of a working theory (see chapter 1). These elements include *(1)* a mechanically semistable volume, *(2)* a supply of cells in the bone-forming chamber, *(3)* neuromuscular input, and *(4)* absence of pathology. Various configurations can meet these parameters, but the construct must also deliver a clinically useful product in a predictable and safe manner.

Fabrication of bone-forming chambers requires recognition of these essential conditions for growth and then specific engineering to incorporate these parameters in the surgical design. The example of coronoid regeneration, which was described in chapter 1, illustrates the theoretical principles from which the engineering guidelines were derived. In that example, the essential elements for regeneration are already in place so that fabrication of the bone-forming construct is unnecessary. After the coronoid process is divided and removed, the bone-forming environment remains. This allows the body to regenerate the structure without surgical intervention.

In clinical practice, patients present with deformities that lack one or more elements essential for bone formation, and surgical fabrication is necessary. The surgical designer must recognize which bone-forming elements are present and with what intensity they will contribute to the bone-forming process. If an element is compromised, a means to augment its effect must be designed into the procedure. If an element is absent, the surgical designer must devise a method to fabricate the missing essential component of the bone-forming construct.

Surgical science has evolved principally in its ability to cut and move anatomical structures. This type of surgery is useful in meeting the requirements to provide a stabilized environment in which bone can grow and organize. Use of bone morphogenetic proteins enables the surgeon to provide a source of cells without resorting to autogenous bone grafting. Antibiotic therapy limits the risk that pathologic bacteria may interfere with bone formation.

The remaining requirement, a source of neuromuscular signaling to regulate cellular activity within the construct, remains a primary challenge. The science of artificial regulatory signaling has not reached a level of practical efficacy; the manner by which the signals are interpreted at the cellular level is still poorly understood. Currently, the best way to satisfy the requirement of neuromuscular input is to recruit an existing natural source. This chapter presents examples of how the major facial muscle systems can be used to direct regulatory signaling to a bone-forming construct.

Genioglossus Muscle in Anterior Mandibular Reconstruction

The anterior mandible is the origin of important muscle systems. The genioglossus muscle attaches to the lingual aspect of the mandibular symphysis. When major bone reconstruction involves this region, this muscle system provides neuromuscular signaling to the healing environment.

Because of its prominent location, this region often sustains damage during facial trauma. Avulsion of the mandibular anterior teeth, alveolar process, and overlying soft tissue is common. In some cases, the symphysis itself is avulsed, resulting in discontinuity of the mandible and a central missing segment. In either clinical situation, replacement of the missing bone is challenged by multiple factors. Without teeth to provide neuromuscular signaling, it is difficult to replace or augment the alveolar ridge in these deformities. Recruitment of the genioglossus muscle attachment to fulfill the requirement for neuromuscular regulation improves the performance of a bone-forming construct at this site.

Displacement of the Genioglossus Muscle for Mandibular Reconstruction

Case description

A 33-year-old woman presented for management of facial fractures and missing teeth resulting from a bicycle accident (Fig 8-1a). Oral examination showed a large avulsion defect of the anterior mandible and maxilla (Fig 8-1b). Seven mandibular teeth and the associated alveolar housing were lost, leaving a large deficiency in bone volume and soft tissue. A radiographic cross section at the mandibular midline showed the osseous symphysis with a narrow ridge crest (Fig 8-1c). In addition to the thin ridge width, the vertical dimension was 10 mm deficient. Onlay bone graft augmentation was not feasible because of the large bone volume needed, the lack of soft tissue, the thin residual ridge, and the lack of teeth to supply stabilizing neuromuscular regulation.

A surgical plan was made to transport an osteotomy segment vertically to fill the defect. Neuromuscular regulation of the bone-forming construct was to be supplied by superior displacement of the genioglossus muscle attached to the distraction segment (Figs 8-1d and 8-1e). At the site where the distraction osteotomy penetrates the lingual cortex of the symphysis, some fibers of the genioglossus muscle attachment are severed. Vertical transport of the distraction segment opens an osseous void that becomes the regeneration chamber. The severed ends of the muscle attachment fibers become aligned with the regeneration chamber and deliver signals into the healing site to stimulate bone formation.[1]

The genioglossus muscle attached to the lingual cortex of the distraction segment tends to pull the bone fragment medially. When the transport segment was prepared, the osteotomies were positioned to provide control and guidance of the segment (Fig 8-1f). The osteotomies established mechanical undercuts to counteract this displacement tendency. The vertical osteotomies converged lingually to prevent lingual displacement of the segment by genioglossus muscle tension. The vertical osteotomies also deliberately diverged apically, creating an undercut and resistance to vertical displacement (Fig 8-1g).

This geometry guided the segment labially as it was displaced coronally. In general, the ridge crest required labial displacement to meet restorative and dental implant position requirements.

Collagen sponges carrying recombinant human bone morphogenetic protein 2 (rhBMP-2) were used to fill the bone chamber

Fig 8-1 Displacement of the genioglossus muscle for mandibular reconstruction.

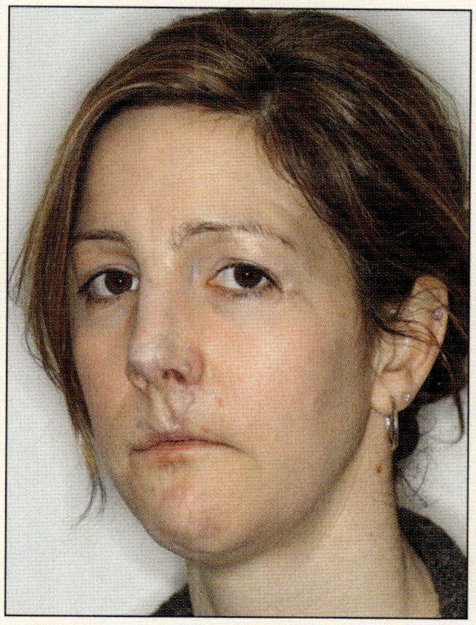

Fig 8-1a A 33-year-old woman fell from her bicycle, sustaining facial fractures and avulsed teeth.

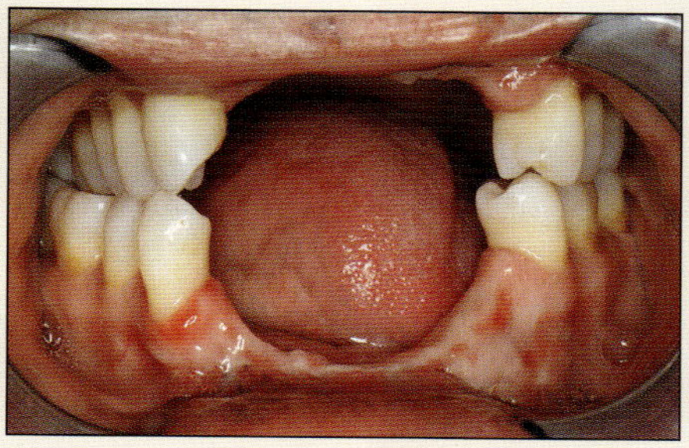

Fig 8-1b Oral examination reveals the avulsion of the mandibular alveolus and seven teeth. Five teeth were lost from the maxilla.

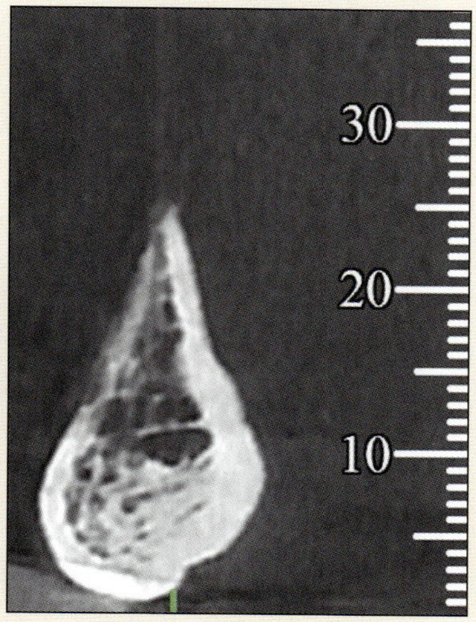

Fig 8-1c A cone beam computed tomogram of the mandibular symphysis shows the thin residual ridge crest.

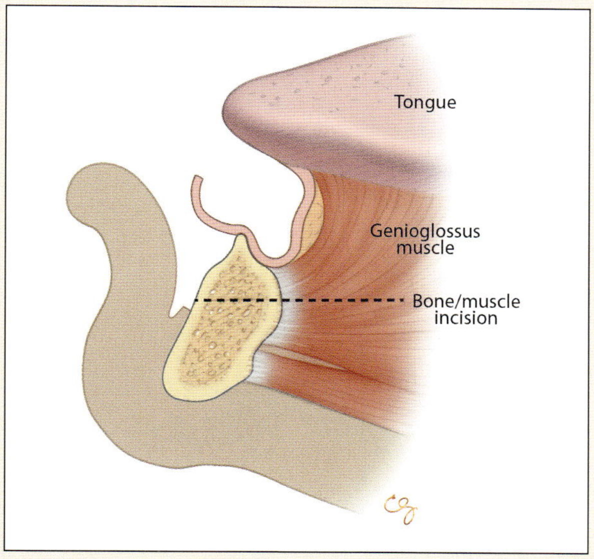

Fig 8-1d The genioglossus muscle inserts on the lingual cortex.

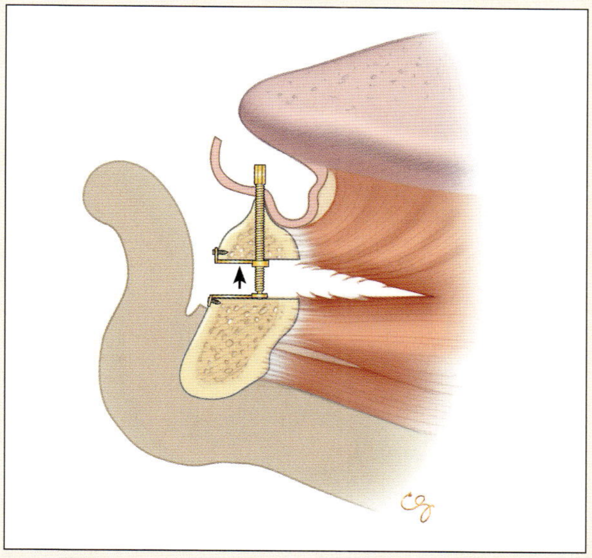

Fig 8-1e Segmental osteotomy allows elevation of the residual ridge into the defect volume. The genioglossus muscle is displaced vertically with the bone segment.

created by the distraction process (Fig 8-1h). As a result of the distraction process, the ridge crest was elevated (Fig 8-1i). The genioglossus muscle and geniohyoid muscle delivered mechanical signaling to their attachment sites on the lingual mandible. These signals were important in the regulation of bone-formation activity in the transport segment and the open distraction chamber.

Discussion

Replacing a large segment of the anterior mandible is challenging because normal bone physiology depends on regulating mechanisms derived from the effect of healthy teeth and their periodontal systems. Sharpey fiber networks extending into the alveolar bone comprise the primary vector to deliver signals that maintain bone morphology in a steady state. Some regulatory input is delivered through penetrating Sharpey fibers from the periosteum. Loss of the teeth, gingiva, and existing alveolar bone pose multiple challenges to establish a bone-forming environment that will meet all of the essential requirements. Recruiting adjacent neuromuscular systems is an important strategy. The genioglossus muscle is important in the maintenance of the mandibular symphysis. This relationship between the muscle and bone is recruited to gain the advantage of a suc-

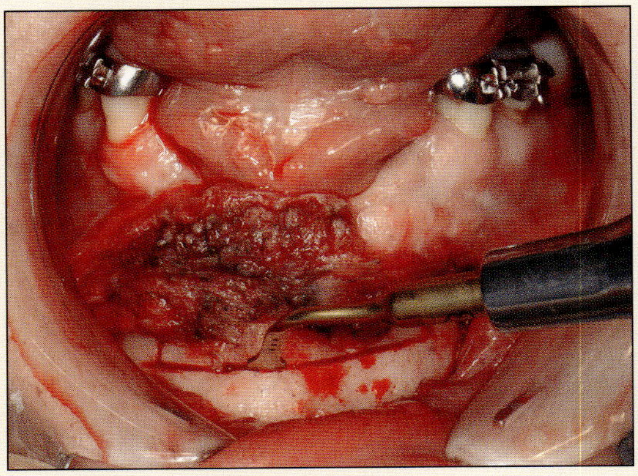

Fig 8-1f Segmental osteotomy is prepared with piezo-electric surgery.

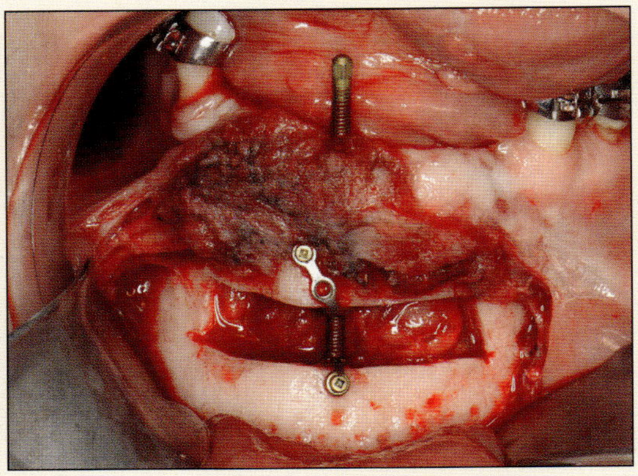

Fig 8-1g The vertical osteotomies converge lingually and diverge apically.

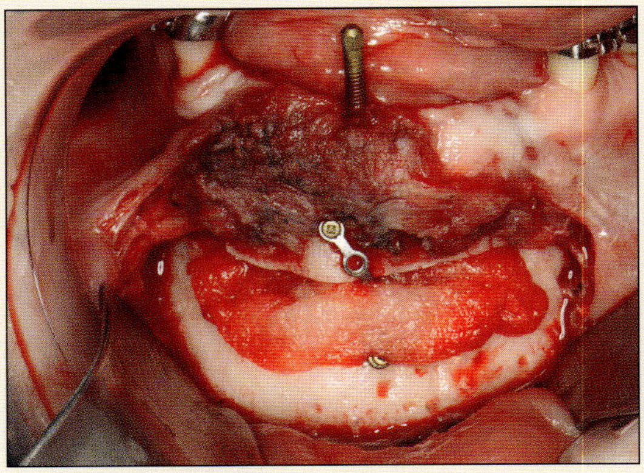

Fig 8-1h Collagen sponges carrying rhBMP-2 fill the osteotomy chamber.

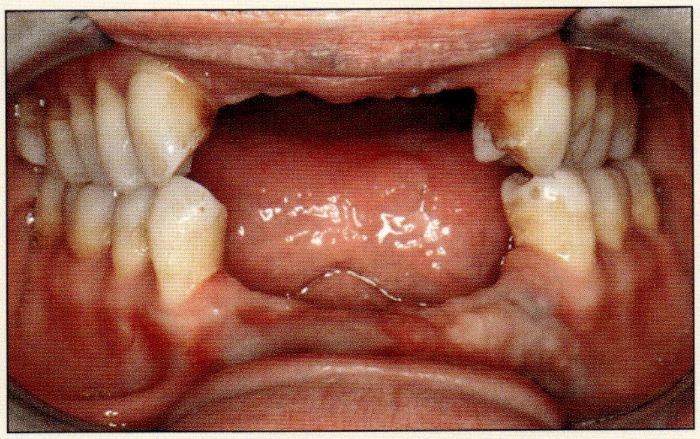

Fig 8-1i Elevation of the ridge crest has provided bone volume for placement of dental implants.

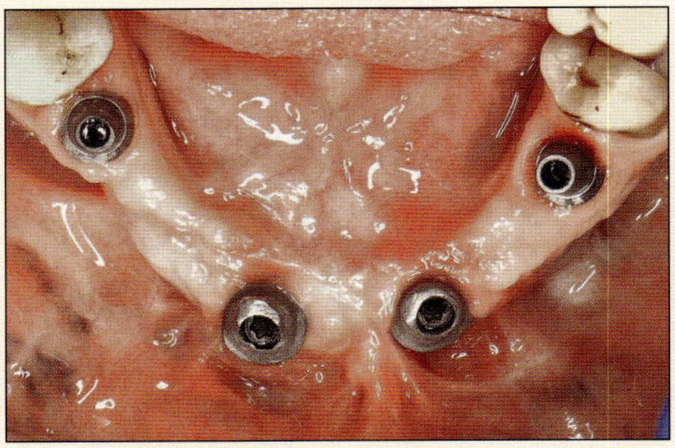

Fig 8-1j Bone developed at the anterior mandible bone-forming construct allows placement of dental implants.

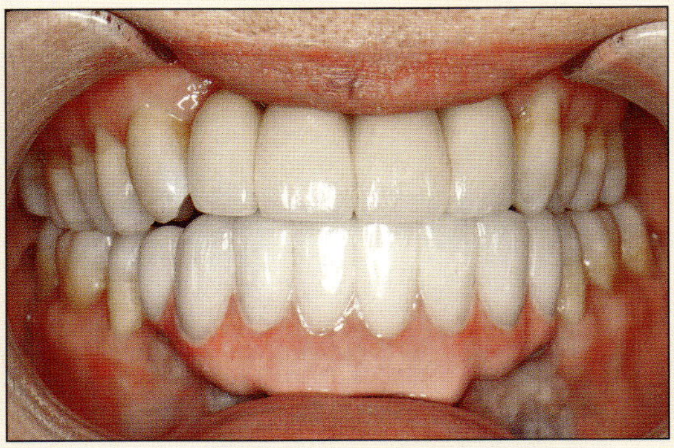

Fig 8-1k A zirconia prosthesis replaces the lost teeth and a portion of the alveolar process.

→

cessful healing response. The transport segment is designed to maintain some genioglossus fibers attached to the lingual cortex. As the transport segment rises, the muscle attachment follows. Maintaining the attachment of the bone segment to the muscle supports the viability of the bone and carries a source of neuromuscular regulation to its destination. Transport of the distraction segment opens a regeneration chamber. Muscle attachment fibers severed from the bone by the osteotomy and adjacent Sharpey fibers displaced as a result of demineralization are available to direct cells in the regeneration to organize into a new bone system. It is also important to recognize the limitation of this type of constructed system. The genioglossus muscle can support the healing of this anatomical replacement but cannot serve as a replacement for the lost teeth and their periodontal systems. The realistic clinical goal is to provide skeletal replacement for the missing structures that can receive dental implants and a dental prosthesis (Figs 8-1j and 8-1k).

In this case, the anterior implants supporting the mandibular prosthesis were anchored in the distracted bone segment. The implants emerged through a gingival graft that covered the

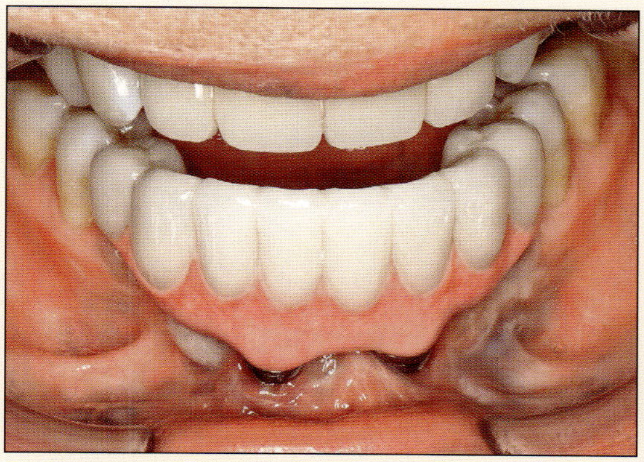

Fig 8-1l The anterior implants emerge through grafted soft tissue.

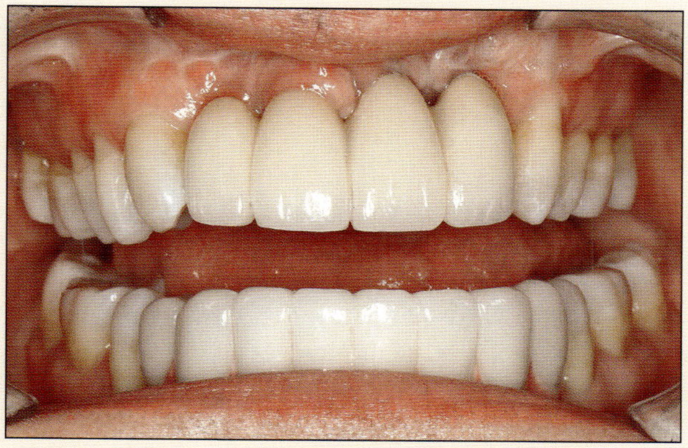

Fig 8-1m Reconstruction of the maxillary defect with a four-piece Le Fort I osteotomy–generated bone volume to place four implants. No onlay bone grafting was done.

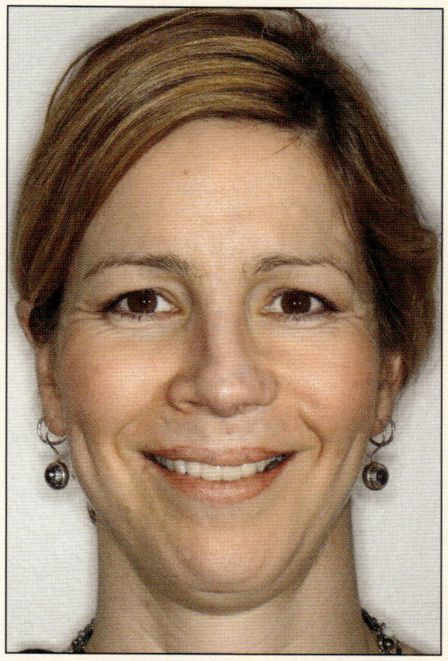

Fig 8-1n A combination of surgery, orthodontics, and prosthodontics has restored esthetics and function.

mentalis muscle attachments (Fig 8-1l). The maxillary defect comprised five lost teeth, including four incisors and the left canine. A segmental Le Fort I maxillary osteotomy repositioned the maxillary left first premolar into the canine position. This decreased the edentulous span to four teeth and transported the periodontal system of the first premolar into the site of the bone construct. Four dental implants were placed to support a fixed prosthesis (Fig 8-1m). A combination of surgery, orthodontics, and prosthodontics restored esthetics and function (Fig 8-1n).

To provide long-term service, dental implants must be placed in a manner so that they are able to gain biologic support from their surroundings. It is not enough to reconstruct the missing bone volume. Neuromuscular regulation is necessary for the new bone to be maintained in a steady state. Bone stability is a prerequisite to stable implant performance. In this case, the premolar implants were positioned in close proximity to the remaining teeth. The periodontal systems of the teeth extended into the adjacent bone and lended regulatory input to the bone that housed the premolar implants. The anterior implants were positioned into the bone that served as the origin of the genioglossus muscle. The muscle attachment provided physiologic stability to the adjacent bone. The portion of the reconstructed segment between the anterior and posterior implants lacked regulatory input from a muscle attachment or teeth. This deficiency would predispose the site to resorption and failure of implants housed within it.

Mylohyoid Muscle in Mandibular Body Reconstruction

Replacement of a lost segment of the mandible is a problem that has challenged maxillofacial surgeons for centuries. Injuries limited to the face were often survivable, even in ancient times. These patients present to the surgeon with disfigurement and functional impairment. If the avulsion defect involves loss of a segment, leaving the remaining mandible with continuity, then reconstruction and rehabilitation can be addressed with a prosthesis or limited bone augmentation. If an avulsion injury results in mandibular discontinuity, lost bone may prevent simple reduction and stabilization.

In the emergency scenario, surgeons may consider replacing the missing mandibular segment with a bone graft. Autogenous bone can be obtained from a variety of locations. Free grafts are commonly obtained from the iliac crest or ribs. Free flaps are generally obtained from the fibula and can be joined to the facial blood vessels with microsurgery.

Although theoretically feasible, logistics and the condition of the patient often prevent use of major reconstructive procedures in the emergency setting. For many reasons, it is often wiser to accept a deformity and focus on stabilizing the patient's physiology first. Delayed reconstruction allows the surgeon to formulate a full scope of treatment options. Each of these approaches can be presented to the patient in a post-trauma setting so that he or she has the opportunity to consider and deliberate over the choices in an environment of relative calm.

This approach is particularly important when use of new technology is considered. Proposing the use of materials and methods that have limited clinical history and that are being applied in an off-label manner carries special responsibility on the part of the surgeon to educate the patient before requesting permission to proceed. This process may involve repeated, prolonged consultation visits prior to surgery. If the patient elects the use of new technology, the surgeon must assemble a team that can address the special range of potential complications related to the use of the techniques. This is particularly challenging given the limited resource of retrospective data addressing issues of efficacy and complications in the off-label environment.

The following case demonstrates the use of rhBMP-2 for reconstruction of mandibular discontinuity defects. Just as important as the surgical technique is the strategy to optimize the morphogenetic protein response and to prepare for potential adverse reactions to the material.

Displacement of the Mylohyoid Muscle for Mandibular Reconstruction

Case description

An 83-year-old woman presented for a fourth surgical opinion for management of a mandibular discontinuity defect and her inability to masticate (Fig 8-2a). One year prior to her presentation, she fell and fractured the right mandible. The emergency repair was done in another center and reportedly involved an open reduction with internal fixation performed through a submandibular external approach. The fracture was reportedly reduced and stabilized with a small bone plate. The bone plate fractured and became infected. A second procedure was then performed to replace the plate, but the fracture did not heal. The second plate was subsequently removed, and the patient was left with a discontinuity defect (Fig 8-2b).

The patient was referred to the local university medical center for evaluation and treatment. She received two treatment recommendations from two different specialty departments. The plastic surgery department recommended reconstruction using a fibula free flap and microvascular anastomosis to available facial or neck vessels. The patient's underlying medical conditions were a concern when such an extensive procedure was considered. The oral and maxillofacial surgery department proposed placement of an autogenous graft from the iliac crest.

The patient was concerned about the potential morbidity involved in iliac crest harvesting. She elected to defer surgical reconstruction and to attempt to accommodate with maxillofacial prosthodontics alone. Dentures were made to function in the presence of the discontinuity.

After 6 months of functioning with the nonunion, the patient presented for a fourth surgical opinion. In addition to the previously proposed treatments, a strategy for reconstruction with rhBMP-2 was presented. The potential risks were explained in detail. The patient elected to proceed with rhBMP-2 treatment.

The treatment team consisted of an oral and maxillofacial surgeon, a prosthodontist, an internist, an anesthesiologist, and an intensive care specialist. The proposed treatment and the potential for unexpected complications that might be encountered when using a novel treatment method were reviewed with each team member. In this case, particular emphasis was placed on the need for heightened vigilance in maintaining the airway given the known increased risk of swelling when rhBMP-2 is used.[2] The patient's age and cardiac status required a plan that would not be likely to overwhelm her diminished reserve.

Experienced users of rhBMP-2 recognize that increased swelling is a consistent response to this material. It is difficult to quantify the amount of additional swelling, but it is clinically apparent. This phenomenon is important to maxillofacial surgeons because of the potential risk of airway embarrassment.[2] The risk of airway obstruction is more concerning in an elderly patient with a limited reserve with which to compensate. When rhBMP-2 devices are placed adjacent to the floor of the mouth, extra attention is required to monitor the postoperative condition. In these cases, patients are monitored in an intensive care unit with one-to-one nursing care.

In a normal, healthy patient, the mandible develops and exists in an environment surrounded by soft tissue. The mylohyoid muscle inserts on the medial aspect of the mandibular body (Fig 8-2c). Muscle insertions deliver important regulatory stimulation to the bone and are important in the maintenance of the bone volume and structure. Teeth deliver similar stimulation to the alveolar portion of the mandible through insertion of periodontal ligament fibers into the lamina dura. The anatomy and mechanics of how the Sharpey fibers of the periodontal ligament transfer forces to the area of insertion are poorly understood.

In this patient, exposure of the mandibular fracture during surgery revealed the discontinuity defect and lack of bone mass on the remaining mandible (Fig 8-2d). The conventional role of the reconstruction plate is to maintain the relative positions of the mandibular fragments. Within the context of the bone-forming construct, the bone plate serves as a method to stabilize the adjacent environment (Fig 8-2e). It participates in the construction of the sheltered environment that will promote bone growth.

Fig 8-2 Displacement of the mylohyoid muscle for mandibular reconstruction.

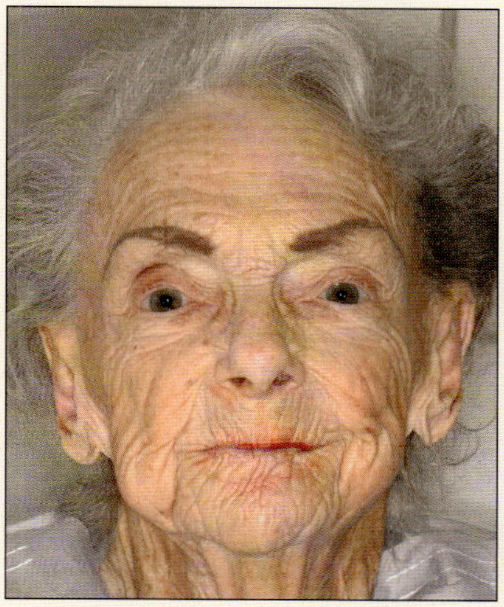

Fig 8-2a An 83-year-old woman presented with an inability to masticate secondary to nonunion of a mandibular fracture. Multiple surgeries had failed to repair the fracture.

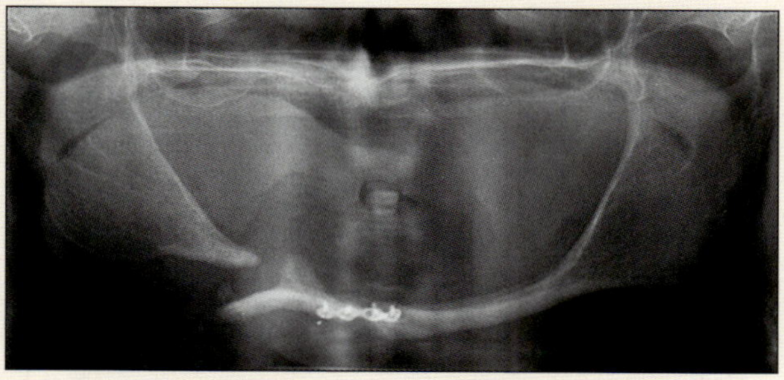

Fig 8-2b The radiograph demonstrates discontinuity of the mandible and displacement of the fragments.

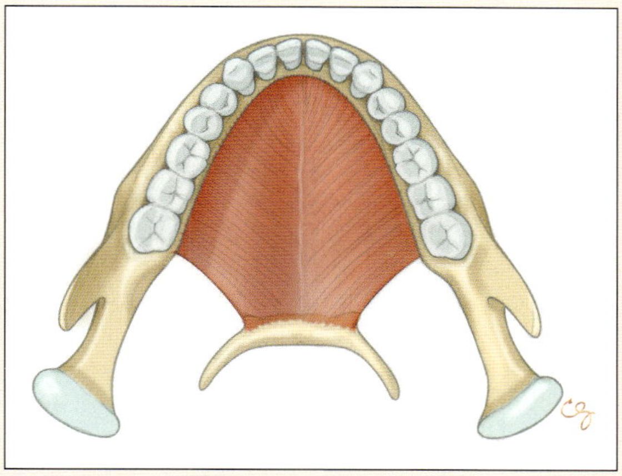

Fig 8-2c Normal functional anatomy of the mandibular body in a dentate patient.

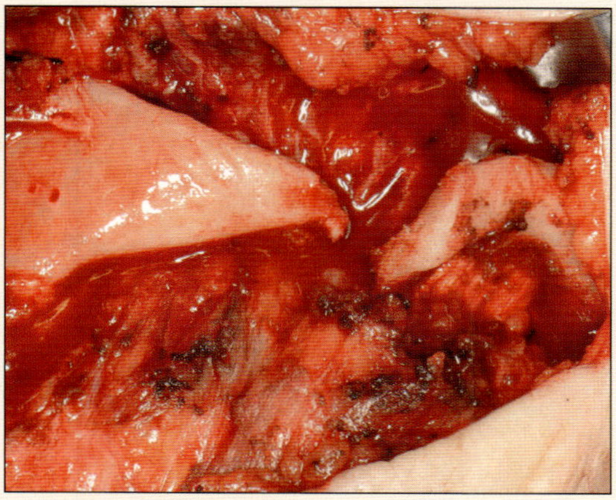

Fig 8-2d Exposure of the mandibular fracture during surgery shows the discontinuity defect and lack of bone mass on the remaining mandible.

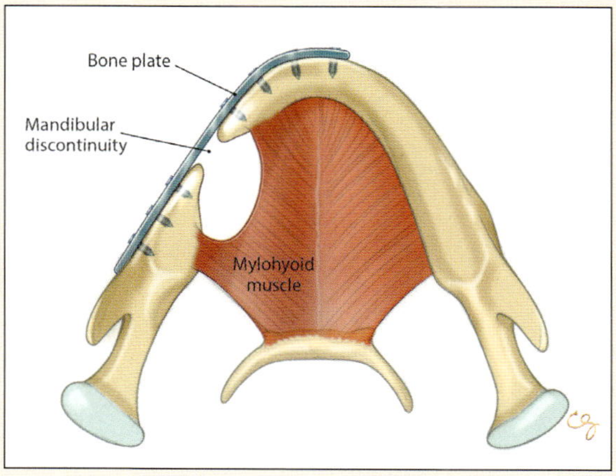

Fig 8-2e After repositioning of the mandible fragments and stabilization with a titanium bone plate, there would not be any native bone at the site of nonunion.

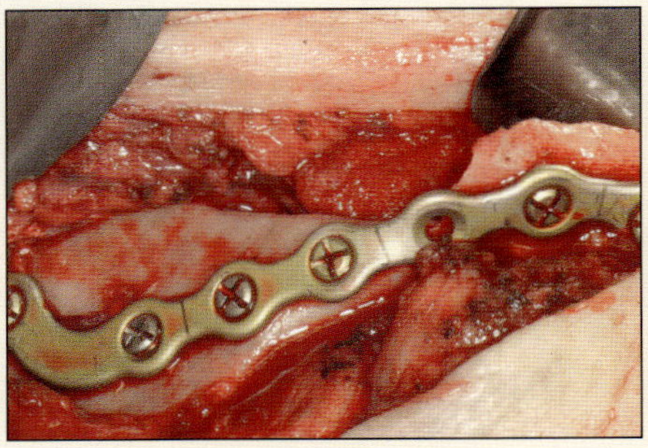

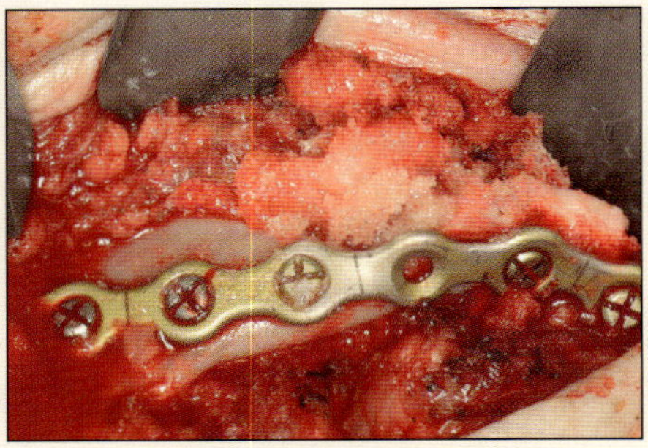

Fig 8-2f *(far left)* The substantial mandibular reconstruction plate is fixed with multiple screws.

Fig 8-2g *(left)* A freeze-dried allogeneic bone graft reconstituted in rhBMP-2 is placed.

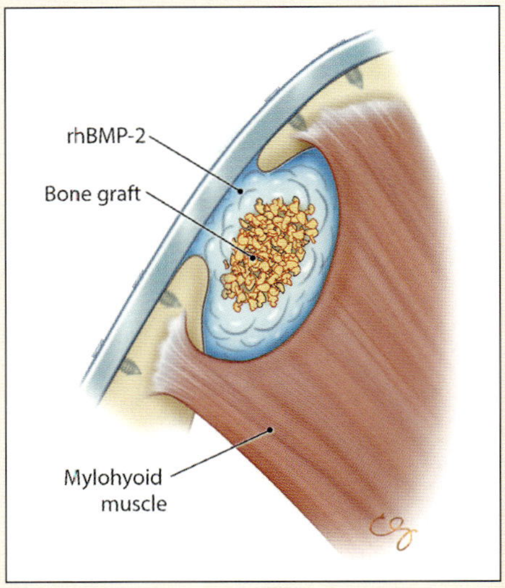

Fig 8-2h In this bone-forming construct, rhBMP-2 collagen sponges surround a volume of freeze-dried banked bone. The mylohyoid muscle is at the medial side of the construct.

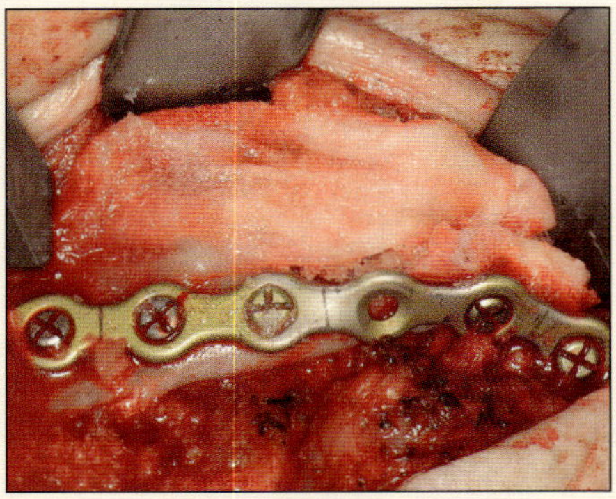

Fig 8-2i Collagen sponges carrying rhBMP-2 surround the volume of cadaveric bone chips.

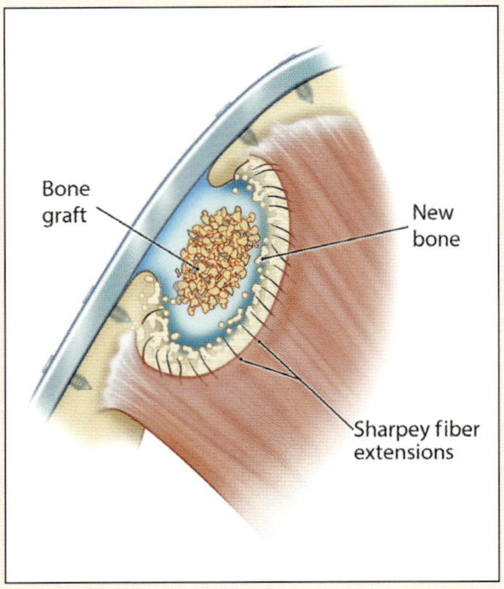

Fig 8-2j Morphogenesis can be expected within the constructed environment.

In the intact mandible, forces travel through the ossicle during normal movement. The pattern of these forces is important in establishing and maintaining the morphology of the mandible. They are also important in the promotion of bone growth and healing at the fracture site. When the reconstruction plate is securely fixed to the mandibular fragments, mechanical continuity is reestablished.

A reconstruction bone plate was formed and affixed to the fragments to establish mechanical continuity (Fig 8-2f). Stabilization of the environment adjacent to the chamber in which the rhBMP-2 device is to function is one of the critical elements of the bone-forming construct. The plate system must be able to maintain relative stability under the substantial stress and flexion of the mandible under function.

Collagen sponges treated with rhBMP-2 were positioned against the medial periosteum. This formed the medial aspect of the regeneration chamber. The sponge-lined chamber was extended to abut the attachments of the genioglossus muscle anteriorly and the mylohyoid muscle medially. Establishment of continuity between the regeneration chamber and the neuromuscular system is an important step in assembling the bone-forming construct.

Crushed cancellous allogeneic bone was soaked in rhBMP-2. The bone was then packed against the medial rhBMP-2 sponges (Fig 8-2g). The purpose of the banked bone graft was to maintain the three-dimensional extension of the regeneration chamber. It was hoped that all of the bone graft would be lost due to resorption. This would leave the maximum potential volume for the remaining chamber to fill with new, living bone.

In the center of the graft site was a mass of allogeneic bone particles. Surrounding the freeze-dried banked bone were collagen sponges containing rhBMP-2 (Figs 8-2h and 8-2i). Lateral to the regeneration chamber was the bone plate. Medial to the regeneration chamber was the mylohyoid muscle. The muscle fibers of the mylohyoid muscle were oriented toward the regeneration chamber.

The details and mechanisms of how the muscle fibers interact with the newly forming bone are poorly understood. Theory suggests that under the direction of the nerves that innervate the muscle, the fibers interact with the tissue and cells of the regeneration chamber to form an attachment. The end result is that bone forms across the discontinuity defect, and the mylohyoid muscle inserts along the medial aspect of the mandible including the newly formed segment.

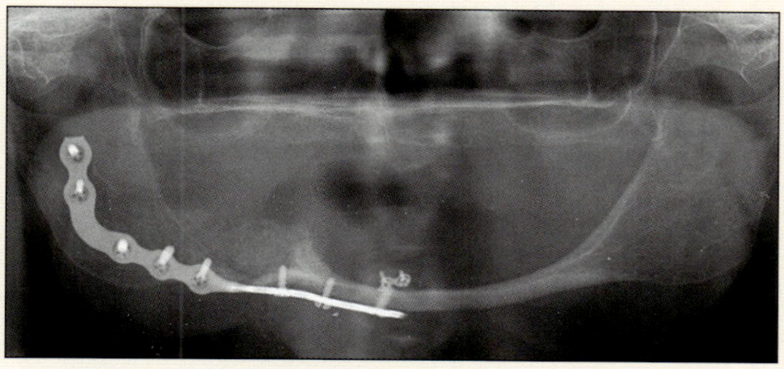

Fig 8-2k A panoramic radiograph taken 2 months after surgery reveals a mass of allogeneic bone.

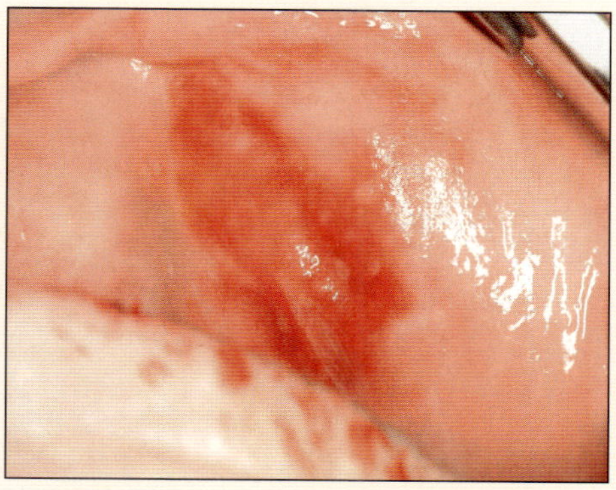

Fig 8-2l Erythema of the oral mucosa overlying rhBMP-2 grafts is a common finding.

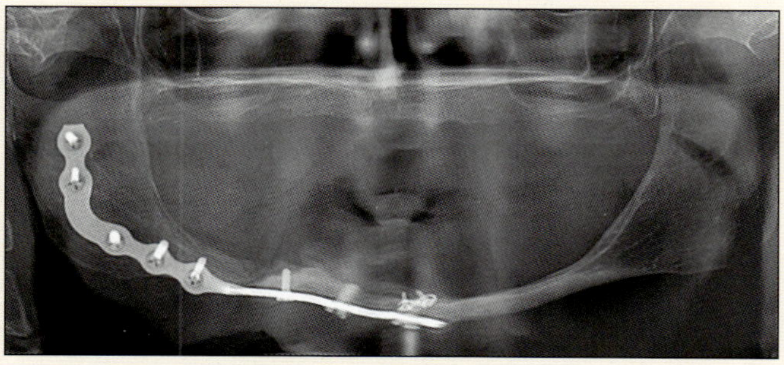

Fig 8-2m Panoramic radiograph taken 6 months after surgery.

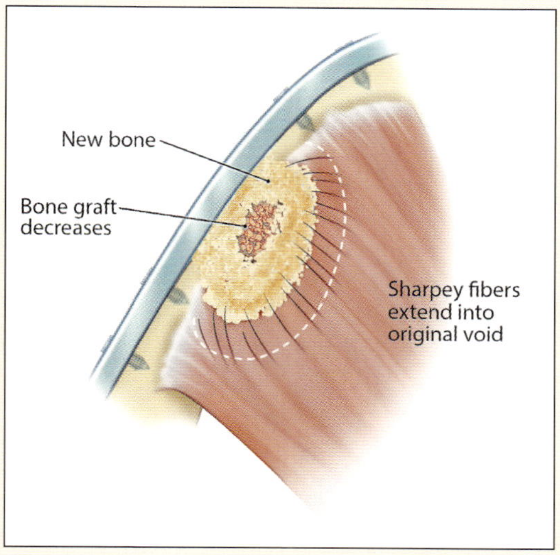

Fig 8-2n Graft consolidation and organization can be expected after 6 months.

→

Collagen sponges with rhBMP-2 were placed to cover the allogeneic graft (see Fig 8-2i). The total dose of rhBMP-2 was 12 mg. The purpose of the lateral sponges was to concentrate bone-forming cells at the periphery of the chamber. As the allogeneic bone resorbed, the chamber would collapse. Bone-forming cells lining the periphery would be carried toward the center of the chamber.

The chamber environment was completed by the introduction of bone-forming cells in large numbers. The rhBMP-2 device collects and concentrates an abundance of bone-forming cells. The regeneration chamber was designed to self-assemble in this manner. The result was an anatomical zone that was mechanically sheltered by the remaining mandible and the reconstruction plate. Continuity of the chamber with the mylohyoid and genioglossus muscles provided the third critical element, neuromuscular stimulation.

Between the laterally positioned bone plate and the free fibers of the mylohyoid muscle was a sheltered region within a soft tissue environment. The rhBMP-2 drew cells with bone-forming potential into the site (Fig 8-2j). The neuromuscular input delivered to the region by the mylohyoid muscle and other adjacent muscle would influence the cells toward bone formation and organization.

Two months after surgery, the allogeneic graft mass assumed a volume that extended well beyond the limits of the mandible's normal morphology (Fig 8-2k). The mucosal tissues had developed erythema, which is a common finding when rhBMP-2 has been used (Fig 8-2l). The mechanism by which this occurs is not completely understood. Inflammation is one possibility, although pain is not generally reported at these locations.

A panoramic radiograph taken 6 months after surgery showed loss of the allogeneic bone mass and incorporation of vital bone into the defect (Fig 8-2m). The volume of the graft mass had decreased. Within the healing site, the nonvital bone graft was being resorbed (Fig 8-2n). The cells that had been recruited by the rhBMP-2 device were forming living bone that was organizing. The neuromuscular input from the inserting mylohyoid muscle was important as a directing and regulating force.

A radiograph taken 17 months after surgery showed incorporation and remodeling of the rhBMP-2–derived bone (Fig 8-2o). Collapse of the chamber continued until the volume of living bone reached a steady state with the anabolic effect of the neuromuscular matrix. If the chamber had not generated living bone, the chamber would have collapsed completely and the discontinuity would have reappeared.

Follow-up evaluation 3 years 8 months after surgery showed that the constructed ossicle was fully integrated into the anatomy and physiology of the site (Fig 8-2p). The morphology of the neo-ossicle was determined by the functional matrix (Fig 8-2q). Its form represented the steady state between resorption and deposition of living bone.

Four years following reconstruction of the mandible with rhBMP-2, the patient developed an oral infection. Examination showed the tip of a screw from the reconstruction plate penetrating the oral mucosa under the denture prosthesis. Two screws were removed through a submandibular incision.

The constructed mandible was found to be in good condition 4 years after repair with rhBMP-2 (Fig 8-2r). Bone had grown over the head of one screw and covered the lingual aspect of the bone plate. The site was directly in the center of the discontinuity defect. The bone overlying the screw head and the plate were removed and subjected to histologic analysis (Fig 8-2s), which revealed that mature vital bone had filled the discontinuity defect. The soft tissue in continuity with the constructed bone volume was also analyzed (Fig 8-2t). Muscle fibers were oriented into the soft tissue attachment to the bone construct.

Discussion

Surgical procedures using bone morphogenetic proteins require adherence to all of the essential elements of bone-forming constructs. In addition to the familiar risks of conventional bone grafting surgery, special attention must be paid to the propensity of the rhBMP-2 collagen sponge system to result in increased swelling in some patients. The location in which the rhBMP-2 device is placed directly relates to the potential risks. Whenever this material is placed adjacent to the floor of the mouth, the potential for airway embarrassment should be considered, and proactive steps should be taken to monitor and manage this problem.

Use of rhBMP-2 is important in achieving the desired result, but it is not the only factor. To obtain predictable results, the surgeon must recognize that rhBMP-2 functions as one part of a complex system. According to the general principles of creating a bone-forming construct, all of the previously discussed essential elements must be in place.

In this patient, a sheltered mechanical environment was established by placement of a substantial reconstruction bone plate. The combination of the titanium plate and the attached remaining fragments of the mandible created a region within investing soft tissue that was sheltered from excessive movement. The miniature plates used in the prior surgeries were unlikely to supply adequate stability. Use of a volume of freeze-dried banked human bone extended the zone that had relative resistance to major movement during mandibular function.

The cell population was enhanced by the placement of rhBMP-2. The banked bone was reconstituted with rhBMP-2 (1.5 mg/mL in water). Collagen sponges carrying rhBMP-2 were positioned against the wound bed before bone grafting material was placed. Additional rhBMP-2–containing sponges covered the volume of bone grafting material before the wound was closed. Bone-forming cells were drawn to the site from the adjacent tissue and the penetrating new vessels.

The neuromuscular input was supplied by the adjacent mylohyoid and genioglossus muscles. The environment also experienced mechanical input from the moving mandible under the control of the muscles of mastication.

Management of pathosis was important. Infection is the primary pathologic risk. External access through a submandibular incision allowed placement of hardware, bone grafting material, and rhBMP-2 without contamination from oral flora. In addition, dissection created a potential space that could be occupied by hardware and grafting materials without compromising the oral mucosa. The surgical design thus addressed all of the essential elements for a bone-forming construct.

The prior, failed reconstruction attempts did not meet the design criteria for a bone-forming construct. Creation and maintenance of a mechanically stable environment is essential to successful bone formation across a mandibular discontinuity defect. Use of small bone plates for fractures with minimal bone contact will not provide the mechanical stability needed. Fracture of the small bone plates also demonstrated that significant forces were delivered to the body of the mandible during normal eating, swallowing, speech, and breathing. These types of forces are important for the maintenance of normal bone physiology. They play a role in the steady state established between resorption and deposition of bone. The same mechanisms direct growth and organization of bone under construction.

Even if the original surgeon had placed a large bone plate, the discontinuity might not have developed a union because of the lack of cells with bone-forming potential. In this case, the atrophy extended well beyond the fracture site itself. To establish a successful union, it was necessary to generate bone both proximally and distally from the fracture site. This required a substantial volume of new bone. Placement of rbBMP-2 allowed delivery of many cells to the site. The application of rhBMP-2 with both collagen sponges and freeze-dried allogeneic bone allowed the introduction of cells while maintaining a potential space for the new tissue to occupy.

Regardless of the volume of graft and rhBMP-2 initially placed, the ossicle will always remodel to occupy the volume dictated by the neuromuscular matrix. Because most patients have symmetric function of the muscles that move the mandible and tongue, the end result of remodeling is an essentially symmetric mandible.

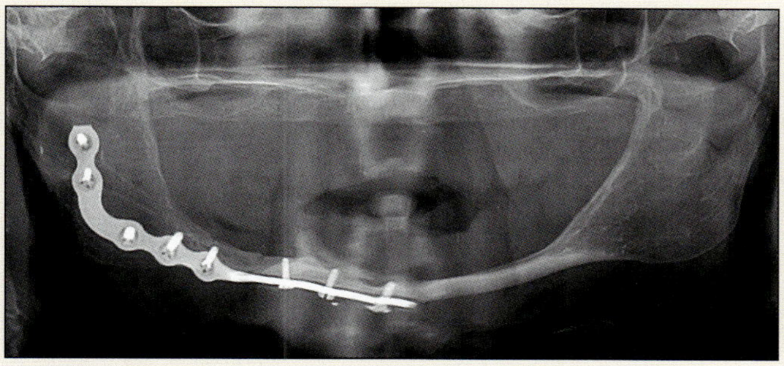

Fig 8-2o Panoramic radiograph taken 17 months after surgery.

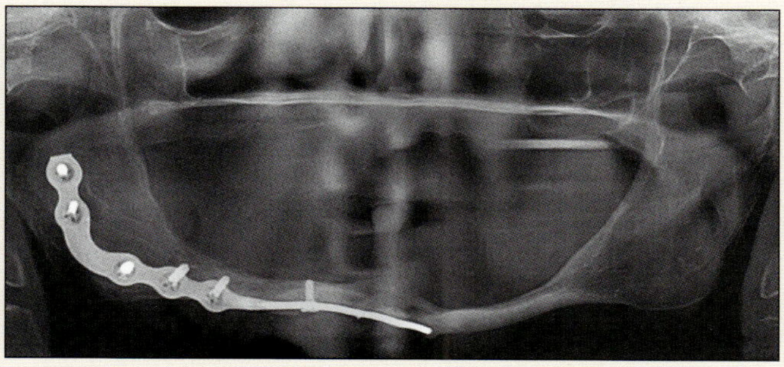

Fig 8-2p Panoramic radiograph taken 3 years 8 months after surgery.

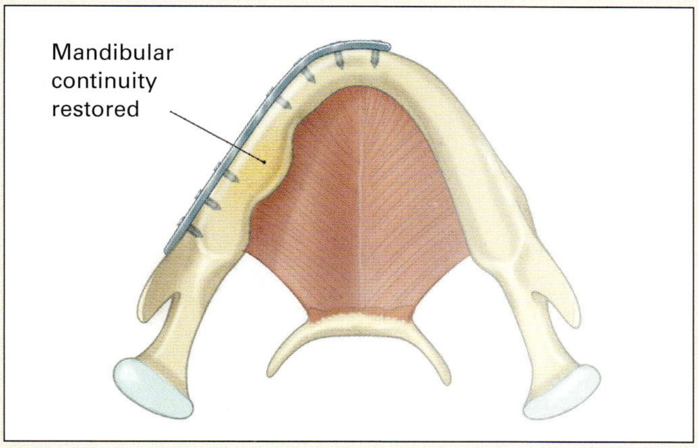

Fig 8-2q By 3 years 8 months after grafting, the newly constructed bone is fully incorporated.

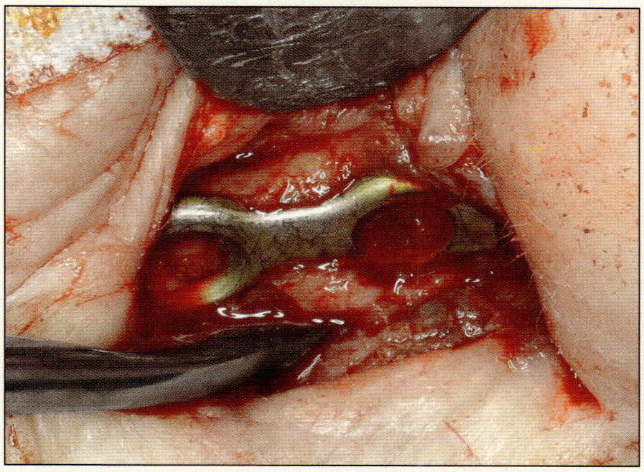

Fig 8-2r Appearance of the constructed mandible 4 years after repair with rhBMP-2.

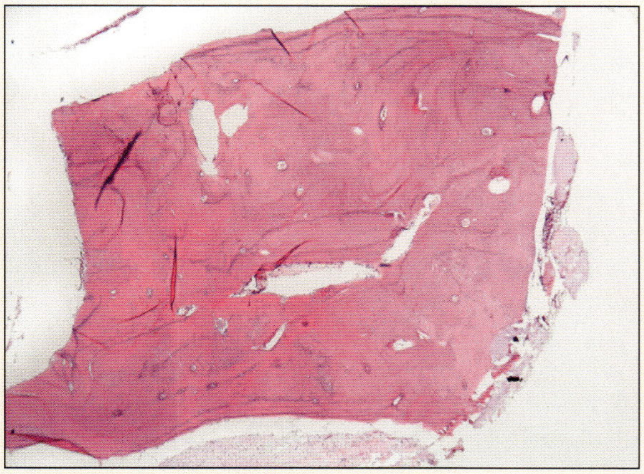

Fig 8-2s Histologic specimen of the bone formed to fill the discontinuity defect 4 years after surgery (hematoxylin and eosin, original magnification ×100).

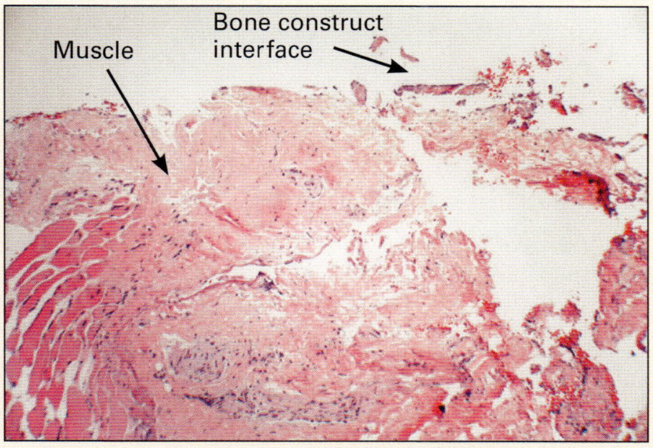

Fig 8-2t Histologic specimen of the soft tissue in continuity with the constructed bone volume. Muscle fibers are oriented to the attachment between the soft tissue and the bone construct (hematoxylin and eosin, original magnification ×40).

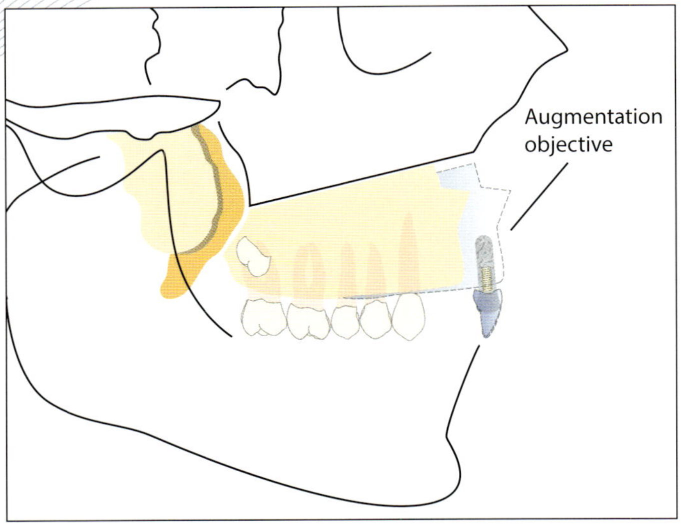

Fig 8-3 Maxillary deformity requires anterior augmentation *(blue shading)*. One option is to fill the volume of the defect with bone from the bone bank or harvest an autogenous graft from the patient. After the bone graft is attached, it must be covered with viable soft tissue. An alternative to grafting is use of the bone-generating potential of the pterygomaxillary junction. This strategy trades the defective healing of the anterior maxilla for the predictable healing site at the pterygomaxillary junction.

Pterygomaxillary Bone-Forming Chambers

The use of maxillary osteotomies to generate bone at the pterygomaxillary junction is particularly useful for the management of a variety of familiar clinical problems. This approach is a versatile tool that can be incorporated in many bone construction designs. An understanding of how this region operates can serve as a prototype for fabrication of bone-forming constructs elsewhere.

Major maxillary anterior deficiencies are common deformities that are difficult to repair (Fig 8-3). They may result from traumatic avulsion, developmental deficiency, or alveolar atrophy following tooth loss. To be successful, the reconstruction must meet the demands of function and esthetics. Staged reconstruction involving onlay bone grafting, soft tissue grafting, implant placement, and dental prosthetics is the common treatment approach. However, the amount of augmentation achievable by these techniques often falls short of the ideal treatment objective. In addition, the questionable long-term stability of bone grafts introduces uncertainty. There is also substantial morbidity associated with the harvesting of large autogenous bone grafts from the iliac crest.

An alternative to augmentation by onlay bone grafting is maxillary osteotomy with protraction (Fig 8-4a). This procedure transports the maxillary fragment into the deficiency to immediately fill the deformity with viable bone, gingiva, and natural teeth. The maxillary unit is a self-contained structure that houses all of the essential elements to grow and maintain bone. It is therefore inherently stable and can maintain itself because it is already integrated into the patient's physiology. Transporting teeth into the deficiency reduces or eliminates the need for implants and dental prosthetics. The presence of natural teeth within the reconstructed segment provides a better restorative solution than implants with fixed or removable prosthetics.

The pterygomaxillary junction joins two primary anatomical units of the head, ie, the cranium and the face. When the surgeon creates a separation between these two important skeletal units, the body launches a vigorous reaction to restore continuity. To be most effective, the separation must be accomplished without damaging the pterygoid plates because these are the muscle origins that deliver neuromuscular signaling to bone precursor cells. Damage to the pterygoid plate displaces the attached muscles and compromises their ability to contribute to neuromuscular input in the bone-forming chamber. It also risks aberrant propagation of the fracture line into the cranial base with possible grave consequences.

Safe maxillary mobilization must avoid damage to the internal maxillary artery and pterygoid venous plexus. Le Fort I maxillary osteotomies and subtotal segmental osteotomies are familiar procedures for maxillofacial surgeons.

The bone-forming chamber is the space between the pterygoid plates and the displaced posterior maxilla (Fig 8-4b). The pterygoid bone-forming chamber is bounded posteriorly by the lateral pterygoid plate, the pterygoid fossa, and the medial pterygoid plate. The anterior wall of the chamber is the posterior maxilla.

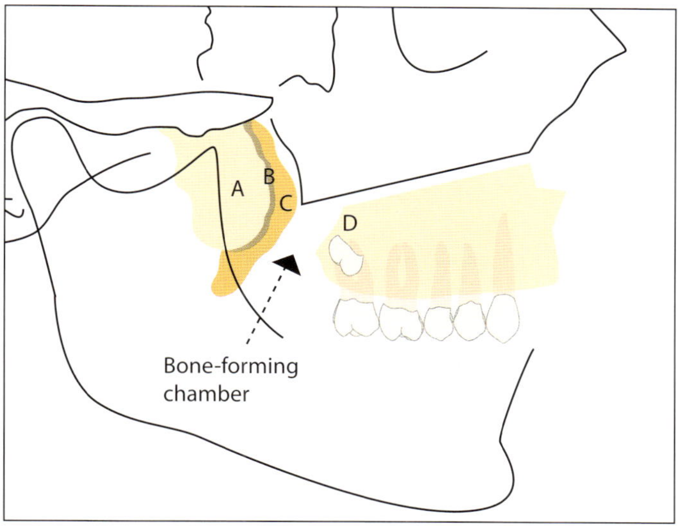

Fig 8-4a Maxillary osteotomy with protraction opens a pterygomaxillary bone-forming chamber. The pterygomaxillary bone-forming chamber is bounded posteriorly by the lateral pterygoid plate (A), the pterygoid fossa (B), and the medial pterygoid plate (C). The anterior wall of the chamber is the posterior maxilla (D).

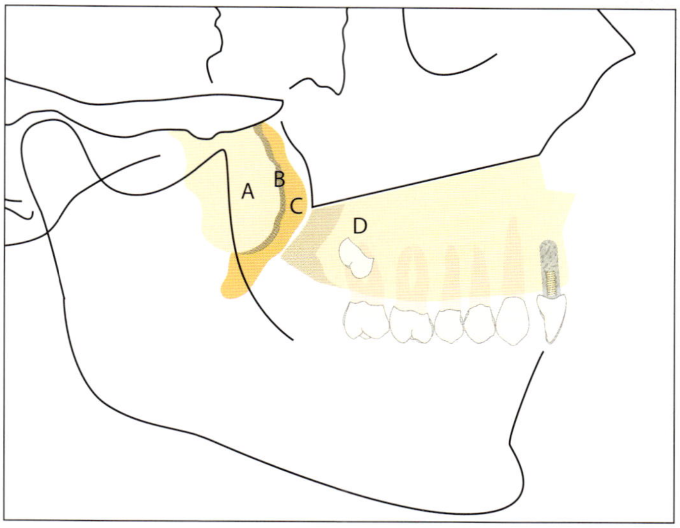

Fig 8-4b The stable, existing portion of the maxilla is transported to fill the anterior defect. No graft consolidation is necessary. The defect between the pterygoid plates and the posterior maxilla created by protraction of the Le Fort I osteotomy heals predictably and without grafting.

Technique for construction of the pterygomaxillary bone-forming chamber

Surgical construction of a bone-forming chamber at the pterygomaxillary junction requires instrumentation at an anatomical site with limited access. Care must be taken to avoid aberrant fractures during the disjunction of the maxilla from the pterygoid plates. The best bone-forming result will be realized when an intact maxilla is separated from undamaged pterygoid plates. Displacement of fractured pterygoid plates displaces the attached muscles and compromises the transfer of neuromuscular signaling to the bone-forming chamber.

Most fractures of the pterygoid plates occur when pterygoid osteotomes are used. These instruments tend to direct force in a superior and posterior vector, resulting in undesirable displacement of the pterygoid plates. In addition to disrupting the origins of the lateral and medial pterygoid muscles, pterygoid plate fractures can extend to the cranial base, resulting in bleeding, optic nerve damage, or intracranial penetration.[3–5]

Following is a clinical example of proper instrumentation to create a pterygomaxillary bone-forming chamber. To prepare the maxilla for disjunction from the pterygoid plates, an osteotomy is created through the lateral maxilla. The osteotomy line descends in the posterior maxilla to the most inferior position possible. Osteotomes are not used to separate the fusion of the maxillary tuberosity and the pterygoid plates. The medial wall of the maxillary sinus and the lateral wall of the nasal cavity are divided with curved osteotomes placed through the maxillary lateral saw cut. The nasal septum is luxated from the maxillary crest with nasal septal osteotomes.

The purchase bars of the midface-mobilizing instrument are positioned to engage the osseous nasal floor. The mobilizing instrument engages the occlusal surfaces of the teeth with an acrylic resin splint that is rigidly mounted to the device (Fig 8-5a). As the screws are tightened, the instrument establishes rigid purchase on the maxilla via this clamping mechanism (Fig 8-5b). Because each bar is independent, their engagement can be positive and stable. As an alternative, Rowe disimpaction forceps may be used to mobilize the maxilla. The objective is to protract the maxilla, creating the pterygomaxillary disjunction without the need to place instruments directly in the site of separation.

After the midface-mobilizing device is mounted for Le Fort I–level pterygomaxillary disjunction (Fig 8-5c), it is activated. The force to luxate the fusion of the posterior maxilla to the pterygoid plates is concentrated by applying pressure on the instrument lever and counterpressure on the forehead (Fig 8-5d). The result of activation is downfracture of the maxilla and luxation of the maxilla from the pterygoid plates (Fig 8-5e). With rigid purchase on the maxilla, the instrument can be used to mobilize and protract the maxillary fragment.

If the posterior extent of the Le Fort I saw cut is placed in the inferiormost position, the fracture propagates through the posterior sinus wall in an inferior orientation (Fig 8-5f).

With expansion pliers deflecting the posterior maxilla inferiorly, the pterygoid plates are shown to be intact and undamaged by the mobilization process (Fig 8-5g). The separation surface shows cancellous bone that will be the source of cells in the bone-forming chamber. Maintenance of intact pterygoid plates preserves the integrity of the muscle attachments and their potential to deliver neuromuscular signaling to the bone-forming chamber. Avoiding fracture of the pterygoid plates reduces the risks of bleeding and damage to the structures of the cranial base and brain.

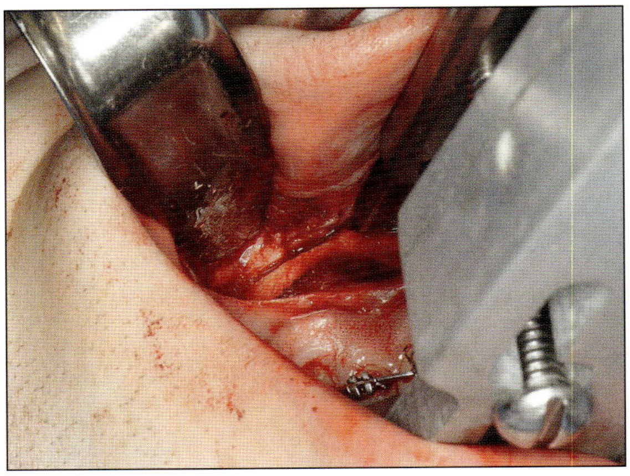

Fig 8-5a The Le Fort I osteotomy has been performed, and the midface mobilizer is placed.

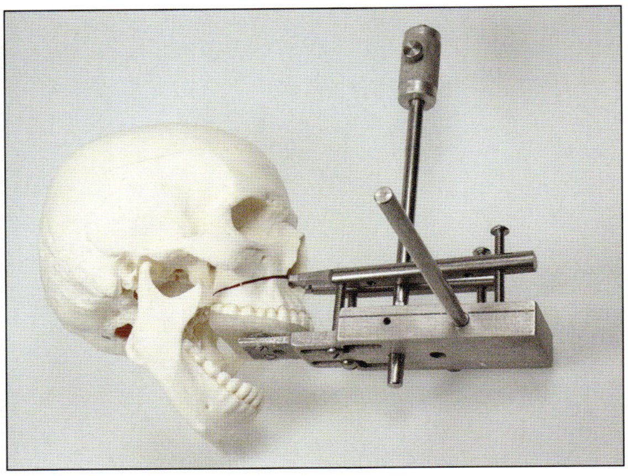

Fig 8-5b The midface-mobilizing instrument is mounted on a Le Fort I osteotomy model.

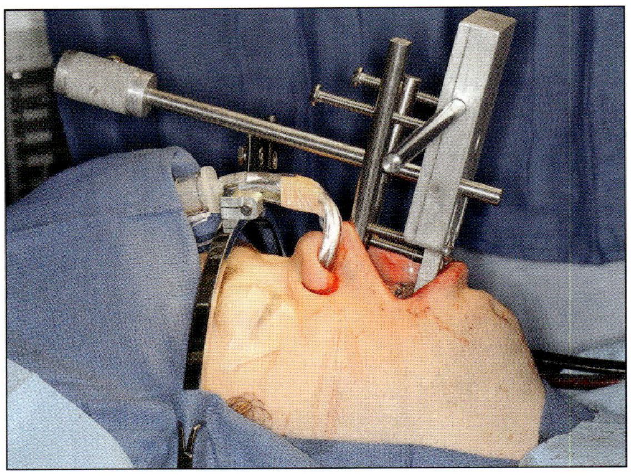

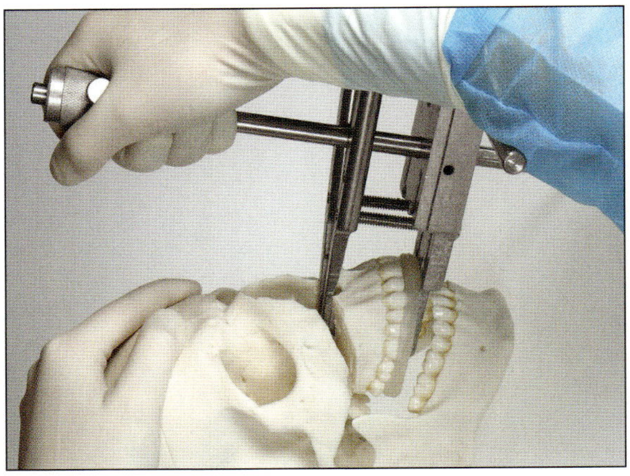

Fig 8-5c *(above left)* The midface-mobilizing device is mounted for a Le Fort I–level pterygomaxillary disjunction.

Fig 8-5d *(above right)* The mobilizing device is activated to separate the pterygomaxillary junction. Counterpressure is applied with a hand on the forehead. The right hand rotates the maxilla inferiorly. The right forearm applies force to the lateral lever from above to protract the left side of the maxilla and from below to protract the right side of the maxilla.

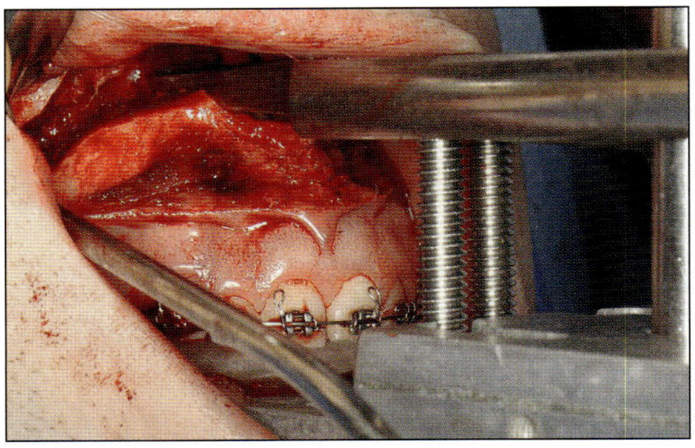

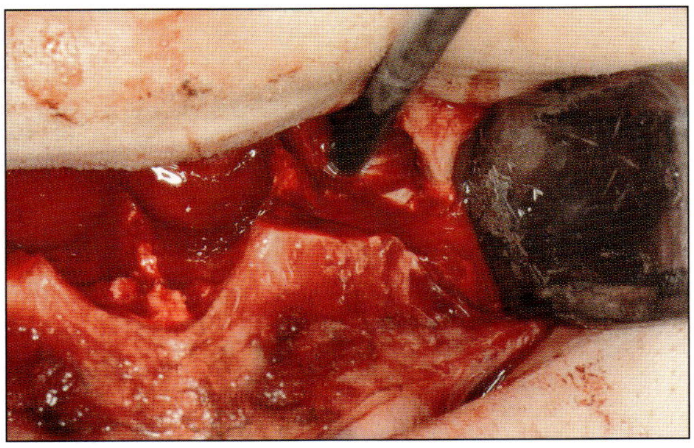

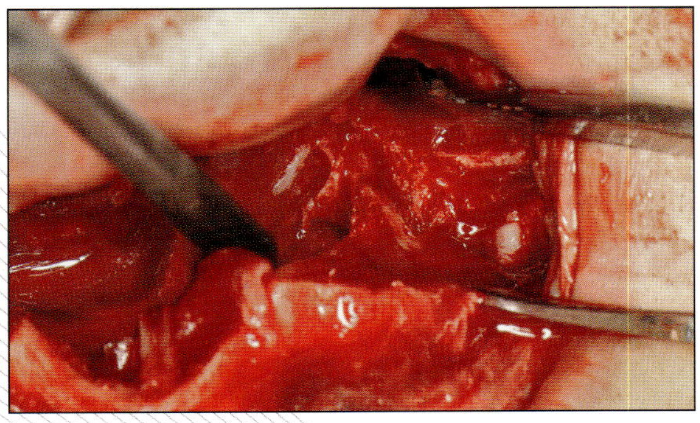

Fig 8-5e *(above left)* With the application of focused and controlled luxation force with the mobilizing instrument, the maxilla is separated from the pterygoid plates. The process minimizes the risk of fracturing one or both of the pterygoid plates.

Fig 8-5f *(above right)* The fracture is propagated through the posterior wall of the maxillary sinus.

Fig 8-5g *(left)* Expansion pliers displace the mobilized maxilla inferiorly, revealing the stable and undamaged pterygoid plate.

The underlying bone-forming potential of the pterygomaxillary system is derived from the divergence of multiple important muscles from this location (Fig 8-6). These muscles originate from the skull base and radiate to their insertions in the facial skeleton. Each muscle and nerve pair connects the cranium to a functional facial structure. The lateral pterygoid muscle, which arises from the lateral side of the lateral pterygoid plate, protracts and balances condylar movements. The medial pterygoid muscle is a principle elevator of the mandible and arises from the medial side of the lateral pterygoid plate. The superior constrictor muscle arises from the medial aspect of the medial pterygoid plate and facilitates swallowing. The tensor veli palatini uses the pterygoid hamulus to change the direction of its fibers into a horizontal vector and functions during speech.

All of these muscles act during breathing. These neuromuscular systems operate, at some level, 24 hours per day and are essential to life. Part of the function of these systems is to maintain and regulate their own morphology. To exist in a steady state, there must be a balance between the anabolic and catabolic processes of bone remodeling. The muscle system is the vector through which the brain delivers regulatory signals to control this process. These mechanisms are the result of millions of years of evolution. Recruiting these processes into surgical designs can greatly improve the patient's response to surgery.

The bone-forming capacity at this site is derived from the high-intensity neuromuscular input from the muscle attaching to the pterygoid plates (Fig 8-7a). In addition, the anterior wall of the chamber houses the maxillary teeth and alveolar process. The teeth are also important sources of bone-forming signals. Bone will fill this chamber and reestablish a union with the advanced maxilla without the benefit of grafting, morphogenetic agents, or slow distraction (Fig 8-7b). The potential of this region to generate bone can bridge very large distances. Protraction of the midface to distances of more than 25 mm over 72 hours will still heal without grafting. Although many implant surgeons are unfamiliar with the use of maxillary osteotomies, the method should be considered when the clinical problem requires it.

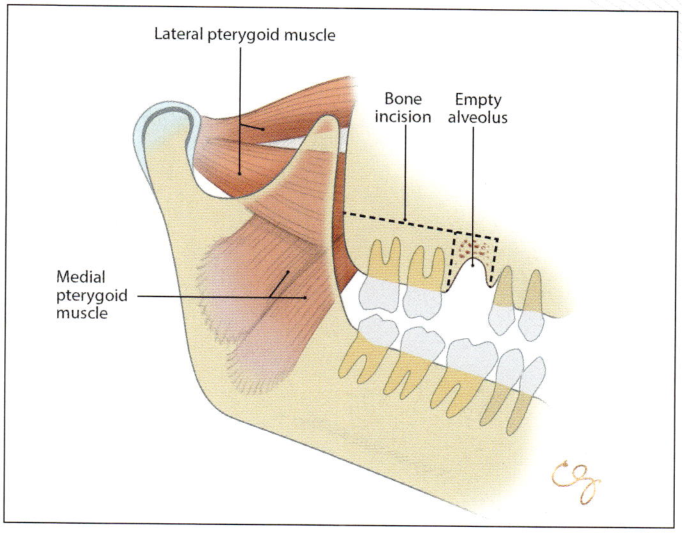

Fig 8-6 Muscle origins from the pterygoid plates.

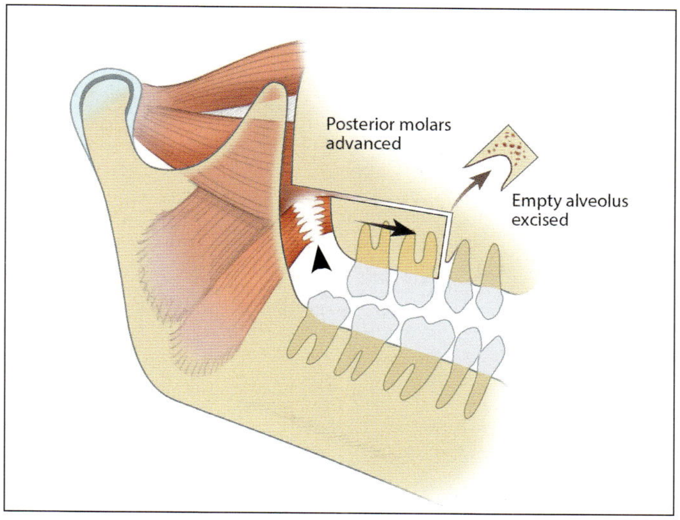

Fig 8-7a Cellular activity within the pterygomaxillary bone-forming chamber *(arrowhead)*.

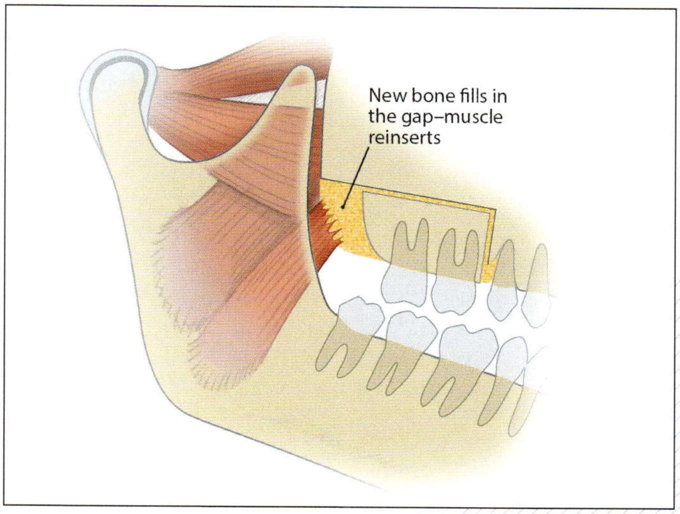

Fig 8-7b Bone fills and organizes in the pterygomaxillary bone-forming chamber.

Fig 8-8 Creation of a pterygomaxillary bone-forming chamber for management of extreme midfacial hypoplasia.

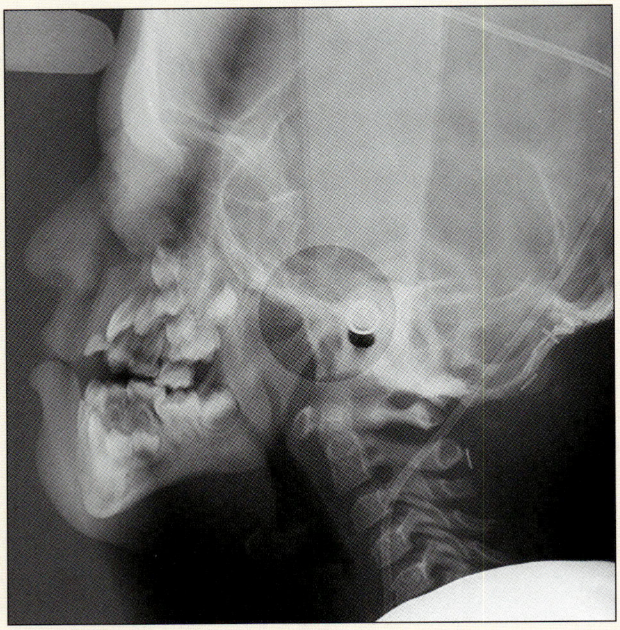

Fig 8-8a The extreme hypoplasia of the midface is related to Crouzon syndrome.

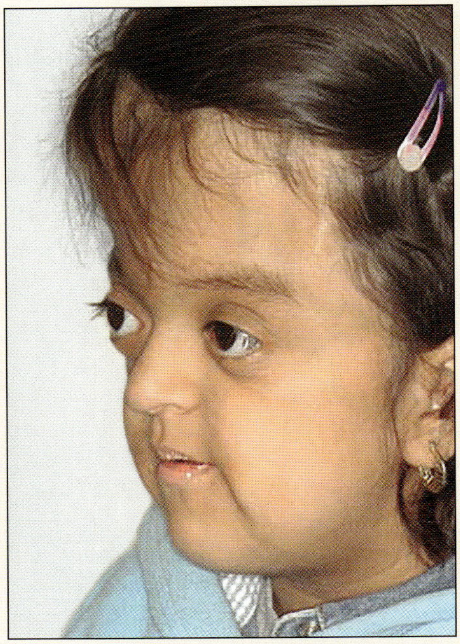

Fig 8-8b Preoperative midfacial retrusion.

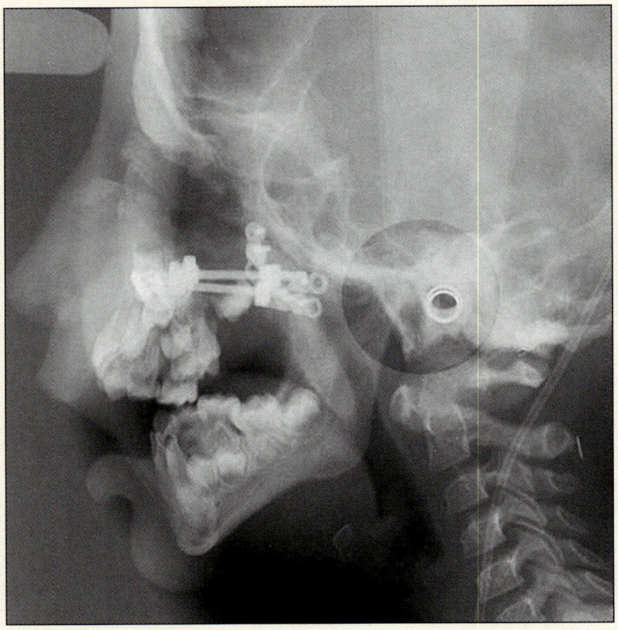

Fig 8-8c The midface-mobilizing instrument has been used to mobilize the maxilla at the Le Fort III level along with the zygoma, inferior orbits, and nose. Internal distraction devices[6] have been used to transport the midface anteriorly, opening a 20-mm pterygomaxillary bone-forming chamber. The anterior fragment contains developing teeth that supply neuromuscular signaling to the bone-forming chamber. The pterygoid muscles attached to the intact pterygoid plates supply neuromuscular signaling from the posterior aspect of the chamber. No bone grafting is necessary.

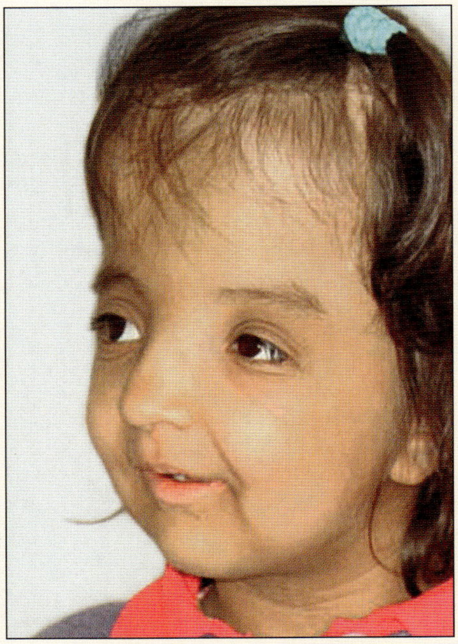

Fig 8-8d The results are satisfactory 14 days after osteotomy and midfacial protraction.

Creation of a Pterygomaxillary Bone-Forming Chamber for Management of Extreme Midfacial Hypoplasia

The purpose of this case presentation is to demonstrate the capacity of pterygomaxillary bone-forming chambers to form bone in large volumes. Craniofacial disorders provide the best demonstration of the bone-forming potential of this anatomical location. Skeletal deficiencies resulting from these developmental disorders may require construction of 20 to 30 mm of bone. Implant surgeons rarely need such a large quantity of bone, but having the potential to deliver structural skeletal units in a predictable manner is valuable. When properly designed, this technique can deliver the quantity of bone needed to complete a reconstruction for most maxillary defects. Regardless of the specific indication and need for bone replacement, the strategy for using the muscle attachment system at the pterygomaxillary junction is the same.

Case description

Extreme hypoplasia of the midface of a 5-year-old girl was related to Crouzon syndrome (Figs 8-8a and 8-8b). The midface-mobilizing instrument was used to mobilize the maxilla at the Le Fort III level along with the zygoma, inferior orbits, and nose. Internal distraction devices[6] were used to transport the midface anteriorly, opening a pterygomaxillary bone-forming chamber of 20 mm (Fig 8-8c). The postsurgery radiograph shows the gap between the pterygoid plates and the posterior maxilla. The anterior fragment contained developing teeth that would supply neuromuscular signaling to the bone-forming chamber. The pterygoid muscles attached to the intact pterygoid plates would supply neuromuscular signaling from the posterior aspect of the chamber. This regeneration chamber would fill with viable bone without the need for grafting. The result is to reestablish a union between the cranial base and the midface. This process advances the maxilla into the deficient facial volume. Fourteen days after surgery, the child's face showed improved convexity from the osteotomy advancement (Fig 8-8d). The maxillary fragment contains a volume of bone, soft tissue, teeth, and their associated periodontal ligament systems. The transported maxilla contains all of the essential components of a bone-forming environment. It is therefore inherently stable and can maintain a steady state long term. For implant surgeons, a transported maxilla housing healthy teeth and their periodontal systems can serve as a supportive environment for osseointegration procedures.

Conclusion

Thoughtful design of surgeries that use bone-forming constructs based on the underlying skeletal physiology can improve healing potential and extend the scope of possible treatment. The cases presented in this chapter required bone formation at sites that do not accept typical onlay bone grafting. Challenges to successful healing may be due to the large volume of bone required, compromised healing potential of the host, or mechanical stress at the repair site. Successful reconstruction requires altering the functional dynamics of the reconstruction site. Controlling the mechanical forces within the bone-forming environment becomes part of the surgical design. Focusing an adequate intensity of neuromuscular signaling into the site requiring bone organization is another essential parameter for the regeneration site. Deliberate design of these parameters into the surgical plan is most important in cases challenged by large volume deficiencies or high-intensity mechanical stress. Using bone-forming constructs that include the major muscles of the facial skeleton are important tools to realize successful outcomes when repairing large defects.

References

1. Harvold EP. The theoretical basis for the treatment of hemifacial microsomia. In: Harvold EP, Vargervik K, Chierici G (eds). Treatment of Hemifacial Microsomia. New York: Alan R. Liss, 1983.
2. US Department of Health and Human Services. FDA Public Health Notification: Life-threatening Complications Associated with Recombinant Human Bone Morphogenetic Protein in Cervical Spine Fusion. Issued 1 July 2008. http://www.fda.gov/MedicalDevices/Safety/AlertsandNotices/PublicHealthNotifications/ucm062000.htm. Accessed 21 October 2014.
3. Cruz AA, dos Santos AC. Blindness after Le Fort I osteotomy: A possible complication associated with pterygomaxillary separation. J Craniomaxillofac Surg 2006;34:210–216.
4. Girotto JA, Davidson J, Wheatly M, et al. Blindness as a complication of Le Fort osteotomies: Role of atypical fracture patterns and distortion of the optic canal. Plast Reconstr Surg 1998;102:1409–1421.
5. Matsumoto K, Nakanishi H, Seike T, Koizumi Y, Hirabayashi S. Intracranial hemorrhage resulting from skull base fracture as a complication of Le Fort III osteotomy. J Craniofac Surg 2003;14:545–548.
6. Chin M, Toth BA. Le Fort III advancement with gradual distraction using internal devices. Plast Reconstr Surg 1997;100:819–830.

9 Controlling the Accuracy of Osteotomy Fragment Repositioning

The role of osteotomies in the management of missing teeth has been discussed in chapters 6, 7, and 8. In some cases, osteotomies are used to establish a volume of bone to place dental implants. In other cases, osteotomies reconfigure the dental arch so that dental implants are not necessary. Osteotomy procedures are capable of moving jaw segments and whole jaws into different positions.

Osteotomies offer the opportunity for dentoskeletal improvement but also involve risk. Surgical repositioning of jaws, teeth, and implants must be accomplished in a predictable and safe manner, because function and esthetics are compromised when the result deviates from the objective. Thus, predictable repositioning of mobilized osteotomy segments is a prerequisite for successful treatment. The objective of this chapter is to examine the factors that govern the accuracy of surgeries involving osteotomies. Having a method that will deliver predictable accuracy of osteotomy fragment repositioning is critical to provide confidence to patients and their surgeons.

Potential Sources of Error in Fragment Repositioning

Modern orthognathic surgery has extended beyond correction of malocclusions and has become an essential tool in reconstructive and regenerative procedures. Osteotomies are essential in the design and fabrication of bone-forming constructs. The combination of osteotomies with tissue engineering technology has broadened the indications for these procedures.

As the complexity of the treatment plans increases, so does the demand for design accuracy in the planning and surgical processes. In the past, errors in osteotomy fragment repositioning were accepted or could be modified with postoperative orthodontic treatment. Today's patients expect higher degrees of predictability even though the procedures have inherent limitations. In addition, patients who undergo osteotomies with implants already in place do not have the option of postoperative orthodontic movement of the prosthesis. This increases the burden on the surgeon to reposition the osteotomy fragment with high precision.

Error is the net discrepancy between the desired objective and that achieved by surgery. *Navigation* is the process by which the surgeon positions the mobilized osteotomy fragments, places fixation devices, and verifies that the result is correct. *Tolerance* is the range of variation that can be expected, given the specific navigation technique used. In the case of orthognathic surgery, multiple aspects of the planning and surgical process can introduce errors and contribute to the tolerance. It is best to examine each of the major factors separately.

Errors can be introduced at any stage of the diagnostic, planning, and surgical process. It is important to know what kinds of errors can be introduced at each step of the treatment sequence. Factors that will lead to fragment repositioning errors must be managed in the design and surgical phases if acceptable accuracy is to be achieved. The method used to plan and execute osteotomies must maintain tolerance at a level that will produce an acceptable outcome. It is critical that the clinician appreciate the limitations of the specific system selected for navigation.

Despite application of a variety of surgical navigation techniques, errors occur during surgical repositioning of mobilized fragments. Most studies claim that variations of 2 to 3 mm in three dimensions can be expected. The source of the discrepancies, however, has never been clear.

Although a standard error of 2 to 3 mm may be within a clinically acceptable range, some outcomes deviate further from the desired result and become new clinical problems. Significant deviation from expected symmetry is the most common source of major patient dissatisfaction. Patients' focus on esthetics, particularly symmetry, often exceeds their concerns about occlusion or even paresthesia. The magnitude of the error typically emerges when the inherent postoperative edema resolves, revealing a result that is unexpected. Complaints about these problems have become more common as patients elevate their expectations. Computer-generated visual projections show ideal depictions of the dentition, skeleton, and soft tissue contours. Even with written disclaimers, patients expect the surgeon to deliver on the projection that was presented.

It is useful to explore the factors that contribute to repositioning problems. The sources of error are complex, multifactorial, and sometimes counterintuitive. Some factors are inherent to the surgical process itself. Other factors are technical and can be improved by modifying the laboratory and surgical technique. This chapter presents planning and surgical techniques that will reduce the risk of error. Before a plan to correct this problem can be created, however, it is important to understand how the error might have occurred.

Sources of error during the design phase

The most common method for studying and planning surgery involving osteotomy fragment repositioning is the use of articulated dental casts. Casts are used to fabricate occlusal splints that guide the repositioning of osteotomy fragments. These devices are important in the surgical process, but underestimation of their limitations can lead to unexpected outcomes. The use of virtual planning is another option that is discussed in chapter 10.

The important sources and means of preventing planning errors are common to both mechanical and virtual planning techniques. It is important to understand the limitations of each planning process. If the errors introduced during cast surgery are not recognized and managed, they are passed on to the surgical planning stage.

Lack of stable landmarks

Conventional surgical planning is done with plaster casts. A facebow is used to mount the casts on the articulator (Fig 9-1). The condylar position relative to the dental arches is approximated by this technique. The relationship between the dental arch and facial soft tissue, however, is lost.

An occlusal registration is obtained with wax or polyvinyl siloxane paste. The intention is to capture the maxillomandibular relationships in centric relation and to use the registration to mount the mandibular cast (Fig 9-2). The belief is that this retruded jaw position can serve as a reference point during cast surgery and then during surgical repositioning of the osteotomy fragments.

The casts are mounted, and index lines are placed. The plaster casts are separated or cut to simulate surgical osteotomies. The fragments are repositioned to meet the treatment objectives of occlusion and esthetics (Fig 9-3). In this example, the occlusal plane cant has been modified by differential impaction of the maxilla. The projection is that altering the occlusal plane in this manner will result in the movement of the chin to the left.

The most critical esthetic structures from a clinical standpoint are the maxillary central incisors. This type of simulation has very limited control of how the central incisors will appear in the final clinical result. This limitation exists because the maxillary incisors lack a point of reference from which movements can be measured. This lack of a stable reference point is a limitation of both the cast surgery setting and the surgical environment.

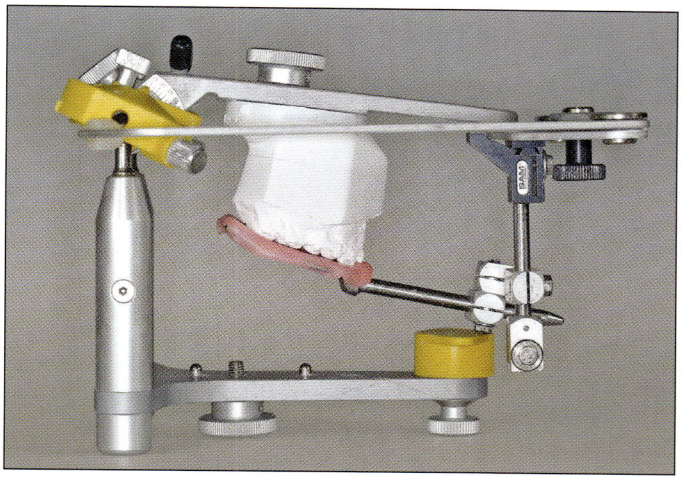

Fig 9-1 Conventional surgical planning begins with facebow-mounted casts on an articulator.

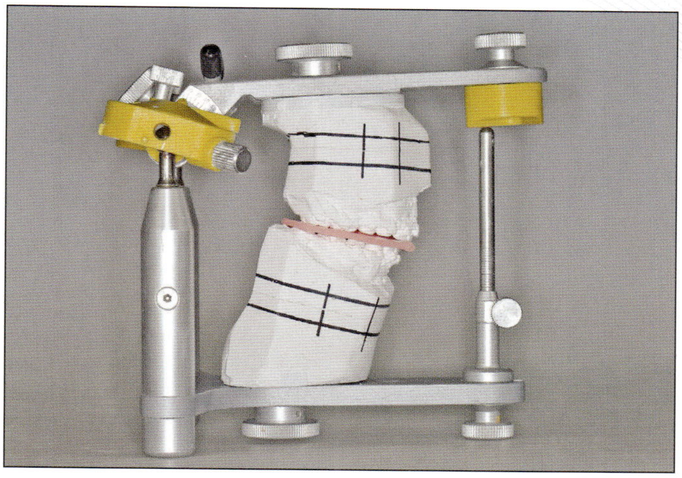

Fig 9-2 An occlusal registration is used to mount the mandibular cast.

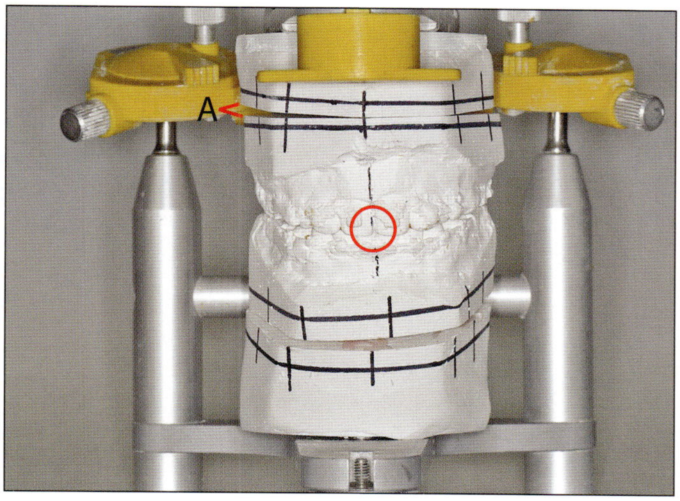

Fig 9-3 The casts are separated from their mountings and repositioned to simulate the desired surgical outcome. Measurements of cast displacement are limited to the index line A, even though the clinically important landmarks are the maxillary central incisors *(red circle)*.

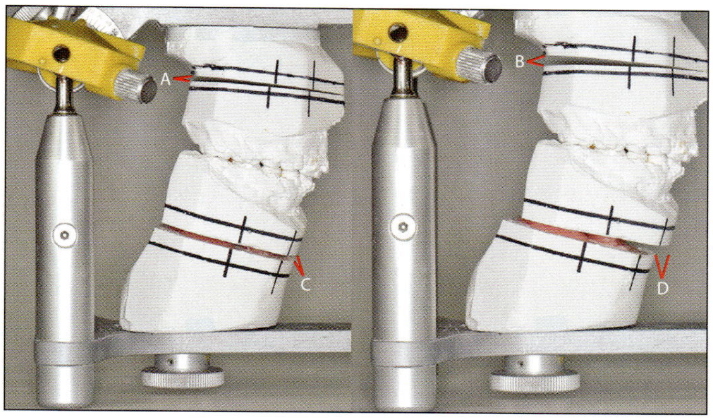

Fig 9-4 From the lateral viewpoint, differences in displacement between A and B, representing maxillary impaction, result in large differences between C and D, representing chin projection.

When viewed by a true lateral axis, it is clear that a difference of 2 to 3 mm in the impaction of the maxillary cast will result in a large difference in the chin projection (Fig 9-4).

To improve the accuracy of the cast surgery process, landmarks can be added to the system (Fig 9-5a) using model-making materials. Square brass tubing and wire (K and S Engineering, Chicago) are affixed with electrical solder to serve as indicators (Fig 9-5b). The mounting base is assembled from a block of acrylic (Plexiglass) and a section of square brass tubing. The minimum number of points to define a plane is three; this enhanced system incorporates three reference points, each representing a point of reference that does not move with the mobilized maxillary cast.

The anterior point defines the point on the facial midline (Fig 9-5c). This is the most important landmark. A pencil mark on the incisor indicates the clinical facial midline. This is the position to which the dental midline should be changed during movement of the maxillary cast. The brass indicator references a point in space that is at the vertical level of the existing incisal edge of the central incisors. Two posterior indicators point to an index mark on the first molar teeth. These indicators guide the correction of the occlusal plane cant. There are gaps between the cast and the tips of all three indicators. These gaps are included to allow space should the desired movement of the cast require anterior movement of the maxilla toward the indicator (Fig 9-5d).

The maxillary cast is repositioned (Fig 9-5e). The clinical objectives to correct the incisor position and the maxillary cant determine how the maxillary cast is repositioned within the articulator frame of reference. In this case, the maxillary central incisors have been advanced 5 mm and impacted 5 mm. This

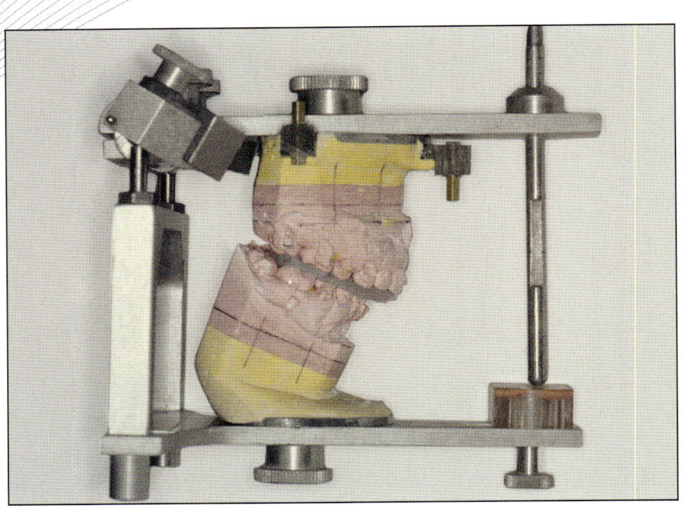

Fig 9-5a A modified articulator mounting incorporates bases to engage indicators to register the position of the dental arch.

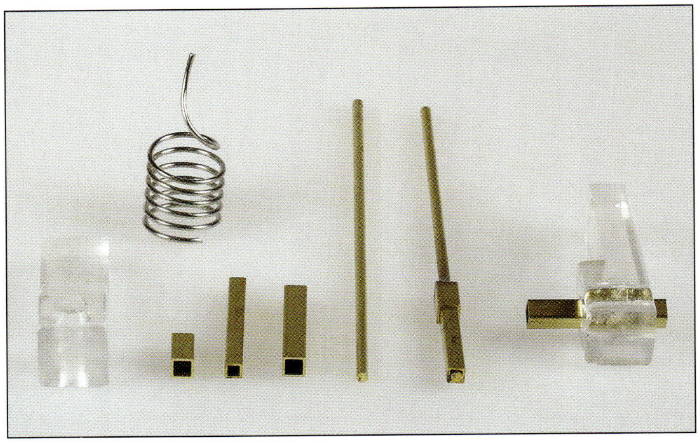

Fig 9-5b Landmark indicators are assembled from square brass tubing and wire joined with electrical solder. The mounting block is a portion of acrylic and a section of square brass tubing affixed with acrylic resin.

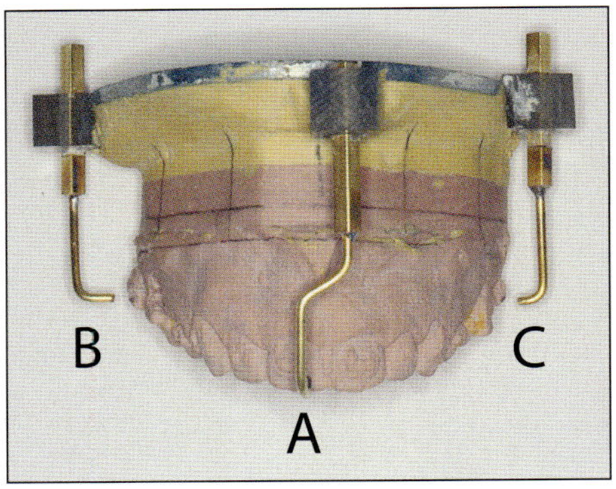

Fig 9-5c Detachable wire indicators record the position of the maxillary central incisors (A) and first molar teeth (B and C) before the cast is repositioned.

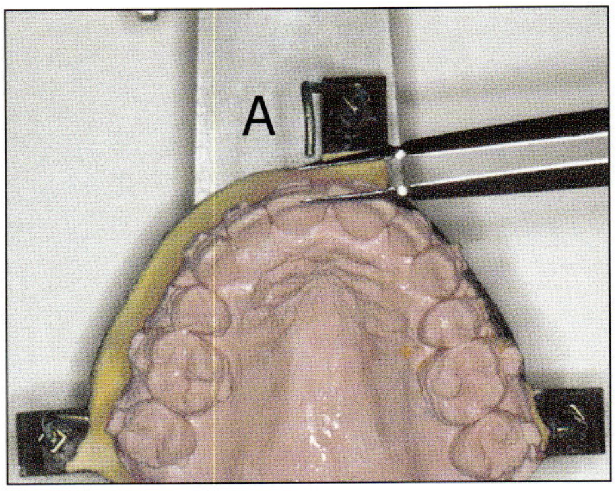

Fig 9-5d In this case, the incisor (midline) indicator A is bent to a position that represents the position of the clinical facial midline. The vertical height of the indicator is set to the preoperative position so that the amount of incisor impaction can be measured directly.

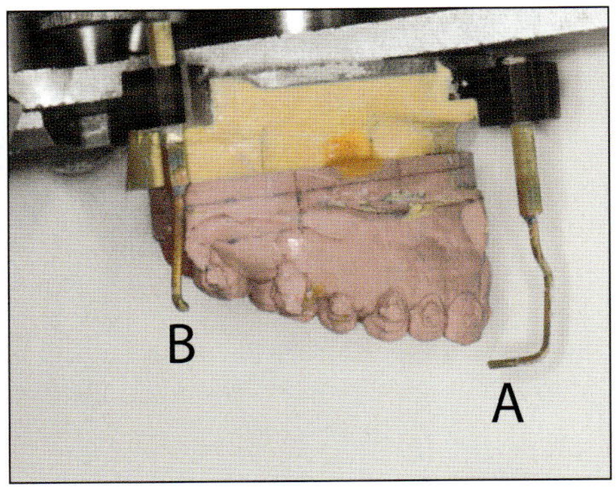

Fig 9-5e After the cast has been repositioned, the vertical displacement at indicator A represents the amount of incisor impaction desired. The incisor has been advanced to be even with the pointer level, indicating that the incisor advancement corresponds to the desired amount set in Fig 9-5d. Indicator B shows the movement of the second molar. This landmark is important when correcting occlusal plane cant disorders.

movement can be verified by the change in the relationships of the indicators and their corresponding marks on the casts. Movement at the plaster osteotomy line, as indicated by the penciled lines, become of secondary importance. The accurately repositioned maxillary cast will be used to fabricate accurate surgical splints.

Sources of error during surgery

Loss of landmarks after osteotomy

Reliance on measurements across osteotomy cuts during surgery is the most common cause of serious fragment repositioning errors. The practice of transferring cast surgery measurements of plaster base displacement across the simulated osteotomy line remains standard practice. Therefore, it is useful to discuss the limitations of using osteotomy landmarks to orient maxillary fragments. These geometric limitations apply to both the cast surgery phase and the surgical phase. Some errors are introduced during cast surgery and are incorporated in the surgical splints. Although the splints are correctly applied during surgery, the error emerges in the final result. Other errors are introduced during surgical repositioning and fixation of the maxillary fragment.

During surgery, the mobilized Le Fort I fragment is elevated into the desired position, and interfering bone is removed to allow proper reduction. The mandible serves as a point of reference through the use of an occlusal splint. The surgeon manipulates the maxillomandibular complex as a unit in a manner that attempts to hold the condyles in their centric relation position. To be valid, the condylar position used as reference during surgery must be the same as that captured on the articulator-mounted cast setup.

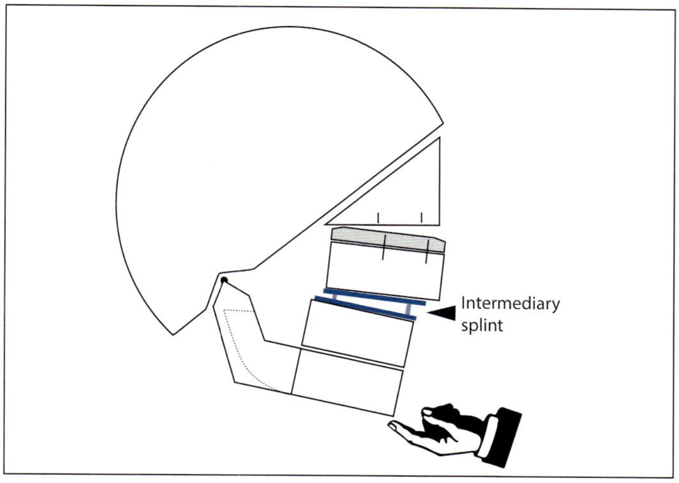

Fig 9-6 During maxillary repositioning surgery, the mandible is used to guide the placement of the maxilla. The mobilized maxilla is fixed to the mandible, and the combined structure is elevated, using the condyles as a rotation axis.

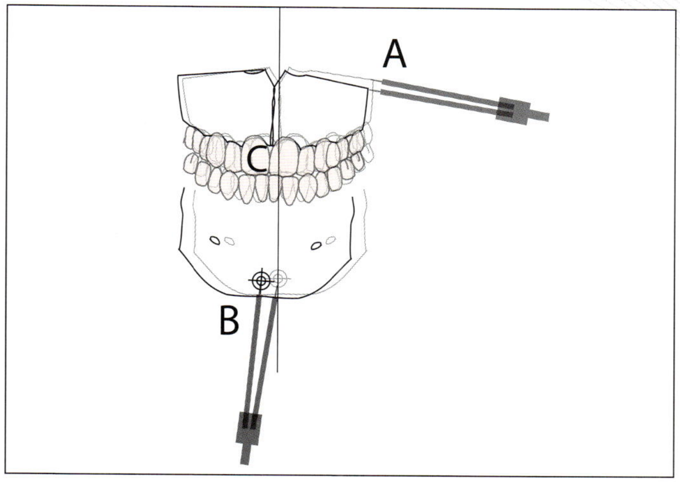

Fig 9-7 In one technique, vertical repositioning of the maxilla is determined by measurements across the lateral maxillary osteotomy (A). Correct positioning of the central incisors (C) cannot be achieved accurately and predictably using distant, poorly defined landmarks. The chin prominence (B) is markedly displaced by small errors at A.

Incorrect assessment of centric relation

Centric relation is supposed to be a unique position of the mandible in relation to the cranial base and maxilla. Because the mandible is a movable structure, occlusion changes depending on how the mandible is positioned in space. The factors that determine the posture and motion of the mandible are complex and multifactorial. The model of mandibular movement depicted on a dental articulator is a gross simplification of how this structure functions in patients.

Gnathologists have studied mandibular movements with sophisticated movement-tracking devices. The data collected are analyzed to gain better insight into this obscure process. Fully adjustable articulators are configured to simulate and reproduce observed movements in individual patients. Even the most rigorous clinical procedures, laboratory techniques, and sophisticated instruments, however, cannot fully capture and reproduce mandibular movements, because the determinants of movement involve a combination of mechanical and neuromuscular factors. Mechanical factors include bone morphology and the mechanics of ligaments and muscles. Neuromuscular factors include the full range of central nervous system control and the afferent and efferent peripheral nervous system. It is important to recognize that both the mechanical and neuromuscular science exceeds current understanding.

The inability to capture and reproduce a reference mandible position is an inherent limitation of the surgical planning process. Errors introduced at this step manifest in the surgical result. All navigation technology that uses centric relation during planning and splint fabrication is vulnerable to these errors. Conventional cast surgery and virtual planning with printed splints incorporate these errors.

Centric relation is thought to be a reproducible position of the condyles. Articulator mounting of casts is supposed to be in centric relation. Centric relation is important because it serves as a reference axis from which surgical splints are created. To be valid as a true reference point, however, the position must be constant and reproducible. Because the splints use centric relation as a reference to orient Le Fort I maxillary osteotomies, any error in centric relation will be manifested in the surgical result.

In conventional practice, the surgeon, attempting to use condylar position to guide the mobilized maxilla, applies force to the maxillomandibular complex to retrude the mandible. The surgeon rotates the mandible around the condyles on an axis that is supposed to be reproducible (Fig 9-6). Any discrepancy between the condylar position captured on the cast surgery setup and that achieved during surgery will result in an error in fragment repositioning. When the surgeon achieves a maxillary elevation position where the surgical osteotomy gap appears consistent with what is expected from cast surgery, the fragment is stabilized with bone plates.

With this system, there is no way to know if the critical landmarks—the central incisors and the occlusal plane—are correctly positioned. Variability ranges from 3 to 10 mm. The net error is the sum of the error at each step. If all of the steps are carefully followed, most results will emerge within a range of error of 2 to 4 mm. The outcomes that demonstrate errors of 7 to 10 mm generally have problems at multiple steps that compound into a major compromise.

Measurements across the osteotomy poorly control the position of clinically important structures (Fig 9-7). These errors can be introduced during the cast surgery, virtual simulation, or surgical procedure. Correct positioning of the central incisors, in the midline of the face, cannot be achieved accurately and predictably using distant, poorly defined landmarks. The chin prominence is markedly displaced by small errors in measurement at the site of osteotomy.

The limitations and hazards of using osteotomy landmarks to orient maxillary osteotomy fragments are due to the inherent anatomy of the region (Fig 9-8a) and the typical geometry required for orthognathic movements. The true lateral view of the skull is the viewpoint used for planning on cephalometrics, virtual simulation, and cast surgery. This view is never seen during surgery.

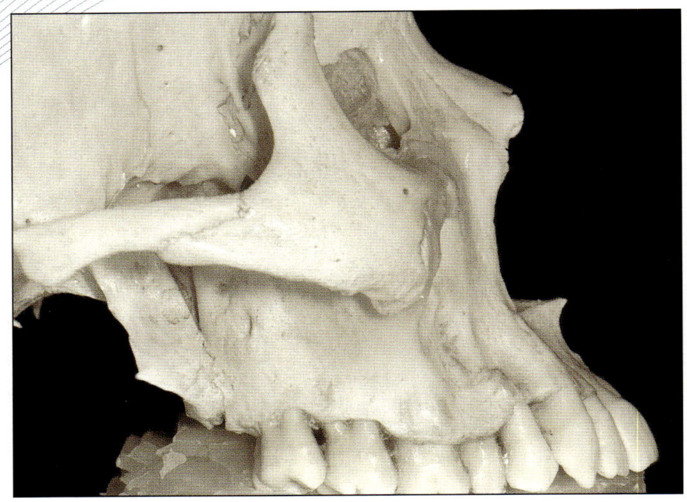

Fig 9-8a The anatomy of available maxillary landmarks limits the accuracy of the technique in which osteotomy landmarks are used to orient maxillary fragments.

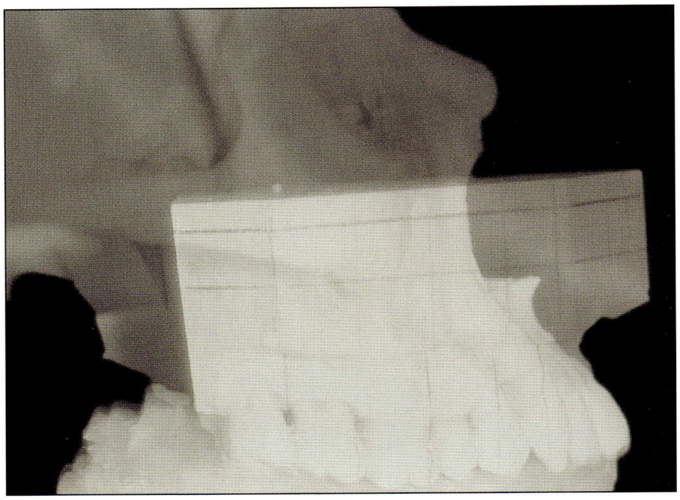

Fig 9-8b Superimposition of a dental cast on a human skull shows that plaster casts do not reproduce the anatomy of the maxilla. The locations on the cast where measurements are taken do not have corresponding anatomical counterparts.

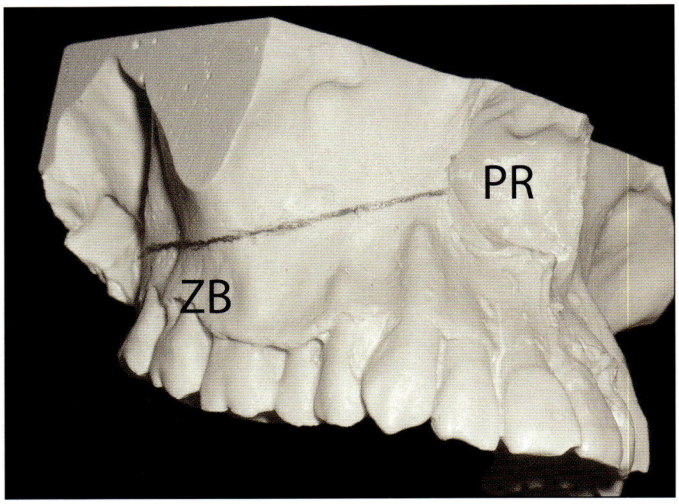

Fig 9-9a When a maxillary cast is oriented in the line of sight available during surgery, the typical osteotomy from the zygomatic buttress (ZB) to the piriform rim (PR) appears as a straight line.

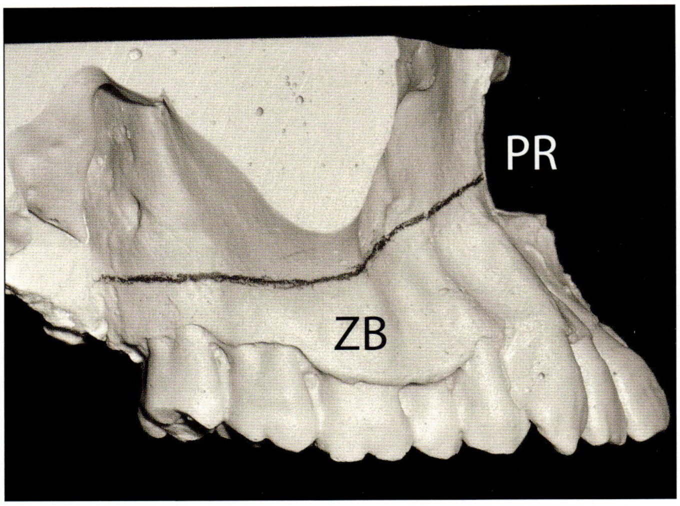

Fig 9-9b The true lateral view of the same cast shows that the osteotomy line follows a nonlinear path and rises markedly in the anterior region.

Superimposition of dental casts on a skull illustrates the limitations of available landmarks (Fig 9-8b). To be useful, measurements derived from the planning phase must be applicable during surgery to reposition fragments. However, measurements taken from conventional dental casts cannot be transferred to the skeleton during surgery because there are no analogous anatomical structures. During surgery, only the osteotomy line from the zygomatic buttress to the piriform aperture is clearly visible. Plaster cast measurements anterior to the piriform apertures and anterior nasal spine have no anatomical analog.

The view and perspective of the surgeon are limited by anatomical access. The surgeon never views the surgical site from the true lateral axis. On reflection of the mucosa during Le Fort I osteotomy, the axis of view is at an oblique angle. The osteotomy is begun at the zygomatic buttress and carried anteriorly to the piriform rim. The osteotomy in the posterior region is superior enough to avoid the molar roots but angled inferiorly to avoid the pterygoid structures. The anterior extent of the osteotomy is angled superiorly to avoid the canine root. The result is a straight-appearing bone cut that is not parallel to the occlusal plane (Fig 9-9a).

When the cast is viewed from a true lateral axis, it is apparent that the line along which the osteotomy fragment will separate is not linear and is markedly canted relative to the occlusal plane (Fig 9-9b). The available skeletal landmarks, the zygomatic buttress and piriform rim, are poorly positioned to control accurate repositioning of the central incisors and the cant of the occlusal plane. The two landmarks are too close together and too far from the clinically important structures to provide useful orientation measurements. At best, measurements made at the zygomatic buttress–piriform rim osteotomy line provide indications of gross error in repositioning.

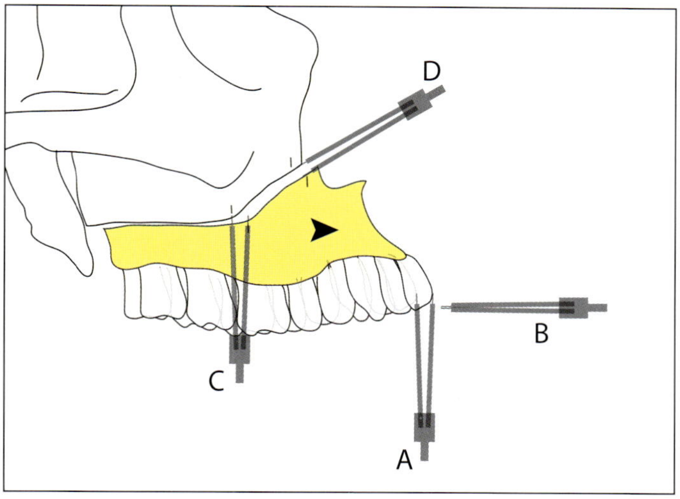

Fig 9-10 Projected movements of the central incisors (A and B) do not correspond to measurements at the osteotomy (C and D).

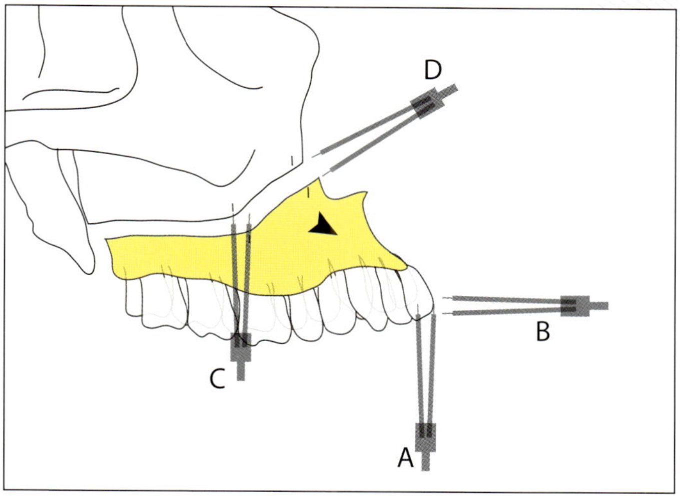

Fig 9-11 Moderate movements to advance (A) and lower (B) the central incisors open large bone gaps across the osteotomy line (D) even though the apparent maxillary protraction at the osteotomy indexes (C) is limited.

True advancement of the Le Fort I segment, parallel to the Frankfort plane, opens an osteotomy gap that does not correspond to the projected amount of movement at the central incisors (Fig 9-10). If the maxilla is deficient in its anterior projection and vertical development, impaction of the dental arch is seldom indicated. Inferior repositioning of the maxillary arch to address vertical hypoplasia opens a large discontinuity across the osteotomy.

Inferior and anterior movements of the Le Fort I segment are commonly needed for patients with skeletal Class III malocclusion, because maxillary retrusion disorders often involve vertical maxillary hypoplasia as well. It is not possible to precisely reposition the maxillary central incisors accurately using measurements across the osteotomy gap. A moderate maxillary advancement for the management of a Class III malocclusion is often combined with a moderate downgraft to address vertical maxillary hypoplasia. These limited movements result in opening a large discontinuity across the osteotomy, even though the apparent maxillary protraction at the osteotomy indexes is limited (Fig 9-11).

Thus, measurements across osteotomies during surgery are of limited use and cannot predict movements to the tolerance demanded by modern orthognathic surgeons, because the critical landmarks that determine clinical success, such as the central incisor position, are distant from the bone cut. Small rotational movements at the osteotomy site produce large movements of the incisors. This inherent geometric relationship limits the usefulness of measurements across the osteotomy regardless of how they are determined. Virtual modeling and conventional cast surgery are equally limited by the basic geometry.

Despite this limitation, the surgical mock-up should still be done in a manner to analyze these movements. This is important because an understanding of the general, expected displacements at osteotomy sites can provide clues to the surgeon when a surgical finding is not what is expected. Ideally, the appearance of bone displacement at the surgical site should be generally the same as that predicted by the surgical mock-up. If there is a significant difference, the surgeon is alerted that there may be a deviation caused by condylar position, unstable internal fixation, or incomplete reduction of fragments into splints.

Changes in centric relation during general anesthesia

Experience has shown that centric relation is difficult to capture on awake patients. Further study has shown that centric relation in the same patient is not the same under general anesthesia as it is in the awake state. Regardless of how carefully a centric relation record is obtained on an awake patient, there is a significant risk that the condyles will assume a different position under general anesthesia.

In an effort to capture a centric relation that would have the best reproducibility, the author studied centric relation in awake and anesthetized patients. First, the best-quality hinge axis was determined. This was done in the awake patient using a Moore axiograph (Fig 9-12). Following mandibular movements in both active and passive ranges of motion, the hinge axis was determined, and a tattoo was placed on the skin on right and left sides so that the position could be referenced during surgery. To further study the mechanical stability of condylar excursive movements, pantographic data were obtained with a pantograph (Pantronic, Denar) and used to program a fully adjustable Denar articulator (Fig 9-13). The position of the hinge axis was confirmed between the axiograph and the pantograph.

The author's other purpose was to investigate possible reasons that some patients exhibit alternative hinge axis locations during surgery. The lateral stability of condylar position near centric relation was evaluated by studying the Bennett shift. Some mandibles show a movement pattern characterized by an immediate lateral side shift on movement from centric relation. Physical characteristics of the temporomandibular joint capsule are

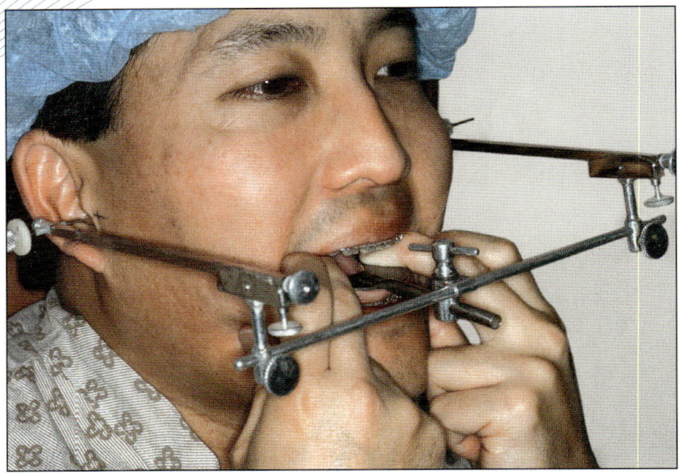

Fig 9-12 The best condylar position in centric relation is captured with an axiograph, and the locations are marked on the skin before surgery.

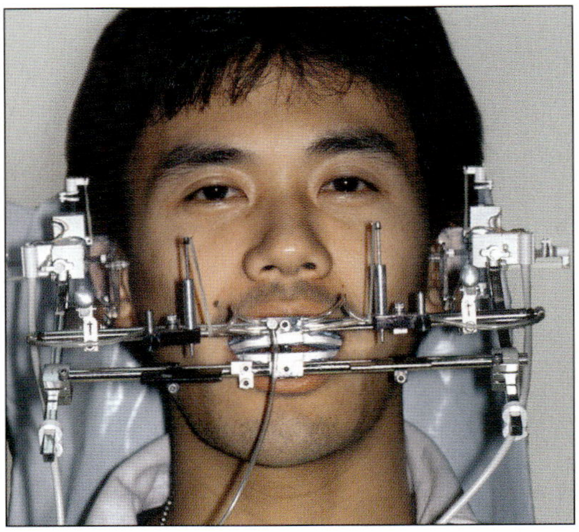

Fig 9-13 A pantograph is used to analyze the active and passive compliance of the temporomandibular joints prior to orthognathic surgery.

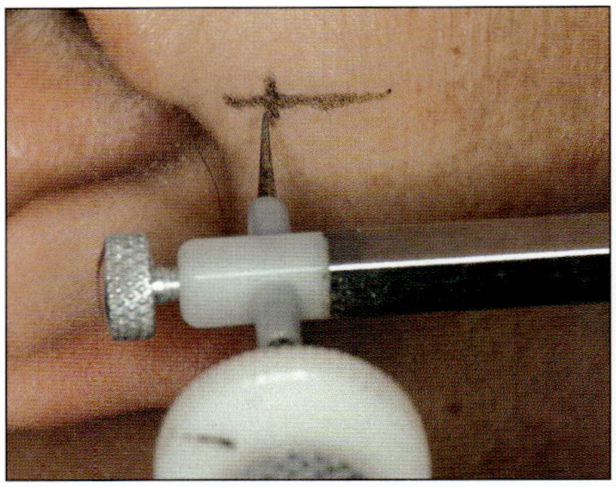

Fig 9-14 Once the patient is under general anesthesia, the axiograph is repositioned to determine if the centric relation captured on the awake patient is reproducible under general anesthesia. In this case, the axiograph points to the hinge axis location on the right side.

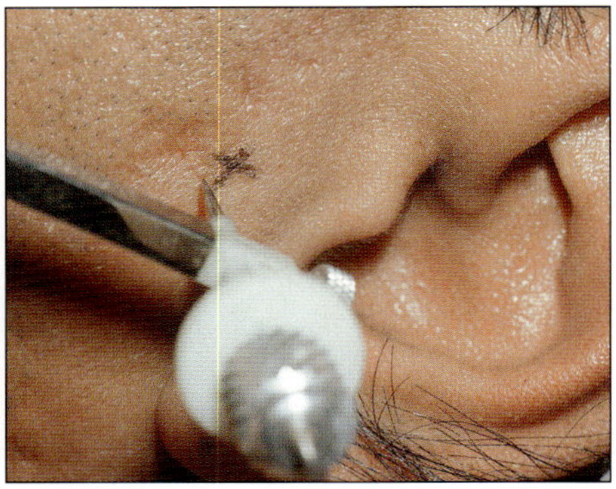

Fig 9-15 This patient shows a unilateral discrepancy between the centric relation taken while awake and that taken under general anesthesia. The left condyle is positioned anteriorly and inferiorly and cannot be manipulated into the awake position.

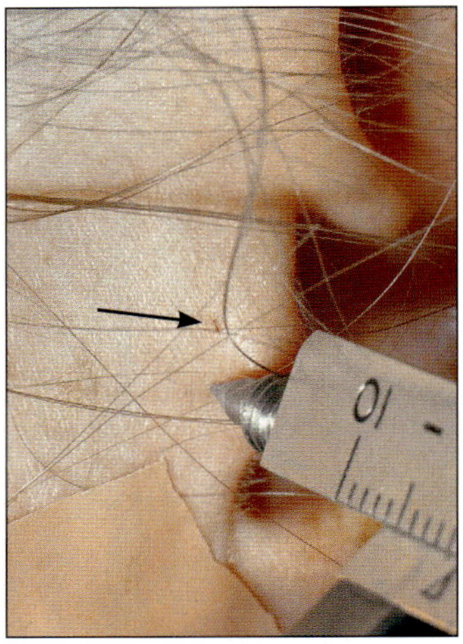

Fig 9-16 This patient shows a 4-mm inferior displacement of the condyle that only manifests while she is under general anesthesia. (*Arrow* points to the position of the condyle when the patient is awake.)

sometimes cited as a cause. Because the vector and magnitude of condylar shift during surgery are unpredictable, it seemed plausible that patients with lax temporomandibular joint mechanics might exhibit rapid Bennett shifts as well as condylar shift under general anesthesia. The results of the preliminary study showed, however, that there was no correlation between the Bennett shift and condylar shift under anesthesia.

The patients were placed on the operating table, and general anesthesia was induced. An endotracheal tube was positioned, which involved use of depolarizing or nondepolarizing muscle relaxants. How the state of anesthesia affected condylar position and the location of the hinge axis was then evaluated. The preset axiograph was engaged on the mandibular arch, and the mandible was manipulated to seat the condyles. The location of the hinge axis, as indicated by the axiograph, was noted (Fig 9-14).

As an example, the patient shown in Fig 9-15 exhibited an inferior and anterior displacement of the hinge axis on the left side. In most cases, the shift of the hinge axis under general anesthesia was not symmetric. Another patient exhibited a 4-mm inferior displacement of the left condyle (Fig 9-16). The right condyle did not show any displacement.

It is important to understand that this shift is not reducible. The mandible cannot be forced into the position captured on the awake patient. Even high-traction pressure on the mandible will not result in movement to the position captured in the awake patient.

A gnathologic pantograph was used to study how preoperative temporomandibular joint laxity affects the degree of discrepancy between awake and anesthetic centric relations. With the patient under general anesthesia, pantographic tracings were obtained. Analysis of the data showed that, under anesthesia,

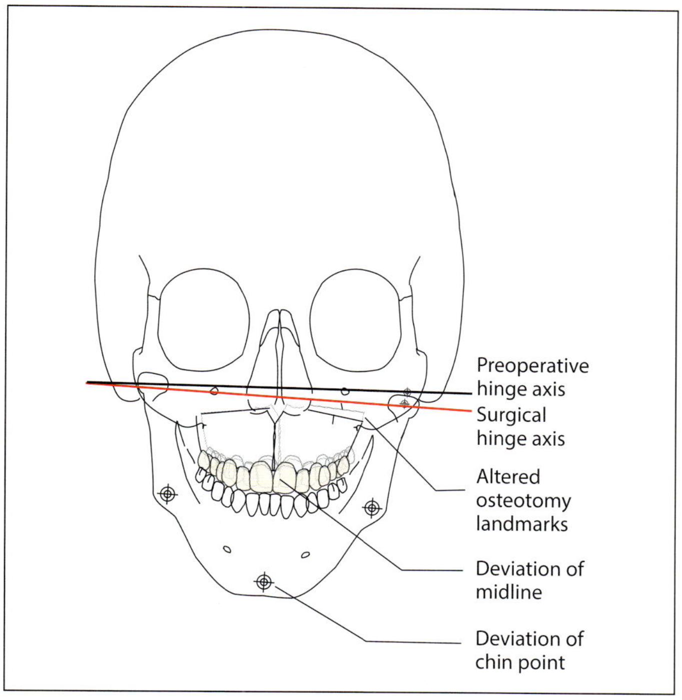

Fig 9-17 Discrepancies between awake and anesthetic centric relations introduce errors in the positioning of critical landmarks.

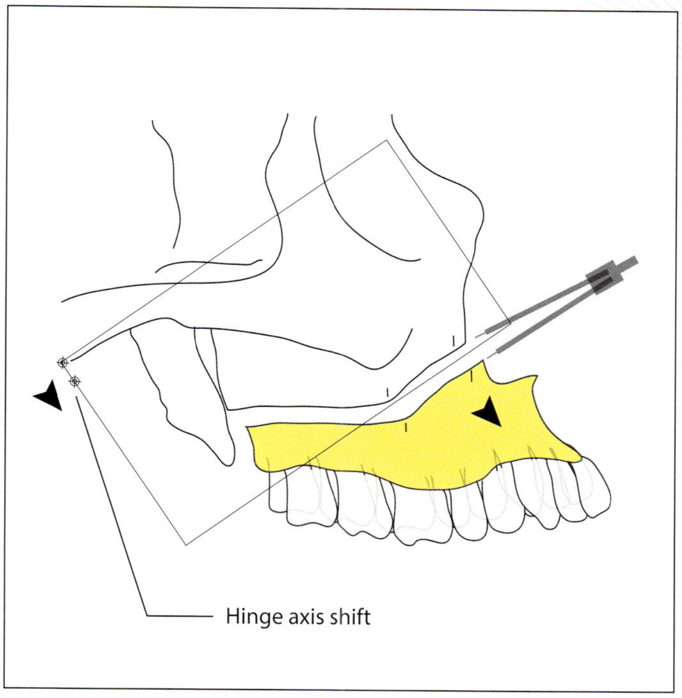

Fig 9-18 The hinge axis shift has an accentuated effect on the osteotomy gap and the position of landmarks.

the mandible did not exhibit accentuated Bennett movements. Joint mechanics and diminished muscle tone are therefore not the primary determinants of mandibular position and movement pattern under anesthesia.

When the patient is in the surgical setting under general anesthesia, the mandible assumes a position that may differ significantly from that captured when awake. The position about which the mandible rotates under general anesthesia may be considered a surgical hinge axis. The surgical hinge axis cannot be manipulated to the position of the awake hinge axis. The deviation of the hinge axis is apparently not related to diminished muscle tone from anesthetic muscle relaxants. It is unknown, however, if the surgical hinge axis changes during the course of the procedure depending on the depth of anesthesia or specific pharmacologic agents used. Clinical results seem to indicate that the condylar positions and hinge axis return to their prior awake positions as the patient recovers from surgery and anesthesia.

Asymmetric vertical shift of the hinge axis. In most cases, the deviation of the hinge axis under general anesthesia is primarily vertical and inferior. This shift has direct and indirect consequences for the course of surgery. Both conventional cast study and virtual planning use clinical centric relation as a spatial reference. The right and left condylar positions in centric relation define the hinge axis. Deviation of the hinge axis that occurs under general anesthesia introduces an error in the repositioning of the osteotomy fragments (Fig 9-17).

The direct consequence is that the midline of the maxillary incisors is displaced to the contralateral side. The indirect effect is that the maxilla assumes a canted orientation, altering the relationship of the osteotomy gap. When the maxillomandibular complex is elevated, the surgeon sees an unexpected gap at the left osteotomy line. To correct this finding, the surgeon most often removes the first contacting bone at the right side. The surgeon continues to remove bone at the right osteotomy until the gap closes on the left side. The result is that the midline is off-center, the maxilla is canted, and removal of maxillary bone on the right side causes the maxillary central incisors to be overimpacted. Overimpaction and midline deviation of the maxillary central incisors can produce a significant esthetic compromise.

Combined vertical and horizontal shift of the hinge axis. Some centric relation displacements involve both vertical and horizontal deviations. The most damaging movement errors involve asymmetric shifts. When the left condyle shifts inferiorly and anteriorly, the problems are compounded. Both direct and indirect consequences are much greater when the centric relation position of the condyle is displaced in this manner. The three-dimensional displacement causes a marked shift of the maxillary central incisors off the midline. The anterior and inferior displacement of the maxilla results in a large gap at the left osteotomy, because the net displacement vector, anterior and inferior, can be nearly perpendicular to the surgical osteotomy line. The shift alters the position of the osteotomy line and index marks placed prior to mobilization of the maxilla (Fig 9-18).

This gap would not have been predicted by surgical simulation on articulated casts or by virtual planning. Trying to accommodate for this finding, the surgeon first attempts to verify seating of the condyles and then rotates the maxillomandibular

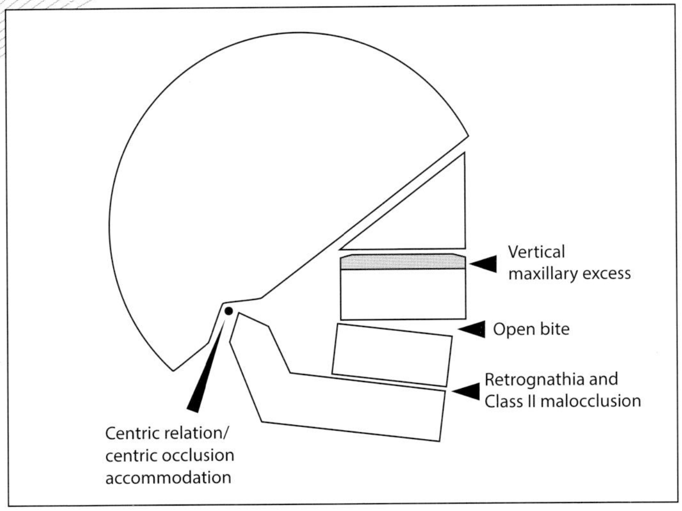

Fig 9-19a Representation of typical facial deformity presenting for orthognathic surgery, in this case long-face syndrome. Patients with long-face syndrome develop vertical maxillary hyperplasia and an open bite malocclusion. In this example, the mandible is deficient. Patients with these deformities optimize their function by accommodating their temporomandibular joint position.

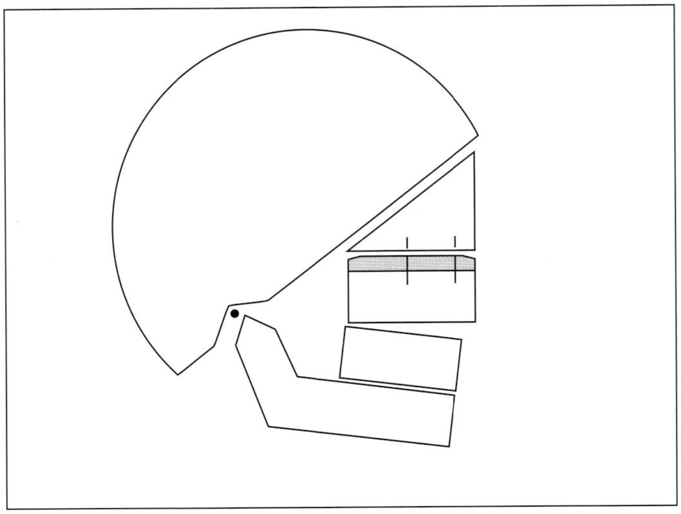

Fig 9-19b Vertical bone indexes are placed prior to Le Fort I downfracture. The conventional technique involves placement of vertical lines with the saw or bur into the lateral maxilla prior to mobilization of the maxilla.

complex stabilized in the splint. The gap remains. Condylar subluxation or hidden bone interference might deflect the attempt to reduce the maxillary fragment, but nothing is found.

When confronted by this discontinuity, the surgeon is usually reluctant to bridge the gap with a graft, particularly if the patient has not previously consented to grafting. The surgeon most often removes bone from the right side to allow bilateral bone contact at the osteotomy line. In the case of single-jaw, Le Fort I surgery, occlusion is verified to be good with maxillomandibular fixation removed. Postoperatively, the patient reveals an open bite on the right side and premature occlusion on the left side as the condyle assumes the position of the awake centric relation.

The surgeon is naturally reluctant to leave the operating room with the patient presenting a malocclusion in the only centric relation that the surgeon has access to. However, it is important for the surgeon to appreciate the amount and in which direction the mandible is likely to shift in the postoperative period due to condylar position accommodation. It is also important to understand what esthetic errors may have been introduced because of the difference between awake centric relation and surgical centric relation.

Methods of Osteotomy Fragment Repositioning

Most surgeons follow a common strategy when approaching the problem of correctly repositioning mobilized jaw fragments. The basic surgical principle is to orient a fragment that is to be repositioned by using an unmoved structure as a reference point. This method works wells when the surgical plan involves only movement of the mandible or only a segment of one jaw. The problem becomes more complex when the reconstruction involves movement of the total maxilla or both the maxilla and the mandible.

If accurate and predictable results are to be realized, the surgeon must understand the inherent limitations of the process chosen to place segments and verify their satisfactory position. Postoperative remodeling and relapse also contribute to discrepancies between the treatment goal and realized result. Thus, correct initial intraoperative positioning of the fragments is a prerequisite to achieving a satisfactory result.

Potential sources of repositioning error have already been described in detail. This section presents a summary of three methods for positioning osteotomy fragments during surgery. Each has inherent limitations and strengths in its ability to correctly reproduce the surgical plan during the surgical procedure. The surgeon must choose a method that has the potential to deliver the level of accuracy the treatment plan demands.

Conventional method of fragment repositioning in maxillomandibular surgery

Technique

Conventional repositioning will be demonstrated using a diagrammatic representation of a patient with long-face syndrome (Fig 9-19a). Patients with long-face syndrome develop vertical maxillary hyperplasia and an open bite malocclusion. In this example case, the mandible is deficient. Patients with these deformities optimize their function by accommodating their temporomandibular joint position.

In a conventional technique, the saw or bur is used to place vertical lines in the lateral maxilla, and the maxilla is mobilized (Fig 9-19b). Le Fort I osteotomy separates the maxilla from the midface (Fig 9-19c). An intermediary occlusal splint is placed between the maxillary and mandibular teeth, and the jaws are stabilized in maxillomandibular fixation (Fig 9-19d).

The surgeon manipulates the maxillomandibular complex to seat the condyles. While the surgeon holds the condyles in the

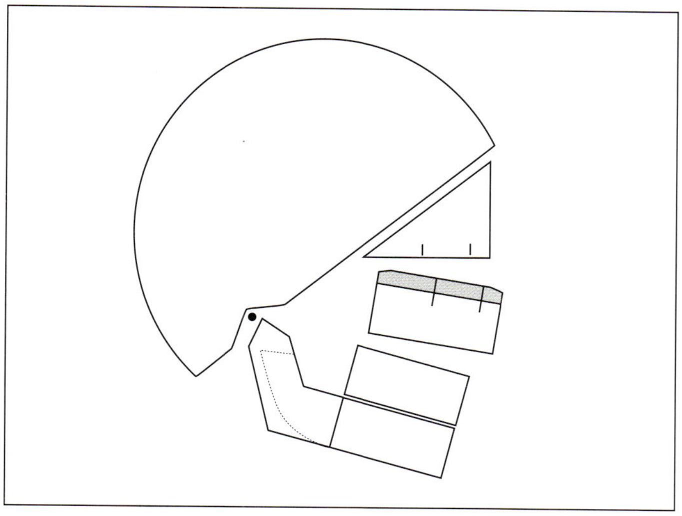

Fig 9-19c Le Fort I osteotomy separates the maxilla from the midface.

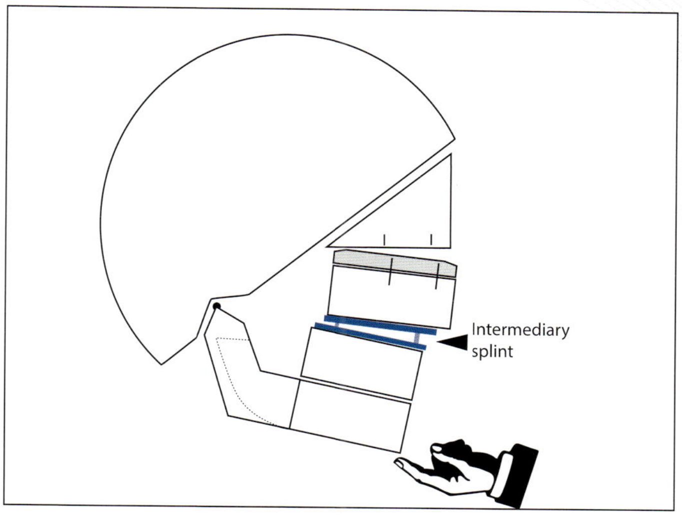

Fig 9-19d The intermediary splint is in place.

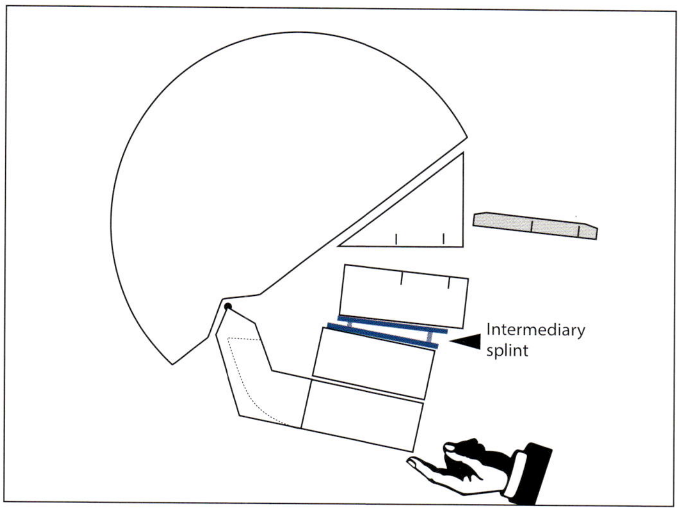

Fig 9-19e Interfering bone is removed.

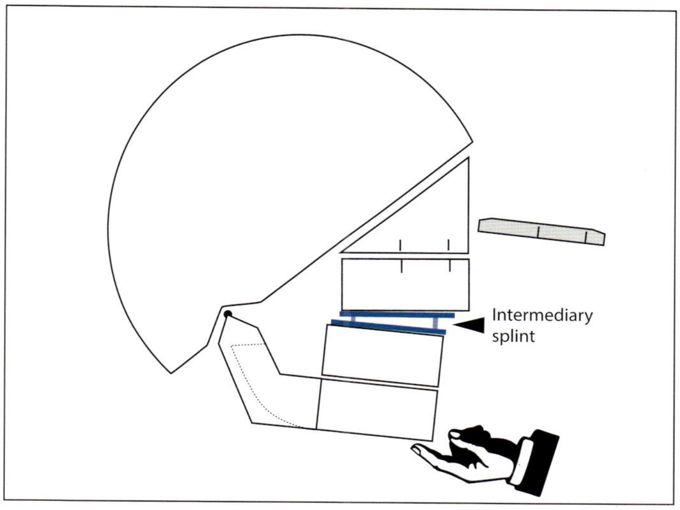

Fig 9-19f The maxilla is elevated into the proper position.

seated position, the maxillomandibular complex is rotated upward. Bone that prevents the elevation of the maxilla into place is removed (Fig 9-19e). The maxilla is then elevated into the proper position (Fig 9-19f).

The most important landmark from an esthetic standpoint is the correct position of the maxillary central incisors. The correct position is dependent on *(1)* correct positioning of the condyle during surgery, *(2)* correct prediction of the amount of bone to be resected at the osteotomy site, and *(3)* correct relationships built into the intermediary splint through accurate cast surgery or virtual simulation. The inherent limitation of this method is that there is no direct measurement of the maxillary central incisor position. Reliance on condylar position and measurements across the osteotomy to correctly position the maxillary central incisors is the most common source of error in orthognathic surgery.

The most common error in maxillary repositioning is incorrect vertical positioning of the maxilla (Fig 9-19g). It is impossible to accurately transfer measurements from the cast surgery or virtual simulation to the osteotomy site. The challenge increases when the maxillary arch is divided into segments, which is often necessary to create sites for dental implants. Small errors at the osteotomy site have a large impact at the incisor position. Both vertical and symmetry errors are introduced at this stage. Options to evaluate or correct the problem are limited with this surgical staging method.

Errors in maxillary repositioning may also be the result of failure to capture an accurate and reproducible centric relation condylar position (Fig 9-19h). The underlying problem is that the method violates the basic surgical principle that the mobilized fragment must be repositioned using a stable structure for reference. The mandible does not meet the requirement of a stable structure because it is naturally mobile. Manipulation of the maxillomandibular complex into an approximate centric relation in the presence of osseous and soft tissue interferences can lead to repositioning errors.

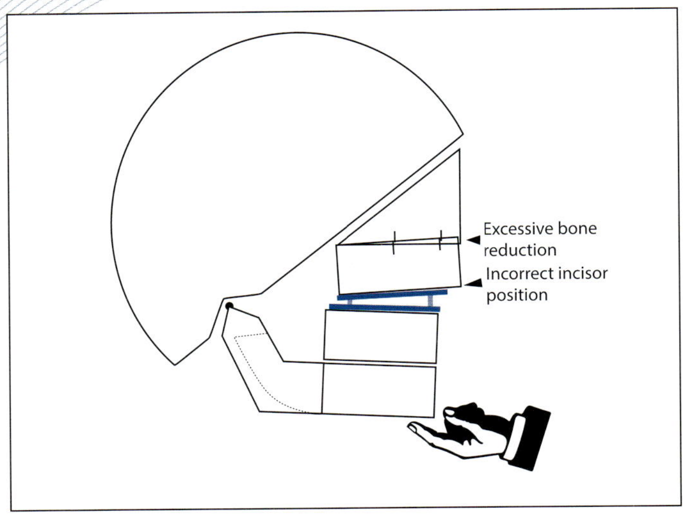

Fig 9-19g Vertical reduction errors are common in Le Fort I surgery. Excessive bone removal at the osteotomy site results in the maxilla being repositioned too far superiorly. The maxillary central incisors then become incorrectly positioned too far superiorly.

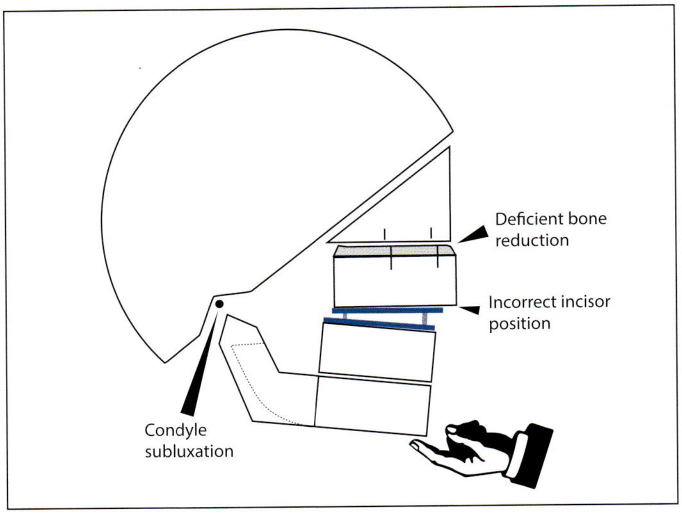

Fig 9-19h Maxillary repositioning errors also may result from condylar subluxation. In addition, insufficient bone reduction at the osteotomy site results in the maxilla and the central incisors being repositioned too far inferiorly.

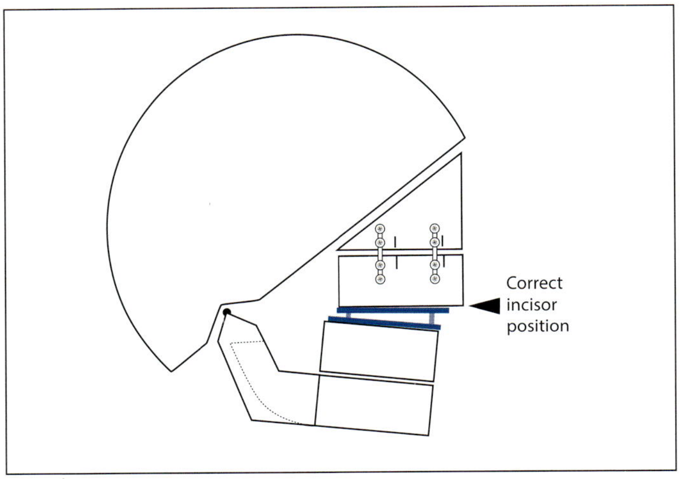

Fig 9-19i The maxilla is fixed with bone plates.

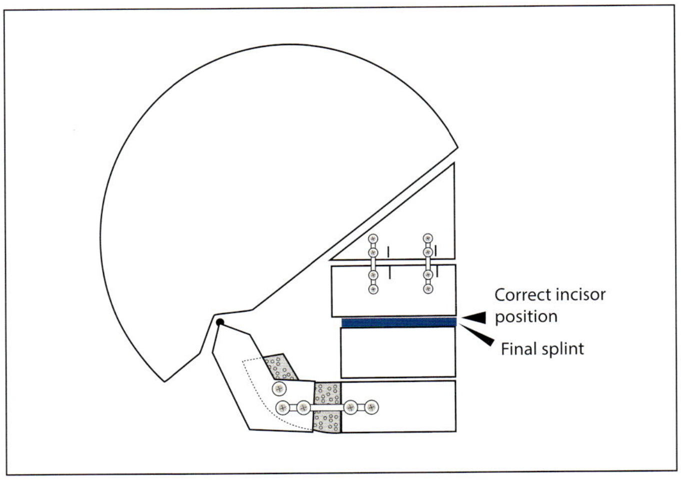

Fig 9-19j The mandible is advanced and fixed.

With the conventional method of repositioning, at some point, the maxilla is judged to be in a satisfactory position. Bone plates are used to secure the maxilla at that position (Fig 9-19i). Bilateral sagittal ramus osteotomies allow advancement of the mancible. If the maxilla was repositioned correctly, the mandible should also be in the correct position (Fig 9-19j).

Discussion

This treatment sequence is the one followed by most maxillofacial surgeons. The technique has limited accuracy and can produce disappointing results. The strategy lacks a method to verify the correct position of the dentition, particularly the maxillary central incisors. When dental implants are already in place, there are very limited options to correct problems of asymmetry or incisor exposure caused by errors in maxillary fragment repositioning. When the procedure is being done as part of a staged reconstruction, significant repositioning errors compromise the ability to place implants and dental prosthetics to best correct the deformity.

Improved method of repositioning to control the vertical dimension

Technique

The same example of typical facial deformity from the prior section will be used to present a method to improve the accuracy of osteotomy fragment repositioning (Fig 9-20a). In this method, two landmarks are established to improve the accuracy of maxillary repositioning (Fig 9-20b). The cast surgery or virtual simulation must be done to incorporate vertical dimension relationships into the intermediary splint. The vertical dimension established on the articulator by the incisal guide pin is then transferred to the surgical setting. To accomplish this, a small

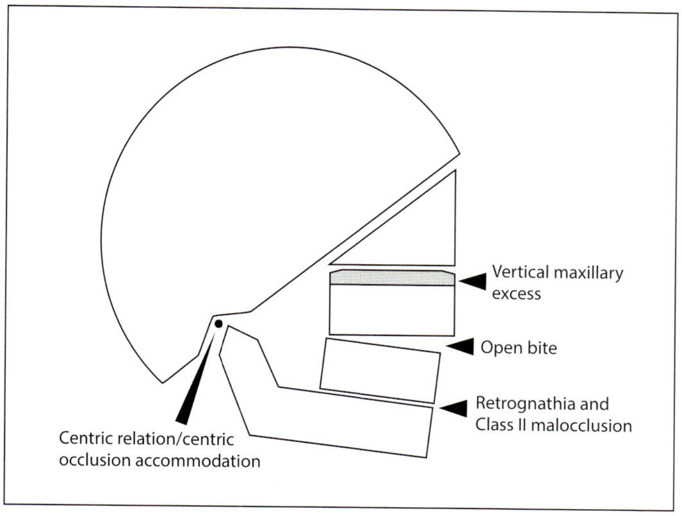

Fig 9-20a The same example of long-face syndrome used in Fig 9-19 will be used to present a method to improve the accuracy of osteotomy fragment repositioning.

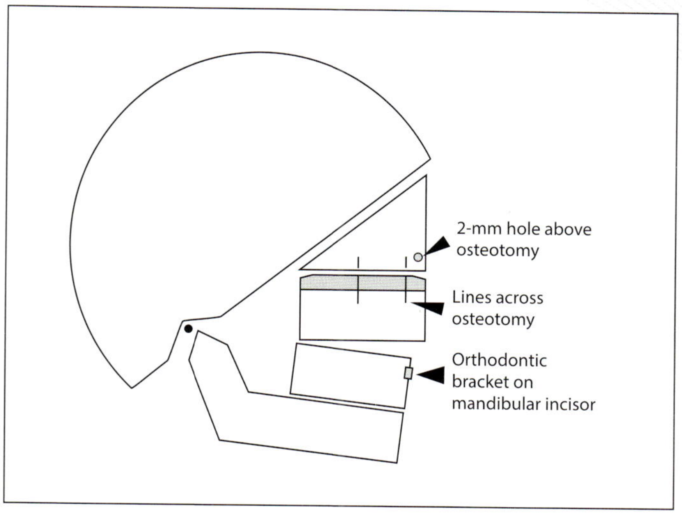

Fig 9-20b Additional landmarks for navigational reference are established. The 2-mm hole is a landmark above the mobilized segments.

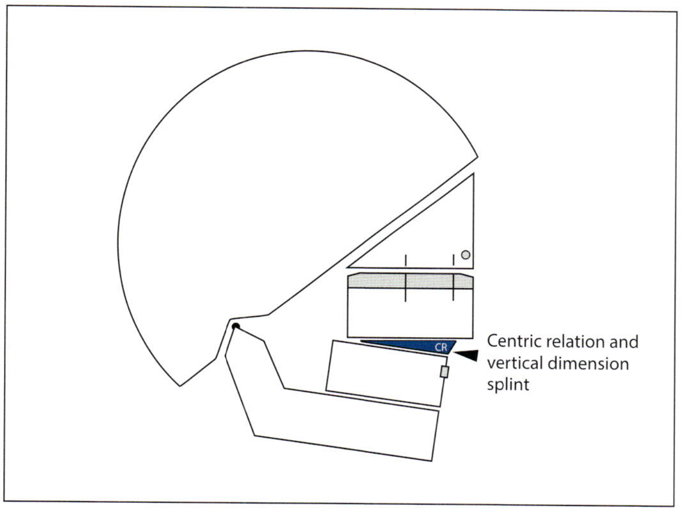

Fig 9-20c A centric relation splint establishes the vertical dimension.

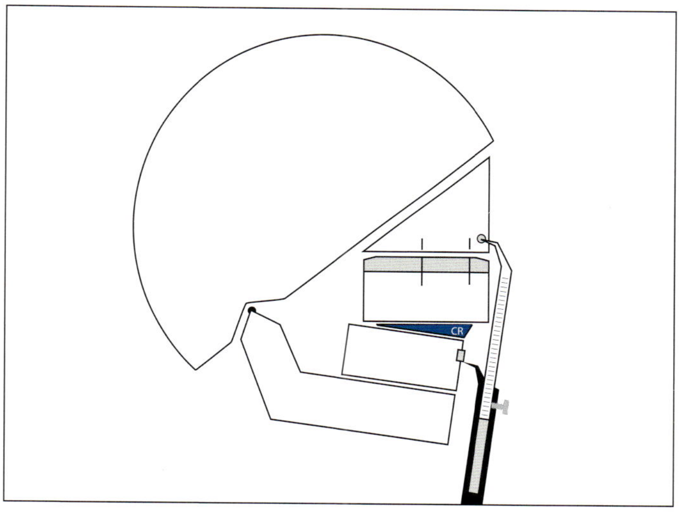

Fig 9-20d The centric relation splint transfers the vertical dimension landmark during surgery using a Thorpe caliper.

hole is drilled in the maxilla above the level of the maxillary osteotomy. This hole is a landmark in the stable, immobilized facial skeleton. A second landmark is chosen on the anterior mandible. This landmark can be a specific orthodontic bracket on a mandibular incisor tooth.

A centric relation splint fabricated on the articulator is used to transfer the vertical dimension landmark to the facial skeleton during surgery (Figs 9-20c and 9-20d). This splint is made before casts are moved on the articulator. It represents the vertical dimension at which the casts were mounted with the centric relation occlusal registration. This measurement is analogous to the incisal guide pin of the articulator. To be accurate, all of the cast simulations must be done at the same articulator dimension. For the intraoperative measurements to be accurate, the mandible must be positioned in the same vertical dimension when osteotomy measurements are taken.

Instead of an incisal guide pin in place at surgery, a measurement is made between the landmarks at the midface and the mandibular incisor bracket while the centric relation splint is in place. The condyles must be in centric relation as well. The vertical dimension of the surgical site is measured with a Thorpe caliper (Fig 9-20e).

Following mobilization, the maxilla is secured in maxillomandibular fixation using the intermediary splint (Fig 9-20f). This splint has been fabricated at the original articulator vertical dimension. Measurement with the Thorpe caliper may indicate that more bone resection is required (Fig 9-20g). If so, additional bone is removed to allow superior repositioning of the maxilla. Again, measurement with the Thorpe caliper may indicate that slightly more bone resection is required (Fig 9-20h). When the vertical dimension indicated by the Thorpe caliper has been reached, the maxilla should be in the correct vertical position (Fig 9-20i). After bone plates have been placed to secure the maxilla, the mandibular osteotomies are completed and fixed (Fig 9-20j).

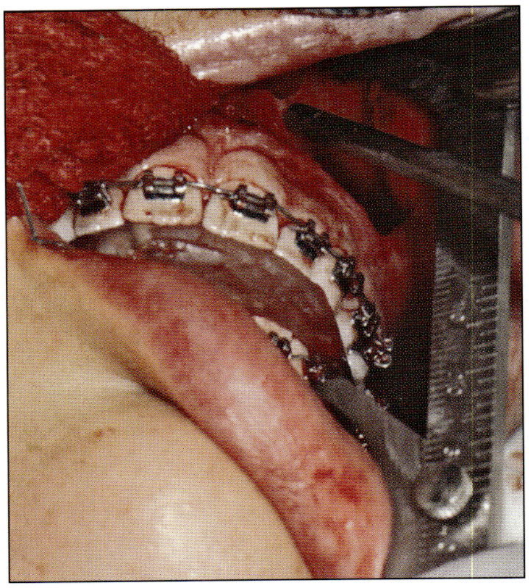

Fig 9-20e The vertical dimension at the surgical site is measured with a Thorpe caliper.

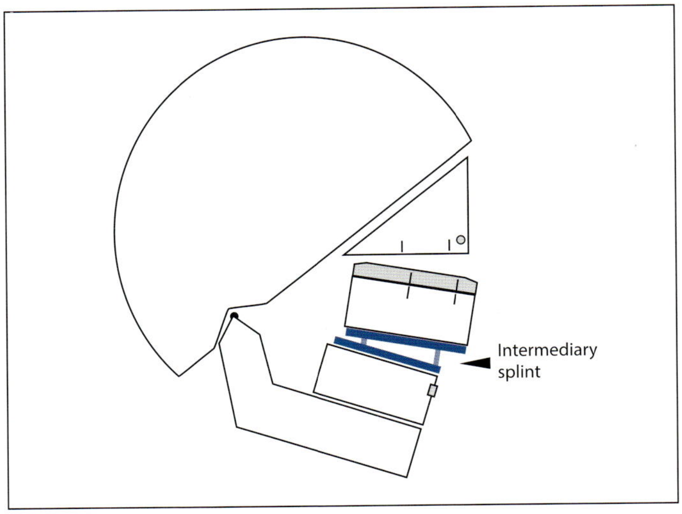

Fig 9-20f The intermediary splint is in place.

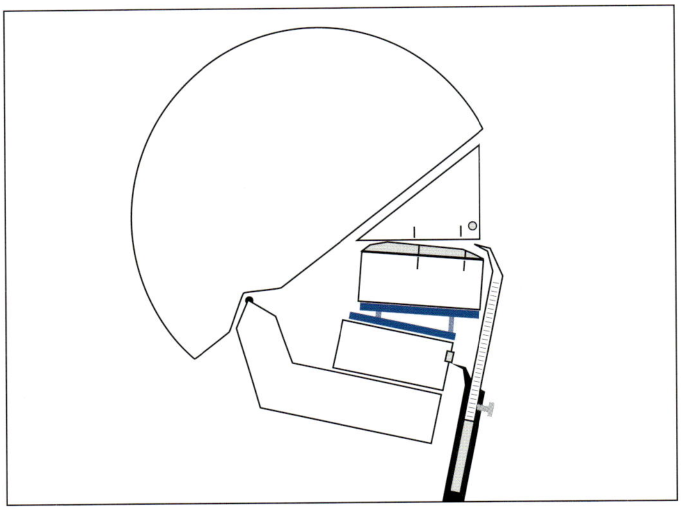

Fig 9-20g Measurement with the Thorpe caliper indicates that more bone resection is required.

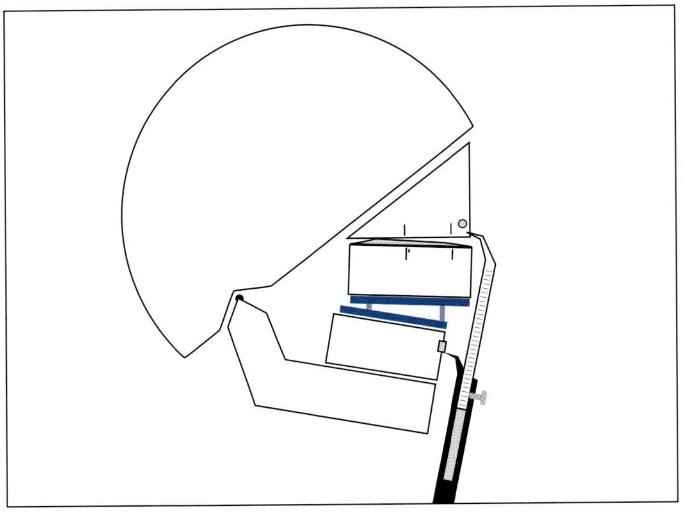

Fig 9-20h After additional bone is removed to allow superior repositioning of the maxilla, the vertical dimension is measured again. Additional resection is required.

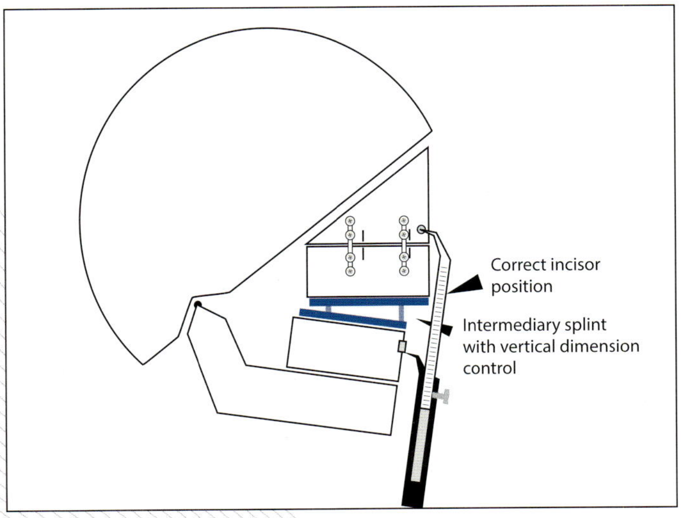

Fig 9-20i The Thorpe caliper indicates that the facial vertical dimension has been reached.

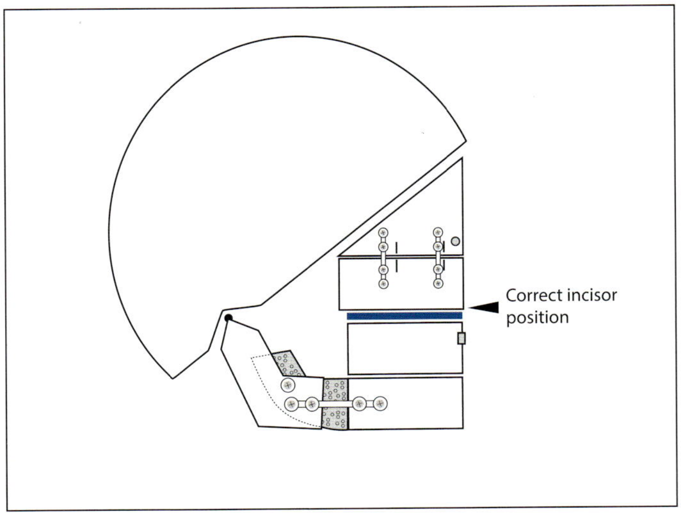

Fig 9-20j The maxilla is fixed, and the mandible is advanced and fixed.

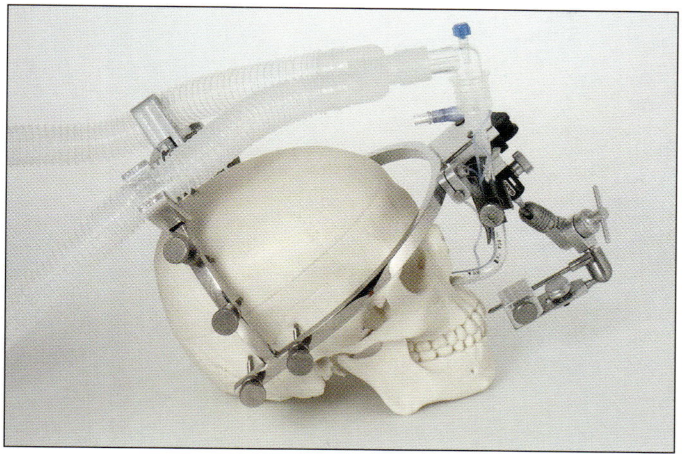

Fig 9-21a Headframe-based navigation provides a frame of reference that is independent of condylar position (ie, the cranium).

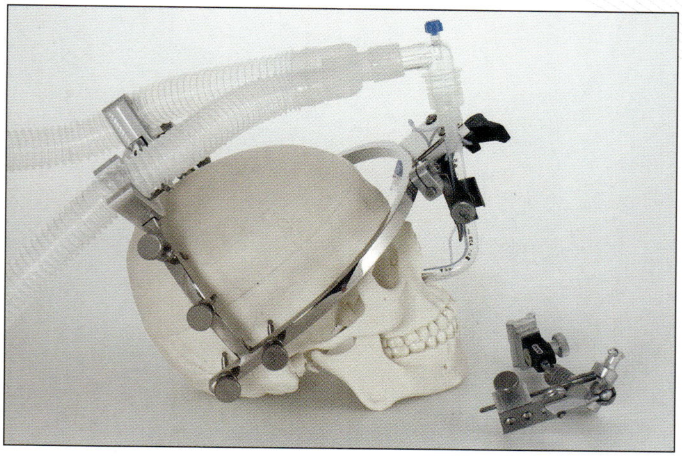

Fig 9-21b The indicator records critical landmarks and is detachable to provide access to perform the surgical procedures.

Discussion

This method offers additional control of orthognathic surgery positioning. The intent is to avoid major errors in vertical position of the maxillary central incisors. These errors can produce the most disappointing results. Even with these additional measurements, errors can occur. The method does not address the inherent flaw of using the mobile mandible as a reference point to reposition the maxillary fragment. This method also cannot directly measure critical maxillary landmarks in real time, and the position of the maxillary central incisors at the end of surgery still cannot be directly verified.

Headframe-based navigation system for orienting osteotomy fragments

To increase the predictability of orthognathic procedures, a frame of reference is needed to allow transfer of planning data to the operative setting. In the previously introduced technique for mounting casts on the articulator, a limited number of additional reference points added to the accuracy of the cast surgery and splint fabrication. In that earlier example, movement of the maxillary central incisors superiorly by 5 mm, anteriorly by 5 mm, and right by 2 mm was determined in the design process (see Fig 9-5). This movement can be verified visually on the patient to be a reasonable plan to meet occlusal and esthetic objectives. The next step is to transfer the movement data to the patient at surgery. The limitations of splints, centric relation, and osteotomy measurements have been discussed. A direct measurement method is needed.

From an engineering standpoint, location of mobile skeletal units must be oriented in relation to a reference frame that does not move. The common use of the movable mandible to guide repositioning of maxillary segments is therefore inherently flawed. The headframe-based surgical navigation system was developed to improve the accuracy and predictability of orthognathic surgery procedures. In the headframe-based navigation strategy, the frame of reference is the cranium (Fig 9-21a). Anatomically, this includes the portion of the skull that is superior to the maxillary osteotomy in Le Fort I surgery.

With this system, measurements are taken from the cranial headframe to important landmarks that are to be moved. After the starting position of the landmark is recorded and stored, the fragment can be repositioned. When the indicator is remounted on the headframe, a precise measurement of the new movement can be made. The indicator mounted on the headframe is analogous to the articulator-mounted indicator. The position of the incisor and the cant of the occlusal plane can be directly transferred.

Like the indicators on the articulator, the devices can be unmounted and remounted. The position is reproducible. This allows direct, unobstructed access to the surgical site. The indicator is safely stored and can be repeatedly remounted and referenced during the surgery (Fig 9-21b).

Because the frame of reference is independent of the mandible, proper maxillary repositioning can be verified even after mandibular osteotomies have been completed (Fig 9-22a). It is important to recheck the position of all repositioned segments after all the bone plates have been placed. If there was a major shift in centric relation when general anesthesia was induced, the surgeon must consider what changes will likely appear in the postoperative period when the patient reverts to an awake condylar position. In some cases, special distraction devices are placed to provide a method to adjust the jaw position in the postoperative period.

The net displacement of the central incisor position in three dimensions is verified to meet functional and esthetic objectives before the patient is awakened from general anesthesia (Fig 9-22b). The correction of the maxillary cant is verified independent of the mandible and centric relation (Fig 9-22c). Use of the orthognathic headframe provides a frame of reference for precise and predictable osteotomy surgery (Fig 9-22d).

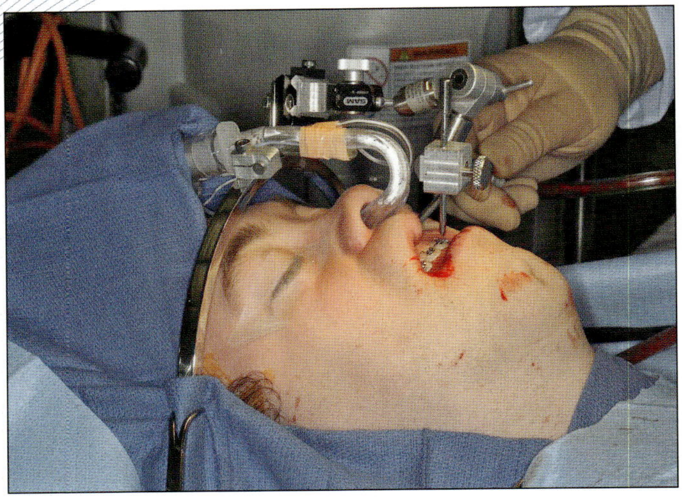

Fig 9-22a During surgery, the indicator is remounted to verify the correct repositioning of any number of critical anatomical structures.

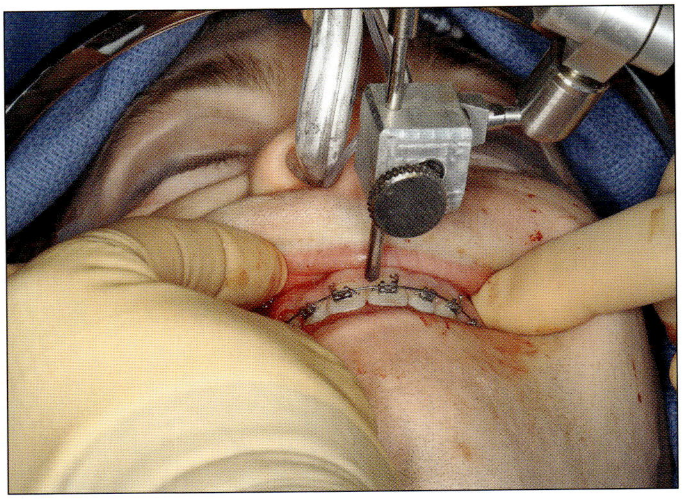

Fig 9-22b The headframe indicators do not depend on the mandible as a frame of reference. At the completion of maxillary and mandibular osteotomies, the indicators are used to verify that the fragment repositioning meets the objectives of the surgical plan.

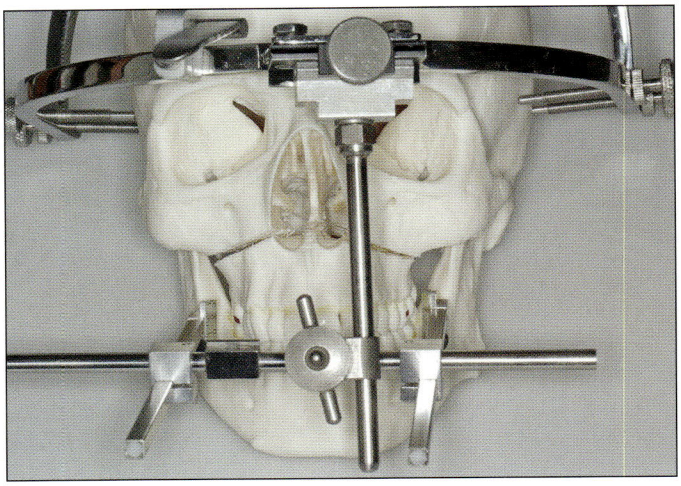

Fig 9-22c Cant-measuring indicator attachments verify that the maxilla has been correctly leveled.

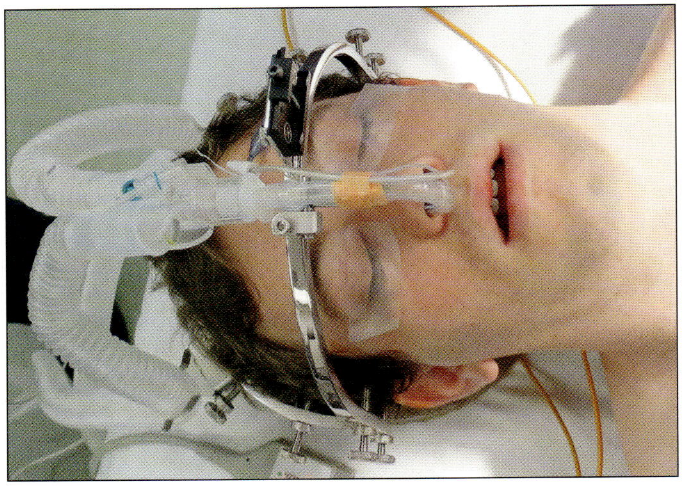

Fig 9-22d The headframe system secures the anesthetic breathing tubes to prevent pressure-related trauma to the nose. The soft tissue drape is also stabilized, avoiding distortion that can alter the appearance of the soft tissue in relation to the dental arch.

Technique

In 1983, an Irby headframe was modified by the author to receive a detachable pointer system that would be used to register the position of the maxillary incisors prior to mobilization of the maxilla with a Le Fort I osteotomy. The Irby headframe was combined with a photographic camera mount, components of an articulator facebow, and a hardware bolt (Fig 9-23a). When assembled, the instrument provided a method of fixation to the skull and a detachable pointer to record anatomical landmarks (Fig 9-23b). This provided a frame of reference that did not move during the course of the procedure. Most headframes intended for facial fractures or distraction osteogenesis can be used to provide a platform for cranial-based navigation. The pointer system allowed direct measurement of the net movement of the maxillary central incisors and assured their correct repositioning with the facial skeleton (Figs 9-23c and 9-23d). Since the first use of the system, the instrumentation has undergone many changes to increase the accuracy and ease of use. The underlying geometric basis has remained the same, however, over 30 years of clinical use.

A representation of the same long-face deformity managed by conventional and enhanced means (see Figs 9-19 and 9-20) will be used to outline how the headframe system is applied to direct correct placement of osteotomy fragments (Fig 9-24a). First, the orthognathic headframe is secured to the calvarium

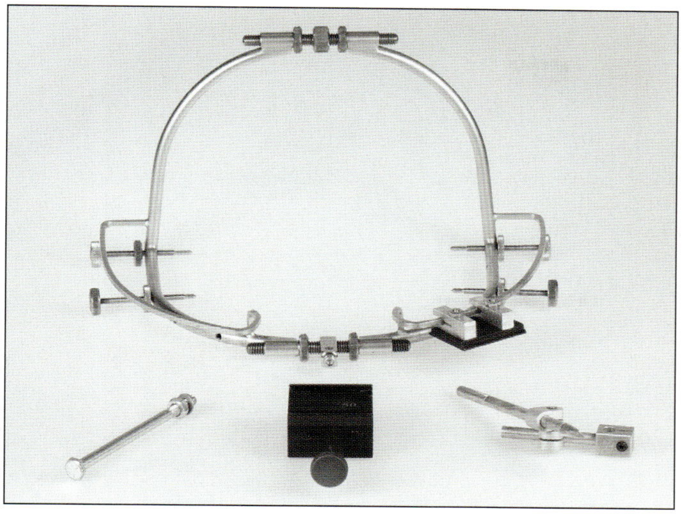

Fig 9-23a An Irby headframe is combined with a hardware bolt, photographic camera mount, and components of an articulator facebow.

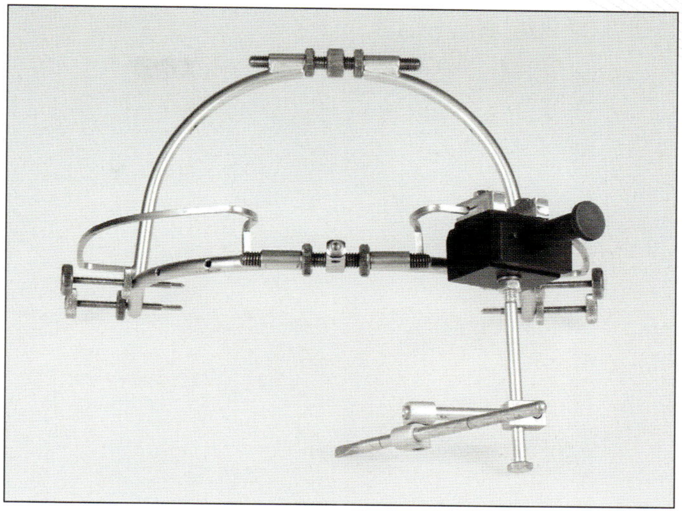

Fig 9-23b The assembled instrument has transcutaneous pins for anchorage into the skull and a detachable pointer to record clinically critical landmarks such as the position of the maxillary central incisors.

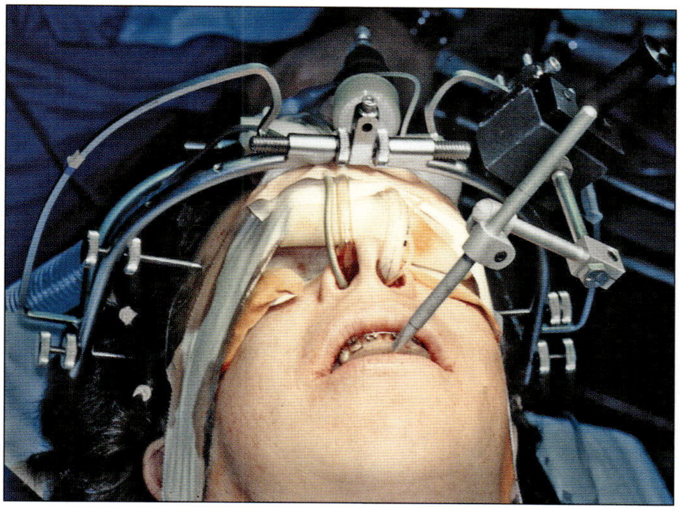

Fig 9-23c Headframe in place during Le Fort I maxillary osteotomy. The indicator shows the position of the maxillary central incisors before the maxilla was repositioned. The maxillary central incisors need to be moved 2 mm to the right.

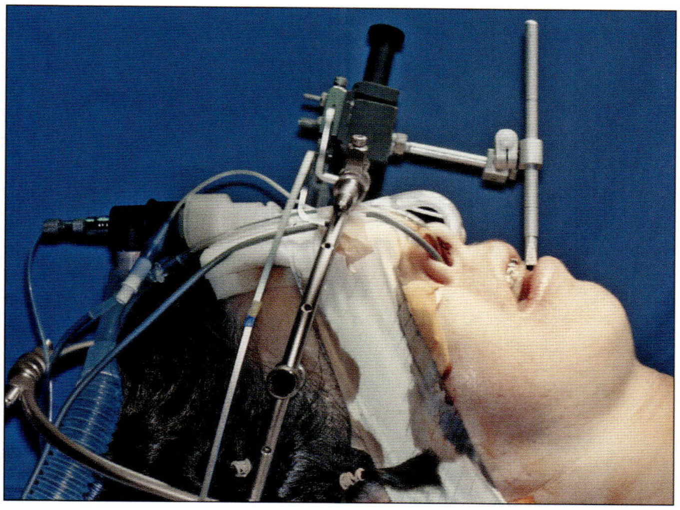

Fig 9-23d The headframe indicator position shows the amount of impaction of the maxillary central incisors as a result of Le Fort I repositioning.

with transcutaneous pins that are positioned within the hairline (Fig 9-24b). Before osteotomies are used to mobilize the jaw fragments, important landmarks, such as the desired position of the maxillary central incisors, are registered by pointer attachments that are engaged into the headframe mount (Fig 9-24c). Any number of landmarks can be registered by the system. In this example, a pointer with two arms is used to register the desired position of the right and left molars in order to correct the cant of the occlusal plane (Fig 9-24d).

After mobilization of the maxilla, it is secured in the intermediary splint. The jaws are placed in maxillomandibular fixation. The maxilla is elevated, and interfering bone is removed (Fig 9-24e). The pointer on the headframe base indicator allows direct measurement of the proper positioning of the maxillary central incisors. The amount of bone removal required to achieve the proper position of the incisors is not determined by cast surgery or virtual simulation. The amount of bone removed is only that needed to achieve the goal of correct incisor positioning (Fig 9-24f).

After it is verified that the maxillary incisors are in the correct position, bone plates are placed to secure the maxillary fragment (Fig 9-24g). Following stabilization of the maxilla with bone plates, the mandibular sagittal ramus osteotomies are completed. The mandible is advanced into the final occlusion splint, and internal fixation of the ramus osteotomies is placed (Fig 9-24h).

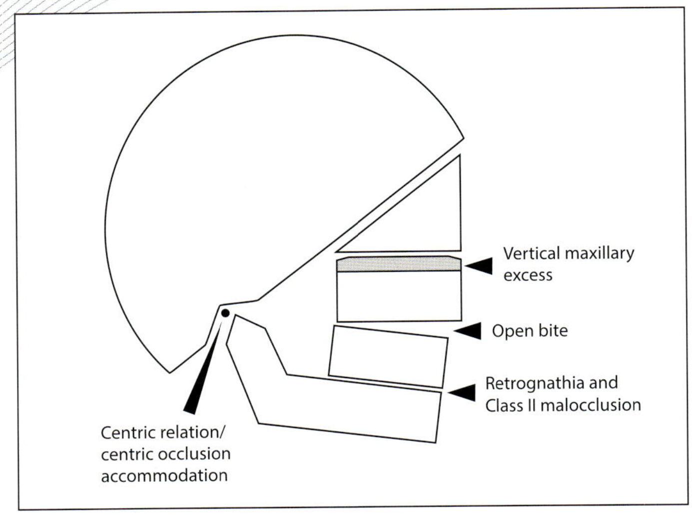

Fig 9-24a The same example of long-face syndrome presented in Figs 9-19 and 9-20 will be used to outline how the headframe system is used to direct correct placement of osteotomy fragments.

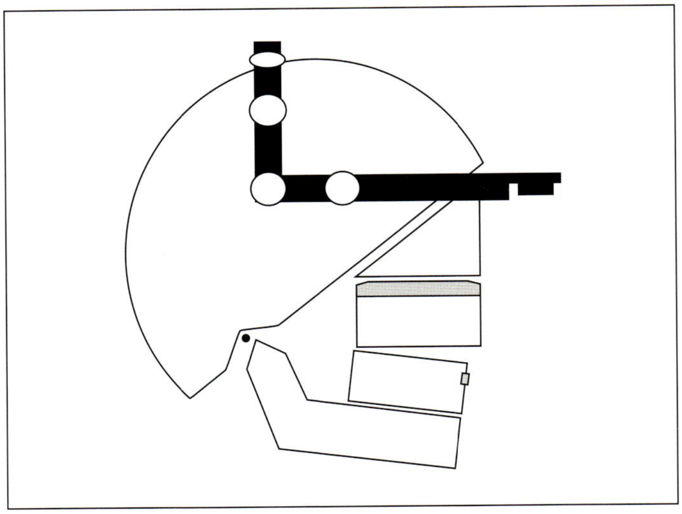

Fig 9-24b The orthognathic headframe is secured to the calvarium using transcutaneous pins that are positioned within the hairline.

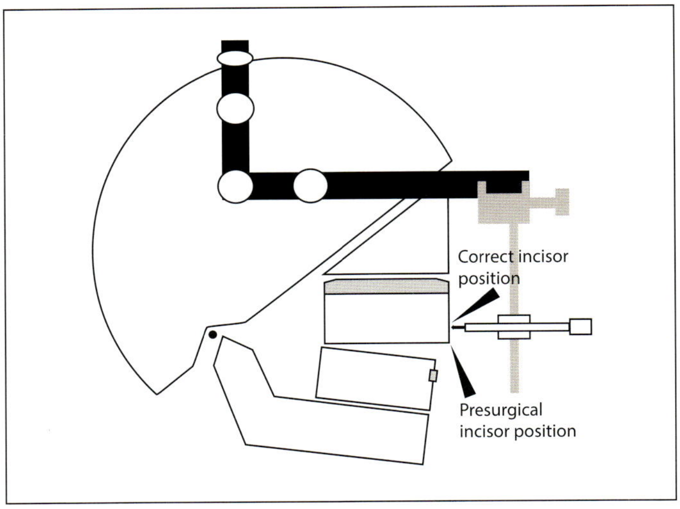

Fig 9-24c Critical landmarks such as the position of the maxillary central incisors are registered first.

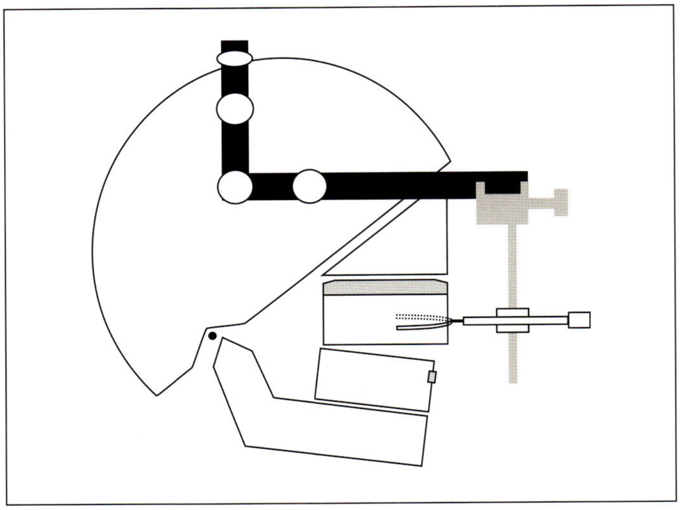

Fig 9-24d Additional landmarks are registered. This fork-shaped indicator is set to the position that represents the corrected cant of the occlusal plane.

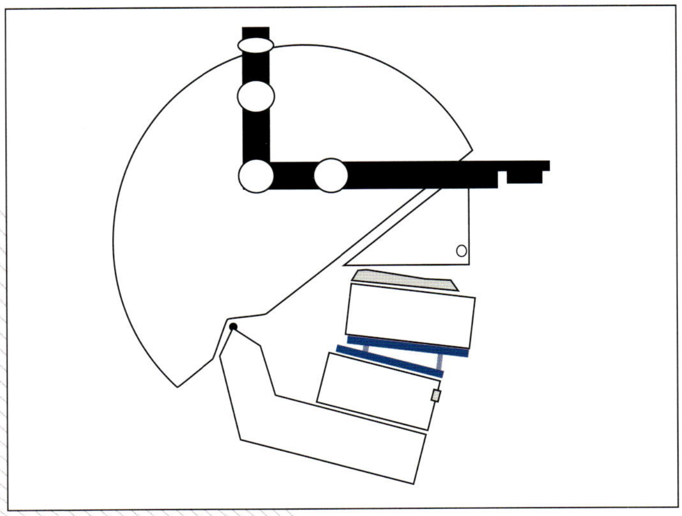

Fig 9-24e The Le Fort I osteotomy is completed, and the intermediary splint is placed. Any interfering bone is removed.

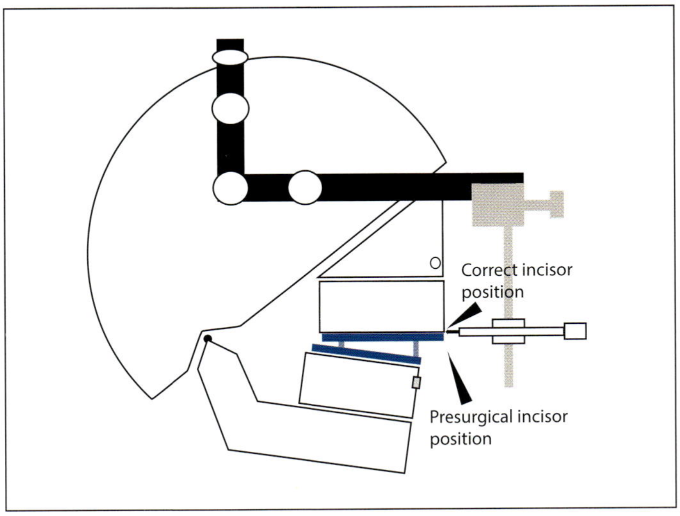

Fig 9-24f The headframe-based indicator guides maxillary positioning.

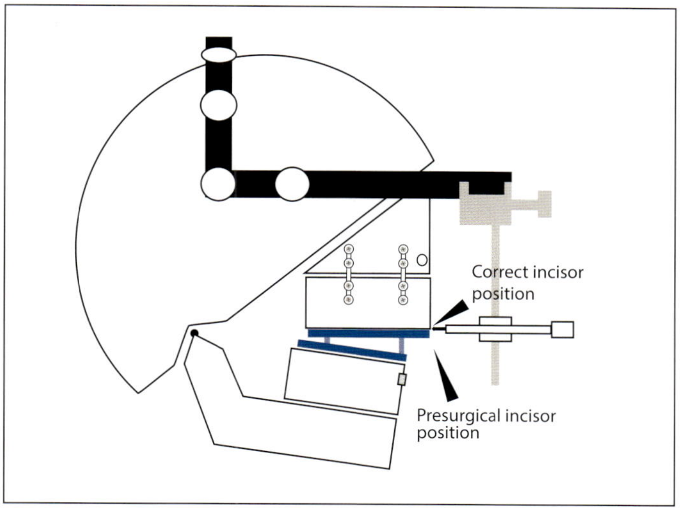

Fig 9-24g Bone plates fix the maxillary position.

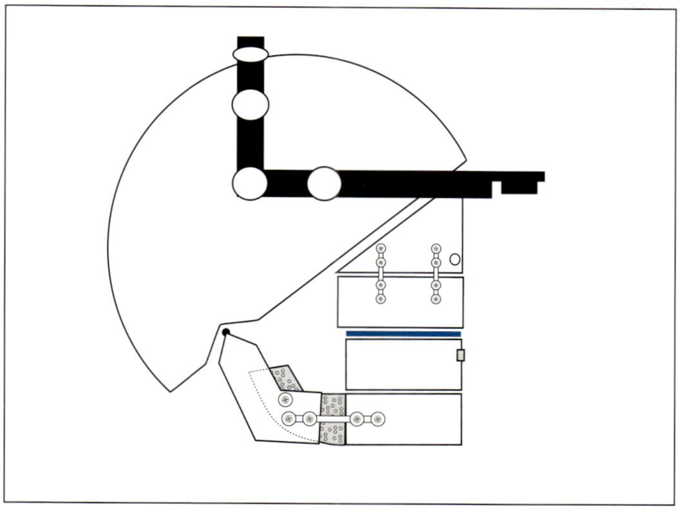

Fig 9-24h The mandibular osteotomies are completed. The sagittal split osteotomy fragments are repositioned using a final occlusion splint. Bone plates and screws establish internal fixation.

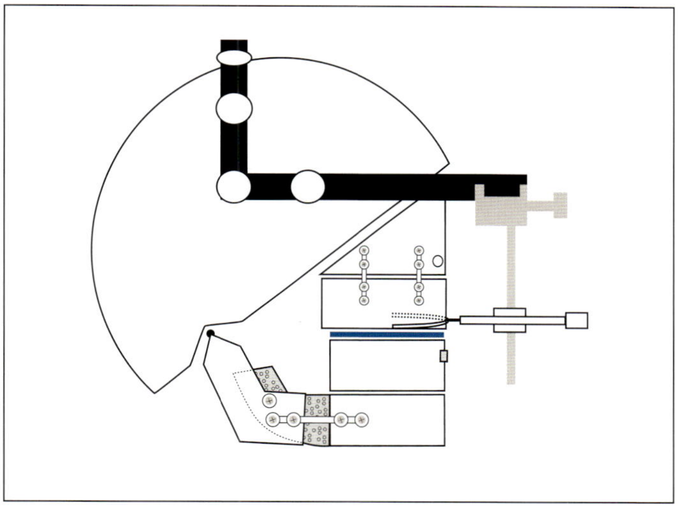

Fig 9-24i Using the fork-shaped occlusal cant indicator that was set earlier (see Fig 9-24d), correction of the occlusal plane is verified.

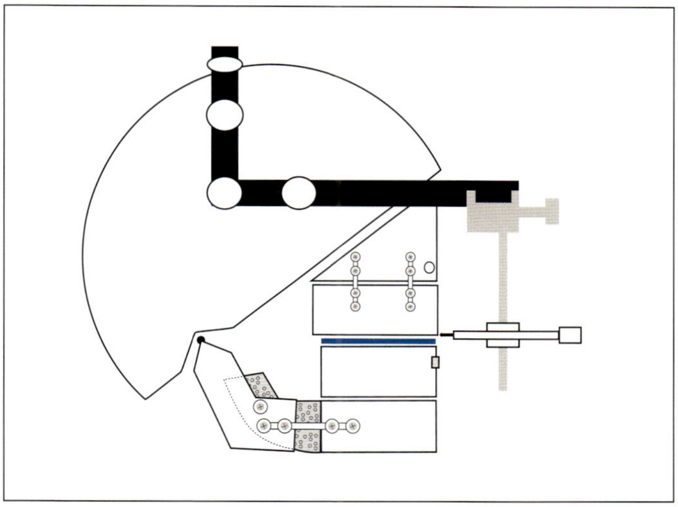

Fig 9-24j Before completing the surgery, the incisor positioning indicator is remounted on the headframe to verify that the central incisors are in the proper position.

The occlusal cant indicator is placed to verify correction of the occlusal cant deformity (Fig 9-24i).

Before completion of the surgery, a final check using the headframe-based indicators verifies that the objectives of treatment have been achieved (Fig 9-24j). If an error is detected at this point, the surgeon can consider whether to introduce a correction. Because the mandible has already been mobilized, the headframe reference points are the only remaining guides from which a correction can be made.

Discussion

The headframe-based navigation system provides a method to accurately reposition osteotomy fragments. The frame of reference remains stable throughout the surgical procedure so it is not vulnerable to errors introduced by condylar position or measurements across the osteotomy line. Because the measurements do not depend on the mandible, the reference remains intact after mobilization of mandibular osteotomies.

Clinical Application of Navigation Techniques

Surgical results that deviate substantially from the planned objective are the most common source of patient dissatisfaction. Patients are most likely to express disappointment when there is a visible esthetic problem that falls short of their expectations. Issues of dental asymmetry and the appearance of the maxillary teeth when smiling are a greater concern to patients than occlusion or even paresthesia. Ideally, these problems would be prevented by control techniques incorporated in the planning and surgical processes. When these problems occur, it is important to analyze and understand how the error occurred and to have a strategy to correct the problem.

The following case report illustrates the common pitfalls that lead to major errors in repositioning of osteotomy fragments. Minor errors occur in most cases and are within the acceptable tolerance of the patient and surgeon. The magnitude of these errors is occasionally unacceptable, however. If the problem is not detected and corrected at the time of initial surgery, it emerges during the early postoperative period. If the error cannot be accepted or mitigated, revision surgery is indicated.

Some surgeons prefer to allow the osteotomies to heal in the incorrect position prior to revision surgery and then to start the planning and surgical process over again. Allowing the osteotomies to consolidate in the incorrect position introduces its own problems because the remodeling process of healing distorts the skeletal morphology into an unpredictable, unnatural form. Limiting the potential for nerve injury is another consideration in timing of revision surgery. If mandibular sagittal split osteotomies have already been performed, revising the positions of the segments carries less potential for nerve damage than repeating the osteotomy on a healed site.

These cases pose a special challenge because the initial orthognathic procedure alters and destabilizes the landmarks surgeons depend on. The familiar sequence for maxillomandibular surgery cannot be followed.

This case demonstrates how major errors occur. Major fragment repositioning errors are almost always the result of both physiologic and planning anomalies. Almost all patients requiring revision surgery demonstrate dual positions of centric relation. If centric relation is captured on the preoperative awake patient, it will often not be obtainable under general anesthesia. The unique and special position centric relation assumes under general anesthesia may deviate in an asymmetric and unpredictable manner. Surgical planning and splints that incorporate awake centric relation introduce an osteotomy repositioning error through this phenomenon.

The problem is compounded when the moderate shift displaces the index marks across the maxillary osteotomy. This alters the osseous landmarks and can disorient the surgeon who is trying to reconcile why the surgical findings differ from those predicted during the planning phase. It is how the surgeon chooses to reconcile these findings that corrects or worsens the problem. Failure to prepare for the situation and lack of a predetermined path to diagnosis and correction of the problem that presents are the basic etiology of these unacceptable outcomes.

The method presented to manage this case can be applied to prevent these problems and increase the predictability of these procedures. The existence of a reliable frame of reference that is accessible in real time can allow rapid fragment repositioning with quantifiable confidence.

The system also allows for deviation from the surgical plan. Most surgeons planning treatment with either virtual or conventional cast surgery methods settle on a single plan. Splints and measurements of projected osteotomy displacement are made with a single objective in mind. The limitation of this approach is that surgical findings often limit the feasibility and safety of performing specific osteotomy movements. Certain cases are predisposed to unexpected obstacles in achieving the desired, projected, and planned movements. The cleft lip and palate patient with a history of multiple surgeries can confront the surgeon with an inability to reposition a fragment because of scar tissue or compromised perfusion.

In these and other situations, the surgeon may wish to change the treatment intraoperatively. Departing from a splint-based surgery plan can make surgeons uncomfortable, particularly when no other frame of reference is available. In addition, issues of pedicle viability, unexpected osteotomy fractures, and vascular anomalies sometimes force the decision to abandon splints. In these cases, it is valuable and reassuring to have a system that can quantify how the change in plan will affect the final result.

Correction of a Repositioning Error

A 20-year-old college student presented with a Class III malocclusion (Fig 9-25a). This case was very typical of the kind that presents every day to maxillofacial surgeons. There were no unusual complicating issues. It was decided that the moderate Class III facial pattern was best treated with a Le Fort I maxillary advancement and mandibular setback using internal fixation (Fig 9-25b). A posteroanterior cephalometric radiograph showed the deformity to be basically symmetric (Fig 9-25c). Presurgical orthodontic treatment coordinated the dental arches for a single-piece Le Fort I osteotomy and a mandibular setback with sagittal split osteotomies (Figs 9-25d to 9-25f).

Three weeks after undergoing orthognathic surgery without cranial-based navigation, the patient presented for a second surgical opinion on the result and the possible need for revision (Fig 9-25g). The primary concern of the patient was unexpected asymmetry. The perception of the patient and his family was that the midline of the dental arch was incorrect and the occlusal plane was canted.

Despite some residual edema, it was clinically apparent that the jaws had been repositioned incorrectly (Fig 9-25h). Although the occlusion was basically Class I, the patient and family would not accept this magnitude of asymmetry. A posteroanterior cephalometric radiograph confirmed that a major asymmetry had been introduced during the fragment repositioning process (Fig 9-25i). The maxilla was canted, and the mandible was repositioned to meet the objective of occlusion. The result was that both jaws were canted. Asymmetric maxillary impaction

Fig 9-25 Correction of a repositioning error in a 20-year-old man.

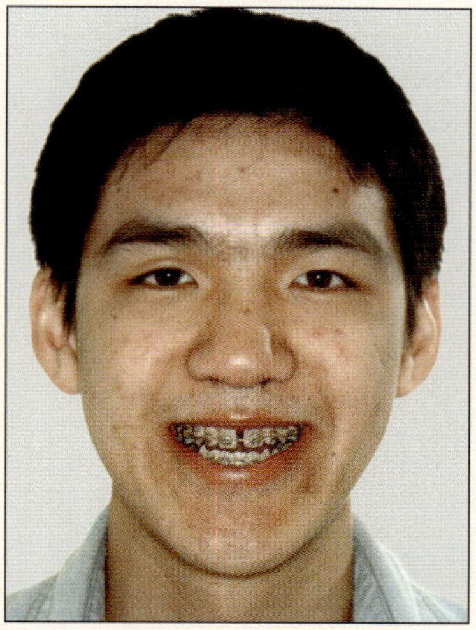

Fig 9-25a Presurgical facial appearance of a 20-year-old man being prepared for orthognathic surgery.

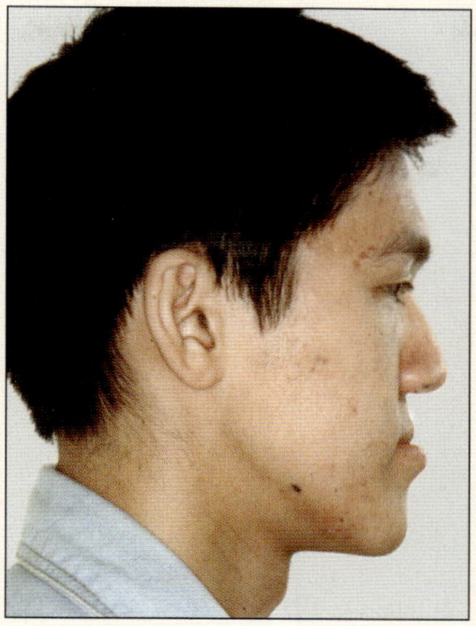

Fig 9-25b A moderate Class III facial pattern is best treated with a Le Fort I maxillary advancement and mandibular setback using internal fixation.

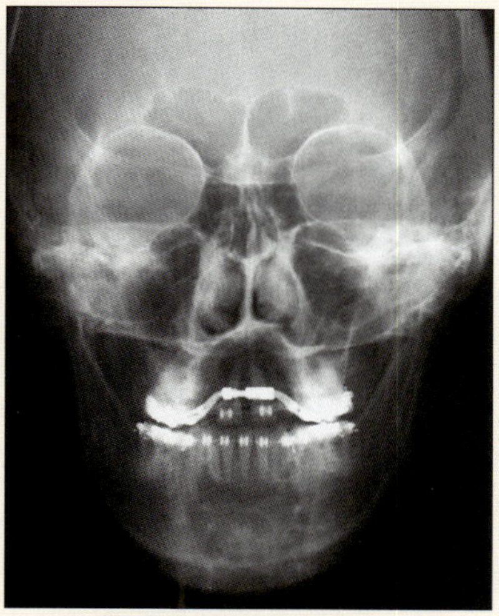

Fig 9-25c The posteroanterior cephalometric radiograph indicates that the deformity is basically symmetric.

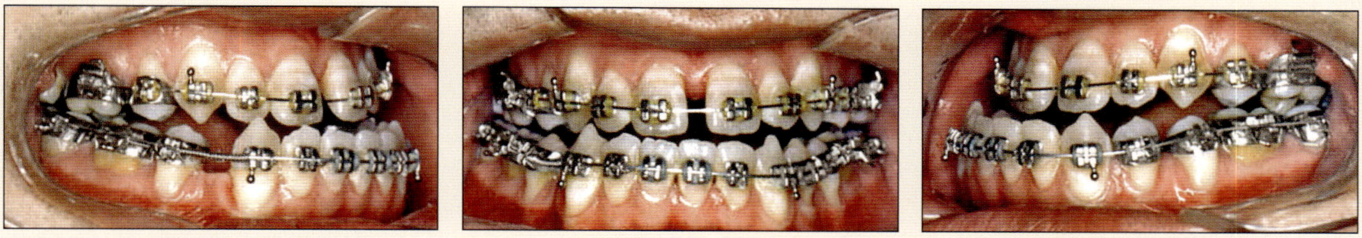

Figs 9-25d to 9-25f Presurgical orthodontic treatment has coordinated the dental arches for a single-piece Le Fort I osteotomy and a mandibular setback with sagittal split osteotomies.

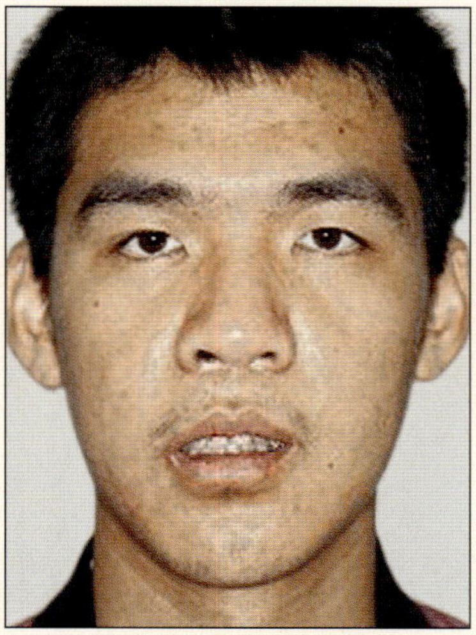

Fig 9-25g Major asymmetry is apparent 3 weeks after maxillary and mandibular osteotomies performed without cranial-based navigation.

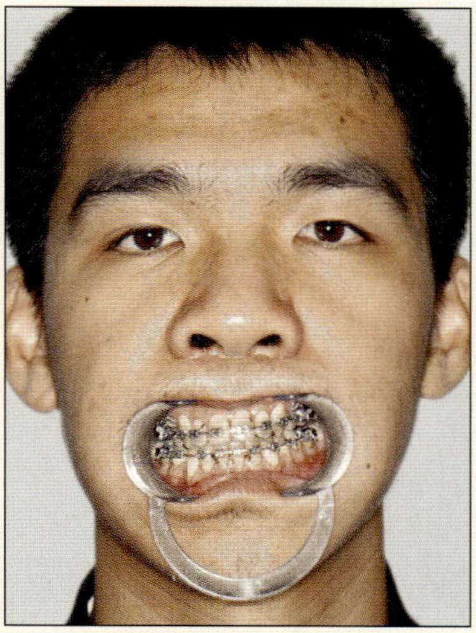

Fig 9-25h A photograph reveals the incorrect repositioning of the maxilla and mandible.

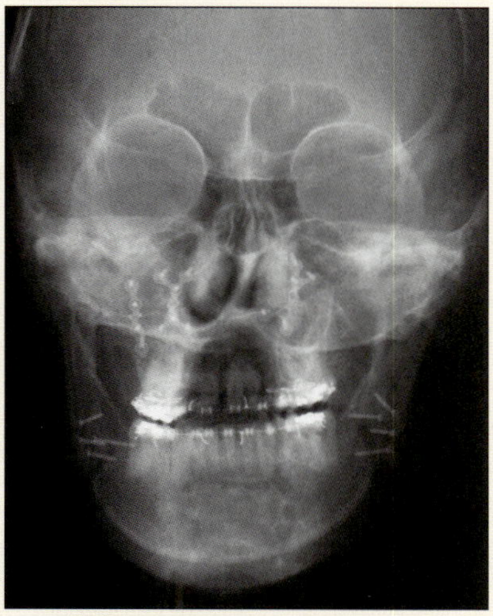

Fig 9-25i Skeletal structures are canted and off the facial midline.

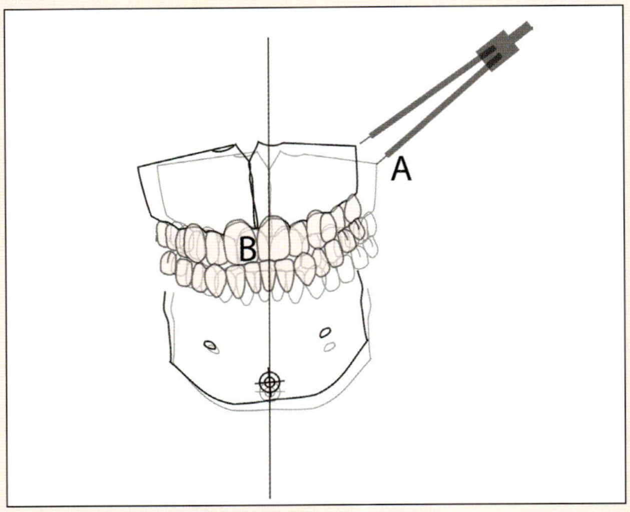

Fig 9-25j The location and magnitude of the repositioning error are analyzed. A combination of left-sided impaction (A) and medial displacement of the maxillary fragment has resulted in an undesirable occlusal plane cant and right-sided displacement of the central incisors (B).

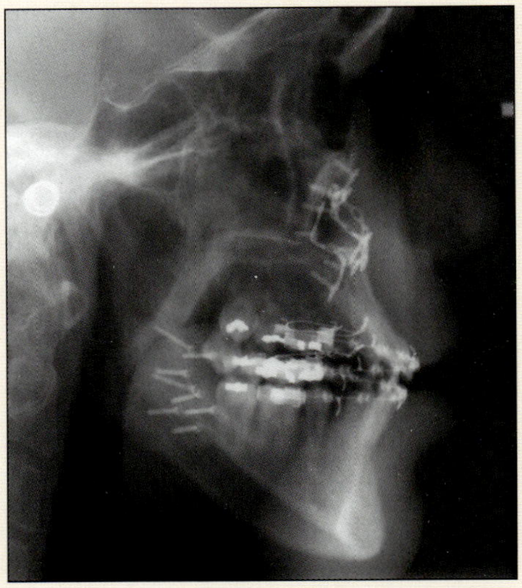

Fig 9-25k The lateral cephalometric radiograph demonstrates that a cant has been introduced during repositioning of the fragment.

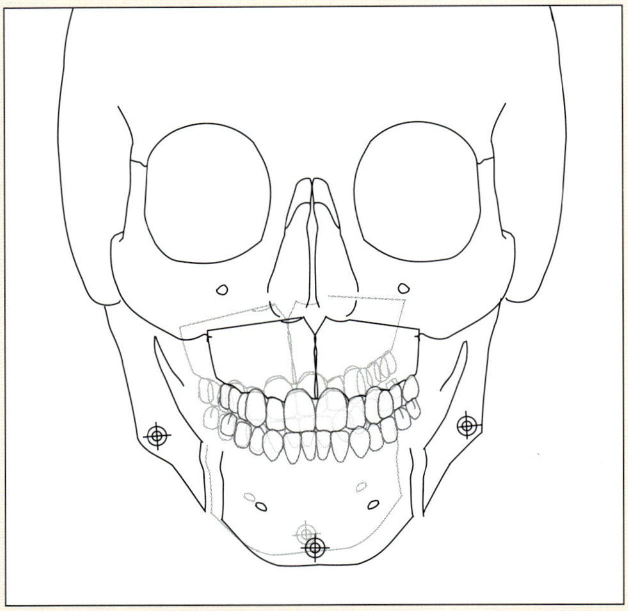

Fig 9-25l The surgical revision strategy shows the magnitude and direction of corrective movements.

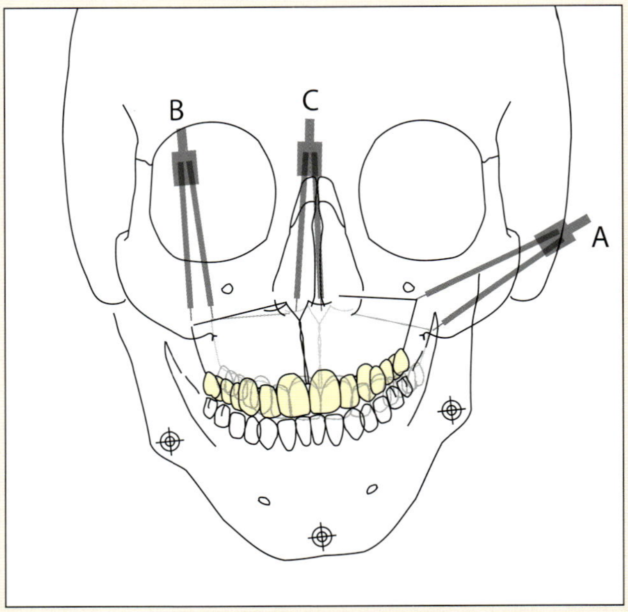

Fig 9-25m A projected 10-mm left maxillary downgraft (A) will require bone grafting. The predicted movement at site B is primarily rotational with medial translation. The objective at site C is to reposition the nasal base toward the left and inferiorly to allow straightening of the nasal septum.

resulted in deviation of the piriform apertures and deviation of the nasal septum.

The use of measurements across the osteotomy to reposition Le Fort I fragments can produce unpredictable displacement of distant structures. In this case, a combination of left-sided impaction and medial displacement of the maxillary fragment resulted in an undesirable occlusal plane cant and right-sided displacement of the central incisors (Fig 9-25j).

The postoperative lateral cephalometric radiograph also demonstrated that a large cant was introduced during the osteotomy repositioning process (Fig 9-25k). The maxillary bone plates were fixed to the stable and accessible sites across the osteotomy. This true lateral radiograph revealed that the distance between the posterior plate and the anterior plate was very short. This reflected the inherent anatomical limitation of the site. The use of landmarks located between the bone plates to orient the maxillary osteotomy and subsequently the mandibular osteotomy is prone to error because of geometry. This is how a moderate error at the maxillary osteotomy line is amplified on distant structures.

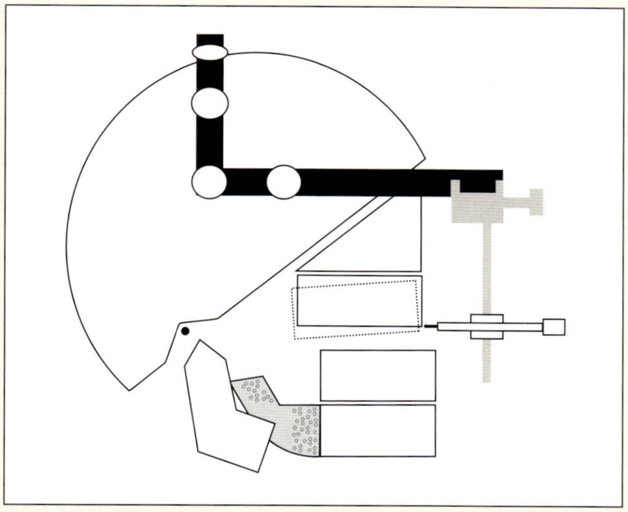

Fig 9-25n The headframe provides a frame of reference independent of the unstable maxilla and mandible. In this case, the osteotomies remained mobile from the prior procedure and could not be used to orient fragments.

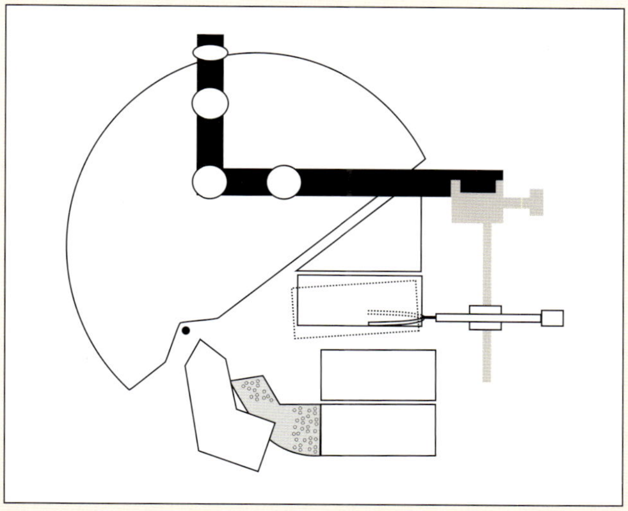

Fig 9-25o The surgical plan includes use of an occlusal cant indicator to guide leveling of the occlusal plane.

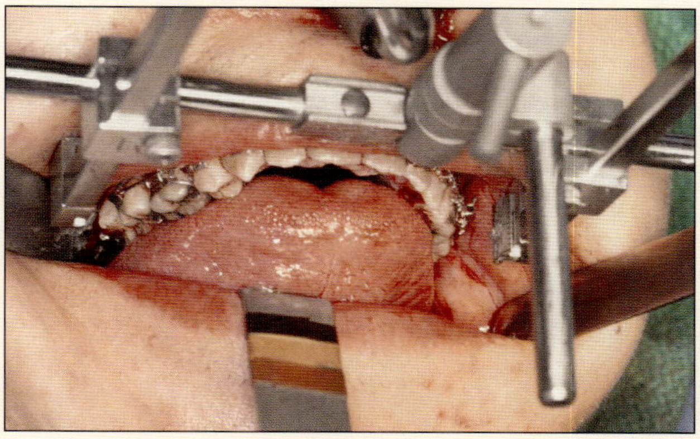

Fig 9-25p After the maxilla is remobilized, the occlusal cant indicator is used to guide the leveling process. The indicator is connected to the headframe above.

To correct the errors, casts were created and mock surgery was performed (Fig 9-25l). The result of the design phase was a surgical plan that involved removing the bone plates and altering the position of the osteotomy fragments before osseous union occurred.

The revision design included repositioning of the maxilla (Fig 9-25m). The left maxillary osteotomy required movement downward and laterally. Cast surgery estimated the resultant gap to be 8 to 10 mm at site A. Because this surgery predated bone morphogenetic proteins, bone grafting was needed. Downgrafting of a hypoplastic maxilla introduces challenges in healing and management of potential relapse. The predicted movement at site B was primarily rotational with medial translation. The objective at site C was to reposition the nasal base toward the left and inferiorly to allow straightening of the nasal septum. The challenge was to manage potential deviation of the nasal septum should the maxillary downgraft fail and relapse.

In a conventional setting, maxillary osteotomies are repositioned with the aid of an intermediary splint and the mandible rotating on a hinge axis. In this case, the mandible had been destabilized by osteotomies and was not a reliable reference source. To establish an accurate, immobile, and accessible frame of reference for repositioning the osteotomy segments, a headframe was placed to allow mounting of location indicators (Fig 9-25n). The headframe was analogous to the upper member of the articulator in cast surgery. This allowed direct transfer of spatial displacement measurements from the articulator indicators to the headframe indicators during surgery.

The most important esthetic landmark was the position of the maxillary central incisors. This position was transferred from the articulator to the headframe with a single pointer. In this case, there was a need to correct the occlusal cant with a left-sided maxillary downgraft (Fig 9-25o).

When the maxilla was leveled, there was a very large gap across the left Le Fort I osteotomy line. Physical measurements across this type of gap are not useful and cannot predict the positions of the occlusal plane or maxillary central incisors. Therefore, a second indicator was attached to the headframe for analysis of cant correction (Fig 9-25p). This indicator was analogous to the two posterior indicators on the articulator. The cant-measuring device showed the position of the maxillary right and left molars before and after revision repositioning. Again, the measurements were independent of the mandible and centric relation. The indicated movement required downgrafting of

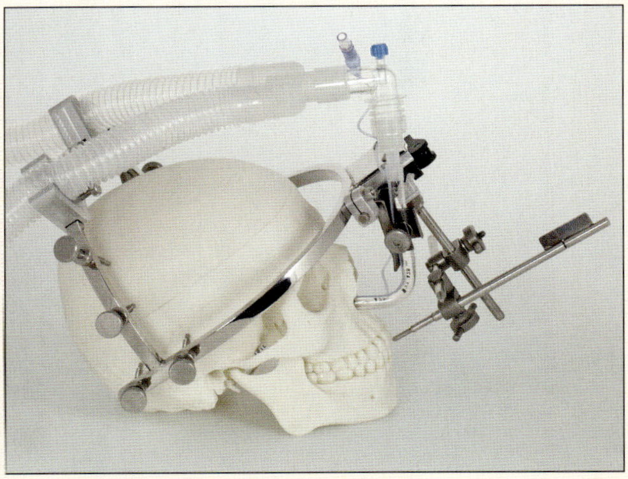

Fig 9-25q The correct positioning of the maxillary central incisors is verified using a single-pointer indicator on the headframe.

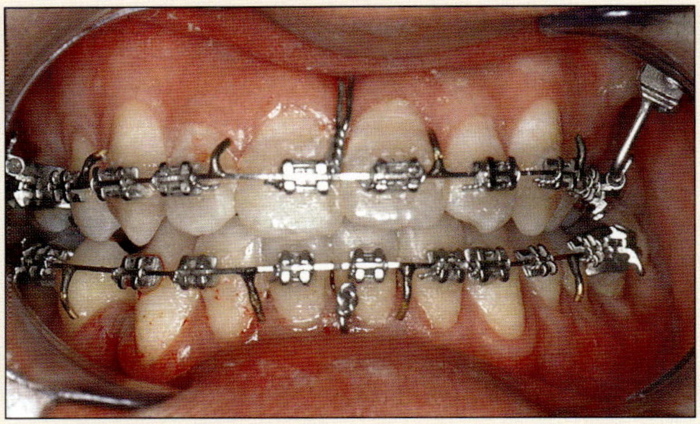

Fig 9-25r After the maxilla has been repositioned, the mandibular osteotomies are mobilized, and internal fixation is placed.

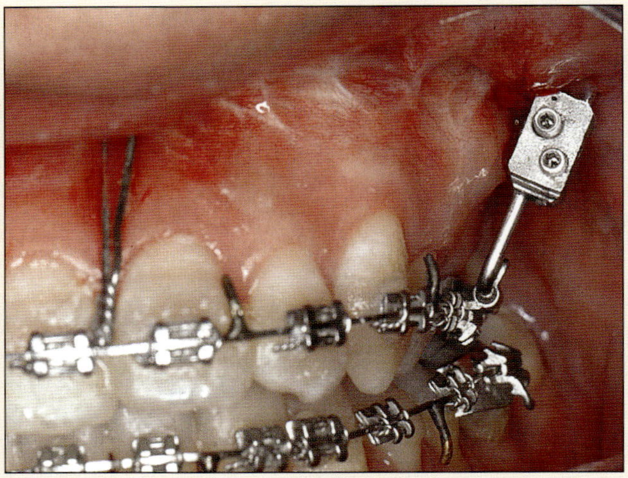

Fig 9-25s A vertical distraction device is placed on the left side to increase the downgraft position as necessary.

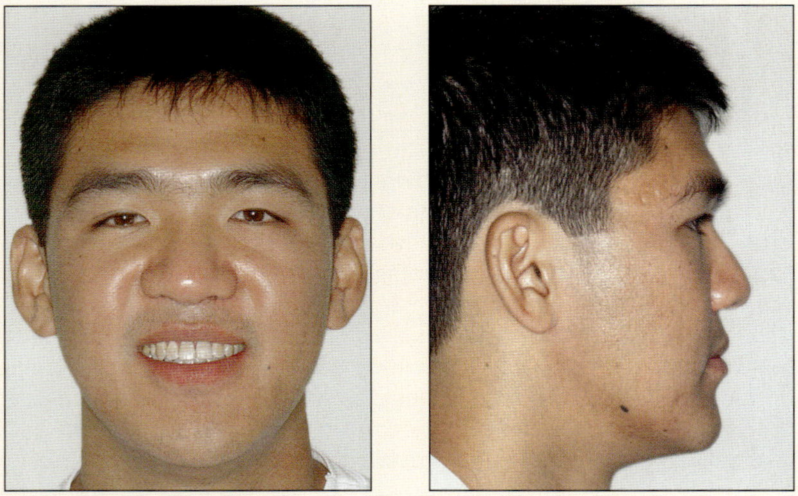

Figs 9-25t and 9-25u Patient's appearance 6 months after revision surgery.

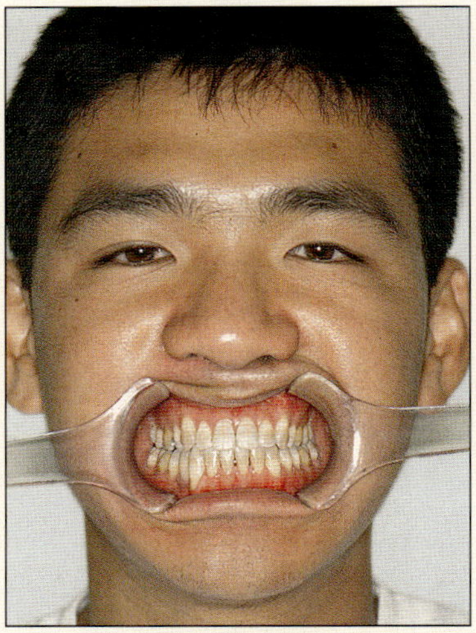

Fig 9-25v Correction of the maxillary midline and occlusal cant at 6 months.

→

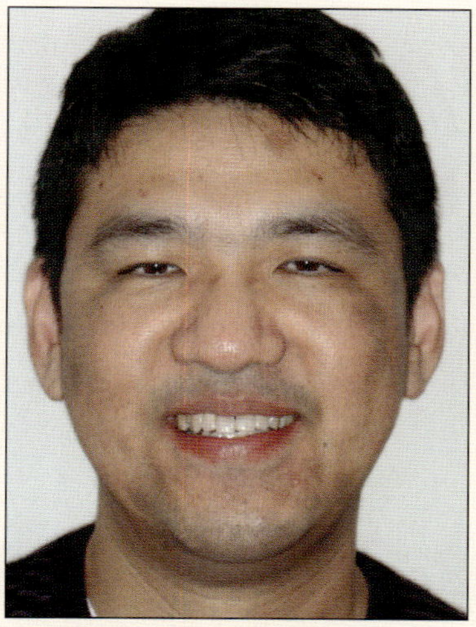

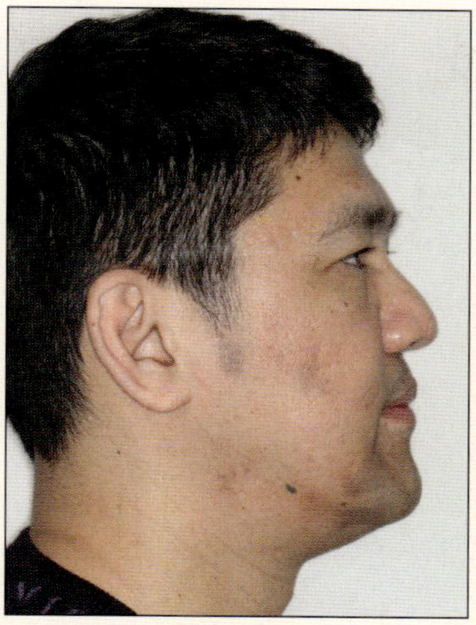

Figs 9-25w and 9-25x Facial appearance at the 20-year follow-up.

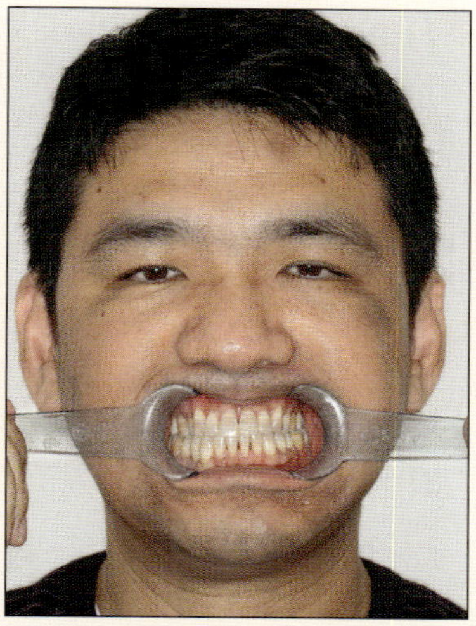

Fig 9-25y Correction of the maxillary midline and occlusal cant has remained stable.

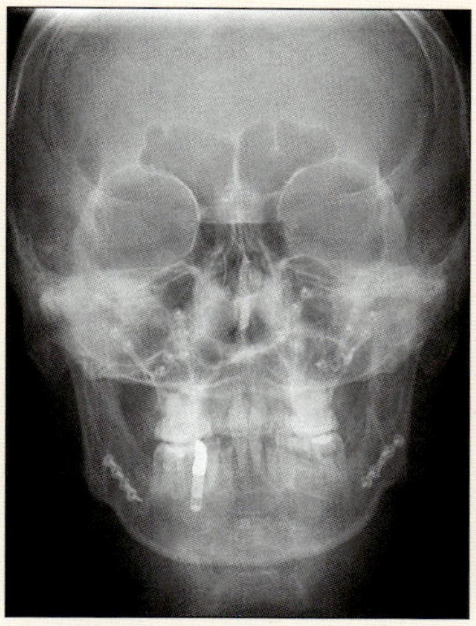

Fig 9-25z A radiograph taken at the 20-year follow-up evaluation shows osseous union across the lateral maxilla and stable correction of the dental midline. The nasal base and nasal septum are at the midline.

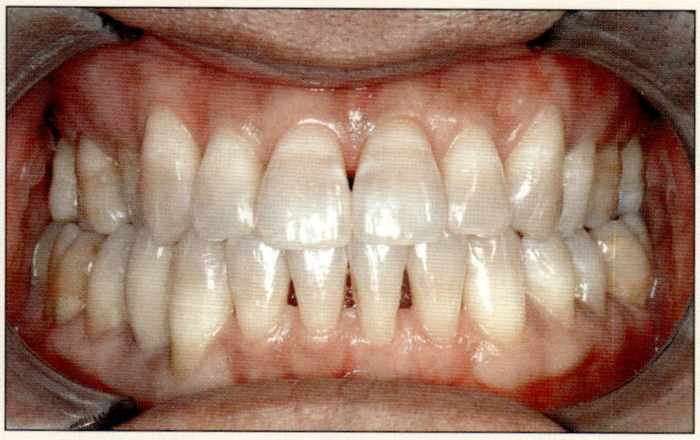

Fig 9-25aa The occlusion has remained stable over the 20 years since revision surgery.

the left maxilla and lateral translation of the posterior maxilla to the left.

Correct positioning of the maxillary central incisors was verified using a single-pointer indicator on the headframe (Fig 9-25q). Figure 9-25r shows the occlusion following revision Le Fort I maxillary osteotomy with bone grafting. The mandibular sagittal split osteotomies were revised by removing the bicortical fixation screws, correcting the fragment positions, and reestablishing internal fixation with bone plates with monocortical screws.

Because some relapse of the maxillary downgraft was anticipated, a distraction device was mounted on the left side (Fig 9-25s). The device was anchored superiorly into the zygomatic buttress and inferiorly into the molar bracket facebow tube. It was an internal device that could be activated transorally. During the postoperative period, some vertical collapse of the left side was observed. The distraction device was activated to compensate for this movement and resist vertical collapse. Follow-up 6 months after revision surgery revealed that the occlusal plane cant and dental midline deviation had been corrected (Figs 9-25t to 9-25v).

Twenty years after revision surgery, correction of the maxillary midline and occlusal cant remained stable (Figs 9-25w to 9-25y). The cephalometric radiograph taken at the patient's 20-year follow-up evaluation revealed osseous union across the lateral maxilla and stable correction of the dental midline. The nasal base and nasal septum were at the midline (Fig 9-25z). The occlusion had remained stable since revision surgery (Fig 9-25aa). The patient had gone to medical school and now practices internal medicine.

Conclusion

Although the literature presents many examples of orthognathic surgery that has produced dramatic and beautiful results, predictability remains a challenge. Providing a consistent result requires a planning and surgical process that has the capability of delivering osteotomy fragment repositioning at a tolerance that is at the level of esthetic restorative dentistry. Techniques that rely on the position of the condyle to orient fragments cannot deliver a consistent result because the mandible assumes a unique and unpredictable position in response to general anesthesia. Creation of articulator-based cast surgery mock-ups with auxiliary landmarks allows fabrication of splints that will meet the objectives of precise maxillary incisor and occlusal cant positioning. The headframe-based navigation system allows rapid and definitive verification that the desired objective of osteotomy fragment repositioning has been achieved.

10 Comparing Mechanical and Virtual Surgical Planning

Osteotomy and repositioning of bone segments are sometimes necessary to establish a successful bone-forming environment. In addition to promoting formation of new bone, the repositioned segments alter the position of teeth and dental implant sites. If a segment is not properly repositioned, the error in the position of the teeth compromises the esthetic and functional result. If the segment contains healed dental implants, the implants in the malpositioned osteotomy segment may be impossible to restore.

Today's patients hold high expectations of the esthetic result of surgery and implant restorations. Achieving a consistent result requires a technique that delivers accuracy within limits acceptable to demanding patients. Both mechanical and virtual planning techniques have strengths and limitations. The purpose of this chapter is to compare and contrast how mechanical and virtual planning are applied to cases involving repositioning of the maxilla, mandible, and jaw segments. In some aspects, neither system can deliver the necessary result. In such cases, an alternative strategy must be in place before the surgery is undertaken.

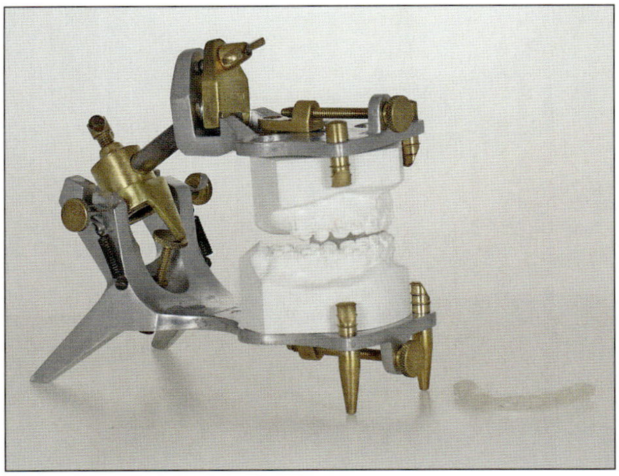

Fig 10-1 Galleti articulator holding dental casts during fabrication of acrylic resin surgical splints.

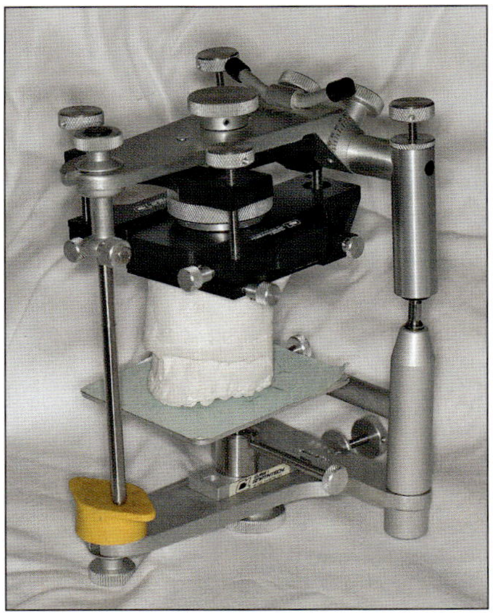

Fig 10-2 Surgical articulator designed by Dr Brian Wong (modified from the SAM articulator system). Multiple micrometers allow repositioning of mounted casts in different axes. How to transfer this information to the surgical setting remains problematic.

Historical Perspective

Mechanical surgical planning has been standard practice for many years. The techniques and instrumentation for early orthognathic surgical planning were adapted from the methods used to plan the repair of facial fractures. Surgical mock-ups used plaster casts mounted on dental articulators.

Early orthognathic treatments were limited to single-jaw surgeries in which the focus was to correct gross malocclusions. Lateral cephalometric radiographs were used to estimate the gross movements necessary to correct the facial deformity and establish a functional occlusion. Splints were fabricated using simple articulators such as the Galleti (Fig 10-1).

Planning grew more complex as maxillomandibular surgery, involving segmental Le Fort I osteotomies and simultaneous mandibular osteotomies, became standard practice. Orthodontists and surgeons sought to meet the challenge by developing more complex articulators. In 1985, Dr Brian Wong developed an articulator that moved the casts with multiple micrometers (Fig 10-2). The system allowed precise measurements of plaster cast movements in three dimensions. The limitation was an inability to transfer the measurements to the surgical site and to verify that the intended jaw movements had been achieved.

In 1986, Contour Medical Systems introduced Cemax, the first system to use computed tomography (CT) digital data to plan surgery. Five prototype workstations were constructed, including the one installed in the author's office to beta test its usefulness for maxillofacial surgical planning (Fig 10-3a). The technique was challenged by the limitations of CT technology, software, and computer processing speed. Its practical use was limited to special applications such as fabrication of custom distraction devices for uncommon craniofacial anomalies. The process allowed fabrication of skeletal models that could be used in mechanical surgical planning (Fig 10-3b). The milled models were also useful in designing custom prosthetics such as distraction devices (Fig 10-3c). Simple skeletal reconstructions could be planned in the virtual environment. The major hurdle to clinical use was difficulty in transferring computer imaging data to the surgical site with convenience and accuracy.

Modern virtual surgical planning uses specialized software to analyze and merge digital data obtained from multiple sources.[2-5] At this time, no single source of image data can adequately represent the patient's clinical condition. CT studies obtained from a medical CT scanner or a dental cone beam CT (CBCT) scanner provide the primary digital data to create a basic three-dimensional virtual image. Optical scanning studies provide data to form a virtual image of the shapes of the teeth. Facial photographs can be merged with the CT data, resulting in a three-dimensional image.

The imaging software allows viewing of a specific subset of the data so that a clinically useful view can be generated. The surface topography of the facial skeleton, for example, can be viewed with the soft tissue digitally removed. The software also allows spatial movement of virtual jaw segments. In the virtual environment, the maxilla can be separated from the midface, simulating a Le Fort I osteotomy. The virtual Le Fort I fragment can be moved within the virtual environment, and the consequence of the movement can be analyzed virtually.

Study of occlusal changes in the virtual environment currently requires optical scanning of plaster casts. The occlusion of the maxillary and mandibular dental arches cannot be evaluat-

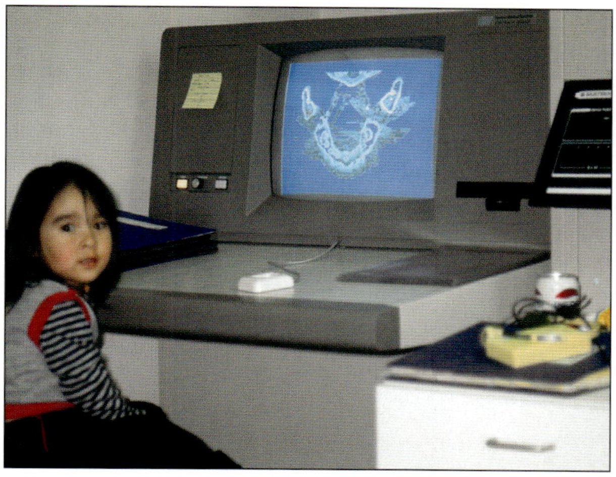

Fig 10-3a Early Cemax workstation during beta testing in 1986.

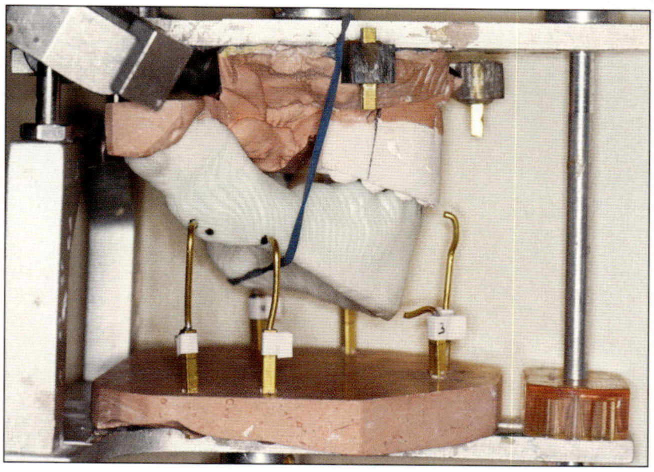

Fig 10-3b Computer-milled mandible from the Cemax 1000 system is merged with dental casts for surgical planning. The patient is a child with hemifacial microsomia. The milled model is embedded into an articulator-based mechanical model surgery in an adaptation of the technique described by Vargervik.[1]

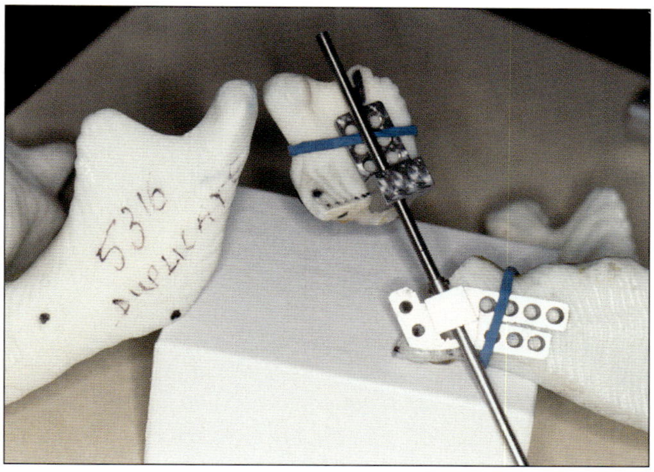

Fig 10-3c Distraction devices are fabricated directly on the mechanical model.

ed with CT image data. Current virtual imaging systems require plaster casts to determine the final occlusion. After virtual surgical planning is complete, three-dimensional printers can fabricate surgical splints directly from digital image data.

The development of new virtual planning tools raises several questions:

- Have these technologic advances made planning in a virtual environment superior to mechanical planning in a clinical setting?
- What are the advantages and disadvantages of each of these surgical planning methods?
- How accurate are the two surgical planning methods?
- What types of errors are inherent to these systems?
- Why do osteotomy fragments end up in unexpected positions?
- Are there methods to improve the precision and predictability of these planning methods?

To compare mechanical and virtual planning, a typical maxillomandibular orthognathic surgery case is presented. The treatment comprised a Le Fort I maxillary osteotomy in two segments and bilateral sagittal split ramus osteotomies.

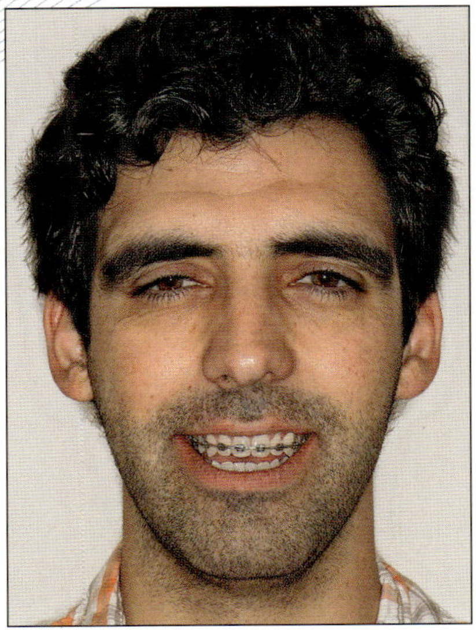

Fig 10-4a A typical patient requiring maxillary and mandibular osteotomies for treatment of malocclusion.

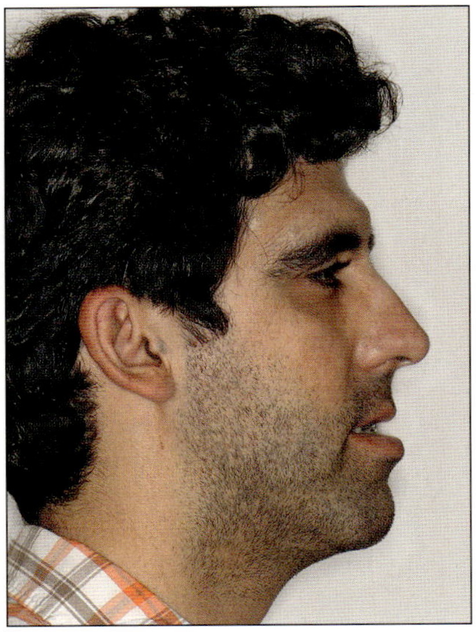

Fig 10-4b The neck form limits the amount the mandible should be set back.

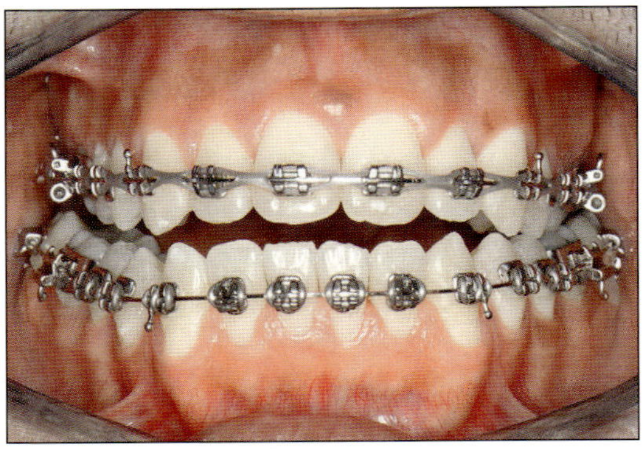

Fig 10-4c Oral examination reveals an asymmetric Class III open bite malocclusion.

Procedures for Surgical Planning

Case description

A 29-year-old man presented with a Class III open bite malocclusion. Initial evaluation suggested that a Le Fort I maxillary osteotomy in two segments and bilateral mandibular osteotomies would likely be needed. The patient underwent presurgical orthodontics to prepare the dental arches for orthognathic surgery.

Evaluation

Whether a case is planned mechanically on articulated casts or in a virtual environment on a computer, the initial evaluation is the same. The chief complaint, history, and physical examination combine to formulate a diagnosis that is the origin of the treatment plan. In this case, the patient desired to have his teeth function with a better occlusion and to maintain basically the same facial form. Examination revealed *(1)* skeletal open bite, *(2)* a 2-mm deviation of the maxillary dental midline to the left side, *(3)* mandibular asymmetry, and *(4)* a slight maxillary cant (Figs 10-4a to 10-4c).

Unless video is a part of the clinical records, the physical examination is the sole opportunity for the surgeon to study and understand how the patient uses the face in motion. Static records and measurements cannot fully capture how the patient has adapted to a specific physical anomaly during mastication and speech. Although mechanical function of the jaws and teeth is an important goal, the patient's ability to maintain or improve his or her social interactive potential is always a major objective. Facial expression patterns and the smile are integral to the communication process. Orthognathic and dental restorative treatments have the potential to alter the underlying dental and facial structure. The surgical process also impacts the posture and range of motion of facial movements. From a functional perspective, standard measurements of anatomical norms do not necessarily meet the objective of an ideal result.

This patient displayed a degree of vertical maxillary hyperplasia. When he smiled, he exposed a greater amount of incisor teeth and gingiva than he wished. He had adapted to his smile and incorporated it into his speech and facial expression patterns. These patterns were not part of either the mechanical or virtual surgery simulation, but these types of relationships must not be overlooked.

Comparison of the mechanical and virtual planning environments

Mechanical surgical planning is accomplished within the physical environment of articulated casts (Fig 10-5). Before the maxillary cast is moved, its position is registered with removable wire pointers. The most important landmark is the position of the maxillary central incisors. The anterior indicator records the position of the midpoint between the central incisors at the level of the incisal edges. This represents a critical landmark against which all other measurements are referenced. Right and left posterior indicators record the positions of the first molars.

The three indicators define a plane that represents the beginning maxillary cant. Casts are mounted according to this protocol in all cases. The technical steps are detailed in chapter 9 and can be undertaken by the surgeon, orthodontist, prosthodontist, or laboratory technician.

Treatment planning in the virtual environment is accomplished with computer-generated graphics. CT or CBCT data are processed to form a three-dimensional computer model. This model cannot be viewed directly. Instead, extraction of a specific portion of the data set allows generation of graphic images.

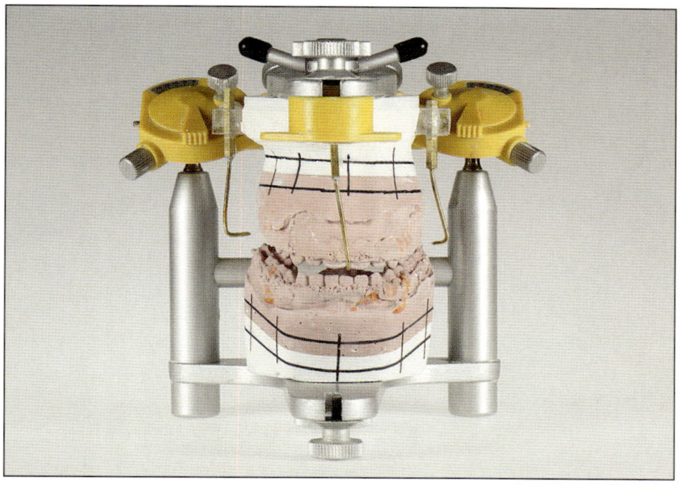

Fig 10-5 Dental casts are mounted on an articulator for conventional mechanical surgical planning. Three indicators have been mounted to guide the repositioning of the maxillary cast.

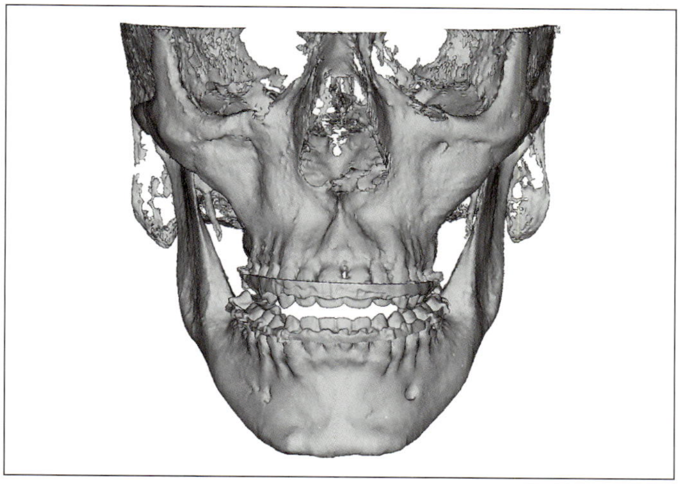

Fig 10-6a Three-dimensional re-formation of CBCT data creates images that can be used for diagnosis and treatment planning.

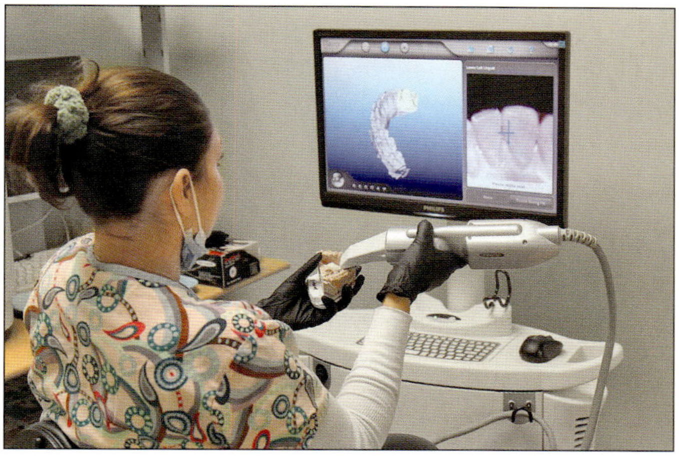

Fig 10-6b An optical scanner obtains data from dental stone casts. This is necessary to create an accurate depiction of the dental anatomy.

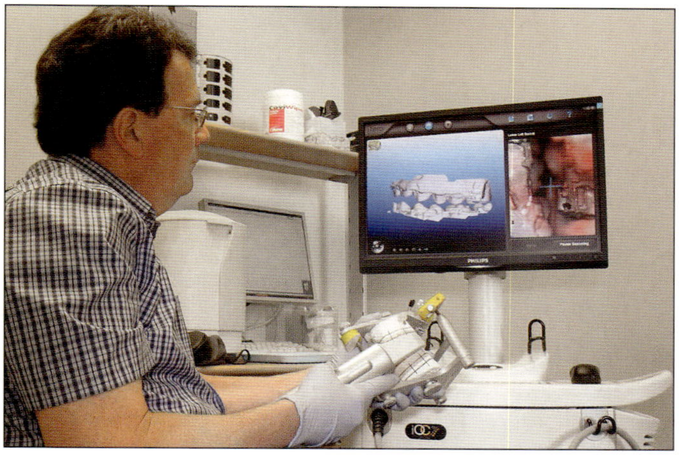

Fig 10-6c An optical scan of the articulator-mounted casts provides data to enable correct orientation of the virtual interarch relationships.

In this case, the surface topography of the skeleton was selected (Fig 10-6a).

Whereas bone morphology can be imaged in this manner, CBCT imaging of the dental occlusion is compromised by artifacts created by metal orthodontic appliances and dental restorations. To compensate for this deficiency, optical scanning of dental casts is undertaken. The digital image data sets from optical scanning of the dental casts are then merged with the tooth positions imaged by CT. The result is a virtual three-dimensional model that is a hybrid of CT data and optical scanning data.

An optical scanner (iTero, Align Technology) gathers image data from a dental stone cast to create a virtual dental model in high resolution that depicts tooth morphology accurately enough to allow fabrication of occlusal splints (Fig 10-6b). Metal orthodontic appliances and dental restorations do not compromise the accuracy of the optical scan. The virtual dental arch derived from optical scanning is merged with the virtual model of the facial skeleton derived from CT or CBCT data.

Optical scanning of the maxillary and mandibular casts that are mounted on the articulator is used to create a digital occlusal registration (Fig 10-6c). The articulator-mounted casts are scanned in their presurgical relationship. This step allows orientation of the optical scans of the maxillary and mandibular dental arches within the virtual model.

Simulation of surgical movements

The maxillary cast is moved to simulate the desired repositioning of the maxilla during surgery (Fig 10-7a). This is the most important step in the surgical planning process. It is this single step that must demand the greatest attention of the surgeon.

Although the movement of the cast appears simple, there are multiple critical factors to consider. The maxillary central incisors are positioned first. Midline correction and incisor show must be determined clinically and then transferred to the cast. In this case, the central incisors are moved 2 mm to the right, advanced 4 mm, and unchanged vertically. These measurements are made in reference to the midline indicator.

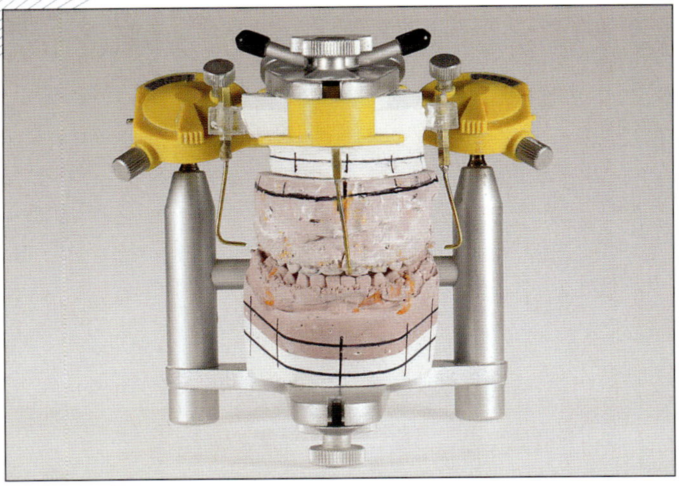

Fig 10-7a In the mechanical environment, the maxillary cast *(pink)* is separated from the plaster mounting base *(white)*. The maxillary cast is divided to simulate a midline osteotomy, and then the two segments are repositioned to meet the clinically derived objectives.

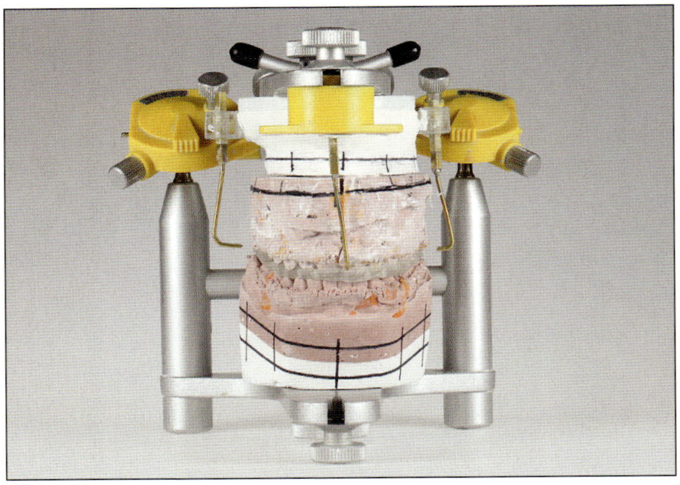

Fig 10-7b An occlusal splint is fabricated on the articulator using autopolymerizing orthodontic acrylic resin. This is the intermediary splint.

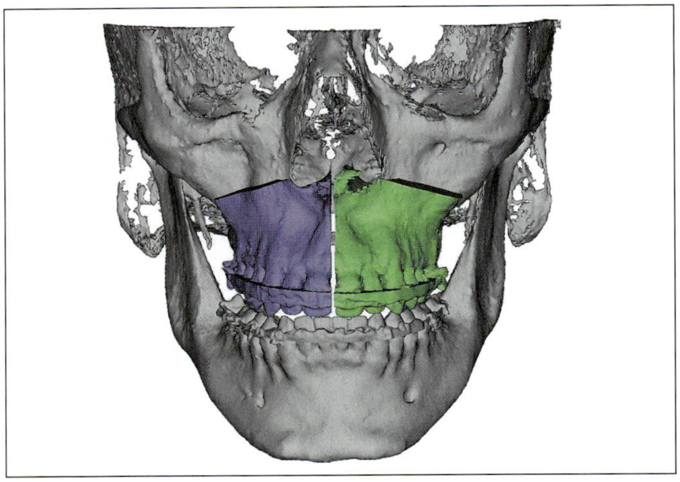

Fig 10-8a In the virtual environment, the maxilla is mobilized and divided at the midline. The two virtual maxillary segments are repositioned by using an optical scan of the segmented dental stone casts.

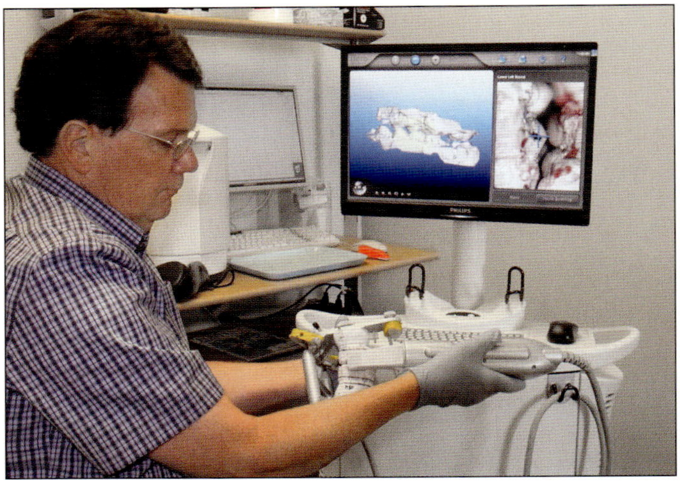

Fig 10-8b The final desired occlusion is determined by repositioning the dental cast segments on the articulator. This cast setup is input into the computer via the optical scanner.

The second movement involves asymmetric impaction of the molars. The posterior left area of the maxilla is impacted enough to allow the mandible to autorotate into an edge-to-edge articulation. Rotation of the mandible occurs along the hinge axis of the articulator. In this position, the maxillary cant is corrected, the central incisor position is maintained, and the mandible can be set back with minimal rotation. The ability to set the mandible back without clockwise or counterclockwise rotation limits the challenge that would otherwise be imposed on the neuromuscular matrix and thus decreases the risk of relapse of the mandibular osteotomy. In the mechanical environment, an intermediary splint is made to relate the Le Fort I movement to the unmoved mandibular arch (Fig 10-7b).

In the virtual environment, the maxillary image is divided at the midline, and a modified maxilla is created (Fig 10-8a). To determine the shape and form of this modified maxillary arch, it must articulate with the mandibular arch in its final position. To accomplish this accurately, an optical scan of the final occlusion is needed. This optical scan is obtained from casts that are mounted on the articulator in the final projected occlusion (Fig 10-8b). The maxillary cast has been divided, expanded, and repositioned. The mandibular cast has been repositioned to articulate with the maxillary cast in the occlusion that would be expected at the time of surgery. The optical scan shows the occlusal registration that would be needed for the expanded, two-segment Le Fort I maxilla to occlude with the mandibular arch. These data are used to guide the virtual segmentation of the maxillary osteotomy.

In the mechanical environment, the mandibular cast is mobilized and repositioned to occlude with the altered maxillary cast (Fig 10-9a). The final splint is made on this articulator setup (Fig 10-9b). In the mechanical environment, the staged movement of the maxillary cast and then the mandibular cast yields the intermediary and final splints (Fig 10-9c).

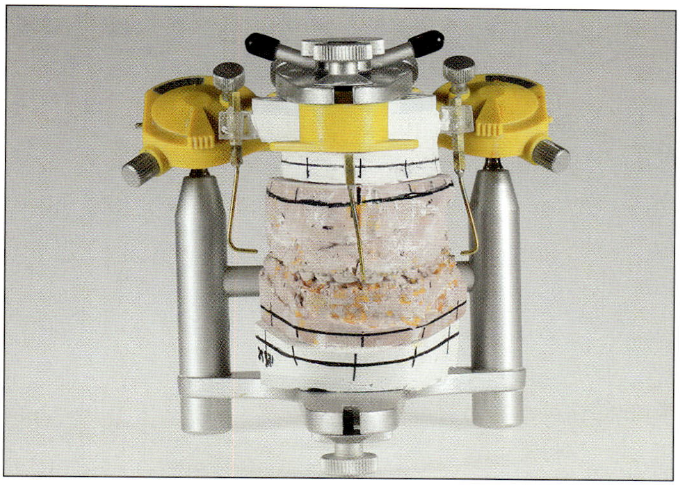

Fig 10-9a In the mechanical environment, the final occlusion is determined, and the cast is fixed in the objective position.

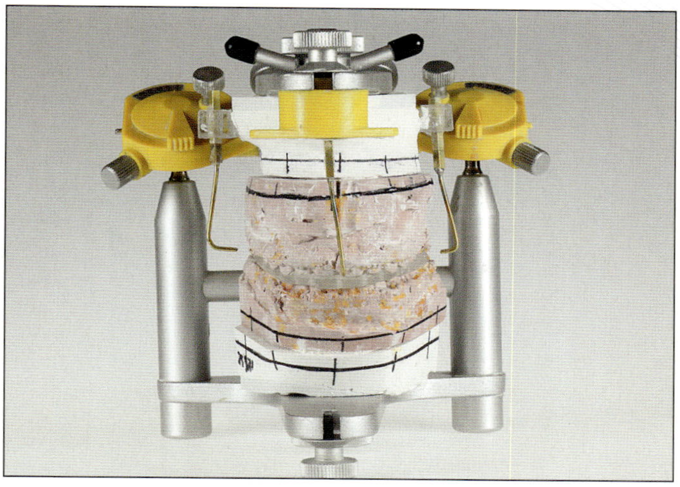

Fig 10-9b An acrylic occlusal splint is fabricated directly on the articulator using autopolymerizing orthodontic acrylic resin. This is the final occlusal splint.

Fig 10-9c The mechanical surgical planning process results in two splints. The intermediary splint is for repositioning of the maxilla. The final splint is for repositioning of the mandible after the maxilla has been stabilized with internal fixation.

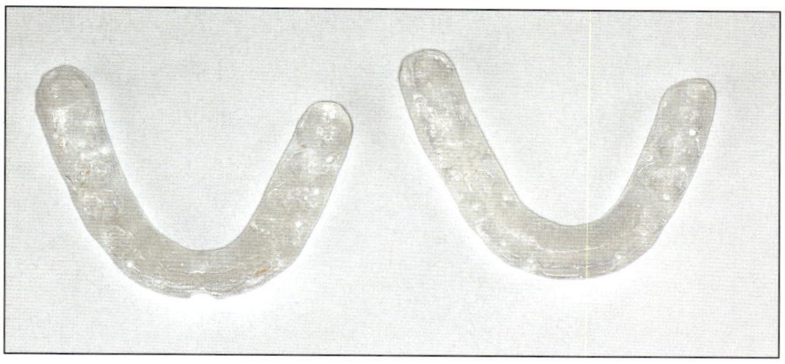

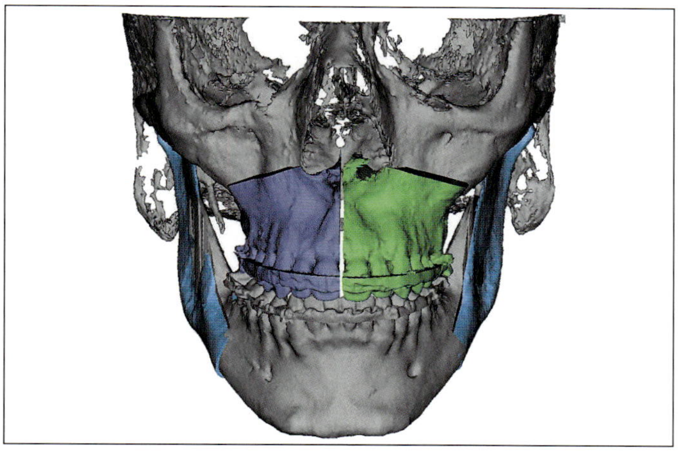

Fig 10-10a In the virtual environment, the ramus fragments of the sagittal split osteotomy are tested for fit at the osteotomy site.

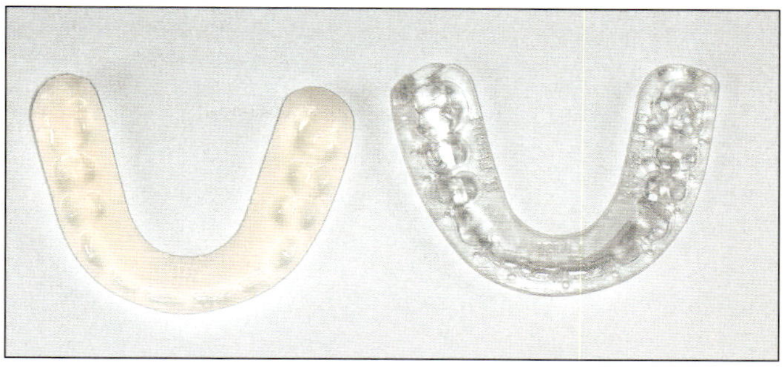

Fig 10-10b Intermediary and final splints are fabricated from the virtual images. Both splints have been created by a three-dimensional printer.

In the virtual environment, the anterior mandibular fragment housing the dental arch is repositioned to conform to the virtual occlusal registration recorded from the articulated casts. The final skeletal movement is made to project the positions of the two ramus fragments. Bilateral sagittal split mandibular osteotomies have been planned. How the ramus fragments fit against the main mandibular fragment is determined by the condyle and fossa, the contour of the osteotomy surface, and the transverse position of the posterior mandible (Fig 10-10a).

The ramus fragments are moved to verify that there are no major interferences. An interference displays graphically as two skeletal volumes assuming the same space. Resolving virtual interferences requires bone removal at the interference site. Another option is to shift the position of the posterior mandible to mitigate the interference. Intermediary and final splints are fabricated from the virtual images. Both splints are created by a three-dimensional printer (Fig 10-10b).

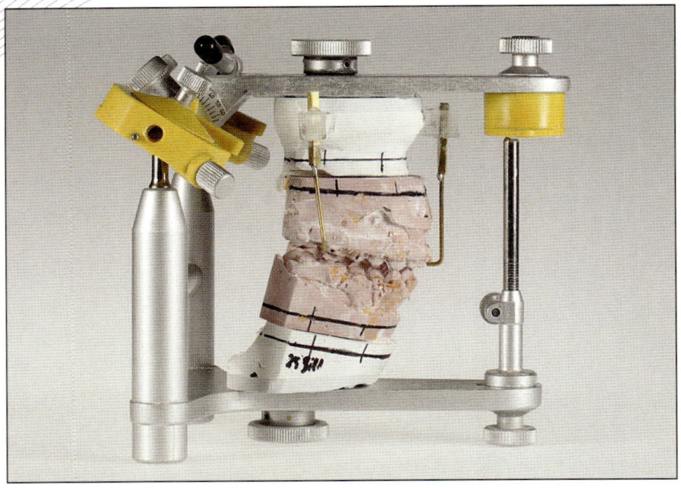

Fig 10-11a Mechanical surgical planning yields measurements of osteotomy site displacement. The indicators show the direct displacement of their respective landmarks in three dimensions.

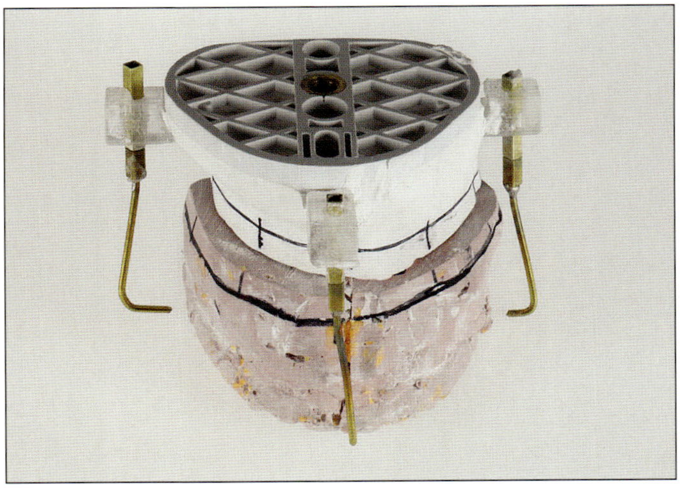

Fig 10-11b The mechanical model shows that the projected maxillary movement would likely create a step at the osteotomy line.

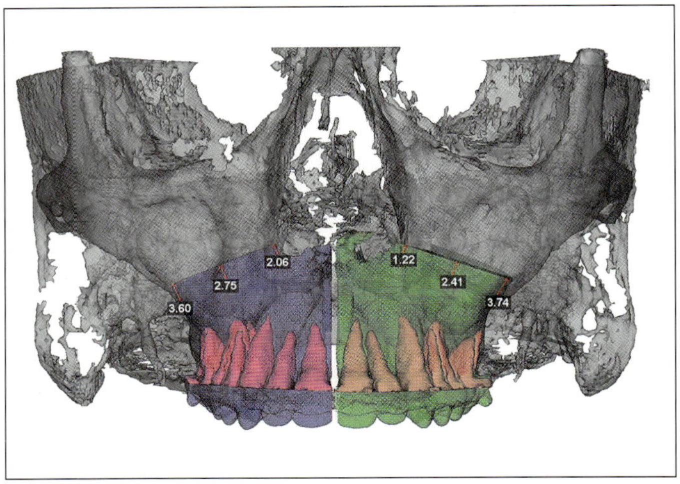

Fig 10-12a Virtual planning produces measurements (in millimeters) at the virtual osteotomy line to guide maxillary repositioning during surgery. Measurement of the displacement of important landmarks such as the maxillary central incisors is also available.

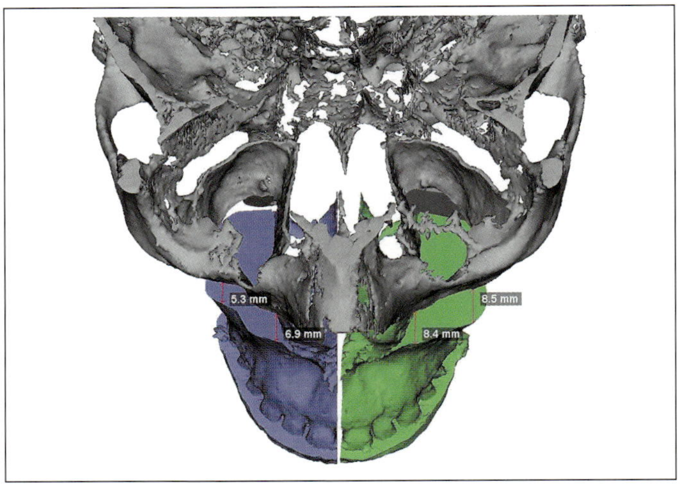

Fig 10-12b The virtual planning gives measurements of the predicted displacement steps at the osteotomy line.

Occlusal splints are important tools to aid in the repositioning of osteotomy fragments during surgery. The proper vertical repositioning of the maxilla is not under the control of the splints. Most surgeons depend on osseous landmarks adjacent to the Le Fort I osteotomy to achieve the desired vertical repositioning of the maxilla. Both mechanical and virtual methods give measurements of the how the osteotomy line is expected to be displaced. This technique, however, is inherently limited. Precise measurement in this region is difficult during surgery. Small errors in assessing how much and in what direction segments have moved will create large errors in the positioning of critical structures. When occlusal splints and osteotomy gap measurements alone are used, the surgeon has no direct control over the pos tion of the maxillary central incisors.

A splint is one method that can be used to guide repositioning of osteotomy fragments during surgery. Direct measurements of the expected horizontal and vertical displacement across the osteotomy are made on the cast mounting base (Fig 10-11a). The mechanical model shows the expected horizontal step at the osteotomy line (Fig 10-11b).

In the virtual environment, projected overlap measurements indicate an amount of fragment telescoping or an amount that must be removed to meet the specifications of the treatment plan (Fig 10-12a). The virtual image also gives a projection of the step expected at the maxillary osteotomy line (Fig 10-12b).

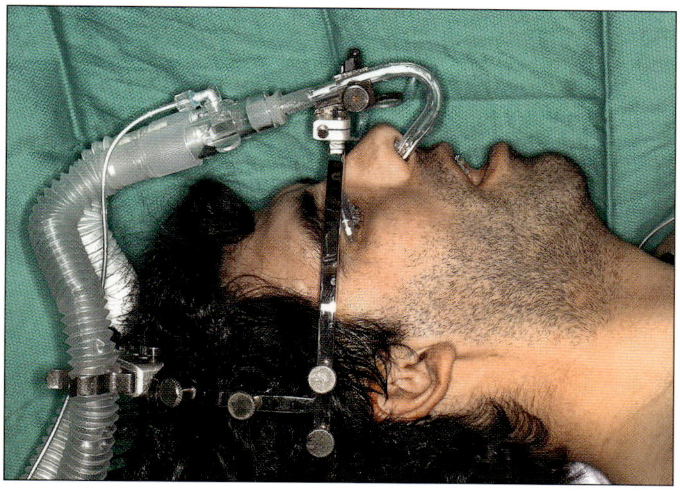

Fig 10-13a A headframe is mounted on the anesthetized patient.

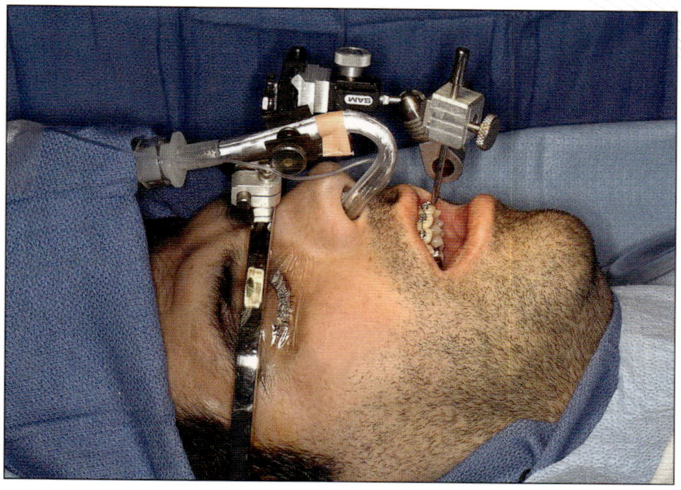

Fig 10-13b The headframe indicator records the position of the maxillary central incisors prior to Le Fort I osteotomy.

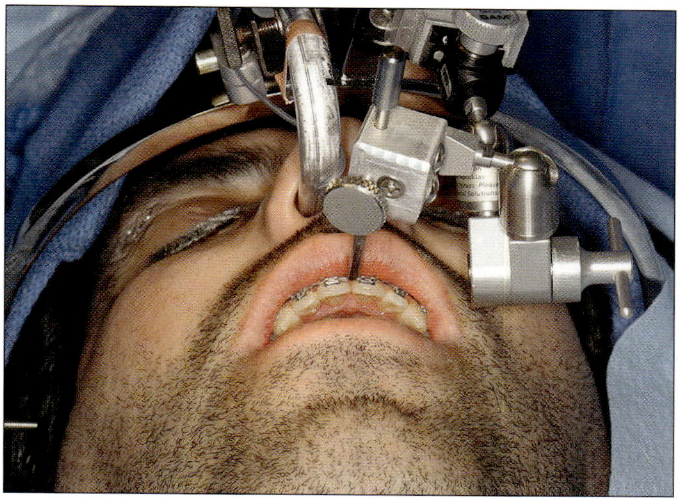

Fig 10-13c Although the position of the maxillary central incisors is the most important landmark, additional indicators can be mounted to record any number of landmarks.

Application of surgical planning guides during surgery

At the time of surgery, a headframe is mounted with eight transcutaneous pins (Fig 10-13a). The anesthesia breathing tubes are secured to the headframe. A detachable pointer device is mounted to the headframe (Fig 10-13b). This instrument is used to record the position of the maxillary central incisors in three dimensions. The reference point represents a coordinate system origin that does not change when the maxilla is mobilized.

The headframe stabilizes the nasal anesthesia tube in the passive position to prevent pressure ischemia of the nostril. The pointer records the beginning position of the maxillary central incisors (Fig 10-13c). This is a critical landmark that verifies when the proper maxillary movement has been achieved.

After the maxillary osteotomy is partially completed, a maxillary mobilizing instrument is mounted (Fig 10-13d). The objective is to mobilize the maxilla without fracturing the pterygoid plates or the piriform buttress. This method of completing the Le Fort I downfracture does not require instrumentation of the pterygomaxillary junction (Fig 10-13e). With the maxilla in the downfractured position, it is divided with a piezoelectric surgical device to allow expansion in the midline (Fig 10-13f).

The maxillary segments are engaged in the intermediary splint to establish the width correction. The dental arches are then placed in maxillomandibular fixation. With the mandible rotating around a retruded condylar position, the maxilla is elevated. Bone across the osteotomy that impedes the desired maxillary elevation is removed. In this case, the maxilla is elevated until the central incisor teeth correspond to the desired vertical position as indicated by the headframe pointer (Fig 10-13g). The headframe pointer indicates that the maxillary central incisors have moved 2 mm to the right and have been repositioned vertically to the original height (Fig 10-13h).

When the correct maxillary position has been achieved as indicated by the headframe pointer, bone plates are adapted to allow passive fixation of the maxillary fragment.

The surgical photograph in Fig 10-13i illustrates the challenge of repositioning maxillary osteotomy fragments without a reference point derived from a headframe. Without an independent reference point, the surgeon uses measurements across the osteotomy to determine the correct vertical repositioning

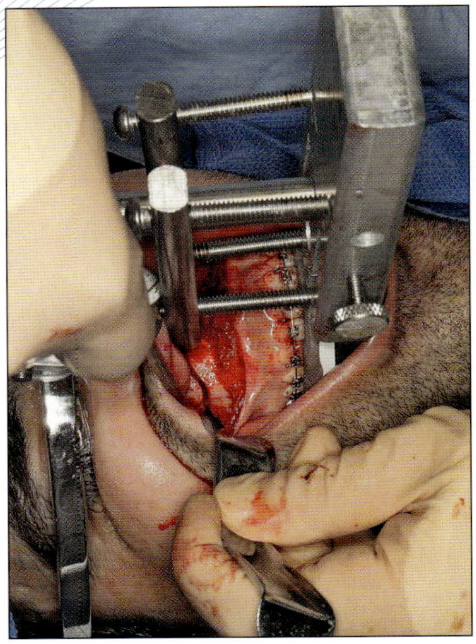

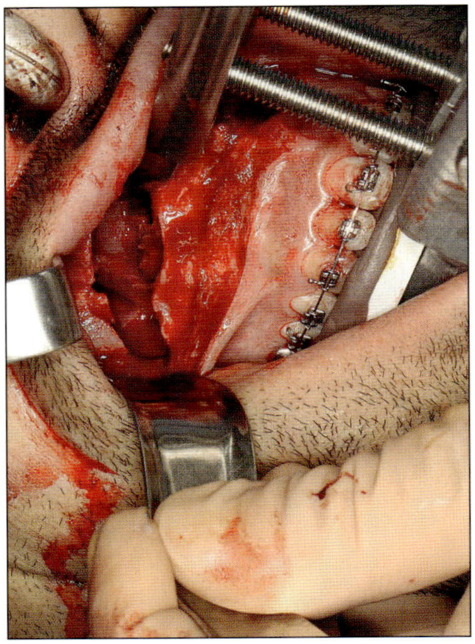

Fig 10-13d *(far left)* After a limited Le Fort I osteotomy is made, a maxillary mobilizing instrument is mounted.

Fig 10-13e *(left)* Protracting force applied by the maxillary mobilizer disengages the maxilla from the pterygoid plates.

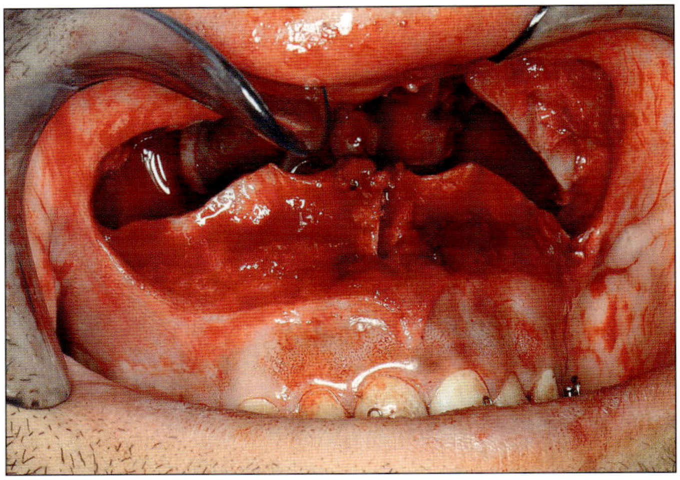

Fig 10-13f With the maxilla in the downfractured position, it is divided with a piezoelectric surgical device to allow expansion in the midline.

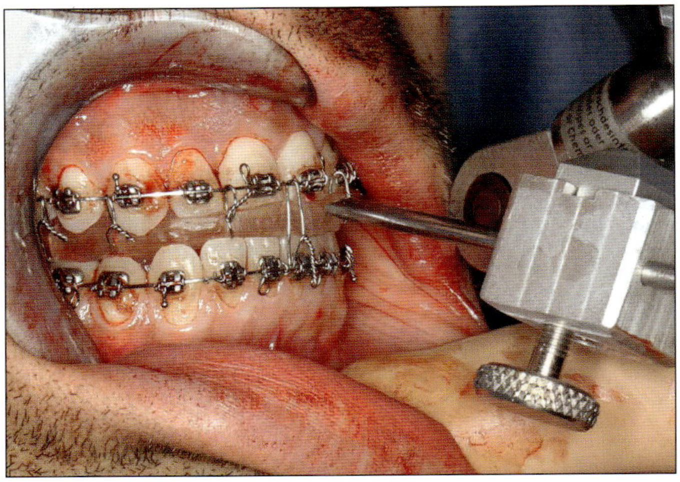

Fig 10-13g The correct repositioning of the maxilla is verified by the headframe indicator.

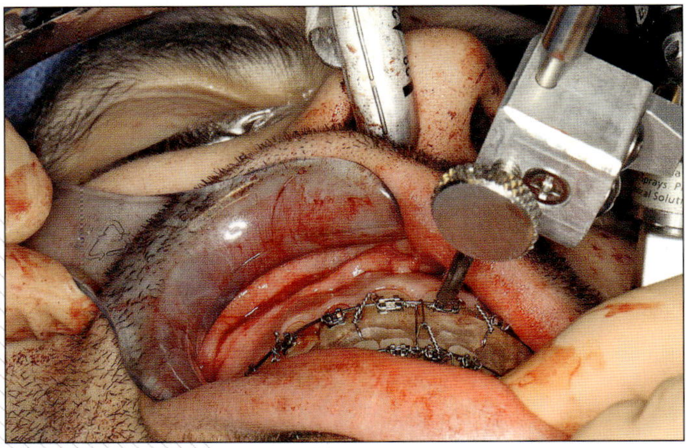

Fig 10-13h The indicator verifies that the central incisors have been moved 2 mm to the right and that the vertical position is unchanged.

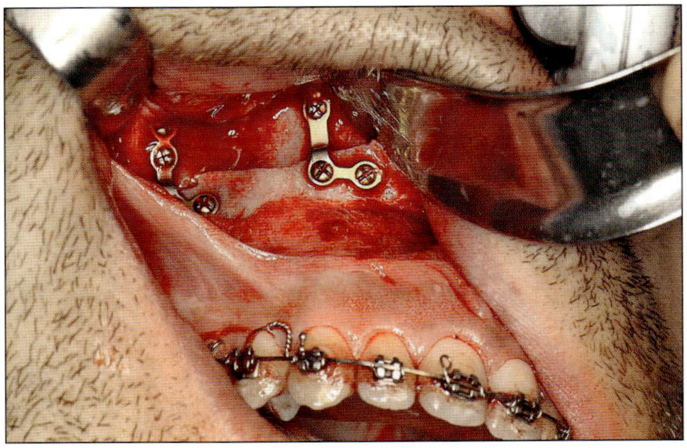

Fig 10-13i The bone step of the maxilla at the osteotomy line does not correspond to the displacement predicted by either the mechanical or the virtual method. Vertical displacement across the osteotomy does not accurately reflect the net movement of the maxillary central incisors.

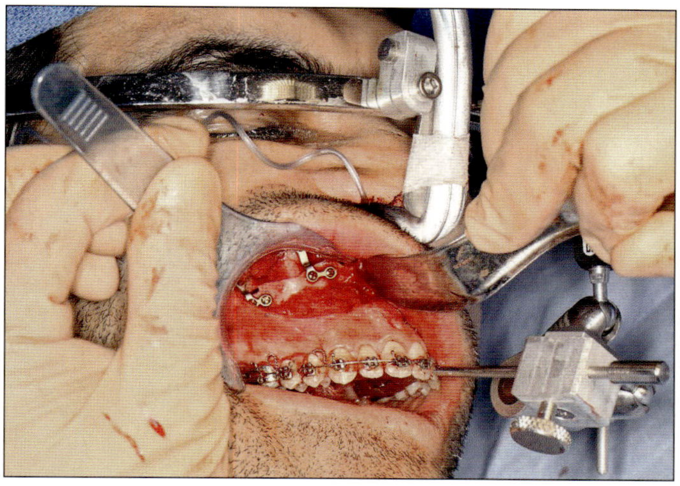

Fig 10-13j The headframe indicator provides a direct measurement of central incisor position. Measurements across the osteotomy are distant from the clinically important landmarks and cannot provide guidance to assure proper repositioning.

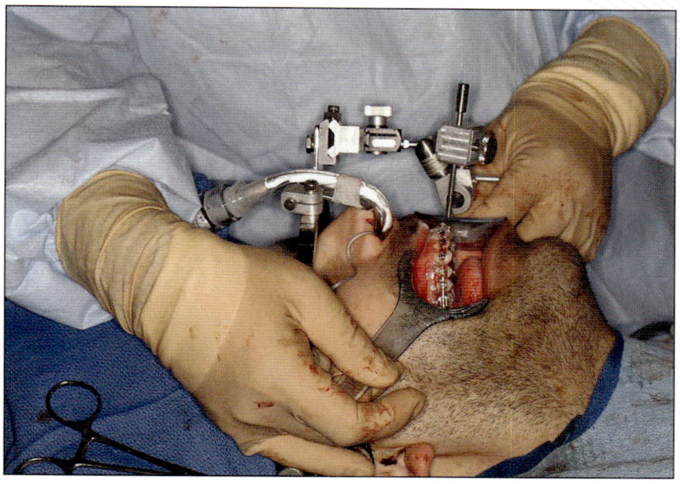

Fig 10-13k Before the surgery is completed and the patient is awakened, each important landmark is checked against a variety of indicators to determine if the repositioning result will meet the desired outcome. If an error is detected, it should be corrected before the patient is awakened.

of the maxilla. Measurements made at the osteotomy site do not directly coincide with the position of the central incisors. As stated earlier, small errors in measuring across the osteotomy result in large errors in the position of the central incisors. In this case, neither the mechanical model surgery nor the virtual planning process accurately predicted the step at the osteotomy. This demonstrates an important limitation in both surgical planning systems. When the surgeon arrives at this step in the surgical procedure, there is no way to verify that the maxillary central incisors are in the correct position. Many errors and unexpected outcomes are the result of an overdependence on measurements across the osteotomy to reposition the maxillary central incisors. Following completion of the mandibular osteotomy and placement of internal fixation, the position of the maxilla is checked again (Fig 10-13j).

The headframe reference point offers a definitive landmark for determining if the surgical result has been achieved. It demonstrates the three-dimensional discrepancy between the planned and the achieved central incisor positions and, equally important, gives the surgeon an opportunity to modify the maxillary position when necessary. The headframe pointer is at the critical esthetic spatial position in an area where there are no other anatomical structures to provide meaningful orientation.

The location of the osteotomy line is distant and is geometrically not well suited to determining the correct maxillary incisor position. This is the most common source of major repositioning errors in orthognathic surgery.[6] Whether the case involves straightforward orthognathic surgery for correction of malocclusion or a complex reconstruction with osteotomies, bone grafting, and dental implants, fragments must be repositioned with accuracy and confidence.

Before the surgery is completed and the patient is awakened, each important landmark is checked against a variety of indicators to determine if the repositioning result will meet the desired outcome (Fig 10-13k). If an error is detected, it should be corrected before the patient is awakened.

Maxillomandibular surgery involves a process that repositions a mobilized jaw using the stable jaw as a guide. The second jaw is mobilized only after the first jaw has been repositioned and fixated. After mobilization of the second jaw, the intermediary splint ceases to be useful. With both jaws mobilized, it is difficult to revise osteotomies with confidence. The headframe reference points remain intact and can be used to guide correction of malpositioned fragments even if both jaws have been mobilized.

Outcome

In this patient, the maxilla was completely mobilized, divided into right and left halves, and then suspended to the midface in the proper position. The mandible was then divided with osteotomies into three segments. The segment bearing the teeth was positioned to place it into a good occlusion with the maxillary teeth. The right and left ramus fragments were positioned to place the condyles in the glenoid fossa of the joints. The position was then stabilized with titanium bone plates and screws.

The jaws were correctly repositioned with the face (Fig 10-14a). The position of the maxillary central incisors met the surgical design objective (Fig 10-14b). The occlusion was positioned to meet the objective determined before surgery (Fig 10-14c). In this patient, some postoperative orthodontic treatment was planned.

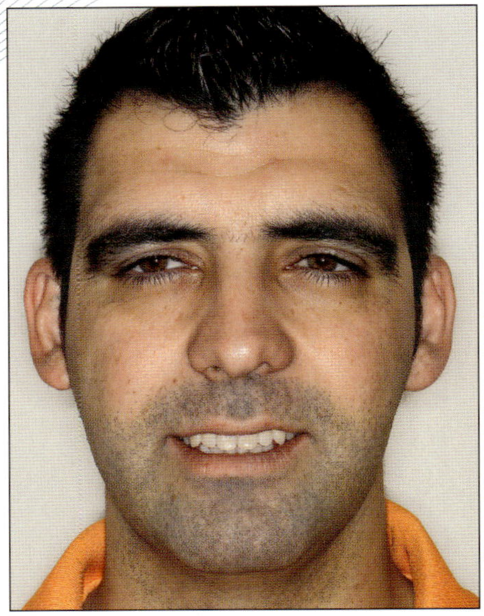

Fig 10-14a Appearance 20 months after orthognathic surgery.

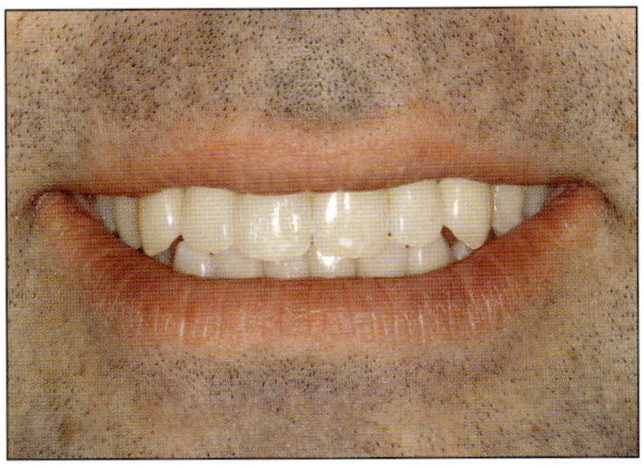

Fig 10-14b Incisor position relative to the upper lip after orthognathic surgery.

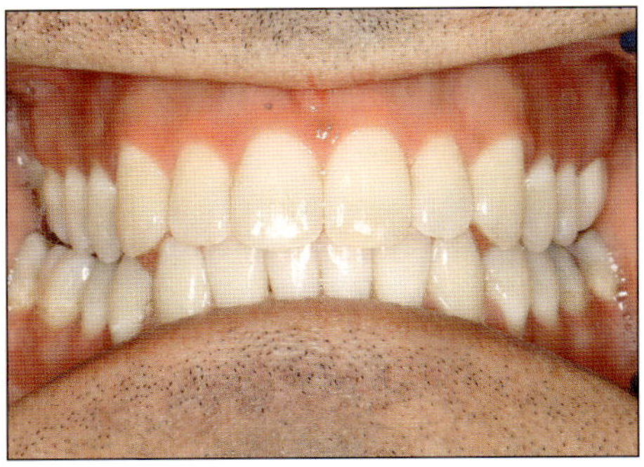

Fig 10-14c Postoperative occlusion.

Analysis of Surgical Planning Methods

Mechanical and virtual surgical planning methods share a common task and objective. The patient presents with a physical deformity and a desire to correct it. The objective is to provide a result that meets the goals of function and esthetics in a predictable and safe manner. It is therefore not surprising that the two methods have more common elements than differences. Each technique has some important benefits that are not shared by the other. There are also limitations that are shared by both approaches. Both techniques must be understood and mastered, but neither solves every planning problem.

Comparison of the strengths of each method

The surgical planning process involves *(1)* understanding the geometry of the deformity, *(2)* creating a projection of the treatment objective, *(3)* providing a method to transfer the treatment plan to the surgical setting, *(4)* providing a method to accommodate for unexpected surgical occurrences, and *(5)* verifying that the desired correction has been realized before leaving the operating room.

Both the mechanical and the virtual planning processes begin with a clinical diagnosis based on the examination of the patient and records. Esthetic deficiencies often direct the course of the treatment plan. Symmetry of the dentition within the face is generally a treatment objective.

The amount of incisor show and projection of the chin prominence require subjective decision-making. Most surgeons rely on clinical observation when determining if the maxillary midline should be shifted laterally. The decision to impact or downgraft the anterior maxilla affects the amount of incisor exposed during speech and in repose. These decisions are best made on the physical patient in a natural, functional setting.

Analysis of asymmetry in the posterior maxilla can be observed in the clinical setting, via articulated casts, and in three-dimensional renderings of the CT or CBCT data. The origins of anomalies in the posterior maxilla are more readily appreciated when viewing the virtual image of the maxilla because it is presented in the context of the entire facial skeleton

Most surgeons use both articulator-mounted casts and a CBCT study for diagnosis and treatment planning. If the preference of the surgeon is to plan orthognathic surgical movements using virtual planning software, the data set required involves optical scanning of the mounted casts. These optical scans of the maxillary and mandibular dental casts are merged into the CBCT data set. The CBCT scan itself is not accurate enough to image the dental occlusion to high precision. Optical occlusal registration scans of both preoperative and postoperative occlusions are taken from the articulator-mounted casts. Intermediary and final occlusal splints based on the optical scanning of the stone casts are then printed.

Limitations of intermediary splints

Establishment of a functional dental occlusion is a primary objective of surgery. Proper occlusion is important not only for mastication but also for its effect on healing of the osteotomy. If the teeth do not occlude well during the healing phase, the neuromusculature is deprived of proprioceptive feedback to guide accommodation of the altered position. Stone dental casts have a clear advantage over virtual images for assessing how osteotomized segments fit with the opposing occlusion. Manipulation of the individual pieces of the segmented maxillary cast is best done in the environment of the dental articulator.

Movements made in the virtual environment allow accurate measurement of the net displacement of each structure compared to the starting point. The effect on maxillary incisor position of a specific amount of maxillary impaction, for example, can be determined. This is an important measurement that is not available on the articulator unless a landmark system is added.

As described earlier, removable wire indicators are added to the articulator mounting to provide reference points to guide accurate cast repositioning. In both systems, this relationship is recorded within the intermediary splint. Both mechanical and virtual planning systems use intermediary splints to guide surgical repositioning of the maxilla during maxillomandibular surgery. The strategy is to use the premobilized mandible held in centric relation as a landmark for maxillary repositioning. This technique was described in chapter 9.

This technique has been employed for many years with variable results. Errors in orthognathic repositioning most often are made at this step. There are several important and often unrecognized flaws in this system. The primary flaw is that the frame of reference—the mandible—is a movable structure. The position of the mandible changes and is not reproducible.[7] The second flaw is an assumption that centric relation is a predictable reference point.[8] The third flaw is the use of measurements across the Le Fort I osteotomy line to control vertical repositioning of the maxillary central incisors. When these errors are additive, predictability is lost and the result may be disappointing.[9]

Advantages of headframe-based navigation

Headframe-based navigation makes it possible to avoid the errors caused by a reliance on intermediary splints and osteotomy gap measurements.[10] The headframe establishes a frame of reference that does not change throughout surgery. Measurements from the headframe are not dependent on centric relation or measurements of osteotomy gaps. This method allows direct measurement of the net movement of any structure. The most important landmarks are the before and after positions of the maxillary central incisors.

Use of the headframe system to depart from a splint-based surgical plan

An independent frame of reference is important when striving to reach a specific, predetermined objective. A reliable constant is critical when unexpected occurrences demand departure from the original plan.

Unexpected problems with compromised perfusion

One situation in which the headframe can be used to guide osteotomy fragment repositioning when the intermediary splint cannot be used is when perfusion is compromised. In one frequently encountered clinical situation, maxillomandibular surgery is being performed on a patient with a bilateral cleft lip and palate who has undergone multiple surgeries. During repositioning of the maxilla guided with an intermediary splint, the surgeon finds that perfusion to the maxilla is compromised due to traction on the pedicle. The decision is made to decrease the maxillary advancement. The reference points on the headframe allow for intraoperative decision-making to choose an alternative maxillary position.

Possibility for greater advancement

Another situation in which the headframe can be used to alter the surgical plan is when greater advancement is desired. For example, the surgeon has chosen a conservative maxillary advancement and mandibular setback for a patient with cleft lip and palate who has undergone multiple surgeries. When the maxilla is mobilized and protracted, it is found that the pedicle will allow for much greater advancement and still maintain its perfusion. If an alternative intermediary splint fabricated for greater advancement has not been made, the maxilla could be advanced under the guidance of the headframe indicators with assurance that objectives of symmetry and incisor show will still be maintained.

Change in occlusion under anesthesia

The headframe can also be useful if the patient experiences changes in occlusion when under anesthesia. Once a patient undergoing maxillomandibular surgery is sedated under general anesthesia, the surgeon places the occlusal registration that was used to mount the casts or to orient the virtual occlusion.[11] The surgeon finds that, under anesthesia, the patient exhibits a mandibular occlusion that is 5 mm lateral to the original position, and the molars are not occluding in the registration of one side. By placing the centric occlusion registration, the surgeon knows that the intermediary splint is not useable because the maxilla would be 5 mm off the midline and canted. In this case, the surgeon can proceed with maxillary repositioning using the headframe reference points to direct the proper three-dimensional movement of the maxilla. After the fragments have been fixated, the headframe is used to verify that the result meets the projected requirements of incisor position and maxillary cant.

Conclusion

Both mechanical and virtual surgical planning processes provide methods to analyze the patient's deformity. Both techniques provide an environment to study the feasibility and potential outcomes of various surgical plans.[12,13] The case presented shows that mechanical and virtual methods each have unique advantages. The case also shows that each technique has important limitations.[14]

Surgical planning begins with an analysis of the deformity. At this stage, virtual planning has an advantage over mechanical planning on plaster casts. The virtual image is based on CBCT digital data. The contour of the facial skeleton can be accurately rendered. This allows the projected position of osteotomies and displacement geometry to be simulated in an accurate anatomical representation. When the positions of osteotomy fragments are altered in the virtual environment, it is possible to accurately measure the three-dimensional displacement of all the structures within the repositioned segment. The net effect of osteotomy displacement on the position of the maxillary central incisors can be measured with this technique.

The limitation of the virtual environment is that manipulation of the occlusion lacks the tactile feedback possible when plaster casts are articulated. This is most significant when the effect of segmenting the dental arch in different patterns is tested.

When surgery is planned on articulator-mounted casts, the contour of the bones is an approximation. Measurements made across index marks on the plaster mounting bases will not accurately correspond to osteotomy displacement measurements at the time of surgery. Attempts to transfer the plaster base measurements to the surgical site will result in unpredictable and often disappointing outcomes.

Movement of plaster casts within the environment of the articulator must start with a stable reference frame that can measure the net movement of important structures such as the maxillary central incisors. To create this stable frame, reference points must be placed with auxiliary indicators so that the original positions of the landmarks can be used for net displacement measurements. Without these auxiliary pointers, the net effect of osteotomy movements on critical landmarks cannot be measured.

Studying how alternative patterns of jaw positioning or dental arch segmentation affect the occlusion is an important capability of cast-based surgical planning. A plan that will yield a good occlusion is important from functional, esthetic, and physiologic standpoints. Deviations from the ideal final occlusion must be managed postoperatively with orthodontics or dental restorations. It is important to know whether or not the projected result can be managed with postoperative treatment. A stable postoperative occlusion also affects the manner in which osteotomy fragments heal. If the surgical plan results in an occlusion that is not stable, the neuromusculature will have difficulty accommodating. If the neuromuscular system assumes an abnormal pattern of posture and movement, there may be a negative effect on the temporomandibular joints and facial muscles.

The limited ability to accurately analyze and plan occlusal changes is a recognized limitation of the virtual environment. Management of this challenge involves merging mechanical planning with the virtual planning process. Currently, virtual planning processes use plaster casts as part of their technique. Optical scanning produces digital images of the mechanical planning models at various steps. The occlusal surface of each dental arch before segmentation is scanned into the database.

To establish the interarch relationship between the two virtual dental arch images, the optical scanner is used to record the lateral occlusion on the articulator-mounted casts. If total-jaw movements are to be done, an optical scan of the lateral occlusion in the final position is obtained and merged into the virtual database. The scan is best obtained on the articulator with the casts moved into their final occlusion.

If the treatment plan involves segmentation of one or both dental arches, the altered occlusion is first determined on the articulator casts that have been segmented and repositioned. Repositioning of fragments of a segmented dental cast can be awkward and is best accomplished on mounted casts within the environment of the articulator. Attempts to alter the arch form of a segmented dental cast without articulator mounting are hazardous because small rotational changes in the fragment position can produce challenges to the vascular pedicle during surgery.

The case presented followed the protocol recommended by the service bureau providing the virtual planning technique. Completion of the process involved using most of the steps of the mechanical planning process.

Splint fabrication is one step that differs between mechanical and virtual planning. In the mechanical technique, self-curing methyl methacrylate resin is used to make splints on the articulator-mounted casts. In the virtual setting, the splints are fabricated by a three-dimensional printer.

Planning itself does not guarantee a successful surgical outcome. In this case, the surgery proceeded with *(1)* occlusal splints from the mechanical and virtual processes, *(2)* osteotomy displacement measurements from the cast surgery and the virtual imaging, and *(3)* a three-dimensional objective on the movement of the teeth, including the maxillary central incisors. The orthognathic headframe was placed as a reference point to measure how well the mechanical and virtual systems performed.

The surgical procedure went well and was without complications. The maxilla was mobilized and segmented, and the fragments were placed in the mechanical intermediary splint. The maxilla was repositioned and suspended under the guidance of the splint and headframe-based reference point (see Fig 10-13j). The splint was removed, and the virtual planning–derived splint was placed. Both intermediary splints guided maxillary repositioning to the same location.

Measurements across the osteotomy line were then compared, with amounts determined by both mechanical and virtual methods. The osteotomy gap and displacement at surgery were not the same as those predicted by either mechanical or virtual methods (see Fig 10-13i). If either measurement set had been used to vertically reposition the maxilla, a substantial error would have been produced. The error in incisor position would only become evident in the postoperative period.

This type of error has multiple sources, including variations in condylar position that cannot be held consistently throughout the diagnostic, planning, and surgical processes. The existence of an orientation point based on a stable frame of reference allows rapid and accurate repositioning of critical anatomical structures. The system also allows the surgeon to study the limitations of other navigation techniques.

References

1. Vargervik K. Appliances utilized in the treatment of hemifacial microsomia. In: Harvold EP, Vargervik K, Chierici G. (eds). Treatment of Hemifacial Microsomia. New York: Alan R. Liss, 1983:139–154.
2. Bell RB. Computer planning and intraoperative navigation in orthognathic surgery. J Oral Maxillofac Surg 2011;69:592–605.
3. Hsu SS, Gateno J, Bell RB, et al. Accuracy of a computer-aided surgical simulation protocol for orthognathic surgery: A prospective multicenter study. J Oral Maxillofac Surg 2013;71:128–142.
4. McCormick SU, Drew SJ. Virtual model surgery for efficient planning and surgical performance. J Oral Maxillofac Surg 2011;69:638–644.
5. Zinser MJ, Sailer HF, Ritter L, Braumann B, Maegele M, Zoller JE. A paradigm shift in orthognathic surgery? A comparison of navigation, computer-aided designed/computer-aided manufactured splints, and "classic" maxillomandibular splints to surgical transfer of virtual orthognathic planning. J Oral Maxillofac Surg 2013;71:2151.e1–21.
6. Polido WD, Ellis E III, Sinn DP. An assessment of the predictability of maxillary surgery. J Oral Maxillofac Surg 1990;48:697–701.
7. Ellis E III. Condylar positioning devices for orthognathic surgery: Are they necessary? J Oral Maxillofac Surg 1994;52:536–552.
8. Rotskoff KS, Herbosa EG, Villa P. Maintenance of condyle-proximal segment position in orthognathic surgery. J Oral Maxillofac Surg 1991;49:2–7.
9. Polley JW, Figueroa AA. Orthognathic positioning system: Intraoperative system to transfer virtual surgical plan to operating field during orthognathic surgery. J Oral Maxillofac Surg 2013;71:911–920.
10. Nattestad A, Vedtofte P. Pitfalls in orthognathic model surgery. The significance of using different reference lines and points during model surgery and operation. Int J Oral Maxillofac Surg 1994;23:11–15.
11. Yaghmaei M, Ejlali M, Nikzad S, Sayyedi A, Shafaeifard S, Pourdanesh F. General anesthesia in orthognathic surgeries: Does it affect horizontal jaw relations? J Oral Maxillofac Surg 2013;71:1752–1756.
12. Xia JJ, Gateno J, Teichgraeber JF, et al. Accuracy of the computer-aided surgical simulation (CASS) system in the treatment of patients with complex craniomaxillofacial deformity: A pilot study. J Oral Maxillofac Surg 2007;65:248–254.
13. Xia JJ, Gateno J, Teichgraeber JF. New clinical protocol to evaluate craniomaxillofacial deformity and plan surgical correction. J Oral Maxillofac Surg 2009;67:2093–2106.
14. Xia JJ, Shevchenko L, Gateno J, et al. Outcome study of computer-aided surgical simulation in the treatment of patients with craniomaxillofacial deformities. J Oral Maxillofac Surg 2011;69:2014–2024.

11 Design and Surgical Technique in Detail: A Clinical Demonstration

Surgeons who are developing new strategies to construct facial structures with living tissue can benefit from understanding how engineers approach the process of design in their discipline. Mechanical and civil engineers are confronted with challenges that are very different from those presenting to facial surgeons. Engineers are trained to follow a sequence of steps that lead to a successful, functioning construct. Their industry standards and the law require that they adhere to this protocol. Safety and predictability are the goals. Each step must be completed to the accepted standards before the next is considered. At each step, multiple engineers analyze the design for its expected performance and potential shortcomings. Although experience may allow the engineer to conceptualize the project in the completed state, the sequence of steps is still followed.

Adherence to a standardized sequence to design a solution has many advantages:

- It allows the engineer to analyze multiple designs and compare the relative benefits before investing in physical construction.
- It enables analysis of the individual components to determine the physical demands on each segment and the consequences of failure.
- It allows multiple engineers to contribute by developing the plan in a format that is understandable to each member.
- It allows theoretical analysis of how the construct may interact with the environment. Students benefit from observing and learning how the thought process results in the development and completion of a project.
- If a problem occurs during or after completion of a project, the sequential process allows retrospective analysis to pinpoint where the weakness in the design occurred.

The process is divided into three basic phases: *(1)* engineering, *(2)* design, and *(3)* construction. Each phase is a special discipline with specific challenges. Success of all of the phases is essential. Civil engineers draw on basic science parameters such as geometry, strength of materials, gravity, and earth science when determining if the construct can exist stably at the site. Designers propose theoretical configurations that can potentially solve the functional objective. Their designs must satisfy the analysis of the engineers, who determine if the materials used in the design have performance characteristics that will meet the stress placed on them. Even if the structure could stand on its own, it is not useful unless it can interact safely with the environment in which it has been placed. Engineers therefore study the potential challenge to the proposed structure from environmental forces such as wind, tidal oscillation, and earthquake. Designers consider the physical arrangement of the components and the method to join them into the end product as well as cost of materials, availability, and esthetics. The third phase is construction. A sound plan that meets both engineering and design standards is not useful if it cannot be built. Technical execution of the engineered design is essential to realizing a safe and durable construct.

Although surgeons are solving fabrication challenges within living systems, lessons can be learned from the methods developed by engineers in their construction projects. Both surgery and civil engineering share a common goal of safety and predictability. However, surgeons generally follow a very different approach to problem-solving than do engineers. In a typical case, the surgeon recognizes that the presenting problem appears similar to ones that have been successfully treated in the past. The surgeon then proceeds with repair using familiar materials and techniques.

This approach yields success when the patient's response to surgery is similar to that experienced by prior patients. However, failure may occur for a variety of reasons. It is possible that the problem being confronted just appears like prior ones but is actually different. The materials the surgeon selects for repair may not heal in the patient in the same manner as in prior patients. The technical execution of the procedure may be deficient so that healing does not occur. As the complexity of the problems increase, so do the risks.

An engineered approach to facial surgery is divided into three phases: *(1)* basic biology, *(2)* surgical planning, and *(3)* surgical execution. The basic science step involves defining the parameters that will regulate the physiology of a surgical incursion. It is necessary to understand and define what elements are necessary for bone to grow at the desired site.

It is just as important to know what parameters are necessary to allow a newly constructed or reconstructed bone segment to be stable over the long term. To reach this goal, it is necessary to understand how a new bone segment can be fully integrated into the biologic environment of the patient in question. It is not enough to simply position bone tissue at a site of deficiency; to achieve long-term success, the newly formed tissue must participate in the biologic systems that regulate facial bone morphology.

The second phase is surgical planning. During this phase, various configurations are considered. There are many alternative approaches to creating a portion of the facial skeleton. Each proposal is analyzed to determine if success is likely if the basic science parameters are met. Does the design incorporate all of the essential elements required for bone formation? If the design results in successful healing, will the result meet the objectives of function, esthetics, and durability?

The third phase is surgical execution. After the design is established and the plan verified on surgical casts or through virtual technology, a method is needed to execute the plan on the operating table. The surgical technique must incorporate the ability to transfer the surgical design to the patient. In the surgical setting, any modifications to the original surgical plan must be made in real-time without compromising critical outcome objectives. The method should optimize accuracy and predictability and minimize potential risks.

In this chapter, surgical management of one patient will be described to demonstrate the general protocol followed for treatment of all facial disorders. The process is divided into three sections: *(1)* diagnosis and engineering, *(2)* surgical planning, and *(3)* surgical technique. This general three-stage approach to surgical treatment can be followed for the full range of deformities. The basic science is common to all deficiencies, whether they involve a small alveolar defect or a major craniomaxillofacial disorder. Successful and predictable management of the full range of patient problems can be optimized by following this logical sequence of steps.

Diagnosis and Engineering

The process starts with thoughtful analysis of the presenting deformity. This evaluation extends further than usual. Clinically obvious deficiencies, such as missing teeth, bone segments, and soft tissue, are the first structures to be placed on a list of replacement objectives.

In addition to the missing structures, the integrity of the neuromuscular system must be evaluated. Because engineering of bone-forming constructs requires neuromuscular elements, it is essential to know the condition of the patient's neuromuscular system as he or she presented. In trauma patients, neuromuscular deficits are most often related to the injury itself. Developmental disorders always include some degree of neuromuscular deficiency that is related to the process that gave rise to the failure of a structure to fully form.

In the case that will serve as an example, the patient presented with both afferent and efferent deficiencies. The sensory deficits included paresthesia of the lower lip and mandibular anterior teeth, probably related to fracture of the mandible. Loss of sensory feedback from occlusion compromised the global neuromuscular regulation of the region. The patient's injury also included fracture of the cervical spine. This resulted in a degree of muscular weakness. Over months of recovery, this weakness diminished.

The process of recovery in patients with nervous system injuries involves compensation through neuroplasticity and is probably not true regeneration. Special caution must be applied to treatment planning for such patients because their ability to compensate further may be compromised. When the neuromuscular system is challenged by general anesthesia and orthognathic surgery, such patients may have difficulty accommodating. This can pose immediate postoperative challenges to swallowing and maintaining the airway. In addition, potential limitations in the neuromuscular regulation may impair the ability of bone-forming constructs to heal. These parameters must be factored into the engineering process.

Figs 11-1a and 11-1b *(right)* A 54-year-old woman presents for treatment 1 year after falling from her bicycle. She had sustained facial fractures, avulsed teeth, and a cervical spine fracture. Medical management of the cervical spine fracture allowed for only limited repair of the maxillary fracture and avulsed portion of the anterior mandible.

Fig 11-1c *(below left)* Malunion of the maxillary and mandibular fractures prevents placement of dental implants or fixed dental prosthetics. A segment of the anterior mandible had been avulsed in the accident, and the labial mucosa had been sutured to the floor of the mouth to close the open fracture.

Fig 11-1d *(below center)* The post-traumatic occlusion on the right side is Class I with a Class III tendency.

Fig 11-1e *(below right)* The post-traumatic occlusion on the left side is Class I.

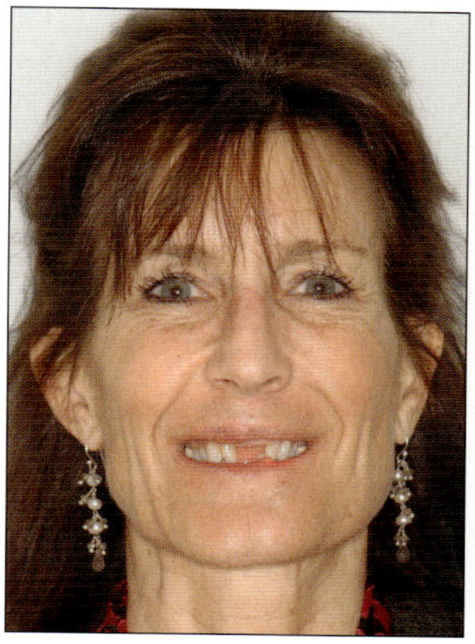

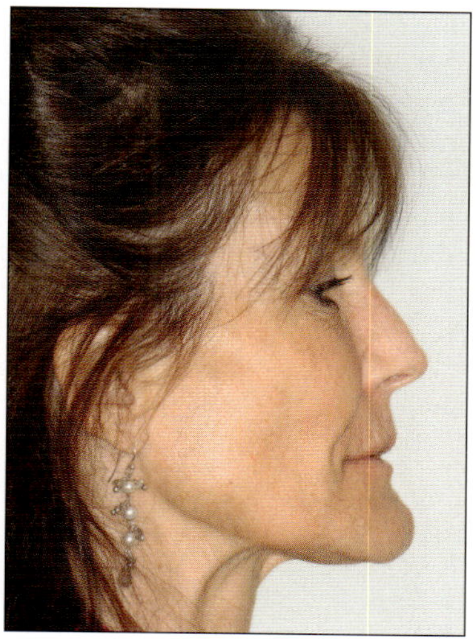

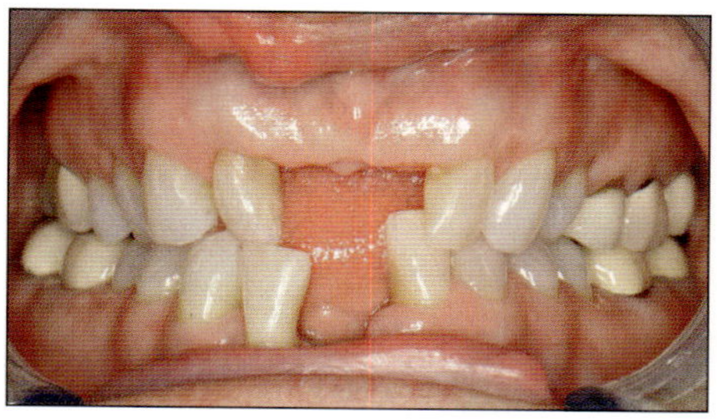

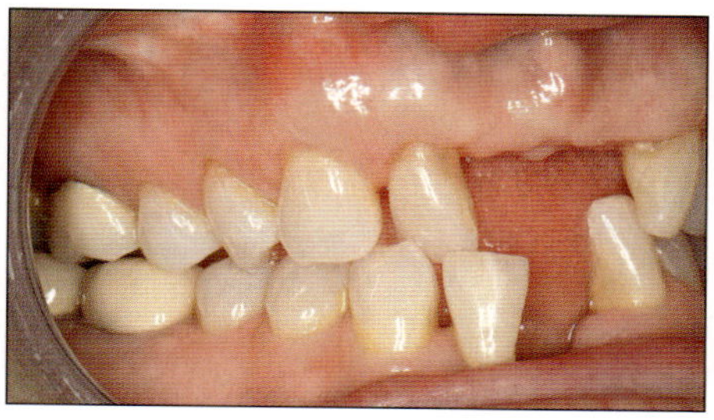

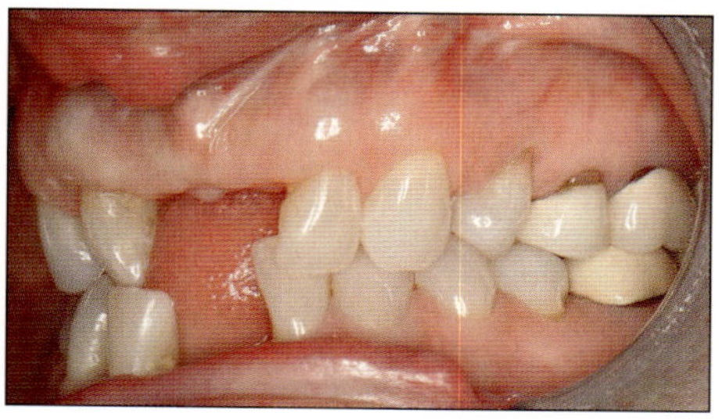

History and evaluation

The patient in this case study presented with a moderate to severe facial deformity resulting from an injury. She was a 54-year-old woman who had fallen from her bicycle, sustaining maxillofacial and neck injuries (Figs 11-1a and 11-1b). The circumstances of the accident were not clear because the patient could not recall the fall. She had sustained facial fractures, including avulsion of maxillary and mandibular teeth. A comminuted midline mandibular fracture resulted in the loss of a segment of the symphysis.

The fractured cervical vertebrae were surgically stabilized. Because of the patient's compromised neurologic status, the facial fractures were stabilized but not reduced or reconstructed. After a period of recovery and rehabilitation, the patient became more aware of her missing teeth and disrupted occlusion. At the time of her initial consultation, the patient desired treatment to repair the malunions at the site of facial fracture and to replace her missing teeth.

A degree of motor weakness remained. The facial lacerations sustained during the accident involved avulsion and damage to the facial muscles of the left side at the lower and upper lips. The findings of motor weakness and direct muscle damage were part of the extended diagnosis. If reconstruction of the facial skeleton and dental arch was to be successful, the underlying neuromuscular deficiency had to be taken into account. Muscle activity and coordination are necessary for function. They are also important for delivery of neuromuscular signaling to newly constructed skeletal segments.

The patient stated that, before the injury, she had a full complement of natural teeth in good occlusion. At her presentation for reconstruction recommendations, her mandibular arch was missing a segment in the midline (Fig 11-1c). This was a challenging reconstructive problem. Repair of the defect would require replacement of the missing volume of bone in the midline. It also required that the two halves of the mandible be repositioned and fixed in the proper three-dimensional orientation relative to the maxilla and the balance of the face. Correct positioning of the temporomandibular joints was another complicating factor. Moreover, the union of discontinuity defects in the mandibular midline is always challenged by movement of the segment that results from powerful muscle activity during movement of the jaw.

In addition, if comprehensive rehabilitation was to be undertaken, the anterior mandible had to be reconstructed so that dental implants could be placed. The edentulous span involved three teeth after the loss of the damaged mandibular right lateral incisor. If a successful and stable mandibular alveolar ridge was to be constructed, a source of neuromuscular regulation had to be introduced into the defect site. Correction of the mandibular width defect would increase the width of the edentulous span and decrease the ability of adjacent teeth to support growth of a new alveolar crest. Finding a source of neuromuscular input to the damaged site was part of the engineering challenge.

There was a deficiency of gingiva in the mandibular midline, and the lower lip mucosa had been sutured to the floor of the mouth mucosa. The right and left hemimandibles were at two different occlusal plane levels. The maxilla was impacted and retruded on the left side. The left hemimandible was retruded even though there was no clear evidence of a fracture in the left posterior mandible. The occlusion was Class I with a Class III tendency on the right (Fig 11-1d) and Class I tendency on the left (Fig 11-1e).

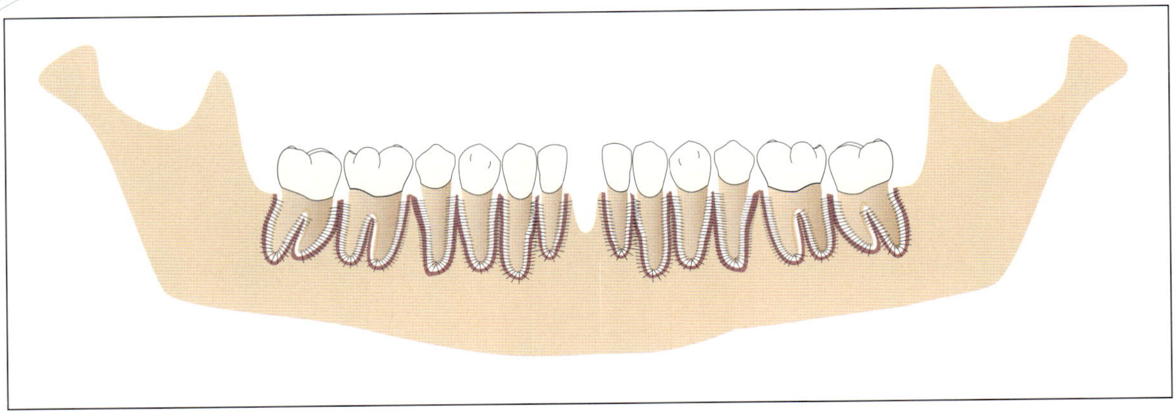

Fig 11-2a The mandibular deficiency includes avulsion of the ridge crest and loss of the central incisor teeth.

Strategy for replacing lost bone in the mandibular midline

The midline defect included avulsion of the ridge crest and loss of the central incisor teeth (Fig 11-2a). The remaining alveolar process at the edentulous site was too thin to house dental implants. Onlay augmentation a deficiency of this width would be expected not to heal because restoration of the mandibular width would open an even larger discontinuity defect, and the site lacked a source of neuromuscular signaling to promote bone growth, long-term maintenance, and osseointegration.

The potential sources for neuromuscular signaling in this region were the periodontal ligament systems of teeth and adjacent muscle attachments. In this case, recruitment of the genioglossus muscle attachment on the lingual aspect of the mandibular symphysis was the best option (Fig 11-2b). The powerful stimulating capacity of the muscle attachment was required to promote bone growth across the large discontinuity defect resulting from restoration of the mandibular width. The midline osteotomy was to be created as outlined in Fig 11-2b. The thin and damaged central alveolar process was to be cut and discarded. A horizontal sliding osteotomy through the inferior border would allow width correction following a procedure described by von Eiselsberg.[1] The damaged alveolar crest segment was to be resected and discarded (Fig 11-2c). The osteotomy would create an independent segment that was pedicled on the lingual side from the genioglossus muscle (Fig 11-2d). The mandible was to be widened at the midline (Fig 11-2e). Expansion instruments would be used to widen the mandible.

When sufficient widening was accomplished, the pedicled symphysis segment would be raised to replace the lost alveolar ridge (Fig 11-2f). This segment would carry the muscle attachment of the genioglossus muscle superiorly during the transport process.

Elevating the transport segment into place would restore the height and width of the alveolar ridge. The interposed bone segment also would provide mechanical resistance to the tendency for the expanded mandible to collapse. Intact gingiva would cover the transport segment. The genioglossus muscle attachment on the lingual aspect of the segment would provide neuromuscular signaling to this surgically created discontinuity of the mandible. During creation and mobilization of the transport segment, some genioglossus and geniohyoid muscle fibers would be separated from their attachments. These detached fibers would become aligned toward the empty bone chamber created when the transport segment was elevated. These free muscle fibers would have the opportunity to deliver regulatory signaling to the bone forming in the regeneration chamber.[2]

To complete the bone-forming construct, the segments required mechanical stabilization and the site needed a source of cells. Stabilization would be achieved by the placement of titanium bone plates (Fig 11-2g). Cells were to be introduced by placement of recombinant human bone morphogenetic protein 2 (rhBMP-2).

Preliminary surgical mock-up

In cases involving complicated deformities, a preliminary surgical mock-up is valuable for understanding how the segments need to be moved to regain the pretrauma objective. Following the general principles of facial fracture treatment planning, the casts were first segmented to reproduce the pattern of the documented fracture locations (Fig 11-3a). This was not a surgical planning mock-up. This step was completed before definitive orthodontic treatment was initiated and was part of the diagnostic process.

To study what effect reducing the midline avulsion defect would have on the occlusion and maxillary position, the articulator was set to allow rotation of the hemimandibular segments around their respective condyles (Fig 11-3b). The method and materials to create this model simulation are shown in Fig 11-9. Because neither the rami nor the condyles were reportedly fractured, this simulation should represent the displacement of the fragments at the time of injury.

The right and left segments of the mandible were rotated laterally until a space corresponding to the width of the two lost incisors was achieved (Fig 11-3c). The maxillary cast was then repositioned to restore the patient to the pretrauma occlusion. This preliminary mock-up showed that simply widening the mandible at the symphysis would not allow the maxilla to be re-

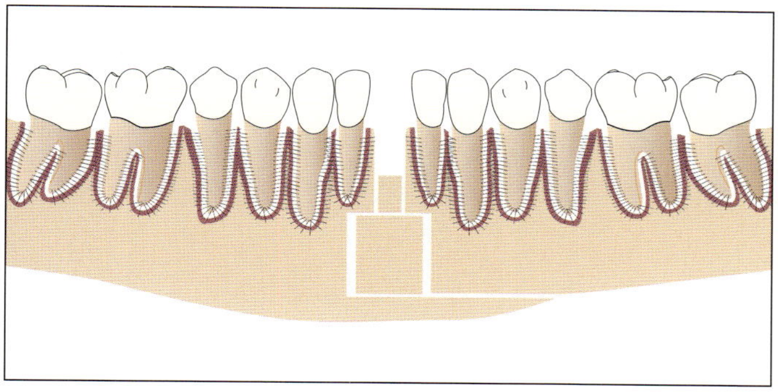

Fig 11-2b In this case, the strategy to provide a source of neuromuscular input into an alveolar bone-forming construct involves recruitment of the genioglossus muscle attachment on the lingual aspect of the mandibular symphysis. The thin and damaged central alveolar process is cut and discarded. A horizontal sliding osteotomy through the inferior border allows width correction.

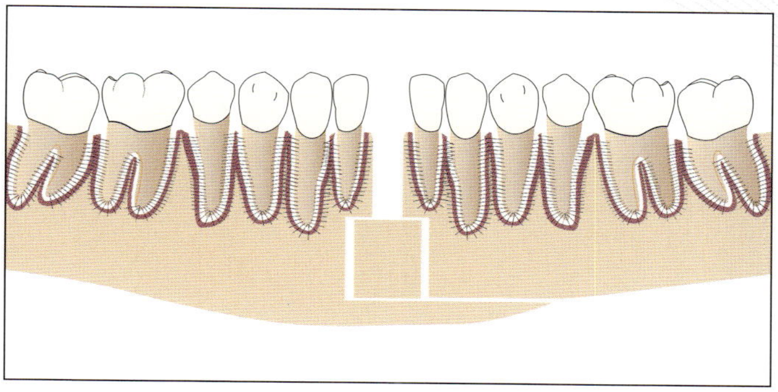

Fig 11-2c The damaged portion of the alveolar ridge is repaired by resection and transposition of a bone flap.

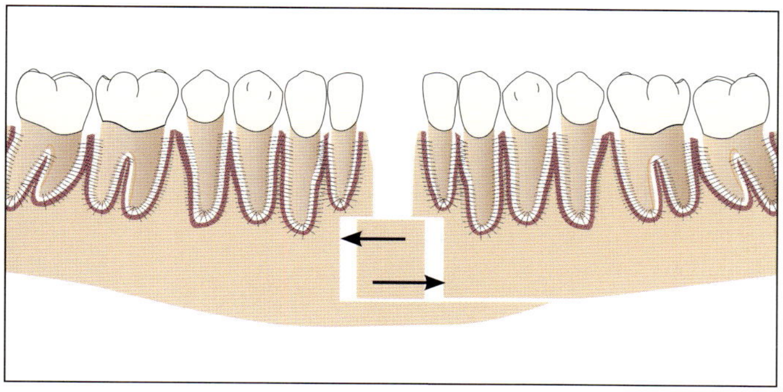

Fig 11-2d The osteotomy creates an independent segment that is pedicled on the lingual side from the genioglossus muscle.

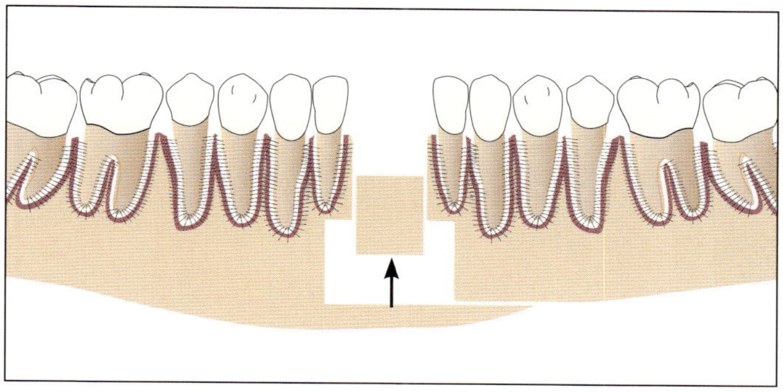

Fig 11-2e The mandible is widened at the midline via expansion instruments.

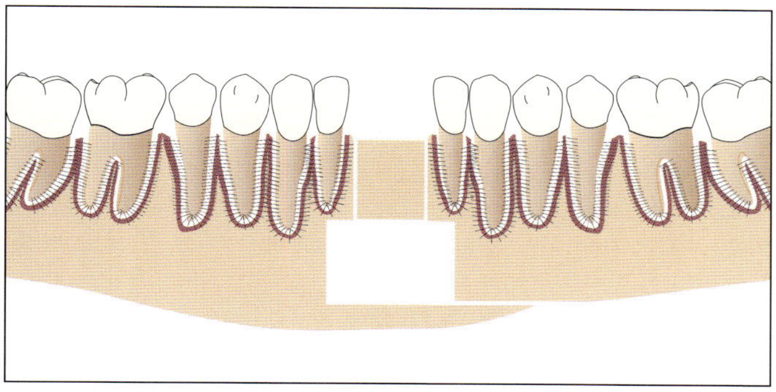

Fig 11-2f The transport bone segment is elevated, restoring the height and width of the alveolar ridge.

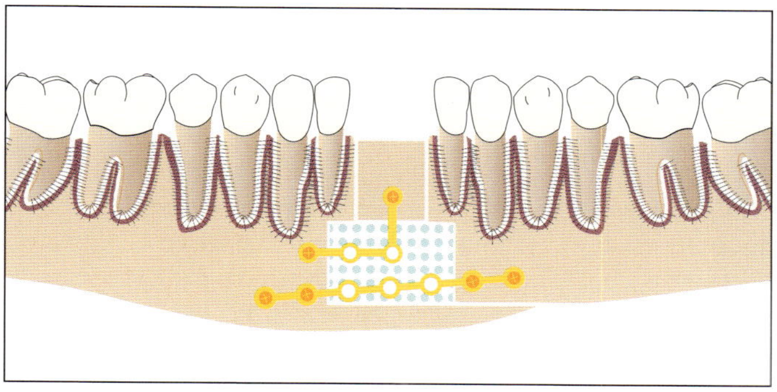

Fig 11-2g Elements of the bone-forming construct. Stabilization is achieved by the placement of titanium bone plates. Cells are introduced by the placement of rhBMP-2.

positioned to meet the requirements of esthetics and function and to restore it to the pretrauma state.

The mock-up was then modified to simulate a two-segment maxilla even though no maxillary fractures occurred. This modification also failed to produce a solution that would meet the requirements of restoring the dental arches to the pretrauma position.

As a third option, the mandibular left segment was released from the orbiting guide to allow advancement. The right hemimandible remained engaged in the orbiting guide. In this configuration, it was possible to reposition the maxilla as a single unit and achieve a pretrauma occlusion with the altered mandible. Achieving these movements surgically would require widening of the mandible at the symphysis and lengthening of the left mandibular body with a sagittal split osteotomy. With this specific surgical plan as the projected treatment, the orthodontist could proceed with the presurgical preparation of the dental arch in anticipation of the specific osteotomy configuration.

In patients with neuromuscular damage, a treatment plan that minimizes the challenge to their ability to accommodate is

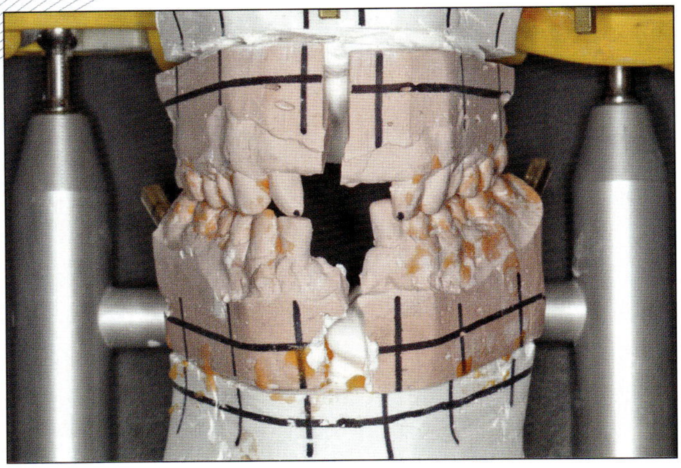

Fig 11-3a The preliminary surgical mock-up reproduces the documented fracture locations.

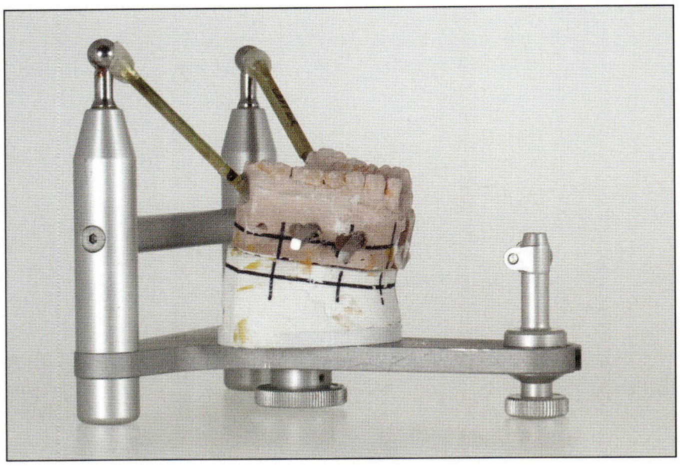

Fig 11-3b Rotation of the hemimandibular segments on the articulator creates a mock-up to simulate the isolated mandibular midline fracture.

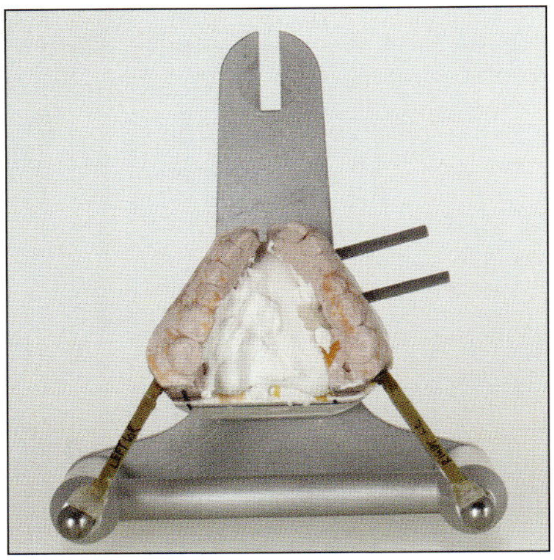

Fig 11-3c The bilateral mandibular orbiting segments are simulated. The square brass tubes restrict each hemimandible to rotate around the ipsilateral condyle.

an advantage. Maintaining the continuity of the mandibular right ramus preserves its structural integrity and avoids damage to its neuromuscular matrix and sensory nerves. In patients with impaired muscular coordination, bone healing of osteotomies is sometimes compromised or predisposed to relapse. Limiting the extent of mandibular ramus surgery reduces the risks of airway compromise and swallowing difficulties in these patients.

The preliminary surgical simulation was performed prior to orthodontic treatment to refine the diagnosis and establish a better working diagnosis. The result of this study demonstrated that the maxilla could not be positioned into a functional occlusion with a reconstructed mandible unless a mandibular left ramus osteotomy was used to lengthen the left side of the mandible (Fig 11-4). The findings of the preliminary surgical mock-up narrowed and refined the diagnosis and working treatment plan. Because the records did not show that the left side of the mandible was fractured, one supposition was that there may have been a preexisting length deficiency. Another possibility was that the temporomandibular joint was already in an accommodated position or was damaged during the injury. Maintaining the integrity of the right hemimandible offered a degree of stability in the presence of the patient's neuromuscular deficiency. Also, maintaining an intact muscular system on the right side of the mandible was important in the general neuromuscular support of the midline and left ramus osteotomies.

As a result of the preliminary surgical simulation, the diagnosis was refined so that a specific presurgical orthodontic plan could be established. The working plan was based on the requirements to reposition skeletal units for functional and esthetic goals. The underlying neuromuscular deficiency from the damage related to the injury had to be considered in projecting how the patient would tolerate the procedure and whether the reconstructed skeleton would be supported by the remaining neuromuscular matrix. The relatively intact neuromuscular system that moves the right ramus would be recruited in the rehabilitation and support of the reconstructed left ramus. The neuromuscular system that was lost when the mandibular anterior teeth were avulsed would be partially restored by vertical elevation of the genioglossus muscle attachment toward the alveolar ridge crest.

The maxillary retrusion deformity was to be addressed by the Le Fort I osteotomy, asymmetric downgraft, and bone replacement with bone morphogenetic protein. The lost maxillary central incisors were to be replaced by two dental implants. This

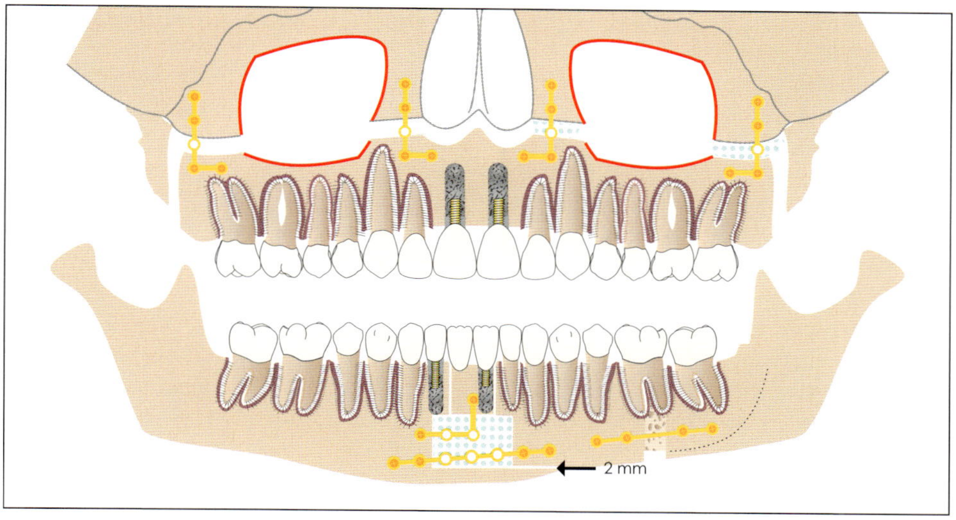

Fig 11-4 Illustration of the skeletal deformity and proposed reconstruction. The maxillary surgery involves a Le Fort I osteotomy, downgrafting, and rhBMP-2 bone regeneration. The anterior maxilla will receive two implants and two implant crowns. The mandible will require a complex midline osteotomy for simultaneous widening and vertical alveolar transport of a pedicled segment. The left ramus will require a sagittal split osteotomy to restore lost length. (Note that after the surgery, the mandibular right lateral incisor was removed because it developed recession and bone loss.) The three lost mandibular incisors will be replaced by two implants and a three-unit implant-supported partial denture.

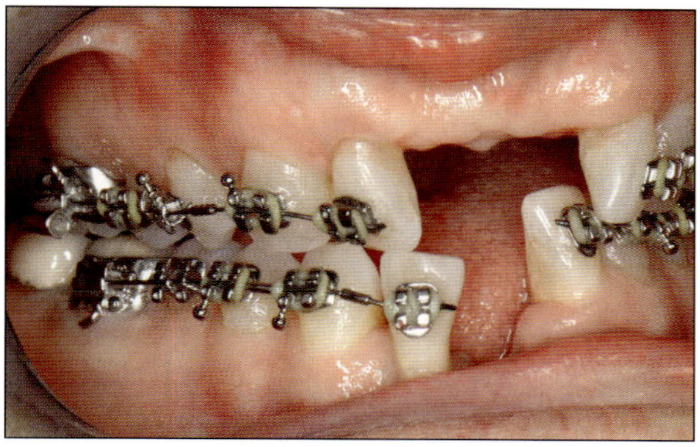

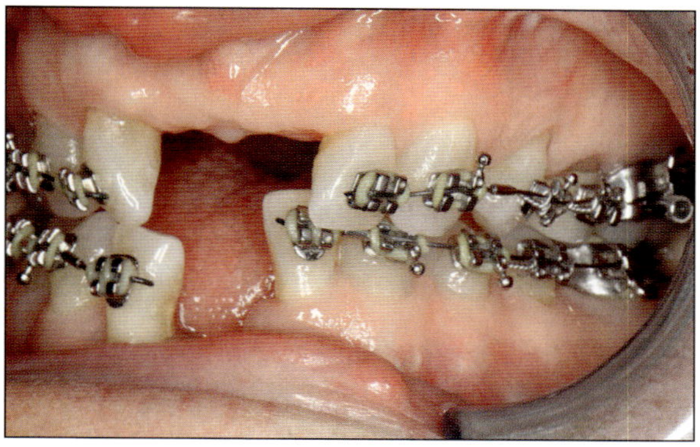

Figs 11-5a and 11-5b Orthodontic treatment is used to prepare the dental arches for the surgical objective.

demanded that the maxilla be repositioned with a corrected occlusal plane and moved to the midline of the face.

The malunion and avulsion of the anterior portion of the mandible were to be repaired by a widening osteotomy. The alveolar process was to be constructed from a pedicled bone segment from the center of the symphysis. The transported bone segment was expected to provide adequate volume to allow placement of dental implants. The deficiency on the left side of the mandible was not the result of fracture. The deficiency may have been preexisting or represented damage to the left temporomandibular joint. A sagittal ramus osteotomy with internal fixation would remedy the length deficiency and have limited long-term effect on the neuromuscular support system that moved the left segment of the mandible. Bone morphogenetic proteins would be used to promote consolidation and union of the discontinuous mandibular symphysis.

Orthodontic treatment cannot be accomplished without a surgical plan. Determining the status of the presurgical orthodontics requires periodic repetition of the surgical simulations. When the surgical simulation of articulated casts shows that the planned movements can be carried out, surgery can be scheduled and the final surgical planning can be done. In this patient, presurgical orthodontics prepared the dental arches for the projected surgery (Figs 11-5a and 11-5b).

Surgical Planning

The objective of the surgical planning phase is to create a specific, high-precision design that satisfies the parameters derived from the engineering phase. Included in the design is a clear strategy that will enable the design to be realized in the surgical setting. Although execution of the design is a part of the surgical phase, the underlying strategy to establish and verify accurate movements begins in the design phase.

In order to be useful, the design must be expressed in a manner that can easily be referenced by the surgeon intraoperatively without increasing the operating time. The accuracy of the measuring or navigation system must substantially exceed the clinical requirements of function and esthetics. After the skeletal fragments have been repositioned and stabilized, the navigation method must include a process to measure how close the result is to the objective. The frame of reference, therefore, cannot be based on structures that are mobile, such as the mandible, or that are mobilized as part of the osteotomy plan.

The diagnosis and engineering phase defines the anatomical and physiologic deficiencies that are to be corrected or mitigated as part of the treatment objective. The design phase refines the general reconstructive strategy yielded by the engineering phase into a surgical process that is specific to the details of the patient's occlusion and esthetic requirements. To deliver a treatment that meets the requirements of successful healing and long-term service to the patient, the reconstruction must meet general requirements of bone healing as well as the specific objectives of occlusion and esthetics. When dental implants are part of the reconstructive plan, the surgical strategy must deliver a result that can receive the implants and a prosthesis and meet the requirements of function and esthetics. The task of the designer is to finalize the occlusal objective and to create a method to guide the surgeon in the repositioning of skeletal segments.

The objective of this chapter is to provide a standardized protocol for orthognathic cast surgery, splint fabrication, and operative navigation that can be used in most cases. The cast surgery process has three phases: *(1)* proper mounting of accurate dental casts, including navigational landmarks, on the articulator; *(2)* repositioning of the casts within the articulator to meet the objectives of occlusion and esthetics; and *(3)* use of the repositioned casts to create splints to guide surgery and stabilize fragments.

The first and third phases of this process are essentially laboratory procedures that can be completed by technicians. The critical decision-making phase is the second phase, when the fragments are repositioned. The surgeon cannot simulate segmentation of jaws without substantial knowledge and experience, because each skeletal fragment involves demands on the vascular pedicle, nerve supply, and visual access that are not apparent in the simulated environment.

The second phase requires the most judgment. Proper positioning of the maxillary central incisors is critical to a successful esthetic result. This position is determined initially during maxillary cast repositioning. The projected central incisor crown positions are set precisely within the reference system of the articulator and embedded surgical indicators. These laboratory landmarks are later transferred to the patient's head during the surgical procedure.

In the present example, the diagnosis and bioengineering phase (including clinical examination and preliminary surgical simulation with articulated casts) indicated that the mandibular surgery would consist of a segmental midline osteotomy and a left sagittal split osteotomy. The maxillary surgery would involve a Le Fort I osteotomy without segmentation (see Fig 11-4).

Preparation and mounting of dental casts

General osteotomy plans are often determined using preliminary records, such as casts made prior to orthodontic treatment, or orthodontic progress records. This process was described in the prior section. Virtual analysis based on computed tomography or cone beam computed tomography can be useful in generating initial plans. In general, the use of dental stone casts is best when definitive surgical plans are being created, particularly when the dental arch requires segmental osteotomies.

Definitive surgical planning begins with dental casts taken specifically for surgical planning. The geometry and theoretical basis of this method is discussed in chapter 9.

Every precaution is taken to ensure that the impressions are accurate and that no tooth movement occurs between the time the impressions are taken and the time surgery is performed. The impressions are taken with a passive archwire in place. This archwire should remain in place and without activation prior to the surgery. Orthodontic tray wax covers the archwire and brackets so that the impression can be removed with minimal force and minimal risk of distortion of the impression material.

The cast base is trimmed at an angle to approximate the maxillary osteotomy, in this case a Le Fort I osteotomy (Figs 11-6a to 11-6c). Although the measurements across the simulated osteotomy are of limited value, general trends in displacement represent useful information. Above the canine root apex, the height of the cast represents the position of the saw cut that will clear the canine root apex, leave enough bone to place the bone plate, and enter the nasal aperture above the nasal rim.

The vertical height tapers downward posteriorly. This is important for the cast simulation and during surgery. The planned osteotomy and the surgical osteotomy must reach the most inferior position as it approaches the junction of the pterygoid plates. This limits the risk of damage to the pterygoid plates and vital adjacent structures. The result is a tapered cast base.

Figure 11-6d shows a Le Fort I maxillary osteotomy fragment created on a dry skull. The dental cast should generally reproduce this shape. There are really only two useful landmarks at the Le Fort I osteotomy on each side: the osteotomy displacement at the piriform rim and at the zygomatic buttress. The anatomy and limited visual access further compromise the use of these landmarks to guide the surgeon during orientation of osteotomy fragments. Reliance on these landmarks is the most common cause of a failure to correctly reposition maxillary fragments (see chapter 9).

After the cast is trimmed, cast surgery indicator mounts are attached to disposable articulator mounting plates (Fig 11-7a). At least three indicators are necessary to define a plane of reference from which the maxillary cast movements will be measured (Fig 11-7b). The mounted indicators are engaged in the grooves of the mounting plate or cemented with cyanoacrylate adhesive. If the maxillary cast is to be divided into multiple segments, additional indicators may be necessary to visualize how cast movements will manifest in the clinical or surgical setting.

The use of a facebow to mount the cast establishes an approximate relationship between the dental arch and the temporomandibular joints (Fig 11-8a). This is important when the

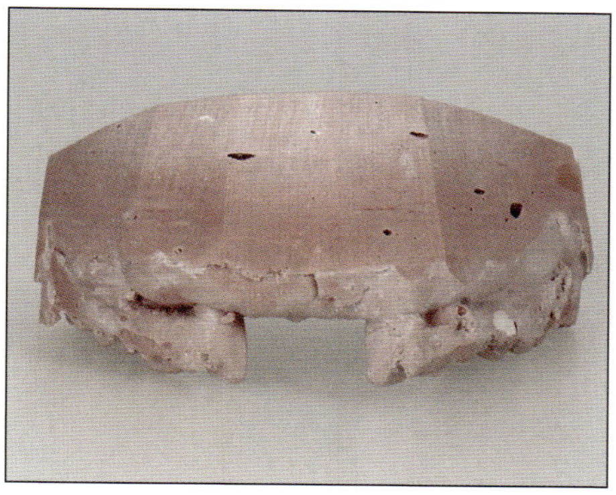

Fig 11-6a *(right)* The surgical cast, prepared with orthodontic appliances blocked out during the impression process, is trimmed.

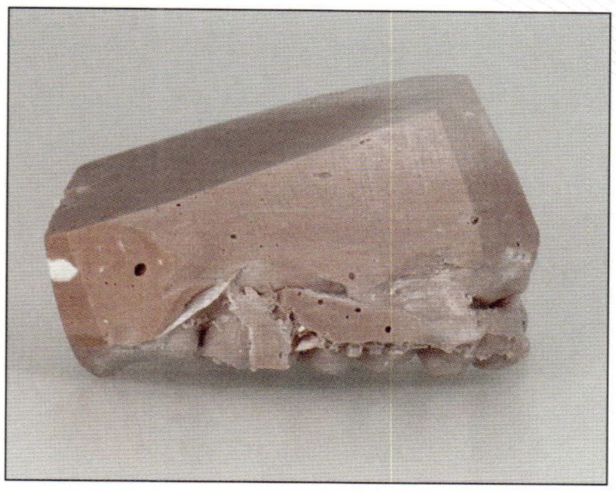

Fig 11-6b *(far right)* The cast base is trimmed to the approximate plane of the osteotomy.

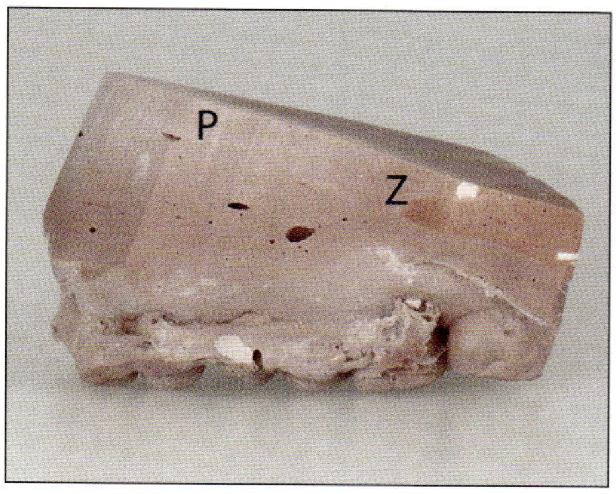

Fig 11-6c *(right)* Cast landmarks have limited usefulness. Only measurements across the simulated osteotomy line between P (piriform rim) and Z (zygomatic buttress) have clinical application.

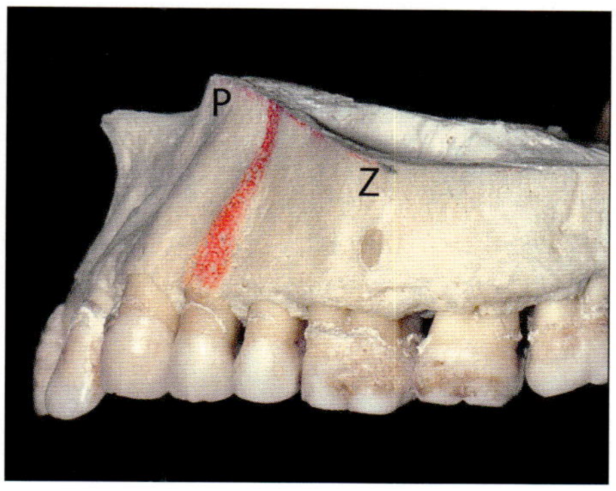

Fig 11-6d *(far right)* A Le Fort I osteotomy created on a skull specimen shows the anatomical limits of landmarks available to reposition the mobilized fragment. The osteotomy extends no further than P, the piriform rim. The osteotomy line is poorly visible posterior to point Z, the zygomatic buttress.

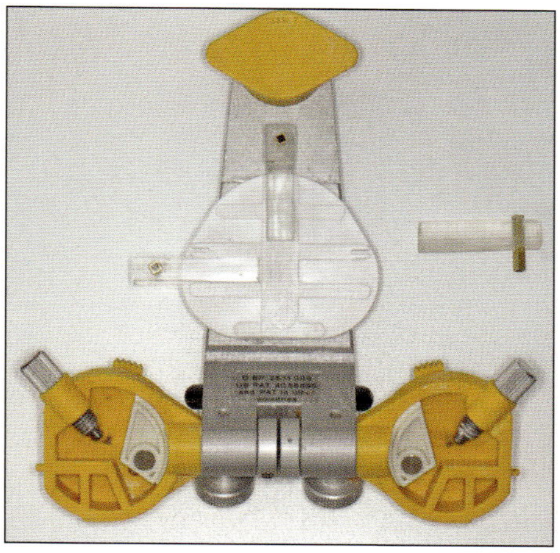

Fig 11-7a *(right)* Cast surgery indicator mounts are attached to disposable articulator mounting plates.

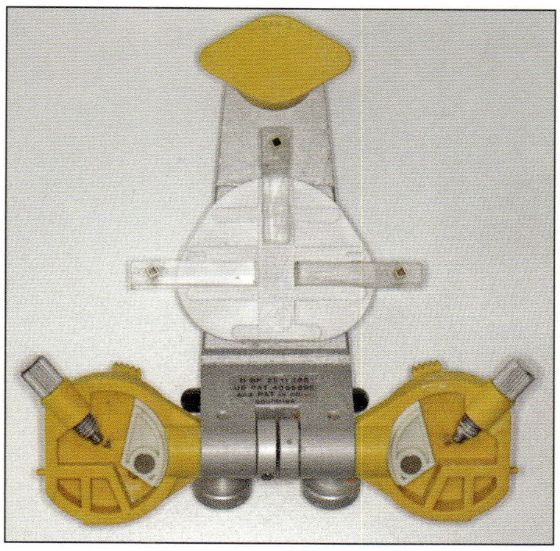

Fig 11-7b *(far right)* Three cast surgery indicator blocks are attached to the mounting plate.

surgical plan involves mandibular osteotomies that maintain ramus continuity. In these cases, the dentition on the orbiting segment must rotate around a condylar pivot. The arbitrary hinge axis transfer of ear-oriented facebows is accurate enough for this purpose.

The second goal of the facebow transfer is to approximate the postural head position. This allows the casts to be oriented within the articulator in a way that simulates the natural head position. In some cases, the ear positions and head cant do not allow a single facebow position. In those cases, the condylar position on the side of the orbiting mandibular fragment is recorded on the facebow. The facebow is displaced at the expense of the ear mount on the side that will undergo mandibular osteotomy. This allows the postural head position and midline to be transferred to the articulator and preserves the condylar position on the side of the mandible that will maintain ramus continuity.

Before mounting plaster is placed, a small amount of separating medium is applied to the cast base to allow separation of the cast and mounting plaster during the cast repositioning phase. Cutting the plaster cast is not necessary. The mounting plaster secures the maxillary cast (Fig 11-8b). The plaster also invests the indicator mounts.

Two vertical lines are placed across the osteotomy line represented by the plaster junction. The anterior line represents the position of the Le Fort I osteotomy as it enters the piriform aperture. The posterior line represents the osteotomy as it passes the zygomatic buttress. From a surgical standpoint, the measurements between these two lines provide the only information to guide the surgeon during repositioning of the maxillary

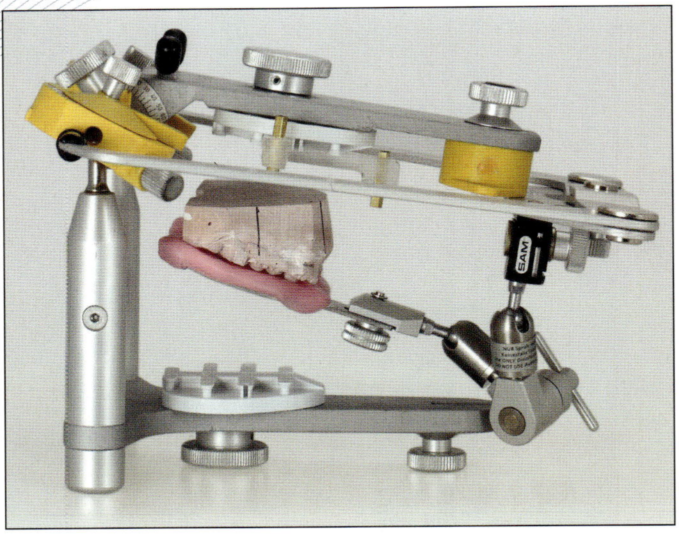

Fig 11-8a A facebow transfer is used for maxillary cast mounting.

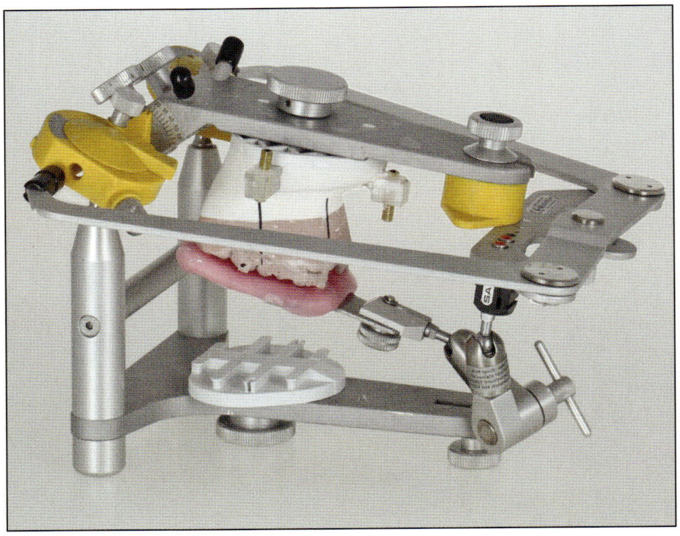

Fig 11-8b After a small amount of separating medium is applied to the cast base, the maxillary cast is mounted with mounting plaster.

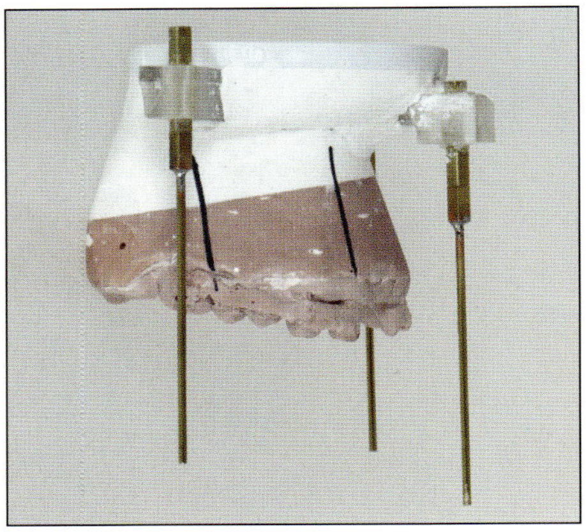

Fig 11-8c Indicator probes are engaged in the mounts.

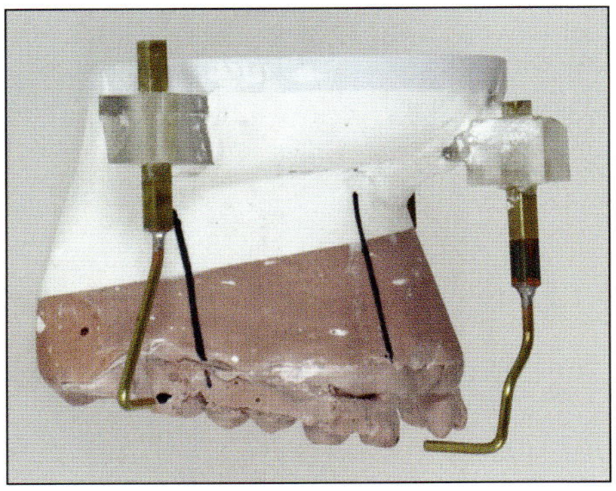

Fig 11-8d The indicator probes are bent and trimmed.

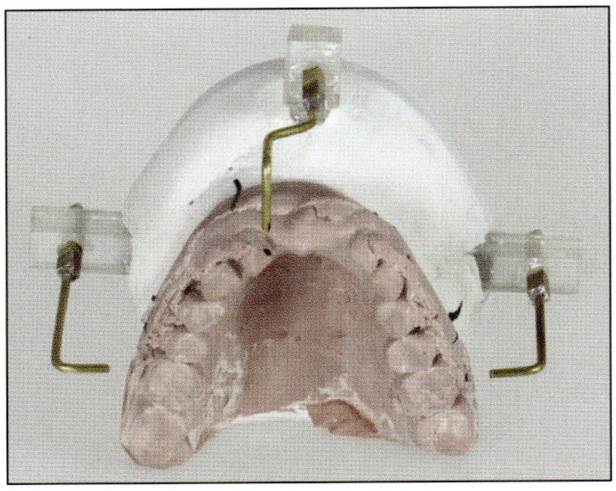

Fig 11-8e Three is the minimum number of indicators needed to define the maxillary plane of reference.

fragment. Anterior to the piriform line is the nasal aperture. No measurements can be made in this region because it has no skeletal analog on the articulator plaster mounting base. The area posterior to the zygomatic buttress line is deep within a soft tissue tunnel and cannot be directly visualized. Measurements within this limited zone cannot accurately orient the maxilla to the precision that modern cases demand.

The three indicators record the positions of essential landmarks (Fig 11-8c). The probes are then bent and trimmed (Fig 11-8d). The most important landmark is the maxillary incisor because it will determine the symmetry of the final restoration and the amount of incisor that is visible. The anteroposterior position of the maxillary incisor must correspond to the limitations of the mandibular orbiting segment. The anterior projection of the incisor will impact the projection of the piriform base. This skeletal unit supports the contour of the face and lip that is critical to the cosmetic result.

The posterior molar landmarks allow orientation of the occlusal cant. These measurements can be transferred directly to the surgical setting using the cranial headframe or indirectly through occlusal splints. Together, the three indicators define the maxillary plane of reference (Fig 11-8e).

In this case, the maxilla will be repositioned as a single unit. The postoperative position of the maxillary right lateral incisor must be accurate if implants placed later to restore the central incisors are to be symmetric. The vertical position of the lateral incisor will determine the amount of anterior teeth visible during smiling and facial expression (Figs 11-8f and 11-8g). If the maxilla were treatment planned for multiple segments, additional indicators might be necessary to orient and verify correct positioning of each fragment

The cast, indicators, and articulator mounting base can be removed from the articulator as a unit without losing their relationships. This allows the case to be referenced for future follow-up and study. The maxillary cast can be separated from the mounting. The indicators remain as stable landmarks. The indicator probes are removed and labeled (Fig 11-8h).

The occlusal registration is used to mount the mandibular cast (Fig 11-8i). The mandibular cast is mounted with orthodontic stone (Fig 11-8j).

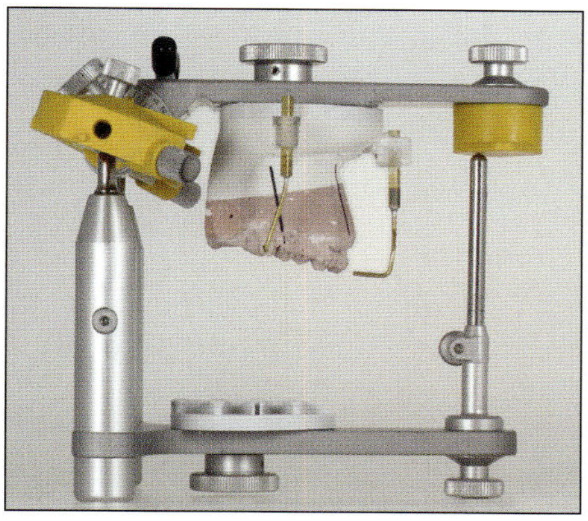

Fig 11-8f The maxillary cast is mounted on the articulator.

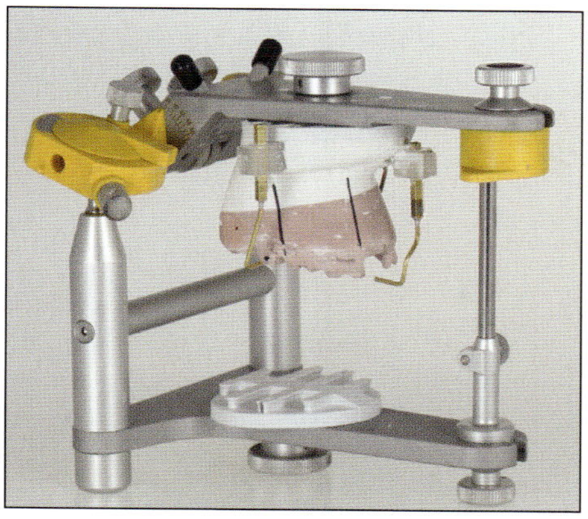

Fig 11-8g The anterior indicator points to the maxillary right lateral incisor because the central incisors are missing.

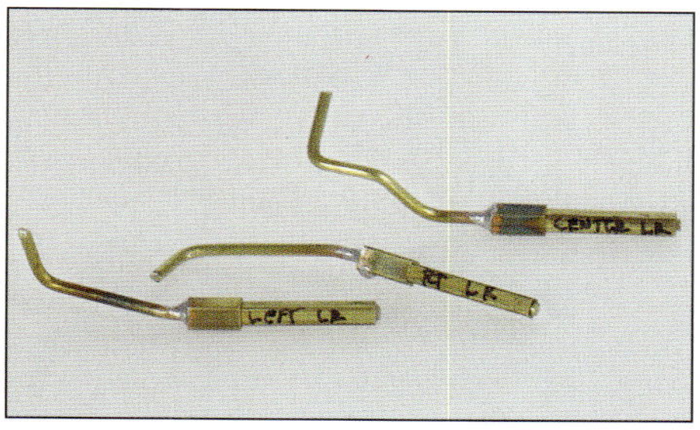

Fig 11-8h The indicator probes are removed and labeled.

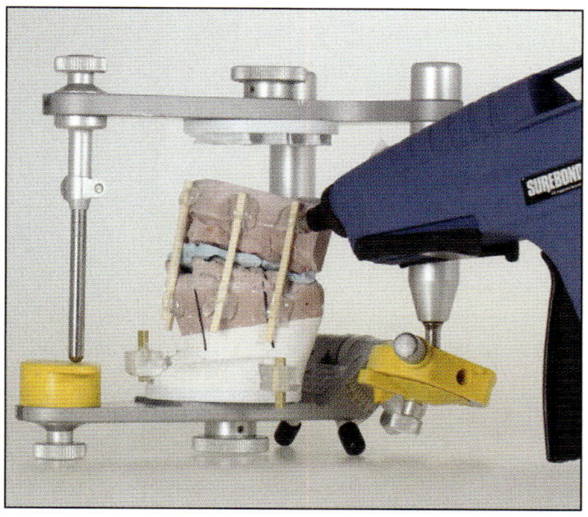

Fig 11-8i The occlusal registration is used to mount the mandibular cast.

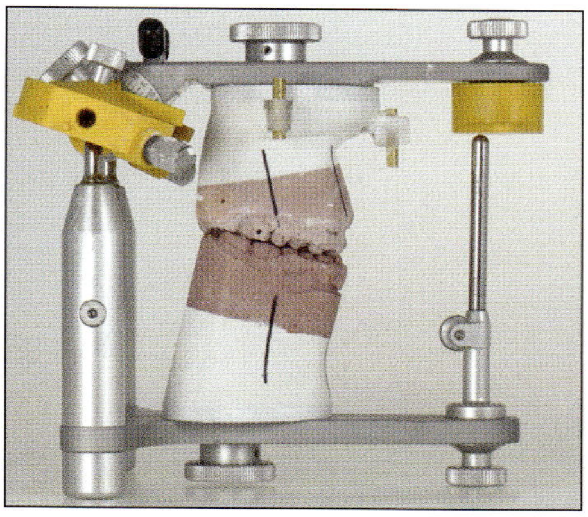

Fig 11-8j The mandibular cast is mounted with orthodontic stone.

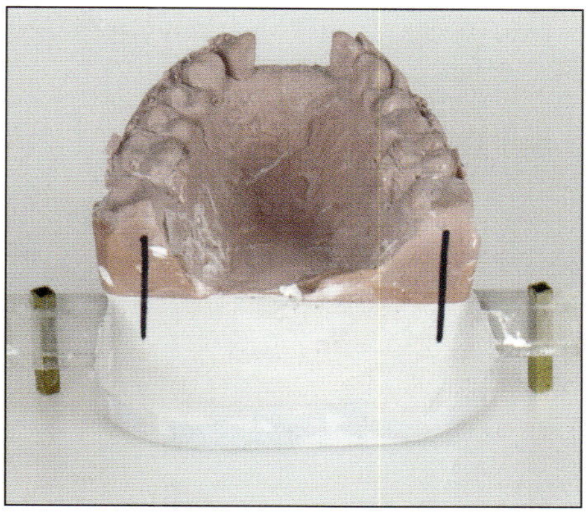

Fig 11-8k Index lines on the posterior surface of the maxillary cast help to assess the lateral rotational displacement introduced during maxillary repositioning.

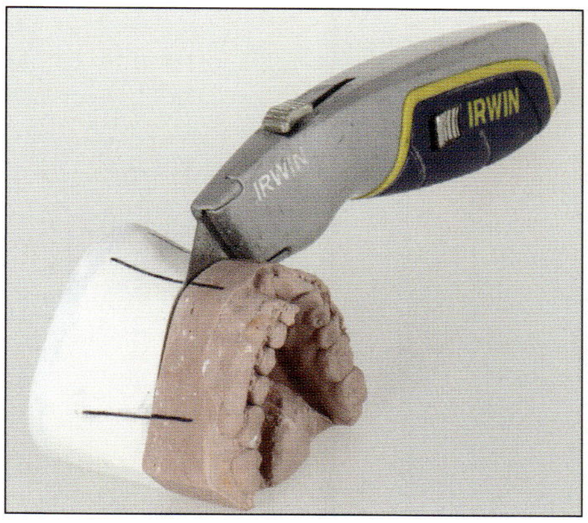

Fig 11-8l The maxillary cast is separated.

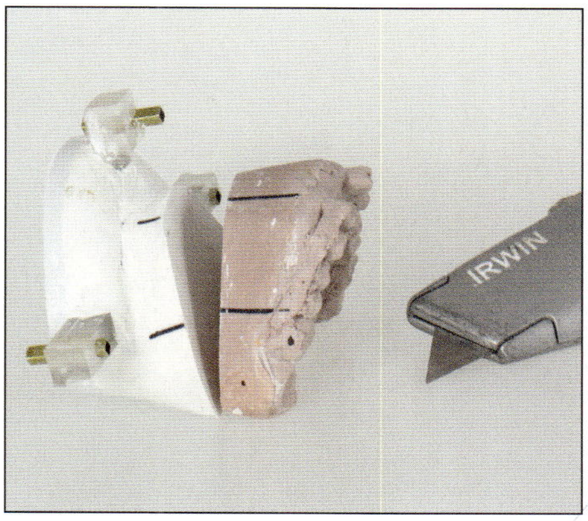

Fig 11-8m The mandibular cast is separated in the same manner.

Index lines created on the posterior maxillary cast help to assess the lateral rotational displacement (yaw) introduced during maxillary repositioning (Fig 11-8k).

The Le Fort I osteotomy is simulated by separation of the cast from the plaster mounting (Fig 11-8l). Because separating medium had been placed, the cast releases with a gentle tap of a utility knife. The mandibular cast is separated in the same manner (Fig 11-8m).

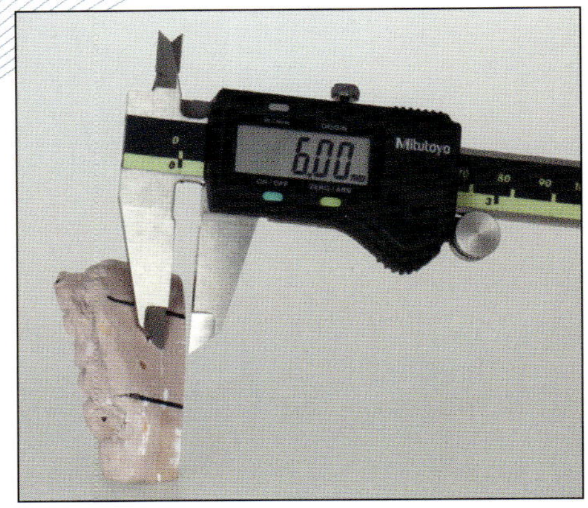

Fig 11-8n A caliper is used for horizontal landmark placement.

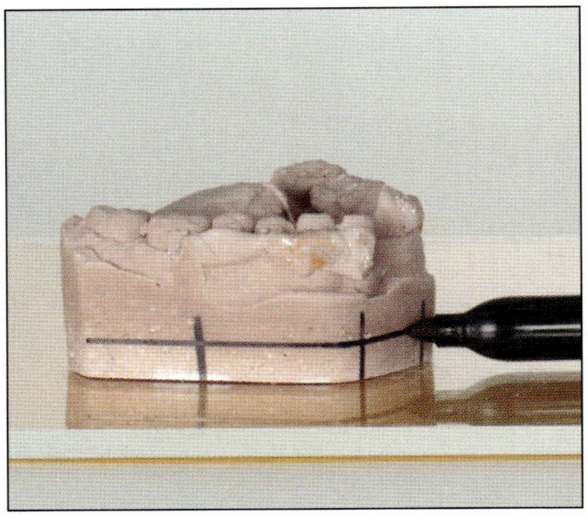

Fig 11-8o A permanent marker is rested on a flat surface, and the cast is rotated, creating a horizontal line.

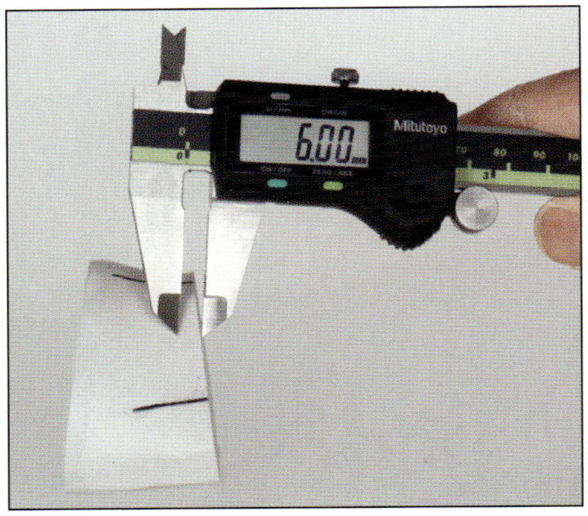

Fig 11-8p The scribe mark is made on the plaster mounting base.

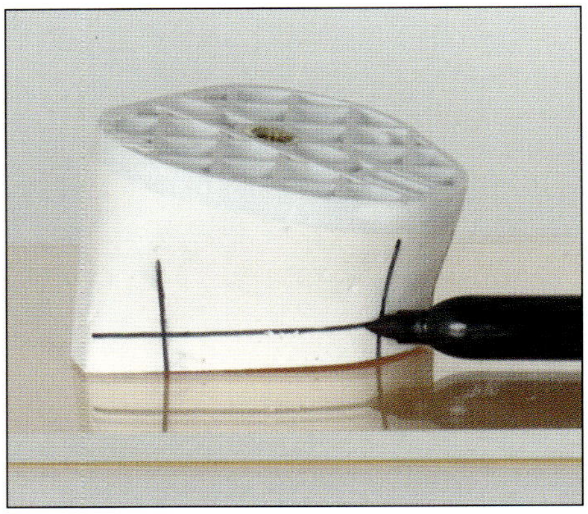

Fig 11-8q A permanent marker is used to place a horizontal index mark.

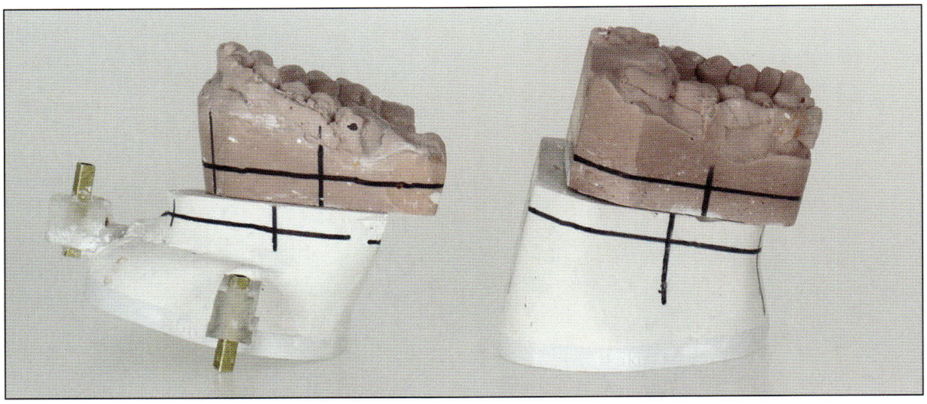

Fig 11-8r The marked casts are ready to remount.

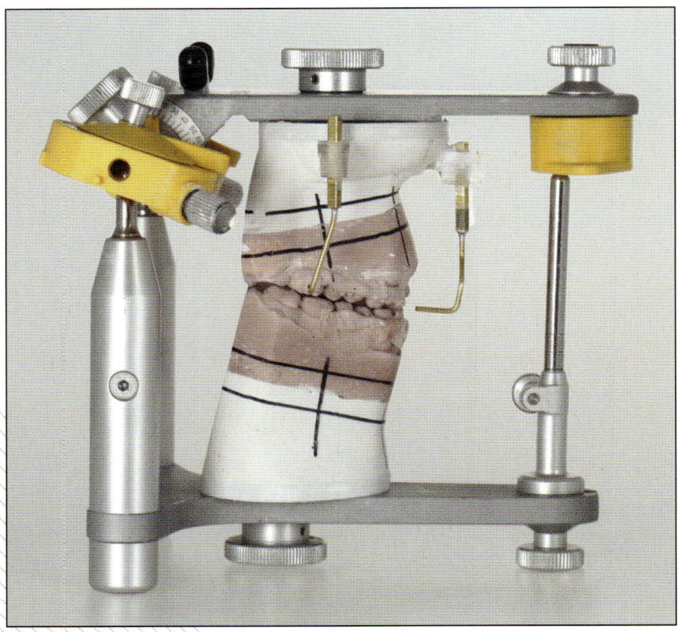

Fig 11-8s The remounted casts are ready for cast repositioning.

A caliper is used to scribe a horizontal line in the cast base (Fig 11-8n). A distance of 6 mm is chosen for two reasons: *(1)* The distance between the lines, 12 mm, is less than the amount usually cut off during cast surgery; and *(2)* more important, 6 mm is the distance resulting from laying a Sharpie marker on its side. A permanent marker is rested on a flat surface, and the cast is rotated, creating a horizontal line (Fig 11-8o). The caliper is used to place a 6-mm scribe mark on the mounting base (Fig 11-8p). Permanent marker is used to place a horizontal index mark (Fig 11-8q). The marked casts are ready to remount (Fig 11-8r). A very small drop of cyanoacrylate glue is applied to remount the casts to their plaster bases.

The articulator setup is ready for cast repositioning if bilateral ramus osteotomies are planned (Fig 11-8s). An additional step is necessary if the surgical plan involves maintaining the continuity of one or both mandibular rami. When the continuity of the mandibular ramus is to be maintained, movement of the osteotomy fragment rotates ("orbits") around the centric relation position of the condyle of the intact hemimandible. Teeth contained within the fragment move in an orbital pattern with the condyle at the coordinate system origin. Two techniques to simulate orbital fragment movements are presented. In the case presentation, a prototype instrument is shown that can be used in multiple cases. The second method uses commercially available materials that are intended for single use.

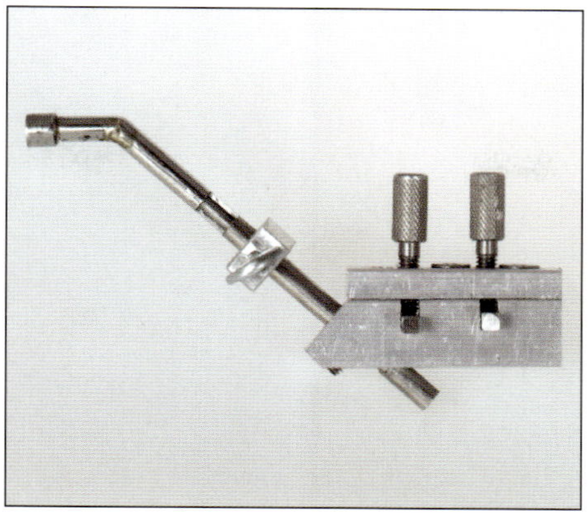

Fig 11-9a *(right)* Instrument to simulate orbiting mandibular osteotomies.

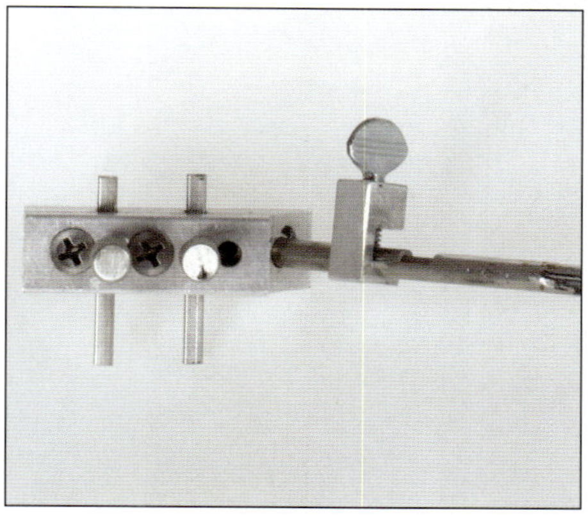

Fig 11-9b *(far right)* Two square keys allow mounting of the instrument onto the mandibular cast segment.

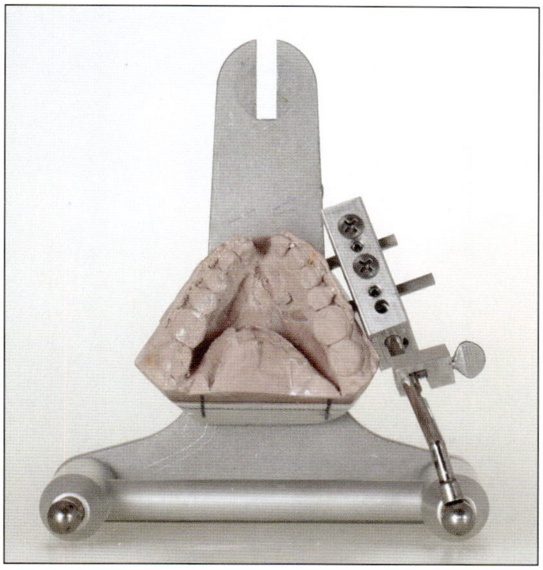

Fig 11-9c The instrument simulates rotation of the hemimandibular segment around the right temporomandibular joint.

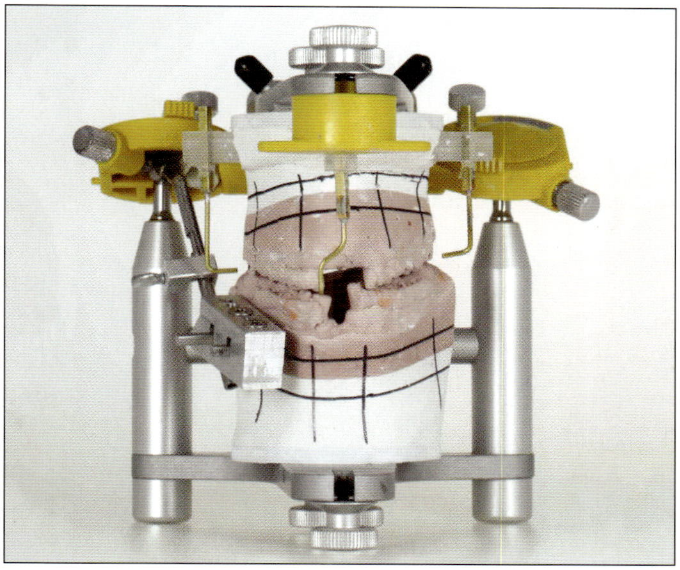

Fig 11-9d Surgical simulation setup for the planned osteotomies.

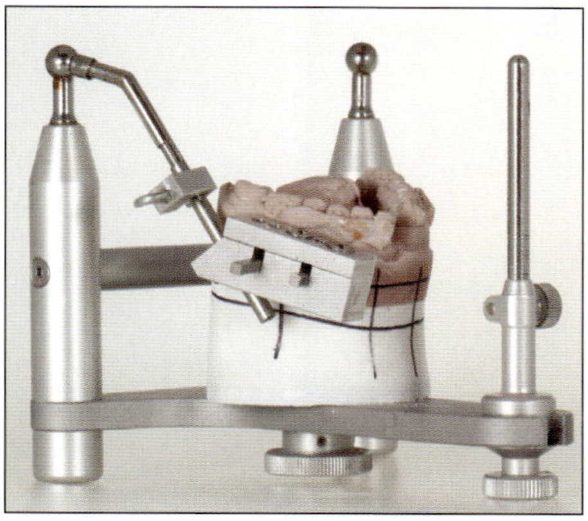

Fig 11-9e *(right)* The orbiting fragment instrument is in place.

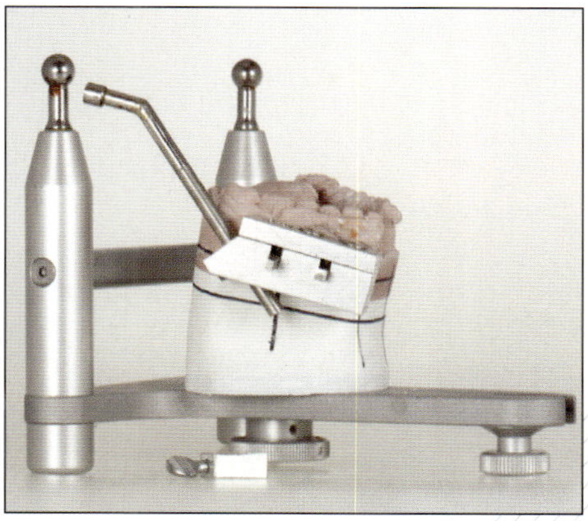

Fig 11-9f *(far right)* The instrument is disengaged so that the cast can be separated.

An orbiting fragment instrument was designed by the author to simulate orbiting mandibular osteotomies. Figure 11-9a shows a prototype of an orbital fragment simulating instrument. Two square keys allow mounting of the instrument onto the mandibular cast segment (Fig 11-9b). The instrument simulates rotation of the hemimandibular segment around the right temporomandibular joint (Fig 11-9c), showing a surgical simulation of the results of the planned osteotomies (Fig 11-9d). When the orbiting fragment instrument is placed, it contacts the articulator condyle element (Fig 11-9e). Before the cast is removed from the articulator, the instrument is disengaged from its articulation with the condylar element (Fig 11-9f).

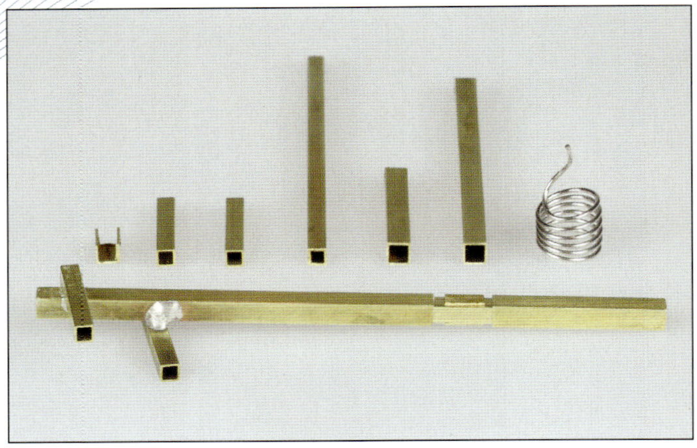

Fig 11-10a Square brass tubing is cut into lengths assembled into the guide device *(bottom)*. The main section components telescope together. The two extensions that engage the plaster cast are affixed to the main body with electrical solder.

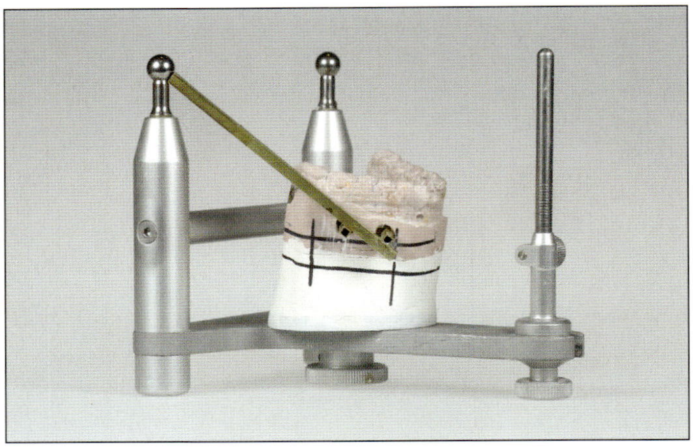

Fig 11-10b Two holes drilled into the plaster cast allow for positioning of the device. Orthodontic resin or composite resin is used to cement the extensions into holes in the cast.

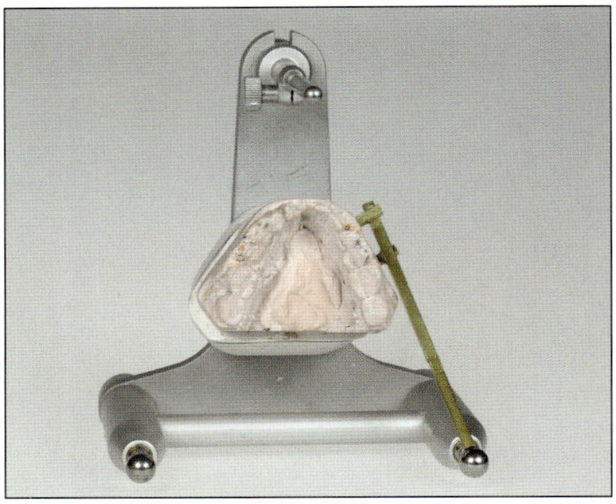

Fig 11-10c The mobilized cast can be moved using the orbiting guide to maintain a fixed radius with the condyle.

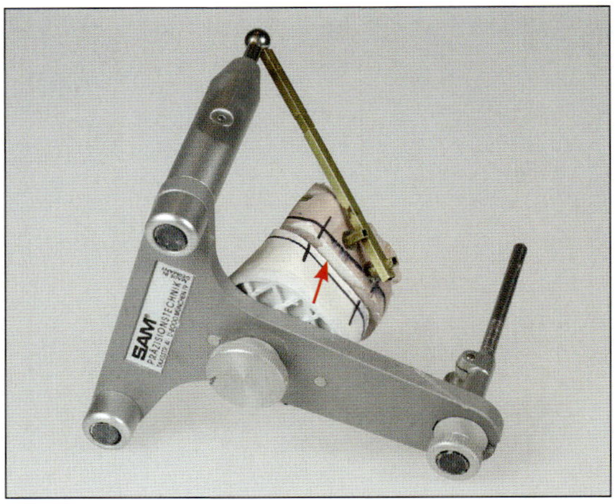

Fig 11-10d The cast movements simulate how the mandibular arch would pivot when surgery spares the right mandible from osteotomy. View of the cast from below shows that the orbiting movement of the mandible results in lateral displacement of the right mandibular body *(arrow)*.

Alternatively, surgical simulation of the results of the planned osteotomies can be created without the use of an orbiting fragment instrument. Sections of telescoping square brass tubing used for model making can be fashioned into a guide to achieve orbiting fragment simulation (K and S Engineering, Chicago). The only fabrication necessary is to join two of the components with electrical solder (Fig 11-10a). Two holes drilled into the mandibular cast accept the anchoring struts (Fig 11-10b). The square tubing mounting extensions are cemented into the cast holes with autopolymerizing orthodontic resin. This configuration allows guided movement of the mobilized mandibular cast around the right articulator condyle (Figs 11-10c and 11-10d).

Repositioning of casts to simulate surgery

When the articulated casts are ready for repositioning, the cast is separated from the plaster base (Fig 11-11a). The mandibular cast is divided at the midline, simulating the planned midline osteotomy (Fig 11-11b). The mandibular right fragment is rotated laterally, using the condylar element as the center of rotation. The fragment is moved so that symmetry is restored with the maxillary landmarks (Fig 11-11c).

Mandibular expansion allows for restoration of a space for two normal incisor teeth (Fig 11-11d). A dental cast obtained prior to the injury verifies the measurement of the width of the lost teeth (Fig 11-11e). The simulation shows the amount of bone that has been lost and will have to be replaced (Fig 11-11f).

The results of repositioning show the planned movements that were developed during the simulation process (Fig 11-12a). The expected occlusion can be evaluated in detail. The specific three-dimensional movements of each segment are shown.

The most important movement from an esthetic standpoint is indicated by the midline indicator probe (Fig 11-12b). The midline indicator shows that, in order to meet the goals of esthetics, occlusion, right temporomandibular joint position, future implant location, and neuromuscular support of the mandibular osteot-

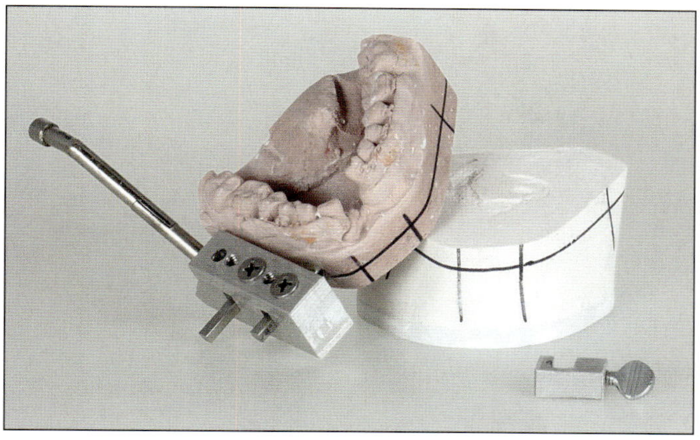

Fig 11-11a The cast is separated from the plaster base.

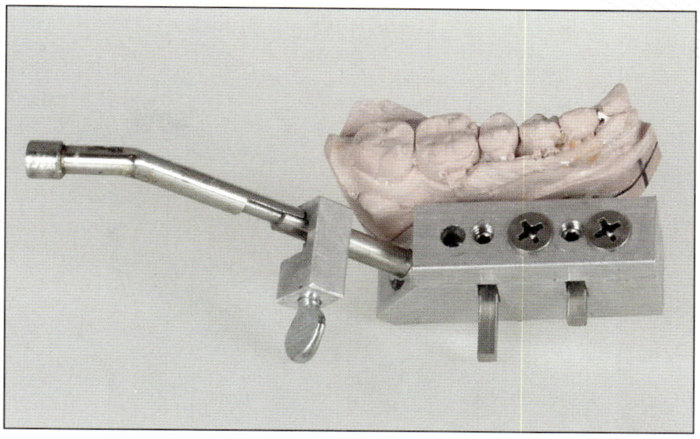

Fig 11-11b The mandibular cast is divided at the midline, simulating the planned midline osteotomy.

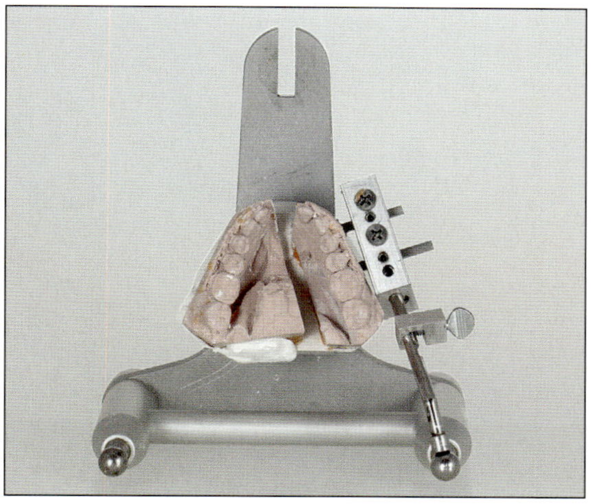

Fig 11-11c The mandibular fragments are repositioned.

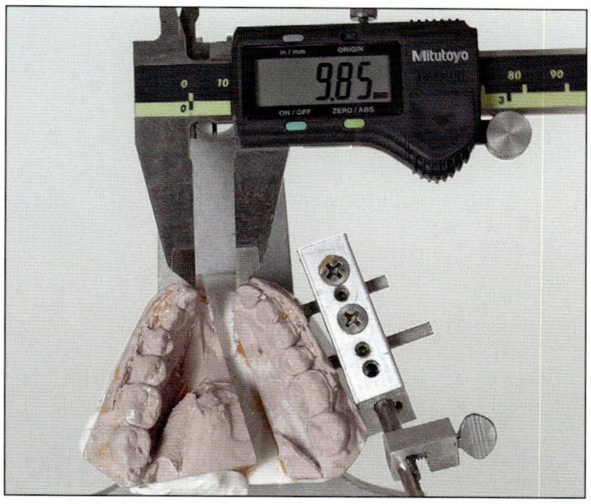

Fig 11-11d Mandibular expansion restores a space for two normal incisor teeth.

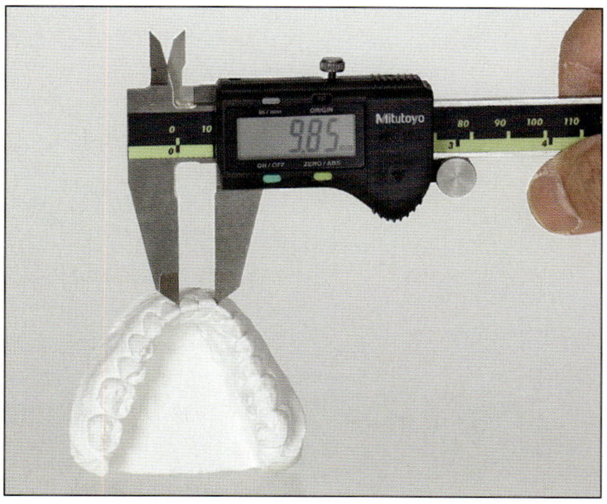

Fig 11-11e A pretrauma dental cast provides the measurement of the width of the lost teeth.

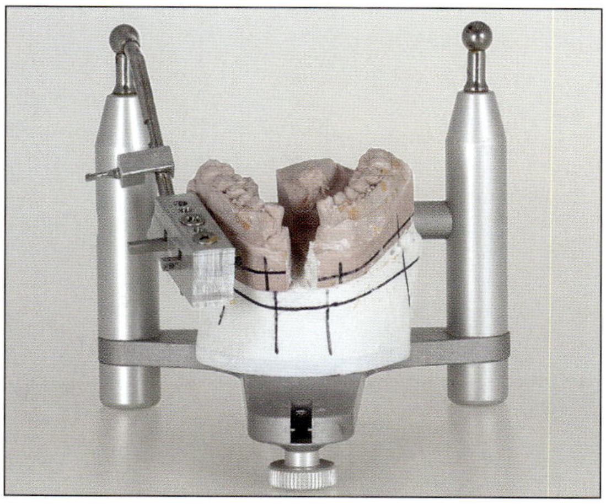

Fig 11-11f Simulation of the mandibular osteotomies shows the amount of bone that has been lost and will need to be replaced.

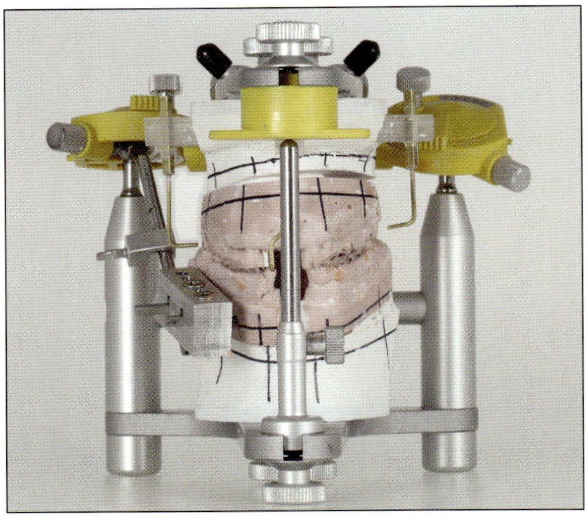

Fig 11-12a Total surgical simulation. The specific three-dimensional movements of each segment are shown. The most important movement from an esthetic standpoint is indicated by the midline indicator probe.

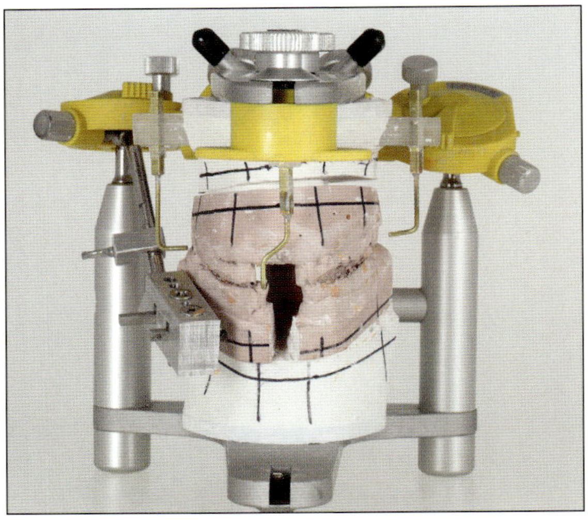

Fig 11-12b The anterior indicator probe defines the critical movement necessary to correct the midline. The mandibular cast shows the amount of bone that must be added to regain the lost width.

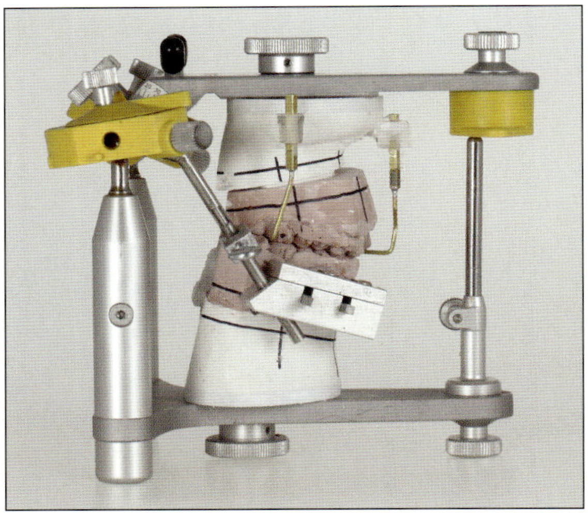

Fig 11-12c The lateral view shows the protraction of the maxillary right lateral incisor.

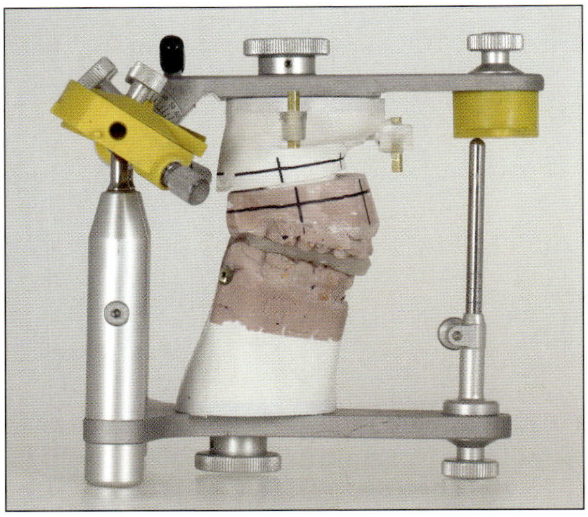

Fig 11-12d The right maxilla shows the need for moderate advancement but not substantial downgrafting. Anterior movement of the maxilla will open a chamber between the posterior maxilla and the pterygoid plates.

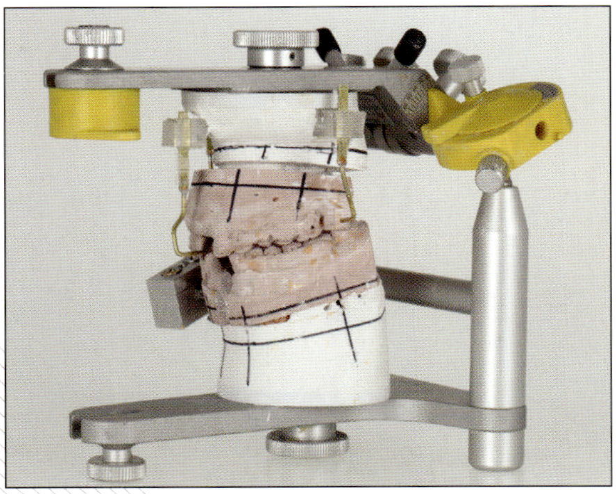

Fig 11-12e The left maxilla requires protraction to correct its traumatic impaction. The movement includes a substantial downgraft that will require internal fixation and management of the predicted discontinuity.

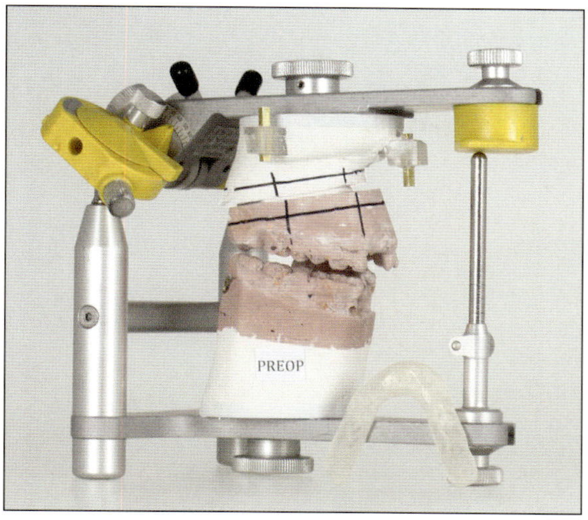

Fig 11-13a An intermediary splint is fabricated to reposition the maxilla.

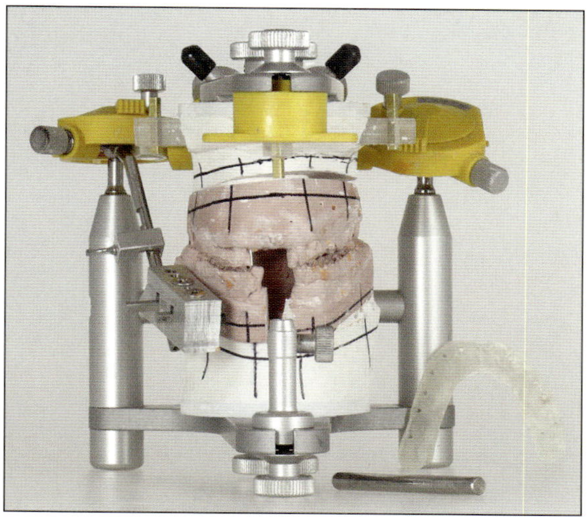

Fig 11-13b A final occlusal splint is fabricated.

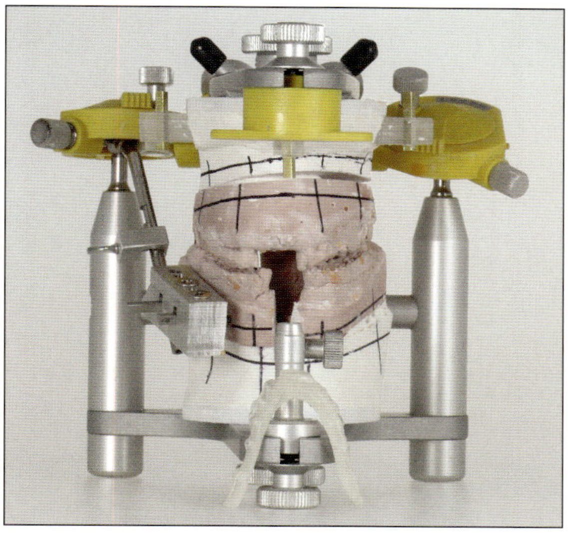

Fig 11-13c A lingual splint is fabricated to stabilize and maintain the mandibular width correction. Use of a lingual splint instead of occlusal splints allows direct evaluation of the occlusion during the postoperative period.

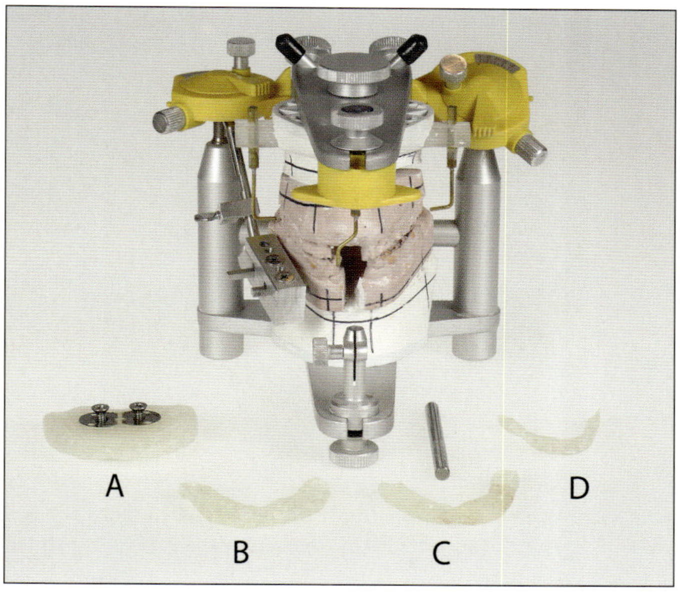

Fig 11-14 Guides used during surgery. Maxillary osteotomy mobilizing splint (A), intermediary splint (B), final interocclusal splint (C), and final lingual splint (D). The articulator brass rod indicators show the net movements to be verified by the headframe-based indicators.

omies, the maxillary right lateral incisor must move laterally 3 mm. For the fragments to be properly positioned, the right lateral incisor must be protracted 4 mm and be maintained vertically with 0 mm of change (Fig 11-12c).

The right side of the maxilla shows the need for moderate advancement but not substantial downgrafting (Fig 11-12d). Anterior movement of the maxilla will open a chamber between the posterior segment of the maxilla and the pterygoid plates. The left side of the maxilla requires protraction to correct its traumatic impaction (Fig 11-12e). The movement includes a substantial downgraft that will require internal fixation and management of the expected discontinuity.

Fabrication of splints

An intermediary splint is fabricated to reposition the maxilla (Fig 11-13a). The repositioned maxillary cast is oriented relative to the unmoved mandibular cast. A final occlusal splint is fabricated between the repositioned maxillary and mandibular casts (Fig 11-13b).

A lingual splint is fabricated to stabilize and maintain the mandibular width correction (Fig 11-13c). Use of a lingual splint instead of occlusal splints allows direct evaluation of the occlusion during the postoperative period. Maintaining a patient in an occlusal splint may obscure an occlusal problem resulting from errors in fragment repositioning or discrepancies in centric relation records. Figure 11-14 shows all of the guides to be used during surgery.

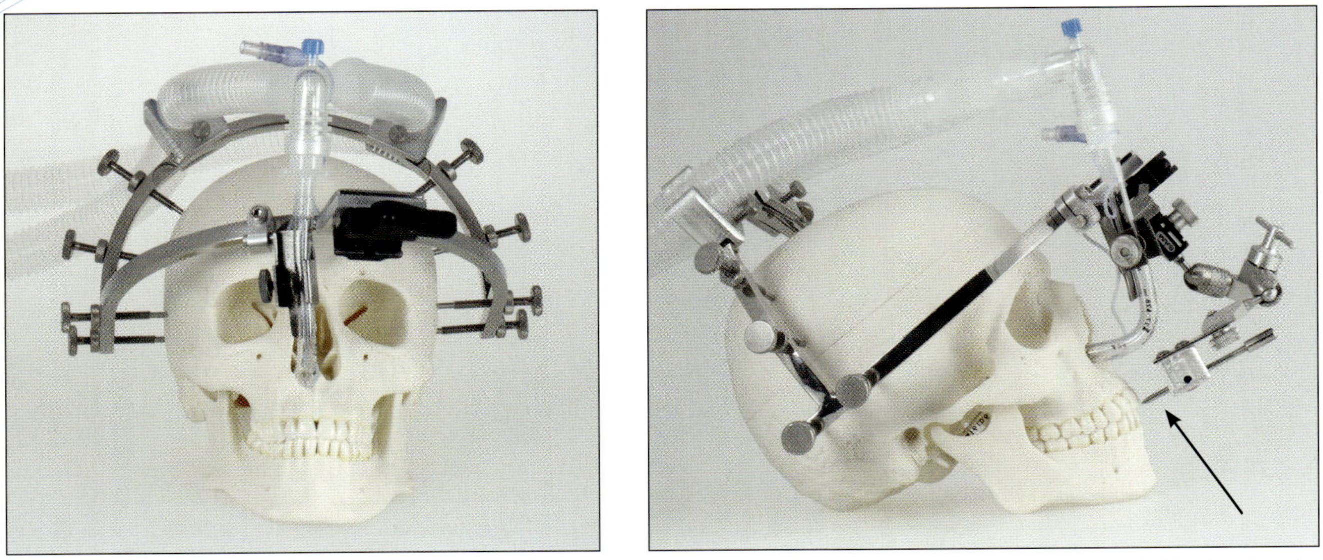

Figs 11-15a and 11-15b Surgical headframe. This instrument has detachable mechanical indicators that register anatomical landmarks prior to their mobilization with osteotomies. Single-tip pointers *(arrow)* are used to register the preoperative position of critical landmarks such as the central incisors or the facial midline. Other indicators may be placed to register the cant of the occlusal plane, the projection of the gonial angle or malar process, or the position of the mental prominence. It is essential that critical landmarks be registered before osteotomies and skeletal movements are performed.

Surgical Technique

The objective of the surgical phase is to apply the design created in the planning phase to the patient in an accurate and safe manner. The mission of the surgeon is to perform the osteotomies, reposition the fragments, and place fixation devices without compromising the integrity of adjacent anatomical structures or the patient's general physiology. Ideally, there is no compromise among accuracy, safety, and expediency. All of the factors that impact accuracy and safety must be balanced in the surgical phase.

The surgical plan must include specific technical procedures that will yield an end result that meets both the functional and esthetic criteria. The ability to deliver predictable fragment repositioning in a consistent and safe manner must be inherent to the procedure design itself. This becomes more important with treatment plans that involve multiple fragments, two jaws, and dental implants. It is not useful to develop surgical plans that cannot be reproduced in the surgical setting.

Real-time surgical navigation must allow the surgeon to assess how the fragments are being oriented. This resource is critical to provide the surgeon information on the accuracy of the skeletal construction. The technique must include a strategy to assess the net effect of the surgery before the procedure is completed and general anesthesia reversed.

The bioengineering phase resulted in a plan that could meet the objectives of function and esthetics for the patient in the case example (see Fig 11-4). The essential elements critical to bone formation and maintenance were included in the proposed treatment plan. Neuromuscular deficiencies related to the injury were considered, and the osteotomies were engineered to accommodate for these challenges to healing. The design phase developed the general surgical plan into a detailed surgical plan. The surgical plan included definition of measurements and creation of devices needed to guide the surgeon in the execution of the design. Implementation of this design is greatly facilitated by headframe-based surgical navigation (see chapter 9).

Headframe-based surgical navigation

The surgeon enters the operating room with surgical casts that together serve as a three-dimensional blueprint of the surgical plan. The cast indicators on the articulator show the desired movements of important landmarks before and after repositioning. The headframe-based indicators should match the articulator indicator measurements, providing verification that the desired maxillary movement has been achieved. The series of occlusal splints guide the sequential repositioning of jaws and jaw segments (see Fig 11-14).

To establish a frame of reference that does not change during the course of surgery, a specially designed cranial headframe is used (Figs 11-15a and 11-15b). This instrument has detachable mechanical indicators that register anatomical landmarks prior to their mobilization with osteotomies. Single-tip pointers engaged on the headframe register the preoperative position of critical landmarks such as the position of the central incisors or the facial midline. Other indicators may be placed to register the cant of the occlusal plane, the projection of the gonial angle or malar process, or the position of the mental prominence. It is essential that critical landmarks be registered before osteotomies and skeletal movements are performed.

The second function of the headframe is to secure the anesthetic breathing tubes. Safe administration of general anesthesia demands protection of the endotracheal anesthetic tube. In addition, undesirable traction of the tube results in trauma

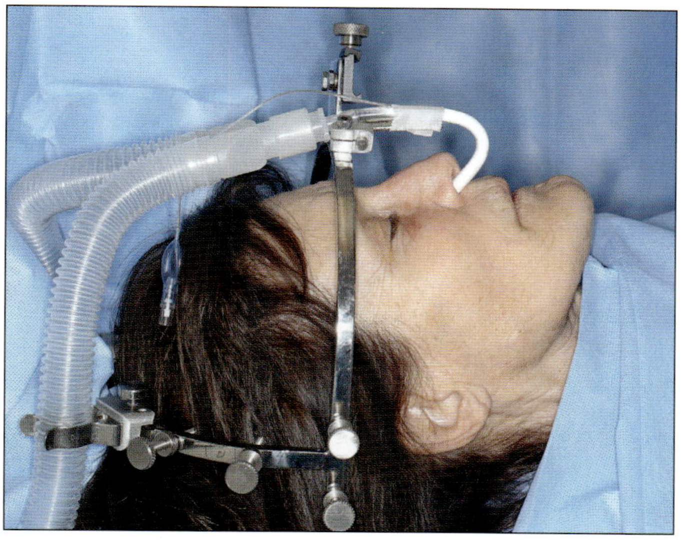

Fig 11-16a The headframe is mounted on the patient under anesthesia, and the anesthesia tubes are secured in a passive position.

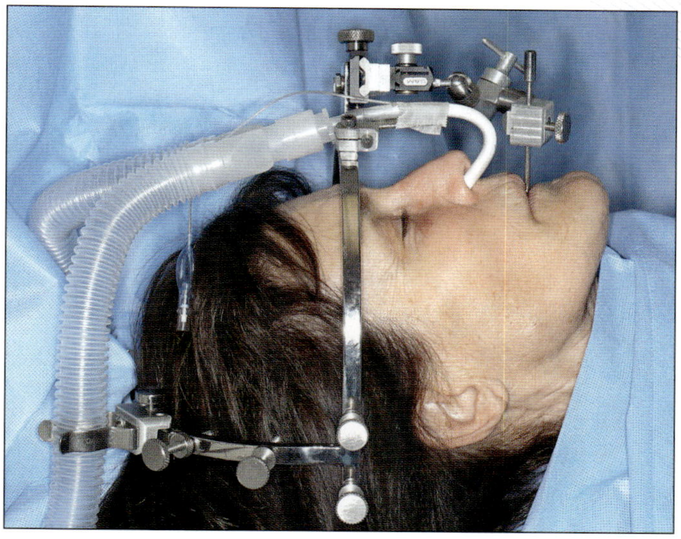

Fig 11-16b A single-tip pointer is mounted on the headframe and used to record the position of the incisor tooth.

to and distortion of the nose. This may result in ulcers of the nostril. Deviation of the nose also distorts the facial soft tissue drape, making assessment of symmetry more difficult.

The headframe establishes a reference point that is anchored to a structure that does not move or change during the procedure. During instrumentation of the osteotomies, the indicator is detached and safely stored. This allows unimpeded access to the surgical site.

The first step is to mount the headframe (Fig 11-16a). This device will serve as a frame of reference from which osteotomy fragment repositioning measurements are made and therefore must be mechanically stable. The headframe is secured by transcutaneous pins within the hairline. Anesthesia breathing tubes are secured to an attachment on the headframe.

An indicator device is engaged into the mounting platform on the headframe. This instrument incorporates a cardanic joint that allows rapid positioning of the indicator probe (Fig 11-16b). The probe is positioned to correspond to the same landmarks established by the articulator indicators. The headframe system allows direct transfer of the measurements from the articulator to the surgical setting.

Osteotomies and repositioning

Headframe-based navigation was critical to ensuring accurate fragment repositioning for the patient in this case, who had complicated traumatic deformities. The Le Fort I–level osteotomy was created through the lateral maxilla with a surgical saw (Fig 11-17a). The osteotomy was extended medially with osteotomes to divide the lateral nasal wall. A nasal septal osteotome was used to luxate the nasal septum from the maxillary crest. The lateral maxillary osteotomy extended posteriorly to the pterygomaxillary junction. The pterygomaxillary junction was not directly instrumented. A maxillary mobilizing instrument (Biomet) was engaged to rigidly purchase the maxilla.

The maxillary mobilizing instrument consisted of a base on which an acrylic resin occlusal splint was mounted (Fig 11-17b). The splint engaged all of the occlusal surfaces of the maxillary dental arch. Following elevation of the nasal mucosa, nasal rods with cleats were placed in the nasal cavity through the right and left nasal apertures. The cleats of these rods rigidly purchased the osseous nasal floor. The screws were tightened to secure the device in rigid purchase on the maxilla. The maxilla was clamped between the acrylic resin splint below and the nasal rods above. Vertical and horizontal levers were engaged on the instrument to apply force that luxated the maxilla and disengaged it from the pterygoid plates. As the levers were activated, the osteotomy opened. Protracting force separated the fusion between the posterior maxilla and the pterygoid plates (Fig 11-17c).

Depressing the mobilized maxilla inferiorly with expansion pliers revealed the intact pterygoid plates behind the mobilized maxilla (Fig 11-17d). Avoiding damage to the pterygoid plates is important. These structures are the origin of the primary neuromuscular system that joins the cranial base to the mandible. Maintaining the integrity of this system results in rapid and predictable bone growth at the pterygomaxillary disjunction. Fracture of the pterygoid plates may result in substantial bleeding. Aberrant fractures that propagate superiorly may damage the optic nerves or penetrate the cranial base.

With the intermediary splint in place, the maxilla was elevated, and interfering bone was removed. With the indicator probe engaged on the headframe, the repositioning was refined and verified to be consistent with the planned movement (Fig 11-17e). When the position of the maxilla was judged to be correct, bone plates were placed to stabilize the fragment.

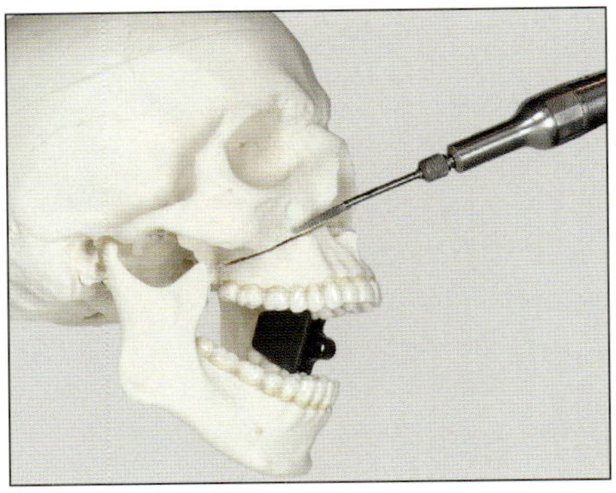

Fig 11-17a The osteotomy is created with a surgical saw.

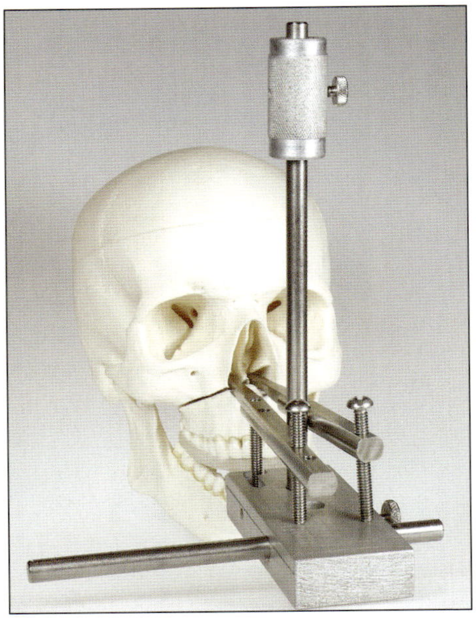

Fig 11-17b The maxillary mobilizer is prepared to separate the osteotomy and disjoin the pterygomaxillary junction.

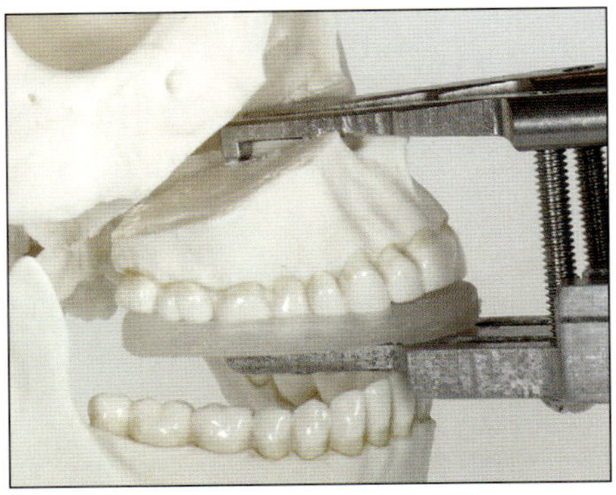

Fig 11-17c The maxilla is downfractured and separated from the pterygoid plates.

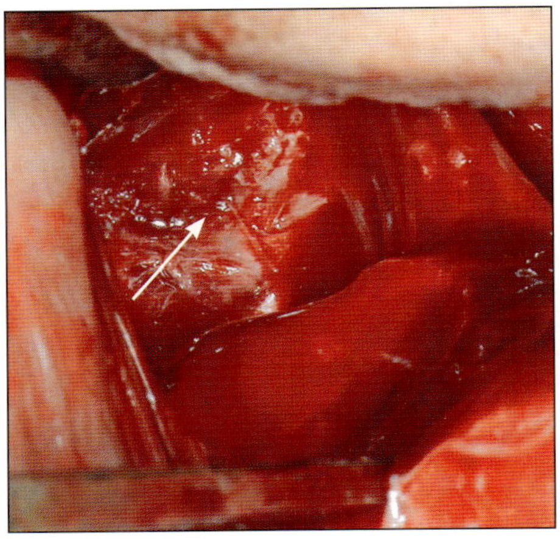

Fig 11-17d When the posterior region of the maxilla is depressed with expansion pliers, the intact pterygoid plates *(arrow)* can be seen.

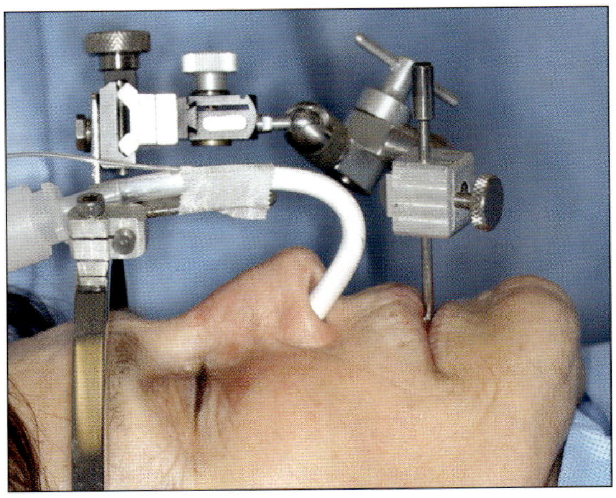

Fig 11-17e The headframe-mounted indicator is used for guidance to reposition the maxilla. After the fixation is in place, the indicator verifies correct placement of the maxilla and dental arch.

On the right side, advancement of the maxilla created a step but no gaps across the osteotomy (Fig 11-18a). This result was verified by comparing the surgical site findings with the surgical simulation. When repositioning was found to be accurate, two bone plates were placed on the right side.

If there is a discrepancy between the results of the surgical repositioning and the surgical simulation, the headframe indicators are used to determine the proper positioning of the maxilla. Measurements made during surgery across the osteotomy cannot predictably orient the maxillary fragment (see chapter 9). Small errors in the perceived repositioning at this osteotomy line may result in major errors in the position of the maxillary central incisors. The use of landmarks across the maxillary osteotomy to orient the fragment is the most common cause of major repositioning errors during orthognathic surgery.

After the fragments were fixated, collagen sponges infused with rhBMP-2 were used to cover the osteotomy line and the degloved portion of the right side of the maxilla (Fig 11-18b). Although osseous union could be expected in this region, rhBMP-2 was placed to promote rapid growth of a volume of bone lateral to the existing maxilla. Because the right ramus had been spared from osteotomy as an orbiting fragment, the vertical dimension of the mandible on the right side was mechanically stable. Promoting early union of the right maxillary osteotomy would support the stability of the left maxillary downgraft.

The left side of the maxilla required inferior and anterior repositioning. This resulted in a discontinuity and a substantial gap across the osteotomy. When the maxillary position was verified to be correct, bone plates provided initial stabilization. The gap was covered by a portion of bone harvested locally (Fig 11-19a).

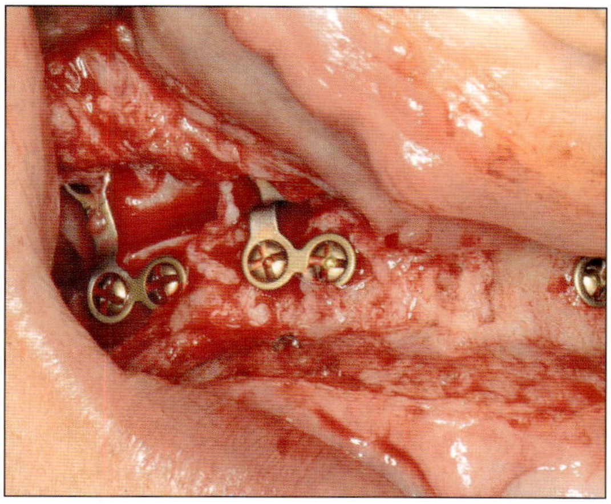

Fig 11-18a On the right side, advancement of the maxilla creates a step but no gaps across the osteotomy.

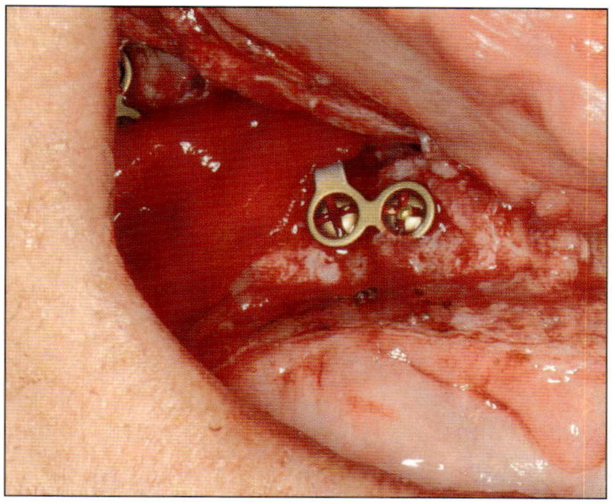

Fig 11-18b Bone morphogenetic protein on collagen sponges is applied.

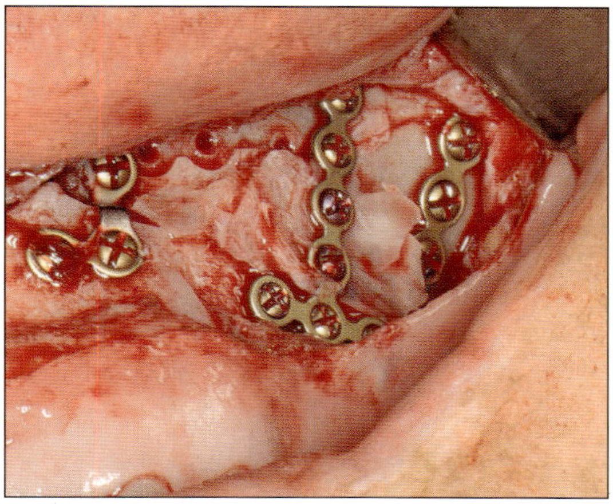

Fig 11-19a The planned maxillary movement has opened a large gap at the left osteotomy. The gap is covered with an autogenous bone graft and stabilized with a T-shaped bone plate.

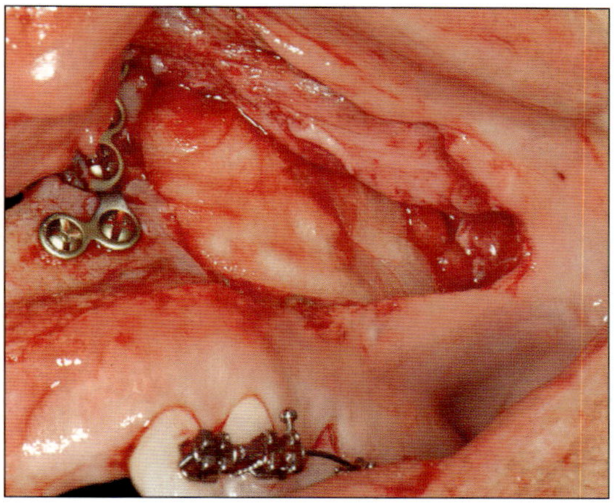

Fig 11-19b Bone morphogenetic protein on collagen sponges is positioned over the lateral portion of the left maxilla.

The purpose of the autogenous bone graft was to control the position of the rhBMP-2 graft and prevent its displacement into the maxillary sinus.

The left sides of the maxilla and mandible were at the highest risk for relapse. Maxillary advancement and downgrafting are inherently unstable. The risk of relapse was increased because the mandibular left ramus required osteotomy to correct a length deficiency. The engineering and design strategy attempted to address this problem by *(1)* maintaining the osseous continuity of the right ramus, *(2)* sparing the mandibular right neuromuscular system from the trauma of osteotomy-related dissection, and *(3)* maintaining bone contact at the right maxillary osteotomy.

On the left side, healing of the maxillary downgraft was supported by placement of a volume of collagen sponges containing rhBMP-2 to cover the entire degloved surface of the left side of the maxilla (Fig 11-19b). In this way, bone formation would not be limited to the thin, cut portions of the lateral maxillary sinus wall; instead, a mass of young bone would form to cover the lateral surface of the maxilla. This mass of bone would eventually remodel into a normal-appearing maxilla. During the initial healing phase, the additional bone volume helped to stabilize the maxilla and prevent relapse.

Following removal of bone plates placed by the original surgeon, it was difficult to appreciate from the surgical findings alone the volume of bone that was missing (Fig 11-20a). The bone at the edentulous alveolar crest was vertically deficient and required reconstruction if dental implants were to be placed. Reestablishment of the pretrauma mandible width required replacement of the bone volume and healing of the discontinuity that would result from the midline osteotomy.

An osteotomy was outlined to address each of the deficiencies (Fig 11-20b). The small rectangular bone segment at the alveolar ridge crest addressed the damaged region by resection. Instead of augmenting the existing deficient site, the strategy was to remove the compromised bone and replace it with a more viable bone mass.

The source of the new bone volume was the large, central rectangular segment. This section of bone was inherently thicker than the alveolar process and could potentially serve as a

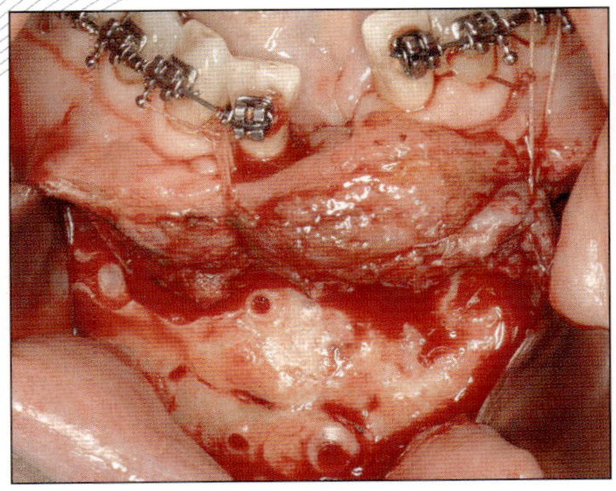

Fig 11-20a Removal of the original bone plates placed immediately after the injury reveals the gross disruption of the normal anatomy.

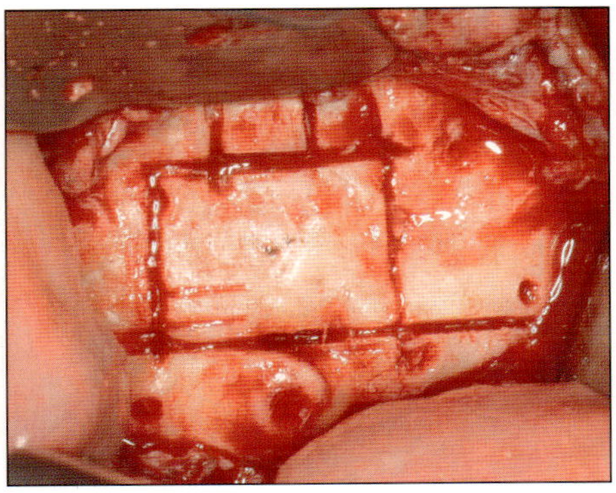

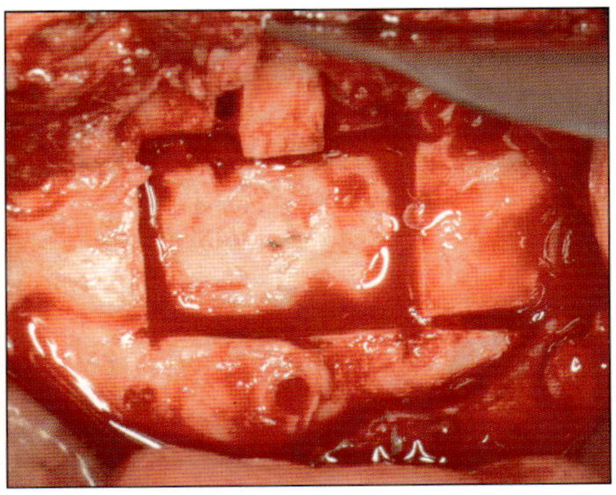

Fig 11-20b *(above left)* An osteotomy is outlined to address each of the deficiencies. The small rectangular bone segment at the alveolar ridge crest addresses the damaged region by resection. The strategy is to remove the compromised bone and replace it with a more viable bone mass. The source of the new bone volume is the large, central rectangular segment. The genioglossus muscle attachment at its lingual cortex can deliver neuromuscular signaling to the bone to which it inserts. The horizontal osteotomy at the inferior border extends through the inferior border on the left side, creating a discontinuity of the mandible that is necessary if widening is to be achieved. The horizontal orientation of the bone cut allows widening without opening of a large bone gap.

Fig 11-20c *(above right)* The damaged ridge crest is resected.

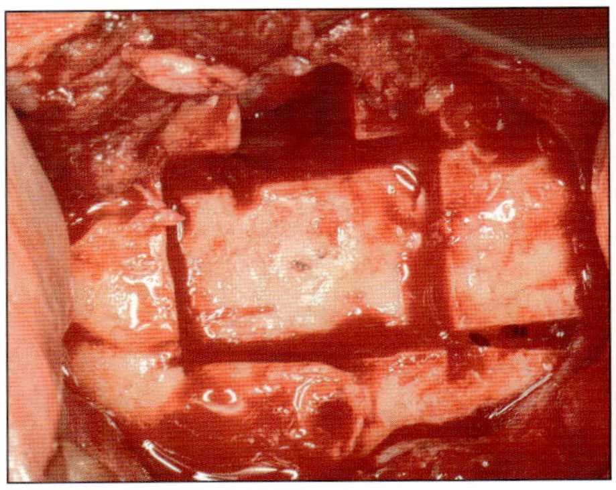

Fig 11-20d The central transport segment is mobilized.

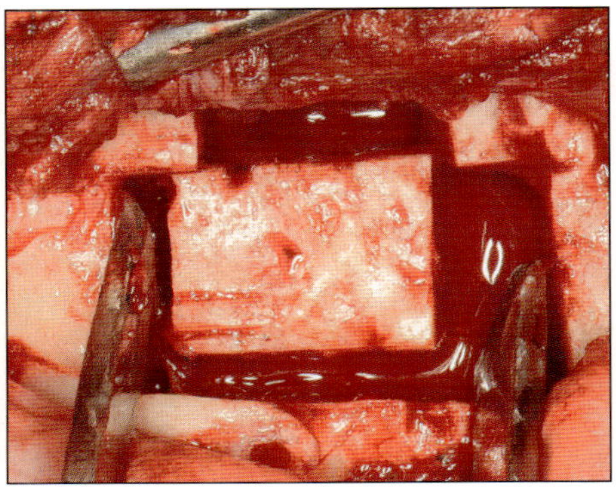

Fig 11-20e Neurosurgical lamina spreaders are used to apply expansion force. The expansion proceeds gradually. At each step of the expansion process, the integrity of and circulation to the overlying oral mucosa are evaluated.

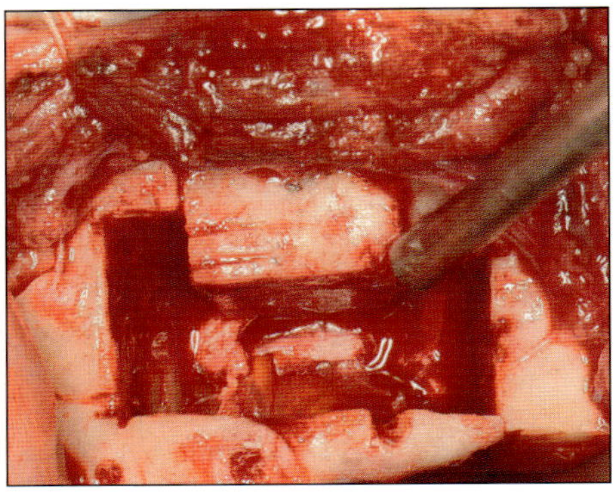

Fig 11-20f The transport segment is elevated into place.

site for implant placement. Just as important as its volume was the genioglossus muscle attachment at its lingual cortex. This muscle attachment would serve to promote and regulate the physiology and morphology of the bone segment. The muscle attachment could deliver neuromuscular signaling to the bone to which it inserted.

The horizontal osteotomy at the inferior border extended through the inferior border on the left side. This created a discontinuity of the mandible that was necessary if widening was to be accomplished. The horizontal orientation of the bone cut allowed widening without opening of a large bone gap.

The damaged section of alveolar ridge crest segment was removed (Fig 11-20c). The overlying oral mucosa and gingiva were not penetrated. The large, central bone segment was mobilized without damaging its attachment to the genioglossus muscle on the lingual cortex (Fig 11-20d). The inferior border osteotomy was completed, creating a midline discontinuity.

Neurosurgical lamina spreaders were used to apply expansion force (Fig 11-20e). The expansion process was done gradually. At each step of the expansion process, the integrity of and circulation to the overlying oral mucosa were evaluated. When the expansion process had regained the width of the anterior mandible, the transport segment was elevated into the alveolar ridge defect (Fig 11-20f).

The large transport segment was used to replace the small, resected piece. The volume of the transport segment greatly increased the width of the alveolar crest (Fig 11-20g). Elevation of the segment restored the height of the ridge. The segment carried the genioglossus muscle attachment superiorly, displacing the neuromuscular signaling source to the level of the alveolar process. This would provide the critical neuromuscular signaling input to this challenging bone-forming environment.

There was now minimal remaining bone contact between the right and left hemimandibles at the left inferior border. Two titanium bone plates were placed in the anterior osteotomy (Fig 11-20h). The 2.7-mm system bone plate (Stryker Leibinger) stabilized the two main sections of the mandible. The 1.7-mm system bone plate (Stryker Leibinger) above held the transport

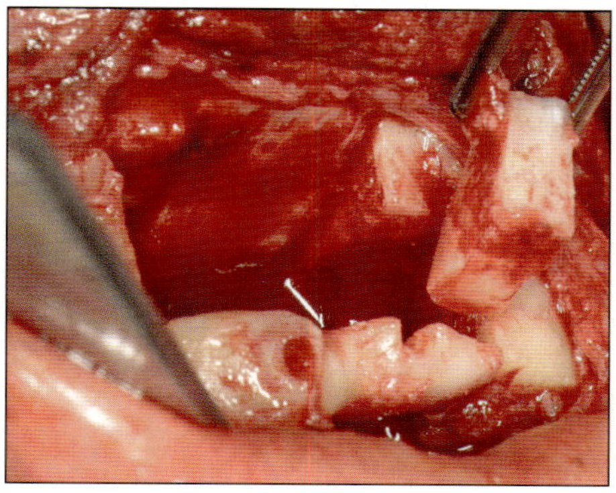

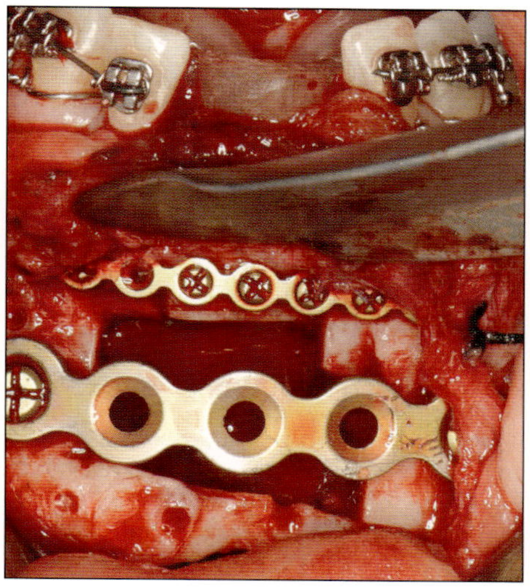

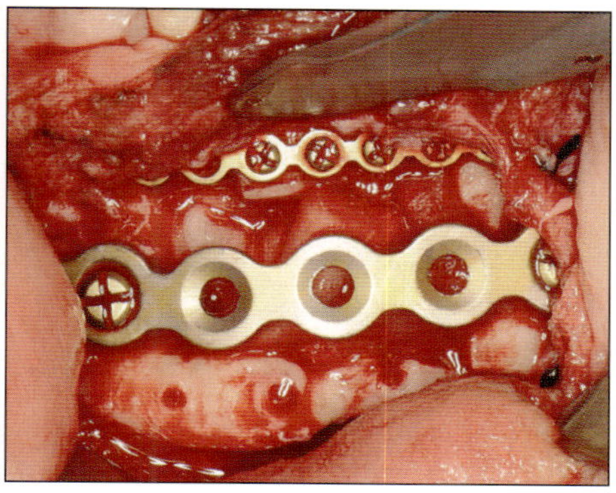

Fig 11-20g *(above left)* Elevation of the transport segment has filled the alveolar ridge defect. The segment carries the genioglossus muscle attachment superiorly, displacing the neuromuscular signaling source to the level of the alveolar process. There is now minimal remaining bone contact between the right and left hemimandibles at the left inferior border.

Fig 11-20h *(above right)* Titanium bone plates stabilize the fragments.

Fig 11-20i Bone morphogenetic protein–infused collagen sponges are placed to deliver a source of cells.

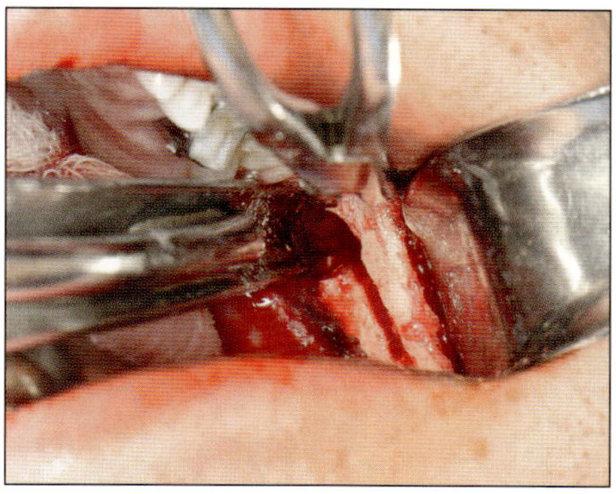

Fig 11-21a During left sagittal ramus osteotomy, gentle handling of the mandibular nerve will limit the potential complication of impaired sensation to the mandibular teeth and lower lip.

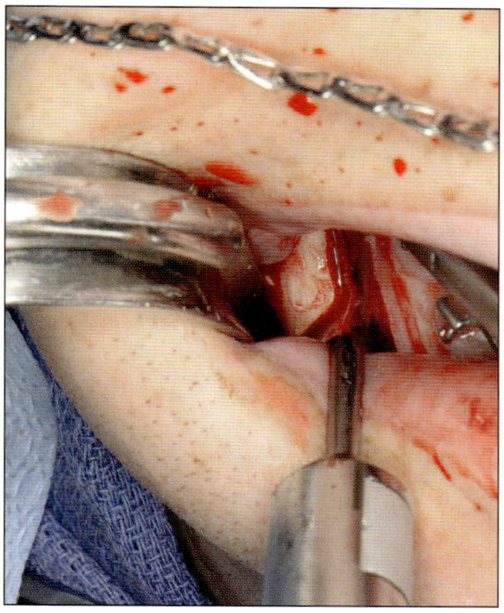

Fig 11-21b The inferior border cortex is cut with a saw. A special upward-cutting blade on the reciprocating saw is used to divide the cortex of the inferior border of the mandibular body.

segment in place. An acrylic resin lingual splint added support at the level of the dental arch.

Cells were delivered to the bone-forming site via collagen sponges containing rhBMP-2 (Fig 11-20i). The wound was closed in multiple layers.

After the midline expansion was completed, a left sagittal ramus osteotomy was performed to lengthen the mandible. Preserving the neuromuscular control of the reconstructed fields is important in any patient. It is particularly important in the patient with preexisting neurologic compromise undergoing facial skeletal reconstruction. Gentle handling of the mandibular nerve will limit the potential complication of impaired sensation to the mandibular teeth and lower lip.

A special retractor was placed to retract the mandibular nerve. An extended horizontal osteotomy penetrated the lingual cortex and extended to the lingula just anterior to the neurovascular bundle (Fig 11-21a). A small saw was used to cut through the superior cortex of the ramus and posterior mandibular body. A special upward-cutting blade on the reciprocating saw was used to divide the cortex of the inferior border of the mandibular body (Fig 11-21b).

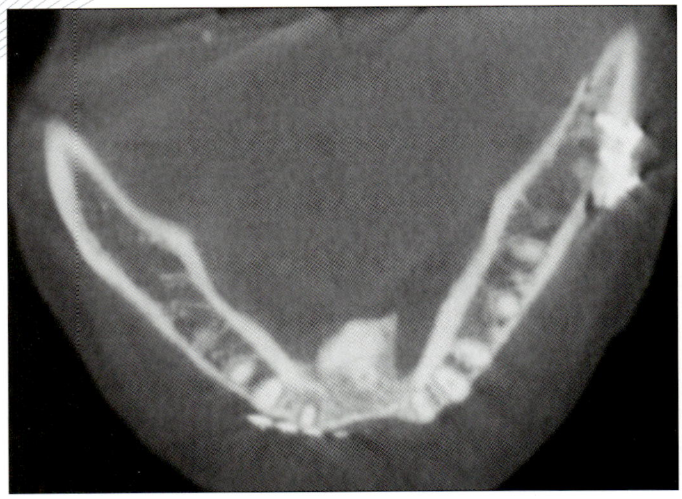

Fig 11-22 Two months after surgery, bone is growing at the site of the genioglossus muscle attachment, as shown radiographically.

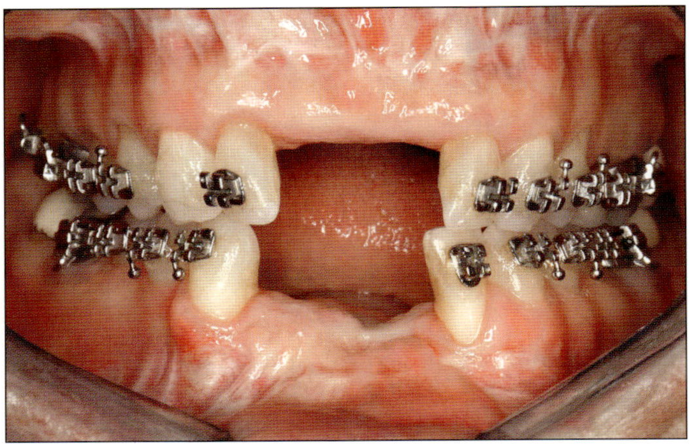

Fig 11-23 Ten months after surgery, the mandibular right lateral incisor and the bone plate fixating the segmental osteotomy were removed.

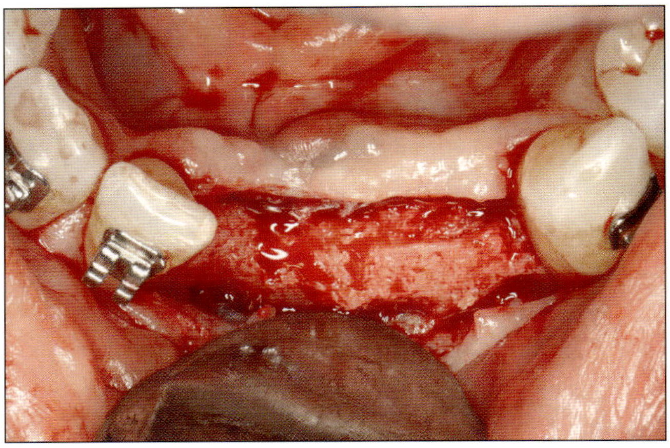

Fig 11-24a Seven months after extraction of the lateral incisor, the site was opened for placement of dental implants.

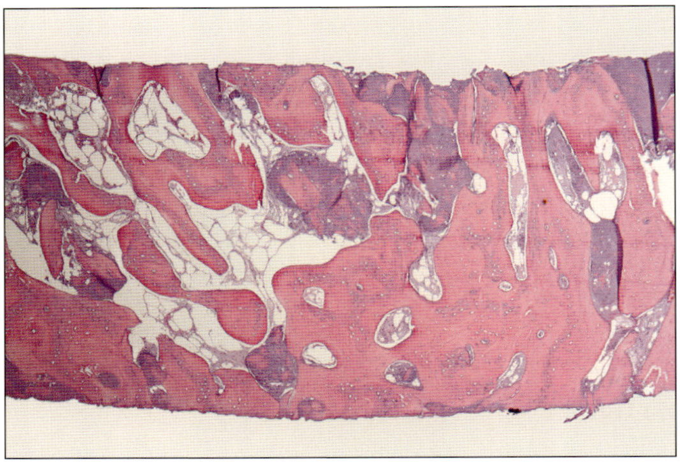

Fig 11-24b At the time of implant surgery, a biopsy showed that bone had developed across the midline mandibular defect grafted with rhBMP-2 (hematoxylin and eosin; original magnification ×40).

Outcome

In response to superior repositioning of the genioglossus muscle attachment and creation of the central discontinuity defect in the anterior mandible, bone formed to fill the regeneration chamber (Fig 11-22). Bone formation extended lingually in the early healing period.

Ten months after surgery, the bone plate fixating the segmental osteotomy was removed (Fig 11-23). The mandibular right lateral incisor was removed because it developed recession and bone loss.

Seven months after removal of the lateral incisor and the bone plate fixating the segmental osteotomy, the site was surgically opened for placement of dental implants (Fig 11-24a). A biopsy specimen was obtained from the regeneration chamber to verify that viable bone had grown. The specimen showed that normal bone formation had occurred (Fig 11-24b). Two implant sites were created (Fig 11-24c), and 3.8 × 13.0–mm implants were placed (Fig 11-24d). Following a period of osseointegration, the two mandibular implants were restored with a three-unit fixed prosthesis (Fig 11-24e).

Two 3.8 × 13.0–mm implants were also placed at the site of the maxillary incisors. The implants were restored with single crowns (Figs 11-25a to 11-25c).

A radiograph of the completed reconstruction showed that the surgical plan was completed as intended in the treatment design (Fig 11-26). Both dental arches were restored to excellent esthetics and occlusion (Figs 11-27a to 11-27f). Through carefully planned and executed surgery, orthodontics, and restorative treatment, maxillofacial function and esthetics were restored (Figs 11-28a and 11-28b).

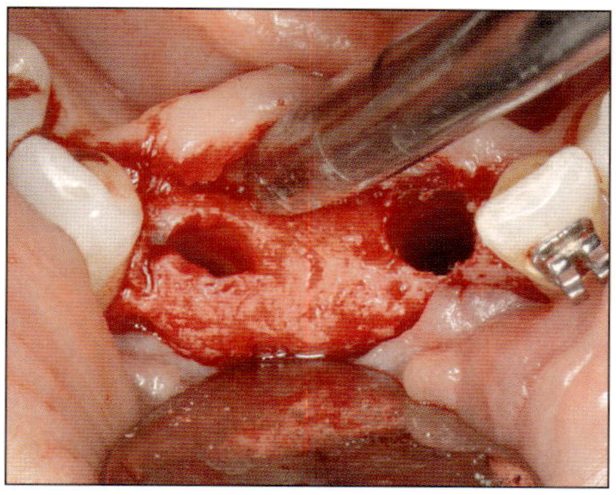

Fig 11-24c Two implant sites are created.

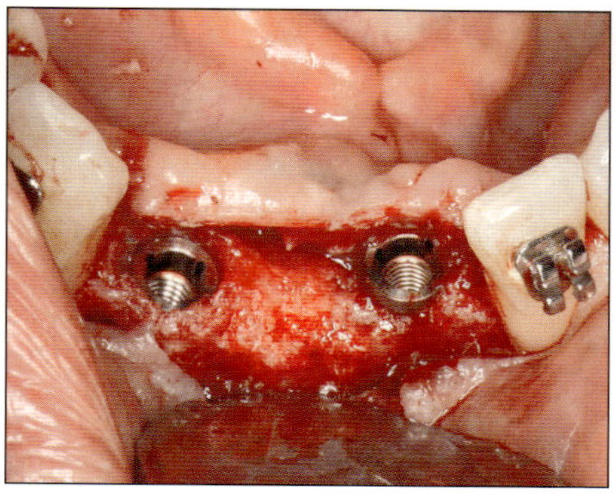

Fig 11-24d Two 3.8 × 13.0–mm implants (Camlog) are placed.

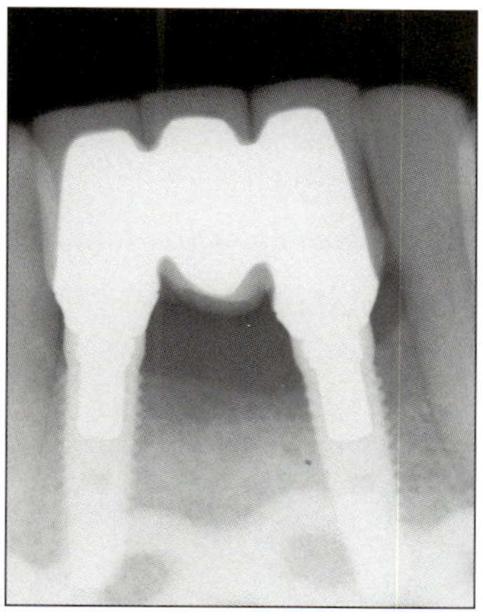

Fig 11-24e Following a period of osseointegration, the two mandibular implants are restored with a three-unit fixed prosthesis.

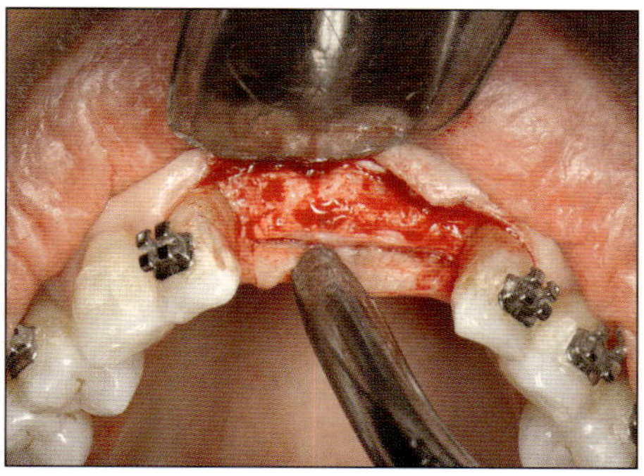

Fig 11-25a Maxillary ridge receiving implants.

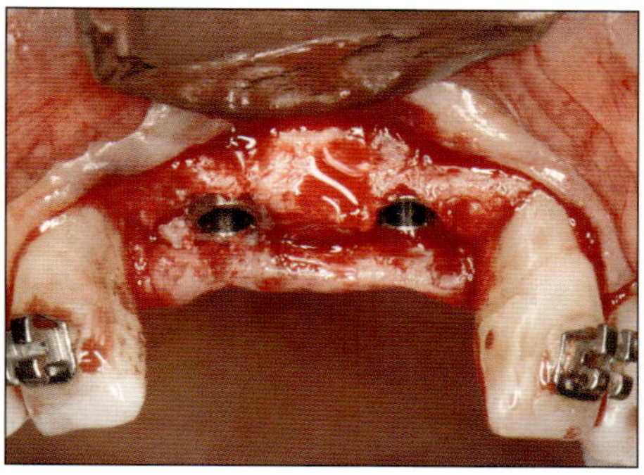

Fig 11-25b Two 3.8 × 13.0–mm implants have been positioned for replacement of the maxillary incisors.

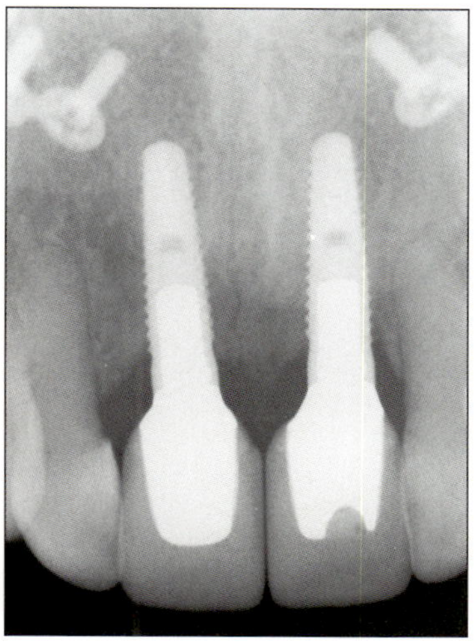

Fig 11-25c The implants have been restored with single crowns to replace the maxillary central incisors.

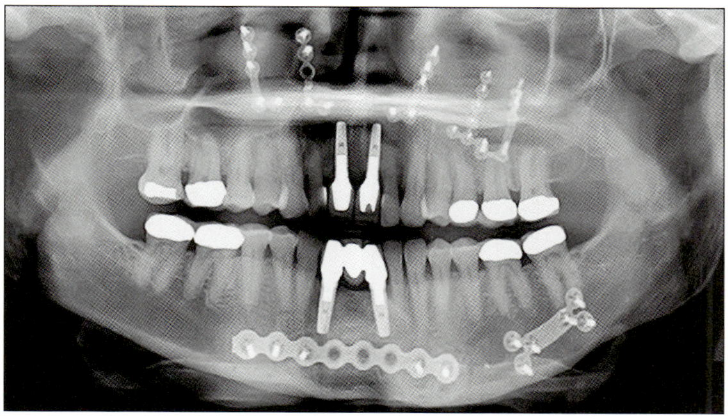

Fig 11-26 A panoramic radiograph of the completed reconstruction reveals that the proposed surgical plan has been implemented successfully (see Fig 11-4).

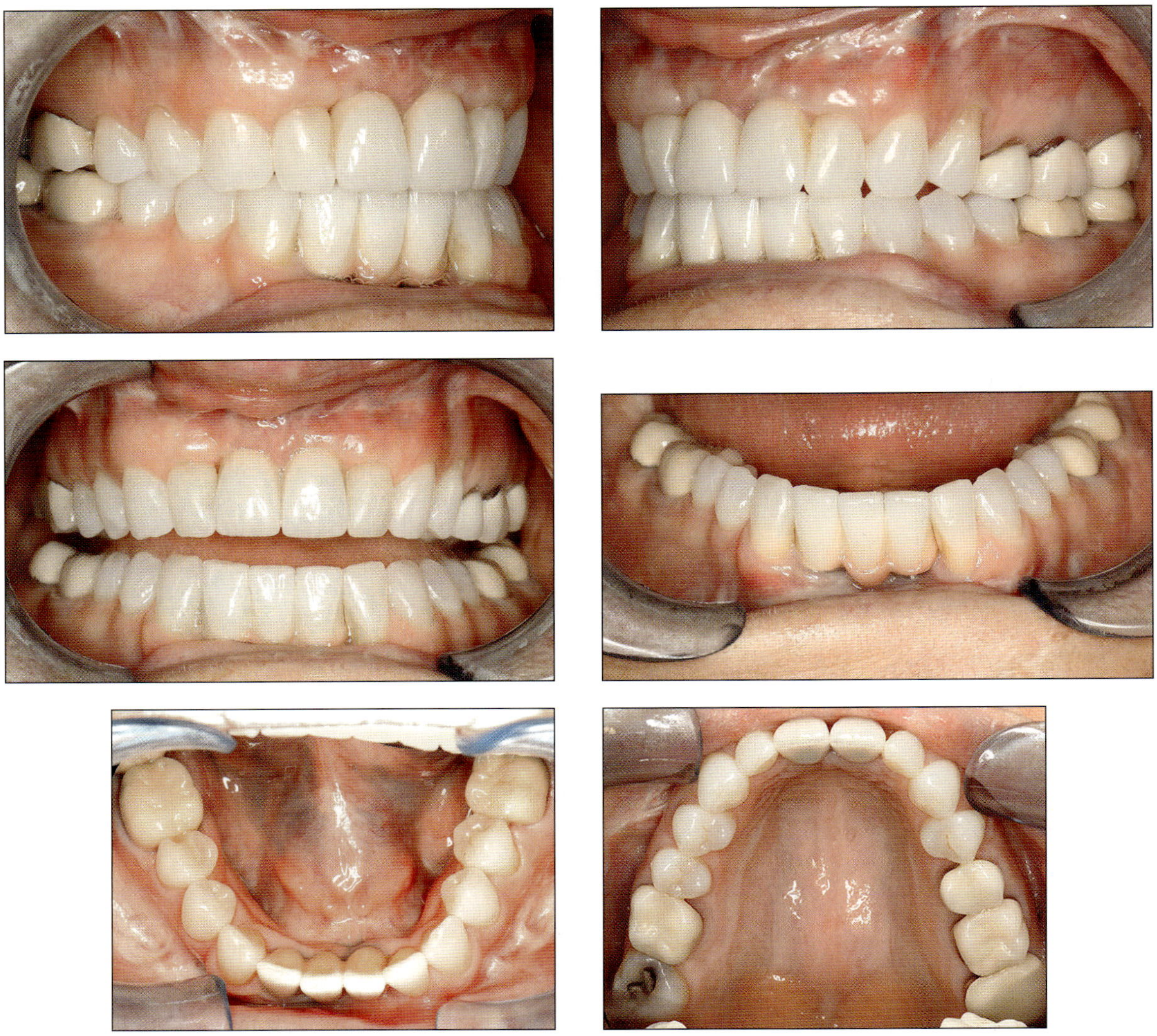

Figs 11-27a to 11-27f The maxillary and mandibular dental arches have been restored to function. The implants in the maxillary central incisor sites have been restored with single-crown restorations. The implants in the mandibular anterior sites have been restored with a three-unit fixed prosthesis.

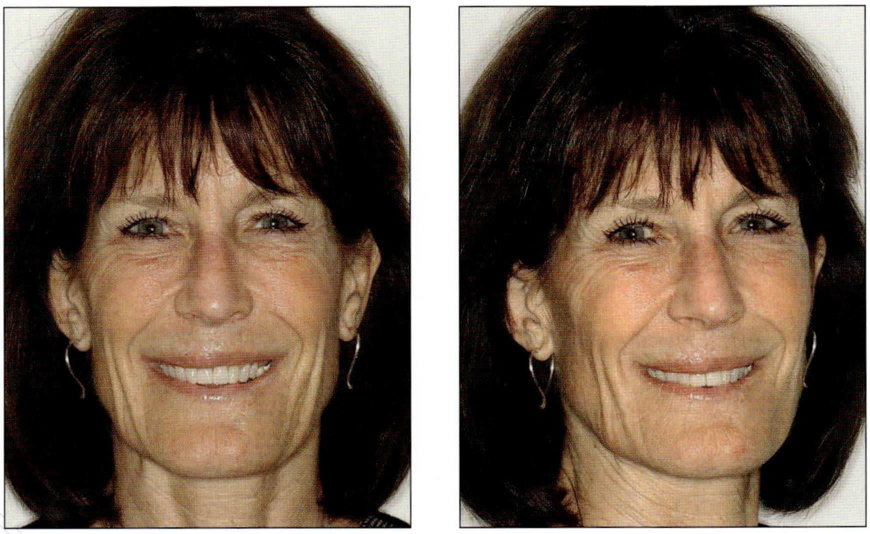

Figs 11-28a and 11-28b The patient's oral and maxillofacial region has been returned to a functional and esthetic state.

Conclusion

The purpose of presenting this case is to demonstrate the stepwise process of treatment planning and surgery in detail. Rather than a theoretical discussion of treatment options, this chapter is a technical instruction document that provides students with guidance in the evaluation, treatment planning, and surgical processes. Experienced clinicians can safely abbreviate some of this treatment sequence.

It is important to recognize the benefits of approaching each case in a deliberate, logical order. Management of this patient's deformity was complicated because it involved multiple physiologic systems and multiple treatment phases. Treatment failure or compromise could have come from many sources. However, careful design, surgical planning, and surgical execution, which were founded on articulator-mounted indicators and headframe-based fragment repositioning, ensured that an excellent outcome was achieved.

As in this case, patients with sensory or motor deficits deserve special attention when major surgical treatments are planned. The response to healing may be impaired because of compromise in the patient's neuromuscular regulatory capabilities. Patients with these impairments may also have difficulty swallowing and breathing when subjected to general anesthesia.

In a typical trauma reconstruction case, the pattern of facial fractures becomes the guide for treatment planning osteotomies to correct malunion. If the objective is to return the patient to the pretrauma state, some clinicians would simply recreate the trauma-related fractures using elective osteotomies and then attempt to reduce the segments into a functional relationship. However, for this patient, clinical evaluation and preliminary cast surgery revealed that a more complicated surgical plan was indicated. The diagnostic step of performing preliminary cast surgery revealed an anatomical deficiency not appearing on the radiographs or in the patient's history. The outcome of the preliminary cast surgery was a refined surgical plan. The projected surgical plan, verified by the preliminary cast surgery, was necessary to allow proper direction of the presurgical orthodontic treatment.

Combining the use of surgical splints and headframe-based navigation allows precise positioning of osteotomy fragments. This technique is particularly valuable when temporomandibular joint stability is in question. Accurate placement of the maxilla and mandible is necessary if dental implants and implant restorations are to meet critical esthetic objectives. Conventional splint-based orthognathic surgery can deliver average position tolerance to no better than 3 mm in three dimensions. In some cases, the deviation exceeds 6 mm or more. If errors of these magnitudes had occurred in this patient, the result would have failed on the esthetic criteria alone. If the result of surgery is to meet the level of tolerance expected in restorative dentistry, headframe-based navigation is necessary.

References

1. von Eiselsberg A. Über Plastik bei Ektropium des Unterkiefers. Wien Klin Wochenschr 1906;19:1505.
2. Harvold EP. The theoretical basis for the treatment of hemifacial microsomia. In: Harvold EP, Vargervik K, Chierici G (eds). Treatment of Hemifacial Microsomia. New York: Alan R. Liss, 1983:1–11.

Index

Page numbers followed by "f" indicate figures; those followed by "t" indicate tables; those followed by "b" indicate boxes.

E

F

G

H

I

P

R

S

T

V

W

Z